1999
YEAR BOOK OF
PATHOLOGY
AND LABORATORY
MEDICINE®

Statement of Purpose

The YEAR BOOK Service

The YEAR BOOK series was devised in 1901 by practicing health professionals who observed that the literature of medicine and related disciplines had become so voluminous that no one individual could read and place in perspective every potential advance in a major specialty. In the final decade of the 20th century, this recognition is more acutely true than it was in 1901.

More than merely a series of books, YEAR BOOK volumes are the tangible results of a unique service designed to accomplish the following:

- to *survey* a wide range of journals of proven value
- to *select* from those journals papers representing significant advances and statements of important clinical principles
- to provide *abstracts* of those articles that are readable, convenient summaries of their key points
- to provide *commentary* about those articles to place them in perspective

These publications grow out of a unique process that calls on the talents of outstanding authorities in clinical and fundamental disciplines, trained literature specialists, and professional writers, all supported by the resources of Mosby, the world's preeminent publisher for the health professions.

The Literature Base

Mosby and its editors survey approximately 500 journals published worldwide, covering the full range of the health professions. On an annual basis, the publisher examines usage patterns and polls its expert authorities to add new journals to the literature base and to delete journals that are no longer useful as potential YEAR BOOK sources.

The Literature Survey

The publisher's team of literature specialists, all of whom are trained and experienced health professionals, examines every original, peer-reviewed article in each journal issue. More than 250,000 articles per year are scanned systematically, including title, text, illustrations, tables, and references. Each scan is compared, article by article, to the search strategies that the publisher has developed in consultation with the 270 outside experts who form the pool of YEAR BOOK editors. A given article may be reviewed by any number of editors, from one to a dozen or more, regardless of the discipline for which the paper was originally published. In turn, each editor who receives the article reviews it to determine whether the article should be included in the YEAR BOOK. This decision is based on the article's inherent quality, its probable usefulness to readers of that YEAR BOOK, and the editor's goal to represent a balanced picture of a given field in each volume of the YEAR BOOK. In addition, the editor indicates when to include figures and tables from the article to help the YEAR BOOK reader better understand the information.

Of the quarter million articles scanned each year, only 5% are selected for detailed analysis within the YEAR BOOK series, thereby assuring readers of the high value of every selection.

The Abstract

The publisher's abstracting staff is headed by a seasoned medical professional and includes individuals with training in the life sciences, medicine, and other areas, plus extensive experience in writing for the health professions and related industries. Each selected article is assigned to a specific writer on this abstracting staff. The abstracter, guided in many cases by notations supplied by the expert editor, writes a structured, condensed summary designed so that the reader can rapidly acquire the essential information contained in the article.

The Commentary

The YEAR BOOK editorial boards, sometimes assisted by guest commentators, write comments that place each article in perspective for the reader. This provides the reader with the equivalent of a personal consultation with a leading international authority—an opportunity to better understand the value of the article and to benefit from the authority's thought processes in assessing the article.

Additional Editorial Features

The editorial boards of each YEAR BOOK organize the abstracts and comments to provide a logical and satisfying sequence of information. To enhance the organization, editors also provide introductions to sections or individual chapters, comments linking a number of abstracts, citations to additional literature, and other features.

The published YEAR BOOK contains enhanced bibliographic citations for each selected article, including extended listings of multiple authors and identification of author affiliations. Each YEAR BOOK contains a Table of Contents specific to that year's volume. From year to year, the Table of Contents for a given YEAR BOOK will vary depending on developments within the field.

Every YEAR BOOK contains a list of the journals from which papers have been selected. This list represents a subset of approximately 500 journals surveyed by the publisher and occasionally reflects a particularly pertinent article from a journal that is not surveyed on a routine basis.

Finally, each volume contains a comprehensive subject index and an index to authors of each selected paper.

The 1999 Year Book Series

Year Book of Allergy, Asthma, and Clinical Immunology: Drs. Rosenwasser, Boguniewicz, Borish, Routes, Spahn, and Weber

Year Book of Anesthesiology and Pain Management®: Drs. Tinker, Abram, Chestnut, Roizen, Rothenberg, and Wood

Year Book of Cardiology®: Drs. Schlant, Collins, Gersh, Graham, Kaplan, and Waldo

Year Book of Chiropractic®: Dr. Lawrence

Year Book of Critical Care Medicine®: Drs. Parrillo, Balk, Calvin, Franklin, and Shapiro

Year Book of Dentistry®: Drs. Meskin, Berry, Jeffcoat, Leinfelder, Roser, Summitt, and Zakariasen

Year Book of Dermatology and Dermatologic Surgery™: Drs. Thiers and Lang

Year Book of Diagnostic Radiology®: Drs. Osborn, Dalinka, Groskin, Maynard, Pentecost, Ros, Smirniotopoulos, and Young

Year Book of Emergency Medicine®: Drs. Wagner, Dronen, Davidson, King, Niemann, and Hamilton

Year Book of Endocrinology®: Drs. Bagdade, Braverman, Horton, Kannan, Landsberg, Molitch, Morley, Odell, Poehlman, Rogol, and Fitzpatrick

Year Book of Family Practice®: Drs. Berg, Bowman, Davidson, Dexter, and Scherger

Year Book of Gastroenterology: Drs. Aliperti and Fleshman

Year Book of Hand Surgery®: Drs. Amadio and Hentz

Year Book of Medicine®: Drs. Klahr, Frishman, Malawista, Mandell, Jett, Young, Barkin, and Bagdade

Year Book of Neonatal and Perinatal Medicine®: Drs. Fanaroff, Maisels, and Stevenson

Year Book of Nephrology, Hypertension, and Mineral Metabolism: Drs. Schwab, Bennett, Emmett, Hostetter, and Moe

Year Book of Neurology and Neurosurgery®: Drs. Bradley and Gibbs

Year Book of Nuclear Medicine®: Drs. Gottschalk, Blaufox, Coleman, Strauss, and Zubal

Year Book of Obstetrics, Gynecology, and Women's Health: Drs. Mishell, Herbst, and Kirschbaum

Year Book of Oncology®: Drs. Ozols, Eisenberg, Glatstein, Loehrer, and Urba

Year Book of Ophthalmology®: Drs. Wilson, Augsburger, Cohen, Eagle, Grossman, Laibson, Maguire, Nelson, Penne, Rapuano, Sergott, Spaeth, Tipperman, Ms. Gosfield, and Ms. Salmon

Year Book of Orthopedics®: Drs. Morrey, Beauchamp, Currier, Tolo, Trigg, and Swiontkowski

Year Book of Otolaryngology–Head and Neck Surgery®: Drs. Paparella, Holt, and Otto

Year Book of Pathology and Laboratory Medicine®: Drs. Raab, Cohen, Dabbs, Olson, and Stanley

Year Book of Pediatrics®: Dr. Stockman

Year Book of Plastic, Reconstructive, and Aesthetic Surgery®: Drs. Miller, Bartlett, Garner, McKinney, Ruberg, Salisbury, and Smith

Year Book of Psychiatry and Applied Mental Health®: Drs. Talbott, Ballenger, Frances, Lydiard, Meltzer, Jensen, and Tasman

Year Book of Pulmonary Disease®: Drs. Jett, Castro, Maurer, Peters, Phillips, and Ryu

Year Book of Rheumatology, Arthritis, and Musculoskeletal Disease™: Drs. Panush, Hadler, Hellman, LeRoy, Pisetsky, and Simon

Year Book of Sports Medicine®: Drs. Shephard, Drinkwater, Eichner, Torg, Alexander, and Mr. George

Year Book of Surgery®: Drs. Copeland, Bland, Deitch, Eberlein, Howard, Luce, Seeger, Souba, and Sugarbaker

Year Book of Urology®: Drs. Andriole and Coplen

Year Book of Vascular Surgery®: Dr. Porter

1999
The Year Book of PATHOLOGY AND LABORATORY MEDICINE®

Editor-in-Chief

Stephen S. Raab, M.D.

Associate Professor, Director of Cytology and Outcomes Research, Department of Pathology and Laboratory Medicine, Allegheny University of Health Sciences, Allegheny General Hospital, Pittsburgh, Pennsylvania

Editors

Michael B. Cohen, M.D.

Professor, Departments of Pathology/Urology; Vice Chair for Research, University of Iowa; Director, Division of Cytopathology, University of Iowa Hospitals and Clinics, Iowa City, Iowa

David J. Dabbs, M.D.

Director of Anatomic Pathology, Department of Pathology and Laboratory Medicine, Allegheny University of Health Sciences, Pittsburgh, Pennsylvania

John D. Olson, M.D., Ph.D.

Professor, Department of Pathology, University of Texas Health Science Center; Director of Clinical Laboratories, University Health System, San Antonio, Texas

Michael W. Stanley, M.D.

Professor of Pathology, University of Minnesota Hospitals and Clinics; Chair, Department of Pathology, Hennepin County Medical Center, Minneapolis, Minnesota

Mosby

St. Louis Baltimore Boston Carlsbad Naples New York Philadelphia Portland London Madrid Mexico City Singapore Sydney Tokyo Toronto Wiesbaden

Mosby
Dedicated to Publishing Excellence

Managing Editor: Gina G. Byrd
Developmental Editor: Laura C. Berendson
Manager, Periodical Editing: Kirk Swearingen
Production Editor: Stephanie M. Geels
Project Supervisor, Production: Joy Moore
Production Assistant: Laura Bayless
Manager, Literature Services: Idelle L. Winer
Illustrations and Permissions Specialist: Steve Ramay

1999 EDITION

Printed in the United States of America
Composition by Reed Technology and Information Services, Inc.
Printing/binding by Maple-Vail

Editorial Office:
Mosby, Inc.
11830 Westline Industrial Drive
St. Louis, MO 63146

International Standard Serial Number: 1077–9108
International Standard Book Number: 0–8151–9723–3

Contributing Editors

Ronald Feld, Ph.D.

Associate Professor of Pathology, Department of Pathology, University of Iowa College of Medicine; Laboratory Director of Chemistry, University of Iowa Hospitals and Clinics, Iowa City, Iowa

Dana M. Grzybicki, M.D., Ph.D.

Assistant Professor, Duquesne University School of Health Sciences, Pittsburgh, Pennsylvania

Michael A. Pfaller, M.D.

Professor, Department of Pathology, University of Iowa College of Medicine; Director of Clinical Laboratories, University of Iowa Hospitals and Clinics, Iowa City, Iowa

Annette J. Schlueter, M.D., Ph.D.

Associate Professor, University of Iowa, University of Iowa Hospitals and Clinics, Iowa City, Iowa

John F. Turner, Jr., M.D.

Assistant Professor of Pathology, University of Iowa; Hematopathologist, Department of Pathology, University of Iowa Hospitals and Clinics, Iowa City, Iowa

Table of Contents

Journals Represented

Mosby and its editors survey approximately 500 journals for its abstract and commentary publications. From these journals, the editors select the articles to be abstracted. Journals represented in this YEAR BOOK are listed below.

Academic Emergency Medicine
Acta Cytologica
American Journal of Clinical Pathology
American Journal of Dermatopathology
American Journal of Emergency Medicine
American Journal of Gastroenterology
American Journal of Hematology
American Journal of Kidney Diseases
American Journal of Nephrology
American Journal of Obstetrics and Gynecology
American Journal of Pathology
American Journal of Roentgenology
American Journal of Surgical Pathology
American Surgeon
Annals of Allergy, Asthma, & Immunology
Annals of Surgery
Annals of Surgical Oncology
Archives of Dermatology
Archives of Internal Medicine
Archives of Pathology and Laboratory Medicine
Arthritis and Rheumatism
Blood
Breast Journal
British Journal of Cancer
British Journal of Haematology
British Medical Journal
Cancer
Clinical Chemistry
Clinical Infectious Diseases
Clinical Orthopaedics and Related Research
European Respiratory Journal
Gastroenterology
Gynecologic Oncology
Human Pathology
International Journal of Gynecological Pathology
Investigative Radiology
Journal of Arthroplasty
Journal of Clinical Microbiology
Journal of Clinical Oncology
Journal of Clinical Pathology
Journal of Cutaneous Pathology
Journal of Infectious Diseases
Journal of Laboratory and Clinical Medicine
Journal of Neurosurgery
Journal of Pathology
Journal of Rheumatology
Journal of Surgical Oncology

Journal of Surgical Pathology
Journal of Urology
Journal of the American Academy of Dermatology
Journal of the American Medical Association
Journal of the American Medical Informatics Association
Journal of the National Cancer Institute
Kidney International
Lancet
Leukemia
Medicine
Modern Pathology
Nephrology, Dialysis, Transplantation
Neurosurgery
New England Journal of Medicine
Obstetrics and Gynecology
Pathology
Pediatric Nephrology
Prenatal Diagnosis
Radiology
Scandinavian Journal of Urology and Nephrology
Science
Seminars in Oncology
Stroke
Thyroid
Transfusion
Transplantation
Urology

Standard Abbreviations

The following terms are abbreviated in this edition: acquired immunodeficiency syndrome (AIDS), cardiopulmonary resuscitation (CPR), central nervous system (CNS), cerebrospinal fluid (CSF), computed tomography (CT), deoxyribonucleic acid (DNA), electrocardiography (ECG), health maintenance organization (HMO), human immunodeficiency virus (HIV), intensive care unit (ICU), intramuscular (IM), intravenous (IV), magnetic resonance (MR) imaging (MRI), and ribonucleic acid (RNA).

Note

The Year Book of Pathology and Laboratory Medicine® is a literature survey service providing abstracts of articles published in the professional literature. Every effort is made to assure the accuracy of the information presented in these pages. Neither the editors nor the publisher of the Year Book of Pathology and Laboratory Medicine® can be responsible for errors in the original materials. The editors' comments are their own opinions. Mention of specific products within this publication does not constitute endorsement.

To facilitate the use of the Year Book of Pathology and Laboratory Medicine® as a reference tool, all illustrations and tables included in this publication are now identified as they appear in the original article. This change is meant to help the reader recognize that any illustration or table appearing in the YEAR BOOK OF PATHOLOGY AND LABORATORY MEDICINE® may be only one of many in the original article. For this reason, figure and table numbers will often appear to be out of sequence within the YEAR BOOK OF PATHOLOGY AND LABORATORY MEDICINE®.

Introduction

Welcome to the 1999 YEAR BOOK OF PATHOLOGY AND LABORATORY MEDICINE! This is the second year for our editorial board and there have been quite a few changes. John Olson moved from the University of Iowa to the University of Texas at San Antonio; Mike Stanley moved from the University of Arkansas to Hennepin County Medical Center; and I moved from the University of Iowa to Allegheny General Hospital. In addition, we have added David Dabbs to the editorial board. Dave is renowned in renal pathology and also has expertise in gynecologic pathology, dermatopathology, soft tissue and bone, and head and neck.

The format of this year's YEAR BOOK is similar to last year's. The amount of new material published in the medical literature is voluminous, and it is no exaggeration that new pathology journals are introduced yearly. As expected, some of the material is excellent, some is bad, and a lot falls in between. We have tried to cull the most recent literature for relevant topics that affect or will affect pathology practice. I hope you find the abstracted articles and our commentary thought provoking and useful. If you wish, please e-mail me your comments (sraab@aherf.edu).

Stephen S. Raab, M.D.

PART I

ANATOMICAL PATHOLOGY

1 Respiratory System and Mediastinum

Reproducibility of Neuroendocrine Lung Tumor Classification
Travis WD, Gal AA, Colby TV, et al (Armed Forces Inst of Pathology, Washington, DC; Emory Univ, Atlanta, Ga; Mayo Clinic, Scottsdale, Ariz; et al)
Hum Pathol 29:272–279, 1998 1–1

Background.—Tumor classification systems are only meaningful if they are reproducible and have clinical significance. The classification of neuroendocrine lung tumors is both complex and controversial. In 1991, Travis et al. (Table 1) proposed a 4-category classification scheme for these tumors, including typical carcinoid (TC), atypical carcinoid (AC), large-cell neuroendocrine carcinoma (LCNEC), and small-cell carcinoma (SCC). Because this approach to classification of pulmonary neuroendocrine tumors has clinical significance, interobserver reproducibility for this classification scheme was investigated.

Study Design.—Forty specimens of surgically resected neuroendocrine tumors of the lung from the files of the Armed Forces Institute of Pathology were examined. One representative slide from each case was circulated among 5 experienced pulmonary pathologists from separate institutions for review, using the criteria described above. Agreement was defined as unanimous if all pathologists agreed, a majority if 4 agreed, and a consensus if 3 agreed.

Findings.—A consensus diagnosis could be achieved in all cases, a majority agreement in 78%, and unanimous agreement in 55% using these criteria. The most common disagreements were between LCNEC and SCC, followed by TC and AC, and AC and LCNEC. The highest level of agreement occurred for SCC and TC.

Conclusions.—Using this classification system, a consensus diagnosis could be reached for all 40 neuroendocrine tumor specimens tested. There is a need for modified criteria to more carefully distinguish TC vs. AC and SCC vs. LCNEC.

Addendum.—Based on the findings of this study and others, the criteria for separation of AC from TC are being revised. Atypical carcinoid will be defined as a tumor with neuroendocrine morphology and mitotic counts

TABLE 1.—Histologic Criteria for Pulmonary Neuroendocrine Tumors

Histological Features	TC	AC*	LCNEC*	SCC*
Organoid, trabecular, palisading, rosettes	Yes	Yes	Yes	Yes
Mitoses	Absent or rare	5 to 10 per 10 HPF	More than 10 per 10 HPF (average, 75 per 10 HPF)	More than 10 per 10 HPF (average, 75 per 10 HPF)
Necrosis	Uncharacteristic	Frequent, usually punctate	Frequent, usually infarct-like	Frequent, usually infarct-like
Nuclear pleomorphism, hyperchromatism	Uncommon	Sometimes	Frequent	Cells are usually small, large pleomorphic cells are rare unless mixed SC/LC
N/C ratio	Moderate	Moderate	Low	High
Nucleoli	Occasional	Common	Very common	Absent or inconspicuous
Nuclear chromatin	Finely granular	Finely granular	Usually vesicular, can be finely granular	Finely granular
Shape	Round, oval, spindled	Round, oval, spindled	Round, oval, polygonal	Round, oval, spindled
Nuclear smear	No	No	Uncommon	Common
Azzopardi effect	No	No	Uncommon	Occasional

*See addendum.

Abbreviations: TC, typical carcinoid; *AC*, atypical carcinoid; *LCNEC*, large-cell neuroendocrine carcinoma; *SCC*, small-cell carcinoma; *HPF*, high-power fields; *N/C*, nuclear to cytoplasmic; *SC/LC*, mixed small-cell/large-cell carcinoma; *Azzopardi effect*, basophilic encrustation of vascular walls from DNA of necrotic tumor cells.

(Courtesy of Travis WD, Gal AA, Colby TV, et al: Reproducibility of neuroendocrine lung tumor classification. *Hum Pathol* 29:272–279, 1998.)

between 2 and 10 per 2 mm^2 of viable tumor (10 high-power fields) or coagulative necrosis.

▶ In this paper, the big boys of neuroendocrine lung pathology throw their hats in the ring and go head to head trying to classify a mix of pulmonary neuroendocrine tumors. If this were Camelot, they'd all agree, but since it is Academia they don't. All 5 pathologists agreed on the diagnosis in only 55% of cases, indicating that at least somebody's disagreeing almost half the time. These pathologists use 4 categories (TC, AC, LCNEC, and SCC), and the areas of disagreement mainly seem to be at the low (TC vs. AC) or high (LCNEC vs. SCC) end. Table 1 depicts the criteria the pathologists supposedly used and is a good reference for those who like the 4-category Travis system. To me, this study means that a pathologist without "expertise" in classifying pulmonary neuroendocrine tumors should not be discouraged if a neuroendocrine tumor sent out for consultation comes back with a diagnosis different from one expected. It also means that if you were to send a case to 5 experts, there is a good chance that not all the experts would agree. One important question that needs to be asked about these interobserver variability data is how does variability in the use of diagnostic categories correlate with treatment for these categories? It would be interesting to investigate how patients were managed and how they did in survival terms for those cases in which one of the expert pathologists was the diagnostic outlyer.

S.S. Raab, M.D.

True Papillary Carcinoma of the Lung: A Distinct Clinicopathologic Entity

Silver SA, Askin FB (Johns Hopkins Med Inst, Baltimore, Md)

Am J Surg Pathol 21:43–51, 1997 1–2

Introduction.—There is controversy over whether papillary adenocarcinoma (PA) of the lung is a specific histologic entity or simply a variant of bronchioloalveolar carcinoma (BAC). A retrospective study was conducted to characterize the morphologic features of PA of the lung that allow its distinction from BAC and other pulmonary adenocarcinomas with papillary features.

Methods.—Cases for review were obtained from the surgical pathology files of The Johns Hopkins Hospital for the period 1981–1993. Slides from 144 of 155 patients with resected primary lung adenocarcinoma specifically diagnosed as having papillary or bronchioloalveolar features were available for review. Also reviewed were 67 randomly selected PAs from the entire group of 825 adenocarcinomas resected during the 13-year study period. Two observers reviewed a mean of 5.4 stained slides of each tumor.

Results.—Thirty-one cases met criteria for true PA, diagnosed when 75% or more of the neoplasm contained papillary structures supported by fibrovascular cores with complicated secondary and tertiary branches.

Marked nuclear atypia was observed in all cases and psammoma bodies in 42%. True PA, unlike BAC, filled and distorted or replaced air spaces in the lung. Patients were 19 men and 12 women with a mean age of 64.5 years. Twenty were asymptomatic and received the diagnosis at a routine evaluation or when seen for other disease. Most patients (86%) reported a smoking history. The neoplasms were solitary in 27 cases and multifocal in 4. Stage I disease was present in 17 cases and stage II in 9. The most common form of treatment was lobectomy (27 patients); 8 patients received adjuvant radiation therapy. At a mean follow-up of 3.2 years, recurrent or metastatic disease had developed in 20 patients (71%). Eleven patients were alive at a median follow-up of 2.8 years.

Conclusion.—Findings of this review indicate that papillary adenocarcinoma of the lung is a distinct clinicopathologic entity. Compared with cases of BAC, cases of PA in this series were seen at a similar age and were as likely to be asymptomatic at diagnosis. The behavior of PA, however, is similar to that of conventional adenocarcinoma of the lung, and morbidity and mortality are considerably worse than that of BAC.

► I am convinced that there are primary adenocarcinomas of the lung with papillary features. I am also convinced that some may confuse these tumors with BACs and that it is important to prevent this confusion. This is because, stage for stage, BACs do better. However, I am unconvinced that PAs are a true entity that should not be combined with conventional adenocarcinomas. Silver and Askin state that PAs behave the same as conventional adenocarcinomas, so why bother separating them? The authors' criteria for PA (papillary stalk and stromal invasion) are convincingly depicted, but I question why anybody who saw these features would classify such a tumor as a BAC in the first place. Using firm criteria, BAC is a relatively rare entity.

I think that the important point of this paper is not that true PAs exist apart from conventional adenocarcinomas, but that we should be careful with our subclassification of BACs. Interestingly, using the statistics presented by Silver and Askin, 14% of conventional adenocarcinomas are true PAs.

S.S. Raab, M.D.

Immunocytochemical Markers in Stage I Lung Cancer: Relevance to Prognosis

Pastorino U, Andreola S, Tagliabue E, et al (Royal Brompton Hosp, London; Univ College Hosp, London; Istituto Nazionale Tumori, Milan, Italy; et al)
J Clin Oncol 15:2858–2865, 1997 1–3

Background.—The search continues to identify factors involved in carcinogenesis so that appropriate treatment decisions can be made and instituted as early as possible. Numerous biological markers were studied to identify their prognostic value in non–small-cell lung cancer (NSCLC).

Methods.—Surgical tumor resection was performed in 515 patients with stage I or II NSCLC, and the median observation time was 64 months (up to 102 months for survivors). Specimens were examined by hematoxylin and eosin stain. Tumor angiogenesis, the proto-oncogene products of c-*erb* B1 and c-*erb* B2, Bcl-2, p53, blood group A and precursors of blood antigens, and the laminin receptor were the immunocytochemical markers examined.

Findings.—In both univariate and multivariate analyses, pathologic tumor grade was the most significant factor in survival and in time to recurrence. Also, the age at diagnosis was a significant predictor of survival in both analyses. However, none of the immunocytochemical markers were of prognostic significance in multivariate analysis, and only Bcl-2–positive tumors had a significantly better prognosis on univariate analysis. Multivariate analyses in a subset of 137 patients classified as pT1N0 revealed that both epidermal growth factor receptor expression and a nonangiogenic type of vascular pattern were significantly associated with poorer survival rates.

Conclusions.—Although many biological markers are found in NSCLC, none of them were found to be of prognostic significance. Perhaps molecular probes may be of prognostic value, but until such time as they are developed, clinical practice need not be changed based on the biological markers investigated.

▶ Wow! It is unusual to see a paper actually conclude that immunocytochemical markers (e.g., C-*erb* B1, Bcl-2, and p53) do not have a prognostic role in NSCLC diagnosis. I am so used to seeing the words "might," "possibly," "in the future," and "could" that I have wondered whether the whole battery of these markers should be used in the workup of non–small-cell lung tumors. Pastorino et al. conclude that cancer stage is the most reliable determinant for prognosis and that, therefore, markers are unnecessary. This does not mean that biological markers that may be developed in the future will not have relevance or that other techniques, such as molecular probes, may not be helpful in predicting patient outcomes. With this paper, the ball is now in the court of those who advocate the use of these markers.

S.S. Raab, M.D.

Utility of 123C3 Monoclonal Antibody Against CD56 (NCAM) for the Diagnosis of Small Cell Carcinomas on Paraffin Sections

Kaufmann O, Georgi T, Dietel M (Humboldt Univ Berlin)

Hum Pathol 28:1373–1378, 1997 1–4

Purpose.—Neural cell adhesion molecule, also known as CD56, can be detected by immunohistochemistry in frozen sections of nearly all small cell carcinomas (SCCs). Monoclonal antibody 123C3 against CD56 has been used for the diagnosis of T/natural killer (NK) cell lymphomas on paraffin sections with suitable antigen retrieval methods. The use of 123C3 was evaluated to distinguish pulmonary and extrapulmonary SCCs from nonneuroendocrine non–small cell carcinomas.

Methods.—The retrospective analysis included 70 SCCs and 344 primary and metastatic nonneuroendocrine carcinomas from different primary sites. Immunostaining with 123C3 was performed in all specimens. The results were compared with those of established neuroendocrine markers such as CD57, ChromograninA, and Synaptophysin.

Results.—Most SCCs showed diffuse staining with 123C3 in a strong membranous pattern, with a sensitivity of 99%. Crush artifacts and decalcification did not reduce the intensity of 123C3 staining. All neuroendocrine markers together were only 44% sensitive for SCCs. Staining with 123C3 was noted in 25% of ovarian carcinomas, 20% of renal cell carcinomas, 20% of endometrial carcinomas, 67% of nonneuroendocrine large cell carcinomas of the lung, 3% of adenocarcinomas, and 8% of squamous cell carcinomas of the lung. No CD56 immunoreactivity was noted for urothelial carcinomas, hepatocellular carcinomas, or squamous carcinomas of the head/neck and uterine cervix, or in adenocarcinomas of the breast, stomach, colon, pancreas, or prostate. Specificity for SCC was 94% for 123C3 and 95% for the combined neuroendocrine markers.

Conclusions.—Monoclonal antibody 123C3 appears to be potentially useful for immunohistochemical differentiation of SCCs and nonneuroendocrine carcinomas on paraffin sections. The results compare favorably with those of other specific neuroendocrine markers. Staining with 123C3 may be particularly useful in small and crushed biopsy specimens.

▶ My opinion: don't add the immunohistochemical antibody 123C3 to your panel to determine if a tumor is an SCC or a non-SCC. My reasons: (1) the data from multiple studies are conflicting with regard to the utility of 123C3; (2) the panel you probably use now (chromogranin, neuron specific enolase, and synaptophysin) is pretty good; and (3) this study was not designed to test the difficult cases. I mean, seriously, why include a whole spectrum of metastatic tumors from the prostate, ovary, liver, etc. (as the authors have) when these aren't even the cases with which we have trouble?

S.S. Raab, M.D.

Cigarette Smoking and Changes in the Histopathology of Lung Cancer

Thun MJ, Lally CA, Flannery JT, et al (American Cancer Society, Atlanta, Ga; Connecticut Tumor Registry, Hartford; Emory Univ, Atlanta, Ga)

J Natl Cancer Inst 89:1580–1586, 1997 1–5

Background.—Adenocarcinoma of the lung is now the most common type of lung cancer in the United States. This increased incidence may be a result of advances in diagnostic technology, changes in cigarette design, or changes in smoking practices. These possibilities were investigated.

Methods and Findings.—Data from the Connecticut Tumor Registry and 2 American Cancer Society studies were analyzed. The incidence of adenocarcinomas increased by nearly 17-fold in women and by almost 10-fold in men from 1959 through 1991. These increases paralleled sex and generational changes in smoking more than advances in diagnostic technology. Compared with data from the Cancer Prevention Study I, which was begun in 1959, data from the Cancer Prevention Study II, begun in 1982, demonstrated a stronger association between smoking and death from lung adenocarcinomas. The relative risks were 19.0 for men and 8.1 for women in the latter study compared with 4.6 for men and 1.5 for women in the earlier study.

Conclusions.—The increase in lung adenocarcinomas since the 1950s appears to be the result of changes in smoking behavior and cigarette design rather than the result of diagnostic advances. These data clearly show that cigarette smoking is the major cause of adenocarcinomas as well as other lung cancers.

► Admittedly, on biopsy specimens and even on excision specimens, I have strayed from subclassifying most lung tumors into categories other than small-cell carcinoma and non–small-cell carcinoma. This is because most non–small-cell carcinomas are treated similarly. Thun et al. and Russo et al.[1] argue that, if we still subclassify non–small-cell carcinomas, using the World Health Organization categories, the incidence of adenocarcinomas has markedly increased compared with the incidence of other non–small-cell carcinomas; furthermore, they argue that adenocarcinomas occur almost as frequently as squamous cell carcinomas. According to the authors, this increase in adenocarcinoma incidence is neither because of our diagnostic ability nor because of the newer technologies that are used to obtain tissues. The authors conclude that the rise in adenocarcinomas is a result of changes in smoking behavior (e.g., deeper inhaling) and cigarette manufacture (e.g., filter tips and low-tar nicotine cigarettes). Carcinogens now reach the periphery of the lung, whereas before the carcinogens mainly acted in the larger airways. Practically, this could explain some of the changes in the specimen types received by pathology laboratories. Over the years, there has been a decrease in sputum samples (good for central lesions) and an increase in fine-needle aspirates (good for peripheral lesions).

S.S. Raab, M.D.

Reference

1. Russo A, Crosignani P, Franceschi S, et al: Changes in lung cancer histological types in Varese Cancer Registry, Italy 1976–1992. *Eur J Cancer* 33:1643–1647, 1997.

The Immunohistochemical Diagnostic Panel for Epithelial Mesothelioma: A Reevaluation After Heat-induced Epitope Retrieval

Riera JR, Astengo-Osuna C, Longmate JA, et al (City of Hope Natl Med Ctr, Duarte, Calif; Universidad de Guadalajara, Mexico; Instituto Nacional de la Salud, Langreo, Asturias, España)

Am J Surg Pathol 21:1409–1419, 1997 1–6

Purpose.—Immunohistochemical studies may be used to distinguish between epithelial mesothelioma and adenocarcinoma. This distinction is currently made using a panel of antibodies to adenocarcinoma-associated antigens, with a few antibodies to mesothelial-associated antigens. With the use of epitope retrieval methods, many antibodies are more sensitive. The mesothelioma/adenocarcinoma panel for immunohistochemical diagnosis was reevaluated using epitope retrieval.

Methods.—A total of 268 paraffin-embedded, formalin-fixed tumor specimens, including 57 epithelial mesotheliomas and 211 adenocarcinomas, were studied. Immunohistochemical studies were performed using an extensive panel of antibodies, both with and without heat-induced epitope retrieval (HIER). The effects of HIER on antibody diagnostic performance were evaluated.

Results.—The use of HIER was associated with a sharp rise in sensitivity for several of the antibodies, with no accompanying decrease in specificity. The antibodies that best discriminated between adenocarcinoma and epithelial mesothelioma were those to carcinoembryonic antigen, BerEp4, and Bg8, all epithelial glycoproteins. Sensitivity and specificity were lower for mesothelium-associated antibodies, including HBME-1, calretinin, and thrombomodulin, although these were still useful in some cases. Cytokeratin and vimentin antibodies aided in assessing the quality of antigen preservation, although they were of little help in differentiating between mesothelioma and adenocarcinoma.

Conclusions.—The immunohistochemical distinction between epithelial mesothelioma and adenocarcinoma is aided by the addition of HIER. Antibodies against epithelial glycoproteins have the highest diagnostic value, whereas antibodies LeuM1, B72.3, and HMFG-2 are a useful secondary panel. With a few exceptions, HIER should be used with the members of the antibody panel.

► During the past year, there have been a number of articles investigating panels of immunostains to separate metastatic adenocarcinoma from epithelial mesothelioma. The articles by Riera et al. and Ordóñez[1] essentially conclude that many of the mesothelial-specific markers are not practically useful in the separation. Others disagree.[2–5] I think Riera et al. imply that we should not purchase these mesothelial-specific markers but should use a tried and true epithelial-specific panel, such as the antibodies of carcinoembryonic antigen, Bg8 and BerEp4. Increased sensitivity may be achieved with heat-induced antigen retrieval.

Although I agree with the conclusions of Riera et al., I still have 2 problems with the methods in all of these studies. First, it is assumed that the tumors used in these studies already have been separated with a 100% sensitivity and specificity into the categories of adenocarcinoma and mesothelioma. But this original separation often was based on immunostains, which is being tested in the current study. There is no true gold standard that can test the "new" antibodies. Second, all of these studies fail to grasp that disease prevalence is critically important in testing sensitivity and specificity. These studies artificially test antibodies in a population with a high mesothelioma prevalence and hope to use these data in a normal population where the prevalence of mesothelioma is exceedingly low. Thus, given the high prevalence of metastatic adenocarcinoma, even if an epithelial panel is negative, there is still a very high posttest probability that a malignancy is an adenocarcinoma, rather than a mesothelioma.

S.S. Raab, M.D.

References

1. Ordóñez NG: The value of antibodies 44-3A6, SM3, HBME-1, and thrombomodulin in differentiating epithelial pleural mesothelioma from lung adenocarcinoma: A comparative study with other commonly used antibodies. *Am J Surg Pathol* 21:1399–1408, 1997.
2. Han AC, Peralta-Soler A, Knudsen KA, et al: Differential expression of N-cadherin in pleural mesotheliomas and E-cadherin in lung adenocarcinomas in formalin-fixed, paraffin-embedded tissues. *Hum Pathol* 28:641–645, 1997.
3. Kennedy AD, King G, Kerr KM: HBME-1 and antithrombomodulin in the differential diagnosis of malignant mesothelioma of pleura. *J Clin Pathol* 50:859–862, 1997.
4. Donna A, Betta PG, Chiodera P, et al: Newly marketed tissue markers for malignant mesothelioma: Immunoreactivity of rabbit AMAD-2 antiserum compared with monoclonal antibody HBME-1 and a review of the literature on so-called antimesothelioma antibodies. *Hum Pathol* 28:929–937, 1997.
5. Sosolik RC, McGaughy VR, DeYoung BR: Anti-MOC-31: A potential addition to the pulmonary adenocarcinoma versus mesothelioma immunohistochemistry panel. *Mod Pathol* 10:716–719, 1997.

The Use of Epithelial Membrane Antigen and Silver-stained Nucleolar Organizer Regions Testing in the Differential Diagnosis of Mesothelioma From Benign Reactive Mesothelioses

Wolanski KD, Whitaker D, Shilkin KB, et al (Queen Elizabeth II Med Centre, Nedlands, Australia; Flinders Med Centre, South Australia)
Cancer 82:583–590, 1998 1–7

Purpose.—For legal as well as medical reasons, it is important to make an accurate diagnosis of pleural lesions. However, it can be difficult to make such a diagnosis from a small, closed biopsy. No test can reliably differentiate between malignant and benign mesothelial tissue. This study evaluated epithelial membrane antigen (EMA) and silver-stained nucleolar organizer regions (AgNORs) for use in differentiating between benign and malignant mesothelial lesions.

Methods.—The study included pleural and peritoneal biopsy specimens collected over a 20-year period. Each specimen underwent immunostaining with EMA and quantitation of AgNORs. Each stain's value in the diagnosis of epithelial malignant mesothelioma was assessed alone and the values were also assessed in combination.

Results.—Immunoreactivity for EMA was noted in 73% of 141 malignant lesions, compared with a 3% rate of equivocal reactions and no positive reactions among 73 benign lesions. The malignant lesions showed a higher average count of AgNORs per cell than benign lesions did. However, the values overlapped significantly. Measuring average AgNOR area produced much less overlap. With a maximum benign AgNOR area of 0.6677 μm^2 as the upper threshold, 64% of cases were correctly identified as malignant. This test had a specificity of 100%, with a sensitivity of 64%. Ninety-five percent of malignant mesotheliomas tested positive for EMA, AgNOR, or both, with no false positives.

Conclusions.—Immunostaining with EMA is of value in the diagnosis of malignant vs. benign mesothelial lesions. When the results are combined with the average area of AgNOR per cell, the diagnosis of epithelial malignant mesothelioma can be made with still greater sensitivity. These tests may have a useful ancillary role in the differential diagnosis of difficult pleural biopsies.

► That old question again raises its head: are there any tests (immunohistochemical, image analytic, etc.) that allow us to tell with certainty that a mesothelial lesion is benign or malignant? The data from this study by Wolanski and co-authors again confirm that the answer is no. As has been shown before, EMA stains positively in the majority of malignant mesothelial lesions, and equivocally in some benign mesothelial lesions, indicating that EMA is helpful, but neither 100% sensitive nor 100% specific. My impression is that AgNOR staining is less helpful, particularly if one does AgNOR counting. Measuring AgNOR area, as the authors did in this study, is neither practical nor definitive.

S.S. Raab, M.D.

Idiopathic Bronchiolitis Obliterans Organizing Pneumonia/Cryptogenic Organizing Pneumonia With Unfavorable Outcome: Pathologic Predictors

Yousem SA, Lohr RH, Colby TV (Univ of Pittsburgh, Pa; Mayo Clinic, Scottsdale, Ariz; Mayo Clinic, Rochester, Minn)

Mod Pathol 10:864–871, 1997 1–8

Introduction.—Idiopathic bronchiolitis obliterans organizing pneumonia (BOOP) and cryptogenic organizing pneumonia (COP) both indicate an inflammatory interstitial process characterized by a patchy distribution of young fibromyxoid connective tissue within airways and air spaces. Most patients have an excellent response to steroid therapy, but 10% to 15% exhibit disease progression. Pathologic predictors of clinical behavior were identified after a review of 19 cases of BOOP–COP.

Methods.—All patients were treated with systemic corticosteroids at doses ranging from 40 to 100 mg/day. Ten patients' disease was steroid-responsive, and the disease of 9 patients (all of whom died of their pulmonary disease) was steroid-resistant. These 2 groups were compared for clinical and pathologic variables.

Results.—The steroid-responsive group had an average age of 67.4 years; 6 were women and 4 were men. Symptoms included coughing, fevers, and shortness of breath. Five patients had patchy bilateral alveolar opacities; 3 had a bilateral mixed alveolar–reticulonodular pattern. At an average follow-up of 26.5 months, all were alive with no evidence of disease. The steroid-responsive group included 6 men and 3 women with an average age of 69.5 years. All had shortness of breath, 5 had coughs, and 3 reported fatigue. Seven patients had bilateral alveolar opacities, 1 had mixed alveolar–interstitial opacities, and 2 had bilateral reticulonodular disease. The average length of survival in this group was 4.2 months from the time of the diagnosis.

Although the 2 groups did not differ significantly in demographic characteristics, symptoms, or radiographic findings, a histologic examination showed scarring and remodeling of the background lung parenchyma in 89% of patients with progressive disease. In contrast, only 10% of patients with steroid-responsive disease who survived exhibited these changes.

Conclusion.—Most patients with the idiopathic form of BOOP–COP respond well to steroid therapy, but, in a minority of cases, the disease is progressive and patients do not survive. A predictor of poor prognosis appears to be the presence of background remodeling of the pulmonary parenchyma with scarring, interstitial fibrosis, and, ultimately, restructuring of the architecture of the lung. This finding may provide a morphological marker of outcome in BOOP–COP.

► This study by Yousem et al. rather convincingly demonstrates that idiopathic BOOP–COP comprises several entities that exhibit different pathologic features that correlate with outcomes. Idiopathic BOOP–COP is rare, and, if we see BOOP-like features, we should first exclude a number of known entities, which is a task that may not always be possible if a history is not provided. Then, besides identifying the BOOP features, we should examine the interstitia to determine the extent of chronic fibrosis. If there is background interstitial fibrosis, these patients' disease may not respond to steroids. I wonder whether these patients with chronic fibrosis really had no symptoms before the BOOP symptoms and when the biopsies were taken in the course of the BOOP symptoms. Nevertheless, the microscopic description should discuss the degree of fibrosis in the interstitia.

S.S. Raab, M.D.

Bronchiolitis: Pathologic Considerations
Colby TV (Mayo Clinic Scottsdale, Ariz)
Am J Clin Pathol 109:101–109, 1998 1–9

Introduction.—Bronchiolitis refers to an inflammatory (cellular) and mesenchymal (granulation-type tissue and scarring) reaction involving the bronchioles. The interaction between these 2 components leads to changes in the lumen size, lamina propria, muscular layer, and bronchiolar adventitia, and thus to various clinical, radiologic, and fundamental patterns of disease. The anatomy and surgical pathology of bronchiolitis were reviewed.

Pathologic Classification.—Bronchiolitis is presented as a spectrum of changes with significant overlap among groups, or evolution from one group to another. The well-recognized histologic changes of asthma lead to luminal narrowing and airflow obstruction, most prominent in the small bronchi but also apparent in the bronchioles. Certain bronchiolar changes are noted in patients with chronic obstructive pulmonary disease, including inflammatory changes, hypertrophy of the bronchiolar smooth muscle, fibrotic narrowing and associated changes, luminal changes, and loss of radial attachments. Cellular bronchiolitis refers to the presence of inflammatory infiltrates of bronchioles; this designation is useful when no cause of the bronchiolitis is apparent. Cellular bronchiolitis may be acute or chronic, with or without fibrosis. Most of the conditions associated with cellular bronchiolitis are airway diseases, although some are interstitial. Bronchiolar necrosis may occur in suppurative bacterial infections and in viral bronchiolitis. Resiratory bronchiolitis, or "smokers' bronchiolitis," affects mainly the respiratory bronchioles, although inflammatory changes of the terminal bronchioles may be seen as well. The major pathologic finding is accumulated tan-brown macrophages in the bronchiolar and alveolar lumina. Respiratory bronchiolitis is usually an incidental finding, although respiratory bronchiolitis–associated interstitial disease may sometimes become pronounced enough to cause clinical disease.

Bronchiolitis obliterans refers to the clinical syndrome of chronic airflow obstruction and radiographic hyperinflation caused by pathologic changes of the small airways. Pathololgically, the term may apply to 2 entities: bronchiolitis obliterans with intraluminal polyps, often associated with patchy organizing pneumonia (bronchiolitis obliterans organizing pneumonia [BOOP]); and the less-common constrictive bronchiolitis, characterized by luminal narrowing caused by scarring. Patients with clinical bronchiolitis obliterans are usually found to have constrictive bronchiolitis on histologic examination. This condition has many causes in common with the BOOP pattern, but the 2 are regarded as distinct clinicopathologic groups. Other forms of bronchiolitis include mineral dust–associated airway disease and peribronchiolar fibrosis/bronchiolar metaplasia.

Discussion.—A practical surgical pathologic classification of bronchiolitis was presented. Some key points to remember when assessing bronchiolar pathology were emphasized, including the presence of a localized vs. diffuse process; whether the bronchiolar lesions are the main lesions; the presence of mild vascular thickening, reflecting pulmonary hypertension; associated changes in the peribronchiolar lung parenchyma; the presence of associated organizing pneumonia; and the presence of subtle bronchiolar lesions in patients with airflow obstruction.

► Colby provides an excellent review article of the different inflammatory conditions of the respiratory bronchioles. This is a "top down" review which, assuming you know the disease process (e.g., asthma, mineral dust–associated airway disease, etc.), provides an explanation of the histologic changes. It is less useful if you don't know what is going on histologically in the first place and you are looking for a differential diagnosis. Colby's description of the types of bronchiolitis obliterans is short and sweet and complete!

S.S. Raab, M.D.

The Histological Spectrum of Chronic Necrotizing Forms of Pulmonary Aspergillosis

Yousem SA (Univ of Pittsburgh, Pa)

Hum Pathol 28:650–656, 1997 1–10

Objective.—Chronic necrotizing pulmonary aspergillosis (CNPA) is a rare, indolent, locally destructive form of pulmonary aspergillosis. The clinical and radiologic findings and biologic behavior of this condition have been well described, but its histopathology has not. A histomorphologic study of 10 cases of CNPA was performed.

Findings.—The patients were 6 men and 4 women, mean age 59 years, with symptoms lasting 2–24 months. All patients met clinical criteria for CNPA. Histomorphologic evaluation revealed 3 distinct types of CNPA. Four patients showed a necrotizing granulomatous pneumonia, which was centered around a zone of infarct-like parenchymal necrosis caused by angioinvasive aspergillus. Four patients had a granulomatous bronchiectatic cavity with a central fungal ball. These cases showed tongues of necrosis and inflammation extending into a thick fibrous capsule and superficially infiltrated lung parenchyma. The remaining 2 patients had a bronchocentric granulomatosis-like reaction, characterized by necrotizing granulomatous bronchitis/bronchiolitis with luminal necrotic debris, with a palisaded histiocytic reaction replacing the mucosa. With antifungal treatment and surgery, all patients survived.

Conclusions.—The study identifies 3 histomorphologic forms of CNPA: a necrotizing granulomatous pneumonia, bronchiectatic cavities with mural invasion, and a bronchocentric granulomatosis-like reaction. Despite these morphologic differences, the responses to treatment are similar. The possibility of CNPA should be considered in patients with chronic infectious granulomatous disease.

► Pulmonic aspergillic infections often are categorized as invasive or noninvasive (aspergillomas). With the invasive variety, the patients usually do poorly, and with the aspergillomas, patients usually do well. In this study, Yousem reminds us that not all aspergillic lung infections can be placed at either end of the spectrum. Chronic necrotizing pulmonary aspergillosis is a rare process that correlates with a specific clinical syndrome (constitutional symptoms, mild immune defects, and often previous disease). Yousem presents an exhaustive differential diagnosis, which is helpful in dealing with patients with aspergillic and granulomatous disease. One take-home message is that we should know the patient's clinical history before subclassifying an aspergillic disease.

S.S. Raab, M.D.

Treated Wegener's Granulomatosis: Distinctive Pathological Findings in the Lungs of 20 Patients and What They Tell Us About the Natural History of the Disease

Mark EJ, Flieder DB, Matsubara O (Harvard Med School, Boston; Natl Defense Med College, Saitama, Japan)

Hum Pathol 28:450–458, 1997 1–11

Introduction.—The serologic antineutrophil cytoplasmic antibody (ANCA) test has almost completely removed the need for lung or kidney biopsies for the diagnosis of Wegener's granulomatosis (WG). Autopsy and biopsy studies have reported changes in the morphological characteristics of treated WG, but the morphological characteristics have never been systematically investigated. The clinical features and pulmonary histories of 20 patients with WG treated with corticosteroids or cyclophosphamide or both were correlated to define morphological changes in treated patients.

Methods.—Surgical and autopsy material from the lungs of patients with WG who were treated with corticosteriods or cyclophosphamide or both for at least 48 hours and at least 48 hours before biopsy or autopsy were assessed by elastic tissue, trichrome, periodic acid–Schiff, reticulin, and iron stains or by a combination of these tests.

Results.—The patient age range was 25–81 years. All 16 patients in whom serum ANCA tests were performed had elevated ANCA levels. The duration of treatment was 6–13 days. Twelve patients (60%) had diagnostic or suspicious extravascular lesions that included palisading granulomas, microabscesses, macronodular necrosis, giant cell nodules, and micronodular scars. One patient had diagnostic bronchiolar lesions, and 13 patients had suspicious lesions, including 3 novel patterns of bronchiolitis fibrosa. Other features included diffuse alveolar damage, alveolar fibrin, interstitial fibrosis, pneumonitis resembling unusual interstitial pneumonitis, and lipoid pneumonia.

Conclusion.—Wegener's granulomatosis has several histopathologic facets involving the arteries, veins, capillaries, bronchioles, interstitium, and pleura. The intrinsic lesion may be collagenous necrosis. Changes in histologic features can be observed after 6 days of treatment. The changes are usually muted and include disappearance of classic histopathologic characteristics; altered, distinctive histologic disease forms; morphological changes within 6 days of treatment; and bronchiolar scarring.

▶ The difficulty with diagnosing WG is that it has many histologic faces. Mark et al. show that there are even more faces of WG after patients have been treated. For example, in their series of 20 patients, only 35% had a granulomatous vasculitis, which is diagnostic for active disease. This indicates that, before we make a diagnosis of WG, we should get a clinical history and ANCA results.

S.S. Raab, M.D.

Pathology of Lung Allografts in Children and Young Adults

Badizadegan K, Perez-Atayde AR (Harvard Med School, Boston; Children's Hosp, Boston)

Hum Pathol 28:704–713, 1997 1–12

Objective.—Heart-lung and lung transplantation are no longer uncommon. Although it is known that disease differences between children and adults result in a higher pediatric mortality rate, these differences have not been well characterized. Posttransplant pathologic findings in pediatric and young adult lung transplantation patients were reviewed.

Methods.—Eleven lung or heart-lung transplantation patients, aged 3.5–20 years, were followed up for a median of 8.3 months. Histopathologic examinations were performed on 98 specimens including 5 postmortem specimens obtained between 1 day and 50 months after transplantation.

Results.—There were 39 acute rejection specimens, including 16 surveillance specimens and 22 problem-related specimens, and all had similar histologic grades. A significant number of biopsy specimens with acute rejection showed lymphocytic bronchitis/bronchiolitis, bronchiolitis obliterans, and focal or diffuse alveolar damage. Chronic airway rejection occurred earlier in patients with bronchiolitis obliterans than in patients without. Accelerated graft vascular sclerosis was associated with chronic vascular rejection. Nonrejection pathology included airway inflammation, vascular changes, acute or organizing pneumonitis, alveolar damage, and focal parenchymal hemorrhage. Infection pathology was characterized by inflammation, alveolar damage, and parenchymal necrosis (Fig 5, C).

C

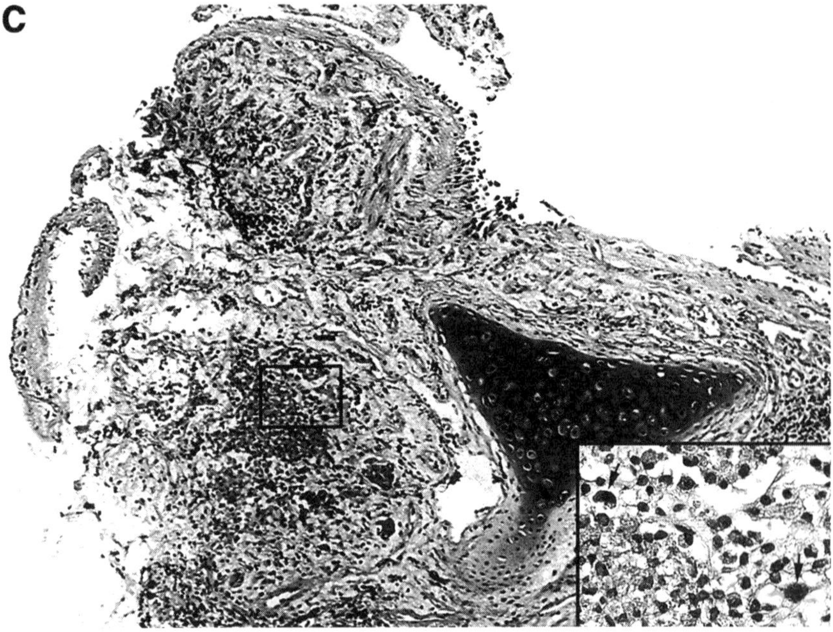

FIGURE 5, C.—Bronchial wall with transmural inflammation and peribronchial microabscess formation. **Inset** shows higher magnification of the periphery of the microabscess with occasional large cells with cytopathic changes consistent with adenoviral infection (*arrows*). (Courtesy of Badizadegan K, Perez-Atayde AR: Pathology of lung allografts in children and young adults. *Hum Pathol* 28:704–713, 1997.)

Conclusions.—Most patients in this age group died of overwhelming infection, in particular adenoviral pneumonia.

► The data regarding pediatric lung allograft pathology has been slowly rolling in over the past several years, and this report by Badizadegan and Perez-Atayde describe the findings in another 11 patients. Compared with other pediatric series,[1-3] there are not any surprises here. There may be some differences in the time course of chronic vascular rejection between children and adults, but the histologic criteria still are the same. Remember that infections may run a rampant course, and therefore it is important to look out for virally infected cells, such as adenovirus.

S.S. Raab, M.D.

References

1. Bejarano PA, Dehner LP, Wick MR, et al: Isolated lung transplantation in children: Pathological diagnosis and incidence of pulmonary complications. *Hum Pathol* 25:1179–1184, 1994.
2. Noyes BE, Kurland G, Orenstein DM, et al: Experience with pediatric lung transplantation. *J Pediatr* 124:261–268, 1994.
3. Kurland G, Noyes BE, Jaffe R, et al: Bronchoalveolar lavage and transbronchial biopsy in children following heart-lung and lung transplantation. *Chest* 104:1043–1048, 1993.

Primary Germ Cell Tumors of the Mediastinum: I. Analysis of 322 Cases With Special Emphasis on Teratomatous Lesions and a Proposal for Histopathologic Classification and Clinical Staging

Moran CA, Suster S (Armed Forces Inst of Pathology, Washington, DC; Univ of Miami, Fla)

Cancer 80:681–690, 1997 1–13

Introduction.—Although most germ cell tumors occur in the gonads, other locations—such as the pineal gland, retroperitoneum, mediastinum, and sacral area—have been involved. Because few comprehensive studies have examined germ cell tumors arising primarily in the mediastinum, researchers analyzed the clinical and histologic features of 322 of these neoplasms.

Methods.—Cases were identified through a search of surgical pathology files for the period 1960 to 1994. Clinical records and hematoxylin and eosin–stained sections were reviewed in all cases. Germ cell tumors of the mediastinum were divided into 2 main categories: teratomatous and nonteratomatous lesions. A system for clinical staging was used to classify the tumors according to extent of invasion.

Results.—All but 2 of the 322 patients were male. The only 2 female patients had teratomatous lesions with additional malignant components. Patients ranged in age from 1 to 79 years, and most were between the ages of 10 and 30 years. Teratomatous lesions accounted for 44% of cases, pure seminomas for 37%, and yolk sac tumors, embryonal carcinomas, and choriocarcinomas for 16%; 3% were combined nonteratomatous germ cell tumors. Clinical staging was completed in 242 cases: 191 (79%) were stage I, 4 (1.6%) were stage II, and 47 (19.4%) were stage III. Stage I tumors were well circumscribed, with or without focal adhesions to the pleura or pericardium but without microscopic evidence of invasion into adjacent structures. Stage II tumors were confined to the mediastinum but had macroscopic or microscopic evidence of infiltration into adjacent structures. Stage III tumors had metastases, either to intrathoracic organs or with extrathoracic spread. In most cases, there was good correlation between clinical staging and clinical outcome.

Discussion.—Primary germ cell tumors of the mediastinum occur infrequently, yet account for approximately 10% to 20% of all neoplasms of this region. Overall, these tumors exhibited demographic and histopathologic distributions similar to those of tumors occurring in the male gonads. Most were teratomatous lesions, but, in contrast to previous studies, mature teratomas accounted for only a minority of tumors in this category. The proposed histological classification and clinical staging may help clinicians to plan therapy and predict clinical outcome.

▶ Three *Cancer* articles, this one and 2 others,[1, 2] form an excellent comprehensive source on primary mediastinal germ cell tumors. Although these tumors are rare, one should consider looking over these articles before making a definitive diagnosis of a primary mediastinal germ cell tumor. In general, the articles reveal no real surprises: (1) patients are overwhelmingly male; (2) the same classification for germ cell tumors exists in the mediastinum as in the gonads; (3) one should look for spread of tumors into surrounding tissues, for this will affect patient prognosis; and (4) nonseminomatous, nonteratomatous germ cell tumors are highly aggressive, and there are frequently metastases at the time of presentation. These articles will become a reference source for future studies.

S.S. Raab, M.D.

References

1. Moran CA, Suster S, Przygodzki RM, et al: Primary germ cell tumors of the mediastinum: II. Mediastinal seminomas. A clinical pathologic and immunohistochemical study of 120 cases. *Cancer* 80:691–698, 1997.
2. Moran CA, Suster S, Koss MN: Primary germ cell tumors of the mediastinum: III. Yolk sac tumor, embryonal carcinoma, choriocarcinoma, and combined non-teratomatous germ cell tumors of the mediastinum. A clinical pathologic and immunohistochemical study of 64 cases. *Cancer* 80:699–707, 1997.

2 Cytopathology

Glandular Cells in Vaginal Smears From Posthysterectomy Patients
Ponder TB, Easley KO, Dávila RM (Washington Univ, St Louis)
Acta Cytol 41:1701–1704, 1997 2–1

Background.—Glandular cells lacking atypical nuclear features are sometimes found in vaginal smears after hysterectomy. Such a finding raises concerns about the development of *de novo* or recurrent vaginal malignancy. The significance of nonatypical glandular cells in vaginal smears from patients after hysterectomy was investigated.

Methods.—Vaginal smears with nonatypical glandular epithelium from 15 patients who had undergone total hysterectomy were identified in a review of records spanning 4.5 years. Mean patient age was 59 years. Cytologic findings and clinical data were correlated.

Findings.—Seventy-three percent of the patients had a history of gynecologic malignancy. Sixty percent had been treated with radiation therapy. All had normal gynecologic examination findings at the time the vaginal smear was obtained. Neither recurrent nor *de novo* vaginal adenocarcinoma developed in any of the patients.

Conclusions.—The finding of nonatypical glandular cells in this patient population apparently does not indicate adenocarcinoma. Most women in this series did not subsequently have vaginal abnormalities. The origin of nonatypical glandular cells in vaginal smears from asymptomatic women after hysterectomy with normal gynecologic physical findings is still not known.

▶ This article discusses an issue that arises for all of us from time to time. This is the largest series of benign-appearing endocervical-type glandular cells on post–total hysterectomy vaginal smears yet published (n = 15). The authors' practice differs from most in that the vast majority of these hysterectomies were perfomred for treatment of gynecologic malignancies. It is not possible to comment further on the relevance of this patient population to the observations made in the paper. The authors do a good job of reminding us about normal anatomical explanations for this finding, and they review studies indicating that adenosis, mesonephric duct remnants, and endometrial implants are more common than sometimes believed. The messages to be taken from this study seem to be the following: (1) even in this cancer-enriched sample of patients, the finding of such cells is usually unaccompanied by a clinically apparent vaginal lesion; and (2) these cells do not herald recurrent or *de novo* vaginal malignancy.

M.W. Stanley, M.D.

Suggested Reading

Bewtra C: Columnar cells in posthysterectomy vaginal smears. *Diagn Cytopathol* 8:342–345, 1992.

Pearce KF, Haefner HK, Sarwar SF, et al: Cytopathological findings on vaginal Papanicolaou smears after hysterectomy for benign gynecologic disease. *N Engl J Med* 335:1559–1562, 1996.

Qualifying the Cytologic Diagnosis of "Atypical Squamous Cells of Undetermined Significance" Affects the Predictive Value of a Squamous Intraepithelial Lesion on Subsequent Biopsy

Genest DR, Dean B, Lee KR, et al (Harvard Med School, Boston)
Arch Pathol Lab Med 122:338–341, 1998 2–2

Objective.—The diagnostic criteria for atypical squamous cells of undetermined significance (ASCUS) in cervical pathology is imprecise and not generally accepted. To test if ASCUS qualifiers may have clinical significance, a 6-month retrospective review of ASCUS smears was undertaken at Brigham and Women's Hospital, Boston, Massachusetts, to define the implications of a diagnosis of ASCUS alone and its subclassification.

Methods.—Between January and June of 1995, 452 Papanicolaou smears were assessed for atypical squamous cells of undetermined significance by 9 cytopathologists. The smears were categorized in 4 groups: (1) favor reactive, (2) not otherwise specified (NOS), (3) favor squamous intraepithelial lesion (SIL) (grade unspecified), or (4) favor high-grade SIL

TABLE 1.—Relationship Between Cytologic and Histologic Diagnoses of ASCUS*

Cytologic Diagnosis ASCUS Qualification	N	Histologic Diagnosis, N (%) No SIL	LSIL	HSIL	Total SIL
Favor reactive	100	93 (93)†	3 (3)	4 (4)	7 (7)
NOS	192	151 (79)	23 (12)	18 (9)	41 (21)
Favor SIL	133	89 (67)	21 (16)	23 (17)	44 (33)
Favor HSIL	27	12 (44)	2 (7)	13 (48)‡	15 (55)
Total	**452**	**345** (76)	**49** (11)	**58** (13)	**107** (24)

*ASCUS indicates atypical squamous cells of undetermined significance.
†$P = 0.04$.
‡$P = 0.00001$.
Abbreviations: HSIL, high-grade squamous intraepithelial lesion; *LSIL*, low-grade squamous intraepithelial lesion; *NOS*, not otherwise specified; *SIL*, squamous intraepithelial lesion.
(Courtesy of Genest DR, Dean B, Lee KR, et al: Qualifying the cytologic diagnosis of "Atypical squamous cells of undetermined significance" affects the predictive value of a squamous intraepithelial lesion on subsequent biopsy. *Arch Pathol Lab Med* 122:338–341, 1998.)

TABLE 2.—Pathologic Outcome for Women With a Diagnosis of "ASCUS, Favor Reactive"*

Cytopathologist	N	Histologic Diagnosis, % Negative	LSIL	HSIL
A	4	75	0	25
B	11	91	9	0
C	15	93	0	7
D	2	100	0	0
E	20	100	0	0
F	8	88	0	12
G	12	100	0	0
H	24	88	8	4
I	4	100	0	0
Total	100	93	3	4

*ASCUS indicates atypical squamous cells of undetermined significance.

Abbreviations: N, number of smears diagnosed as "ASCUS, favor reactive"; *HSIL*, high-grade squamous intraepithelial lesion; *LSIL*, low-grade squamous intraepithelial lesion.

(Courtesy of Genest DR, Dean B, Lee, KR, et al: Qualifying the cytologic diagnosis of "Atypical squamous cells of undetermined significance" affects the predictive value of a squamous intraepithelial lesion on subsequent biopsy. *Arch Pathol Lab Med* 122:338–341, 1998.)

(HSIL). These qualified readings were compared with histopathologic results obtained within 3 months.

Results.—SIL was diagnosed in 108 (24%) of the smears (Table 1). Low-grade SIL and HSIL accounted for 11% and 13%, respectively. There were 100 (22%) smears categorized as favor reactive, 133 (29%) smears as favor SIL, and 27 (6%) smears as favor HSIL. There were 192 (42%) smears categorized as NOS. Biopsy-proven SIL was moderately frequent in the favor SIL smears (33%) and NOS smears (21%) and most frequent in the favor HSIL group (55%). Biopsy-proven HSIL was found in 4% of the favor reactive smears and in 48% of the favor HSIL smears ($P = 0.00001$) (Tables 2 and 3). There was a significant association between a favor

TABLE 3.—Pathologic Outcome for Women With a Diagnosis of "ASCUS, Favor HSIL"*

Cytopathologist	N	Histologic Diagnosis, % Negative	LSIL	HSIL
A	2	100	0	0
B	5	60	0	40
C	5	40	0	60
D	1	0	0	100
E	7	43	14	43
F	0	...	...	...
G	5	40	20	40
H	1	0	0	100
I	1	0	0	100
Total	27	44	7	48

*ASCUS indicates atypical squamous cells of undetermined significance.

Abbreviations: HSIL, high-grade squamous intraepithelial lesion; *N*, number of smears diagnosed as "ASCUS, favor HSIL"; *LSIL*, low-grade squamous intraepithelial lesion.

(Courtesy of Genest DR, Dean B, Lee KR, et al: Qualifying the cytologic diagnosis of "Atypical squamous cells of undetermined significance" affects the predictive value of a squamous intraepithelial lesion on subsequent biopsy. *Arch Pathol Lab Med* 122:338–341, 1998.)

reactive smear (94%) and a benign biopsy finding and between a favor HSIL smear and a biopsy finding of HSIL (53%, $P = 0.00001$).

Conclusion.—Qualifying cytologic diagnoses of ASCUS provides a meaningful risk stratification system for SIL.

► These authors have divided ASCUS into 4 grades that correlate with subsequent histologic evaluation on a trend basis. There remain inevitable undercalls and overcalls when an SIL is suggested. For example there is a small group of smears called ASCUS-favor reactive in which a high-grade SIL will subsequently be detected. Furthermore, about half of ASCUS-favor reactive high-grade SIL cases will not harbor such a lesion. After reciting standard TBS criteria for ASCUS, the nine cytopathologists are said to use a "subjective impression" for further subclassification; I think that we all do this. While criteria for this subclassification are not set in stone, the utility of these interpretations for predicting the histologic outcome are obvious. I suspect that we will be asked to use this type of ASCUS grading system to an increasing extent. However, those requesting this information must be educated regarding the subjective nature of such interpretations as well as the limitations in diagnostic accuracy.

M.W. Stanley, M.D.

Suggested Reading

Collins LC, Wang HH, Abu-Jandeh GM: Qualifiers of atypical squamous cells of undetermined significance help in patient management. *Mod Pathol* 9:677–681, 1996.

Darey DD, Naryshkin S, Nielson ML, et al: Atypical squamous cells of undetermined significance: Interlaboratory comparison and quality assurance monitors, *Diagn Cytopathol* 1:390–396, 1994.

Williams ML, Rimm DL, Pedigo MA, et al: Atypical squamous cells of undetermined significance: Correlative histologic and follow-up studies from an academic medical center. *Diagn Cytopathol* 16:1–7, 1997.

The Cost-Effectiveness of Cervical–Vaginal Rescreening

Raab SS (Univ of Iowa, Iowa City)

Am J Clin Pathol 108:525–536, 1997 2–3

Objective.—Although rescreening of 10% of cervical–vaginal smears to detect false-negative diagnoses is practiced by most laboratories, the cost-effectiveness of this and other rescreening practices has not been evaluated. The clinical usefulness of various rescreening strategies in a population of normal risk women who had a negative cervical–vaginal smear was retrospectively evaluated using decision analysis for life expectancy, cost-effectiveness, and false-negative and false-positive rates.

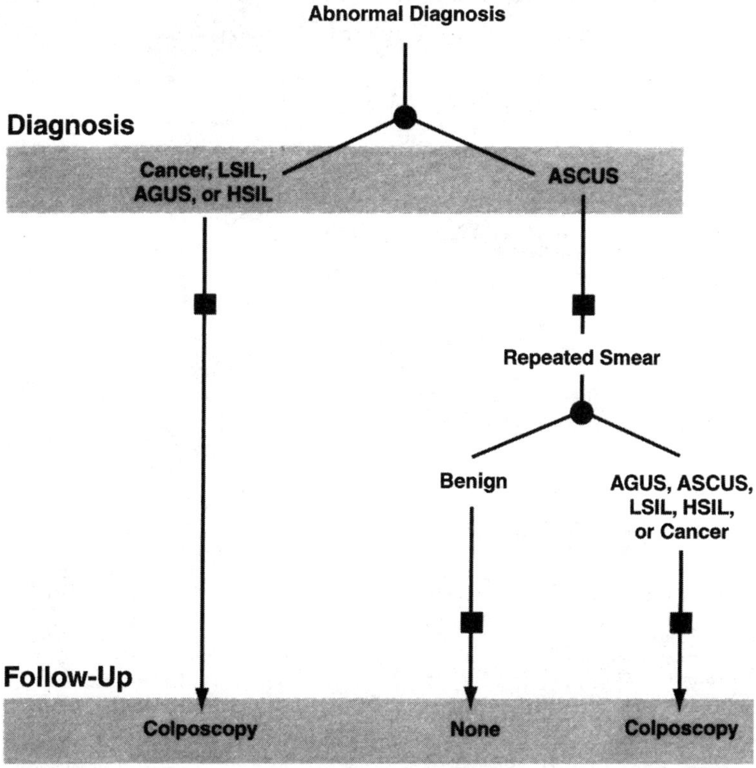

FIGURE 1.—Decision tree showing the workup of a patient with an abnormal cytologic diagnosis. A patient with a cytologic diagnosis of low-grade squamous intraepithelial lesion (LSIL), high-grade intraepithelial lesion (HSIL), atypical glandular cells of undetermined significance (AGUS), or cancer underwent colposcopy. A patient with a diagnosis of atypical squamous cells of undetermined significance (ASCUS) had a repeated cervical-vaginal smear in 3 months. If the repeated smear was interpreted as benign, the patient received no additional follow-up. If the repeated smear was interpreted as AGUS, ASCUS, LSIL, HSIL, or cancer, the patient underwent colposcopy. (Courtesy of Raab SS: The cost-effectiveness of cervical-vaginal rescreening. *Am J Clin Pathol* 108:525–536, 1997. Copyright 1997 by the American Society of Clinical Pathologists. Reprinted with permission.)

Methods.—Using the decision-model reference case of a 30-year-old white woman with a normal risk for development of cervical cancer and having a negative cervical–vaginal smear, 3 options were tested: (1) have the smear rescreened according to 1 of 7 strategies; (2) have a repeat cervical–vaginal smear; or (3) have no rescreening or repeat smear. A rescreened or repeated smear was assigned a diagnosis of benign or abnormal and worked up according to the decision tree (Fig 1). The number of false-negative, false-positive, and cancer diagnoses was calculated for each strategy per 10,000 women (Table 2). Probabilities based on these variables were calculated (Table 3).

Results.—Rescreening detected more false negatives than no rescreening, but was cost-effective only if the cost of rescreening was low (Table 5). Although 100% rescreening increases life expectancy and was cost-effec-

TABLE 2.—Probabilities Used in Decision Model

Probability Variable	Value
False-negative result as a result of misinterpretation[15-23,46]	
Epithelial abnormality	0.048
ASCUS	0.033
LSIL	0.010
HSIL	0.003
AGUS	0.002
False-negative result as a result of sampling error in comparison with total false-negative results15–19	0.50
Cytologic diagnosis on repeated smear after an ASCUS diagnosis[47-59]	
Benign	0.50
ASCUS	0.13
AGUS	0
LSIL	0.30
HSIL	0.07
Carcinoma	0
Carcinoma stage after "normal" detection[60]	
Local	0.51
Regional	0.33
Distant	0.08
Unstaged	0.07
Carcinoma stage after "early" detection[61,62]	
Local	0.80
Regional	0.20
Missing a lesion on repeat cervical-vaginal smear[15-23]	0.096
Progression[67-86]	
LSIL to invasive carcinoma	0.01
HSIL to invasive carcinoma	0.10
Progression in 1 yr[67-86]	
LSIL to invasive carcinoma	0.25
HSIL to invasive carcinoma	0.50

Abbreviations: ASCUS, atypical squamous cells of undetermined significance; *LSIL*, low grade squamous intraepithelial lesion; *HSIL*, high-grade squamous intraepithelial lesion; *AGUS*, atypical glandular cells of undetermined significance.

(Courtesy of Raab SS: The cost-effectiveness of cervical-vaginal rescreening. *Am J Clin Pathol* 108:525–536, 1997. Copyright 1997 by the American Society of Clinical Pathologists. Reprinted with permission.)

TABLE 3.—Probability of Disease on Colposcopy After Cytologic Diagnosis

	Final Diagnosis After Colposcopy				
Cytologic Diagnosis	Benign	LSIL	HSIL	SCCA	Adenocarcinoma
ASCUS × 2	0.49	0.48	0.03	0.0	0.0
LSIL	0.0	0.70	0.30	0.0	0.0
HSIL	0.0	0.09	0.90	0.01	0.0
SCCA	0.0	0.0	0.0	1.0	0.0
AGUS	0.5	0.2	0.2	0.0	0.1

Abbreviations: LSIL, low-grade squamous intraepithelial lesion; *HSIL*, high-grade squamous intraepithelial lesion; *SCCA*, squamous cell carcinoma; *ASCUS* × 2, two consecutive diagnoses of atypical squamous cells of undetermined significance; *AGUS*, atypical glandular cells of undetermined significance.

(Courtesy of Raab SS: The cost-effectiveness of cervical-vaginal rescreening. *Am J Clin Pathol* 108:525–536, 1997. Copyright 1997 by the American Society of Clinical Pathologists. Reprinted with permission.)

TABLE 5.—Number of False-Negative Results, False-Positive Results, and Cancers, and Life Expectancies of Competing Rescreening and Repeated Cervical-Vaginal Smear Strategies

Strategy	FN Results per 10,000	FP Results per 10,000	Cancers per 10,000	Life Expectancy (y)	Gain if Life Expectancy (d)
1 (100% rescreen)	284	196	17.78	19.2276	0.66
2 (10% rescreen)	540	20	29.45	19.2260	0.07
3 (100% rescreen and repeated CV smear)	16	381	11.59	19.2287	1.08
4 (100% rescreen and repeated CV smear*)	8	387	11.08	19.2288	1.09
5 (repeated CV smear)	32	370	17.24	19.2281	0.84
6 (10% rescreen and repeated CV smear)	31	371	17.08	19.2281	0.84
7 (none)	568	0	30.75	19.2258	Reference

*With 100% automated rescreening.

Abbreviations: FN, false-negative; *FP*, false-positive; *cancers*, cancers developing over lifetime; *CV*, cervical-vaginal.

(Courtesy of Raab SS: The cost-effectiveness of cervical-vaginal rescreening. *Am J Clin Pathol* 108:525–536, 1997. Copyright 1997 by the American Society of Clinical Pathologists. Reprinted with permission.)

tive if the cost was low ($2 to $10), the gain in life expectancy was less than 1 day when compared with repeated smears.

Conclusion.—Although rescreening detects more false negatives than no rescreening, it is only cost-effective if the cost is low.

► Most of us agree that a random rescreen of 10% of cervicovaginal smears is not a very effective quality control device, but we are not sure now to replace this strategy. This fascinating paper offers the type of outcomes analysis that increasingly drives allocation of health care dollars, public policy, and practice guidelines. It is obvious that creation of any such model requires that we adopt a number of essentially statistical assumptions about patients, laboratory testing, disease progression, and life expectancy. These are clearly delineated, with adequate references and allow us to ask the inevitable "what if" questions. We clearly need to move toward a more effective (and perhaps cost effective) means of quality control in this area. This study adds considerable momentum to a ball that has been rolling slowly for some time. My own impression is that the bottom line remains little altered; more patients getting more Pap smears more often would do more for the public good than most of our quality control efforts.

M.W. Stanley, M.D.

Suggested Reading

Burns KR, Allen KA, Radio SJ: Efficiency of the 10% rescreen of negative gynecologic smears as a quality control measure. *Acta Cytol* 40:1050–1051, 1996.

Hutchinson ML: Assessing the costs and benefits of alternative screening strategies. *Acta Cytol* 40:4–8, 1996.

Melamed MR: Rescreening for quality control in cytology. *Acta Cytol* 40:12–13, 1996.

The Value of Repeat Pap Smear at the Time of Initial Colposcopy

Spitzer M, Ryskin M, Chernys AE, et al (Queens Hosp Ctr, Jamaica, NY)

Gynecol Oncol 67:3–7, 1997 2–4

Background.—It is standard practice in the United States to perform a repeat Pap smear at the time of initial colposcopy. The author's experience was reviewed to determine whether the clinical benefit of this repeat Pap smear justifies its cost.

Study Design.—A record review was performed for all patients who had an initial colposcopy at Queens Hospital Center between 1984 and 1995. A repeat Pap smear was defined as clinically valuable if it would have changed patient management.

Findings.—The study group consisted of 2,969 women who underwent initial colposcopy at this institution during the study period. Of these women, only 139 (5%) had no repeat Pap smear. Based on the triage

TABLE 1.—The Correlation Between the Indications for Initial Colposcopy and the Pap Smear at the Time of Colposcopy Among the 2830 Patients in Whom the Pap Smear Was Repeated

Indication for colposcopy	Pap at the time of colposcopy: Negative	ASCUS	LGSIL	HGSIL	MCS	Total
ASCUS	305	476	101	7	0	889
LGSIL	324	347	480	57	0	1208
HGSIL	38	59	51	195	1	344
MCS	5	0	0	4	8	17
Vulvar warts (negative Pap)	82	78	23	2	0	185
Positive cervicography (negative Pap)	45	23	6	0	0	74
Positive cervicography (ASCUS Pap)	38	56	10	1	0	105
HIV	5	1	2	0	0	8
Total	842	1040	673	266	9	2830

Abbreviations: ASCUS, atypical squamous cells of undetermined significance; *LGSIL,* low-grade squamous intraepithelial lesion; *HGSIL,* high-grade squamous intraepithelial lesion; *MCS,* malignant cells seen; *HIV,* patient with seropositivity for HIV with negative Pap smear.

(Courtesy of Spitzer M, Ryskin M, Chernys AE, et al: The value of repeat Pap smear at the time of initial colposcopy. *Gynecol Oncol* 67:3–7, 1997.)

protocols of this institution, the comparison between their referral Pap smear and their repeat Pap smear at the time of initial colposcopy on the remaining 2,380 women would have indicated a need for cone biopsy in only 1.1% and a more careful follow-up in 1.6% of these patients (Tables 1 and 2). No cancers would have been missed in the absence of repeat Pap smears. The cost savings of skipping the repeat Pap smear would have been $24.23 per patient or $68,580 for the entire study group. At the national level, skipping the repeat Pap smear would save more than $24,000,000 per year.

Conclusions.—In this large study of the usefulness of the repeat Pap smear at initial colposcopy, repeated cytology provided little additional information. A Pap smear just before colposcopy may interfere with the colposcopic examination. Considering its cost and the limited clinical

TABLE 2.—Comparison of Colposcopically Directed Biopsy and Pap Smear Done at the Time of Colposcopy When That Pap Is a Higher Grade Than the Referral Pap

Biopsy result	Pap at colposcopy: ASCUS	LGSIL	HGSIL	MCS	Total
Normal	63	44	14	0	121
LGSIL	35	77	17	0	129
HGSIL	4	20	36	1	61
Cancer	0	1	0	0	1
Total	102	142	67	1	312

Abbreviations: ASCUS, atypical squamous cells of undetermined significance; *LGSIL,* low-grade squamous intraepithelial lesion; *HGSIL,* high-grade intraepithelial lesion; *MCS,* malignant cells seen.

(Courtesy of Spitzer M, Ryskin M, Chernys AE, et al: The value of repeat Pap smear at the time of initial colposcopy. *Gynecol Oncol* 67:3–7, 1997.)

benefit provided, the practice of a routine repeat Pap smear before initial colposcopy does not appear to be justified.

▶ This is one of those articles that critically examines a widespread practice. Clearly most of the costs these authors describe for the Papanicolaou smear represent losses from our laboratories, as low-cost smears continue to be underwritten by other, less labor-intensive testing. This article makes a strong case for not performing repeat smears at the time of colposcopy in the majority of women.

M.W. Stanley, M.D.

Suggested Reading

Schechter CB: Cost-effectiveness of rescreening conventionally prepared cervical smears by Papnet testing. *Acta Cytol* 40:1272–1282, 1996.

Young NA, Naryshkin S, Bowman RL: Value of repeat cervical smears at the time of colposcopic biopsy. *Diagn Cytopathol* 9:646–649, 1993.

Evaluation of the ThinPrep Pap Test in Clinical Practice: A Seven-Month, 16,314-Case Experience in Northern Vermont

Papillo JL, Zarka MA, St John TL (Univ of Vermont, Burlington)

Acta Cytol 42:203–208, 1998 2–5

Background.—Clinical trials have shown that the ThinPrep technique of sample preparation significantly increases the detection of cervical cancer precursors and improves specimen adequacy compared with conventional cervical cytologic smear. The performance of this method in clinical prac-

TABLE 2.—Cytologic Diagnoses in the Cohort Population Using Bethesda Diagnostic Classification

Diagnostic category	Conventional smear (n=18,569)	ThinPrep Pap Test (n=8,541)	% ThinPrep change	*P* value
WNL	13,799 (74.31%)	6,551 (76.70%)	+ 3.22%	< .001
BCC-infection	1,004 (5.41%)	580 (6.79%)	+ 25.51%	< .001
BCC-reactive/repair	1,801 (9.70%)	637 (7.46%)	− 23.09%	< .001
ASCUS/AGUS Rx	1,058 (5.70%)	352 (4.12%)	− 27.72%	< .001
ASCUS neoplastic	572 (3.08%)	204 (2.39%)	− 22.40%	< .01
LSIL	160 (0.86%)	138 (1.62%)	+ 88.37%	< .001
SIL/AGUS NOS	92 (0.50%)	23 (0.27%)	− 46.00%	< .01
HSIL/AIS/CA	83 (0.45%)	60 (0.70%)	+ 55.14%	< .01

Abbreviations: WNL, within normal limits; BCC-infection, benign cellular changes infectious agent present; *BCC—reactive/repair*, benign cellular changes reactive/reparative process; *ASCUS/AGUS Rx*, atypical squamous cells of undetermined significance and/or atypical glandular cells of undetermined significance favor reactive; *ASCUS neoplastic*, ASCUS favor neoplastic; *SIL/AGUS NOS*, squamous intraepithelial lesion and/or AGUS not otherwise classified due to poor preservation or other limiting factors; *AIS*, adenocarcinoma in situ; *CA*, invasive carcinoma.

(Courtesy of Papillo JL, Zarka MA, St John TL, et al: Evaluation of the ThinPrep Pap Test in clinical practice: A seven-month, 16,314-case experience in northern Vermont. *Acta Cytol* 42:203–208, 1998.)

TABLE 3.—Specimen Adequacy in the Cohort Population

Diagnostic category	Conventional smear (n=18,613)	ThinPrep Pap Test (n=8,574)	% ThinPrep change	*P* value
SAT	16,039 (86.17%)	8,013 (93.46%)	+ 8.46%	< .001
SBLB/UNSAT	2,574 (13.83%)	561 (6.54%)	+52.71%	< .001

Abbreviations: SAT, satisfactory; *SBLB*, satisfactory but limited by . . . ; *UNSAT*, unsatisfactory.
(Courtesy of Papillo JL, Zarka MA, St John TL, et al: Evaluation of the ThinPrep Pap Test in clinical practice: A seven-month, 16,314-case experience in northern Vermont. *Acta Cytol* 42:203–208, 1998.)

tice may be determined by comparing its diagnostic results to those of historical conventional smear data from identical patient populations.

Methods.—During a 7-month period, 16,314 ThinPrep Pap Tests were processed and evaluated at 1 center. The cytologic diagnoses and specimen adequacy of a subset of 8,574 tests were compared with those of the historical conventional cervical cytologic smear data from the cohort population. A 3-tiered diagnostic system was used, in which results were classified as within normal limits (WNL), atypical squamous cells of undetermined significance (ASCUS)/atypical glandular cells of undetermined significance (AGUS), or low-grade squamous intraepithelial lesion and higher (LSIL+).

Findings.—The ThinPrep technique increased the percentage of specimens that could be diagnosed definitively as WNL by 1.71%. This technqiue also reduced the number of ambiguous or borderline cases diagnosed as ASCUS/AGUS by 26.6% and increased the number diagnostic of LSIL+ by 52.2%. Further analysis showed that identification of infectious agents increased by 25.5%, and the detection of high-grade squamous intraepithelial lesion/carcinoma increased 55.1%. Diagnoses of benign cellular changes declined by 23.1%. Cases reported as "unsatisfactory/limited by . . ." declined by 52.7%. The ThinPrep method also decreased the number of patients with subsequent benign biopsy specimens by 31.7%. The number of ThinPrep patients with histologically confirmed cervical intraepithelial neoplasia (CIN) 1 and CIN 2/3 rose by 16.3% and 9.3%, respectively (Tables 2 and 3).

Conclusions.—Clinical implementation of the ThinPrep Pap Test significantly improves diagnostic yield and specimen adequacy. The current data support the claim that this technique is significantly more effective than conventional smear in clinical practice.

▶ This is a very large, recent study by very good investigators. The message from this and other articles seems to be clear—that in experienced hands, this type of monolayer preparation for gynecologic cytology has the following benefits: (1) lower unsatisfactory and satisfactory but limited by rates (an apparent typesetting error in Table 3 notwithstanding); (2) lower ASCUS rates; and (3) improved identification of squamous intraepithelial lesions. Why is this technology not more widely available? The answer seems to turn almost entirely on reimbursement issues. I don't know about your area of the country, but in my hospital, the materials cost alone for this test exceeds our per–Pap smear reimbursement by 30%. We await with interest lawsuits that will force the courts to decide who is at fault for not making this test more widely available. Another interesting point raised by these authors is the effects of patients' risk profile on changes in diagnostic yield.

M.W. Stanley, M.D.

Suggested Reading

Lee KR, Ashfaq R, Birdsong GG, et al: Comparison of conventional Papanicolaou smears and a fluid based, thin-layer system for cervical cancer screening. *Obstet Gynecol* 90:278–284, 1997.

Linder J, Zahniser D: ThinPrep Papanicolaou testing to reduce false-negative cervical cytology. *Arch Pathol Lab Med* 122:139–144, 1998.

Roberts JM, Gurley AM, Thurloe JK, et al: Evaluation of the ThinPrep Pap test as an adjunct to the conventional Pap smear. *Med J Aust* 167:466–469, 1997.

Sheets E, Constantine N, Dinisco S, et al: Colposcopically directed biopsies provide a basis for comparing the accuracy of ThinPrep and Papanicolaou smears. *J Gynecol Technol* 1:27–33, 1995.

The AutoPap System for Primary Screening in Cervical Cytology: Comparing the Results of a Prospective, Intended-Use Study With Routine Manual Practice

Wilbur DC, Prey MU, Miller WM, et al (Univ of Rochester, NY; NeoPath Inc, Redmond, Wash; SmithKline Beecham Clinical Labs Inc, St Louis; et al)
Acta Cytol 42:214–220, 1998 2–6

Background.—The AutoPap System, a computerized scanning device, is used to analyze conventionally prepared cervical cytologic slides. The efficacy of this system in detecting abnormal and normal cervical smears was assessed when used in a primary screening/quality control mode.

Methods.—Slides obtained prospectively were processed first in a routine manner, with cytotechnologist screening followed by 10% random quality control rescreening. Slides were then processed on the AutoPap System. About 25% of the lowest ranking slides were placed in the laboratory archives as being within normal limits, and the rest were screened manually. About 15% of the highest ranking slides were rescreened for quality control.

Findings.—Compared with routine analysis, the AutoPap System–assisted analysis was superior in identifying abnormal slides at the level of atypical squamous cells of undetermined significance and above (ASCUS+), low-grade squamous intraepithelial lesion (LSIL), and higher LSIL+. AutoPap System–assisted practice was comparable to routine practice in identifying unsatisfactory and satisfactory but limited by slides. The

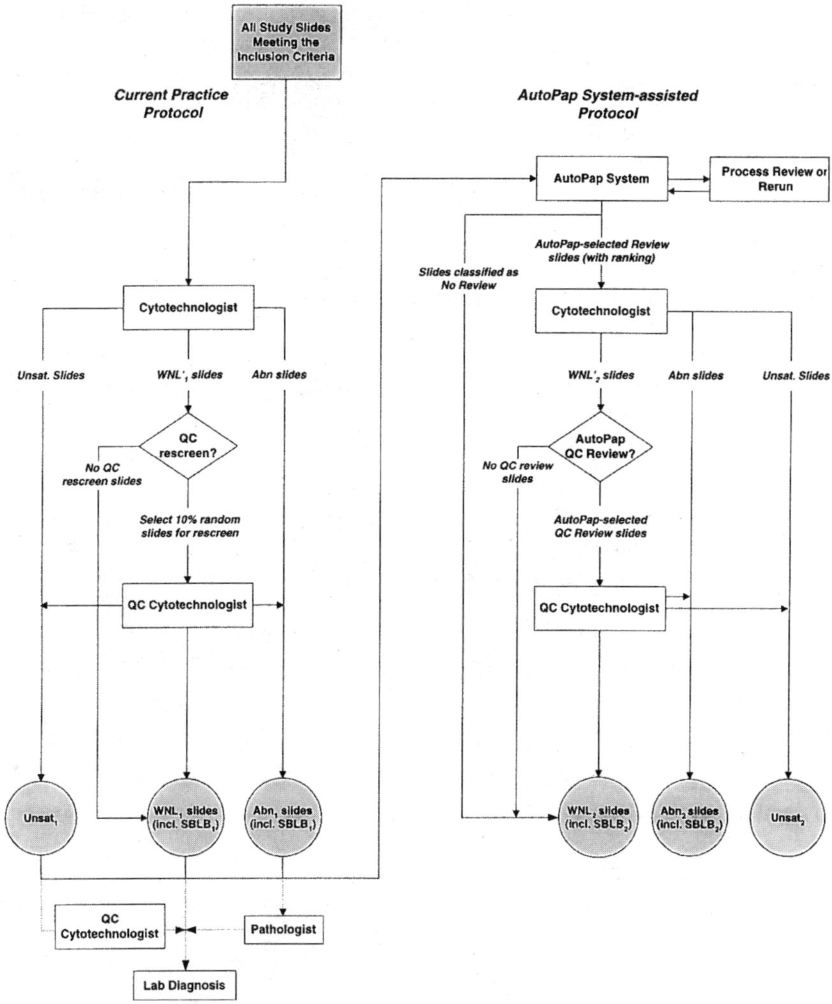

FIGURE 1.—Study work flow. (Courtesy of Wilbur DC, Prey MU, Miller WM, et al: The AutoPap system for primary screening in cervical cytology: Comparing the results of a prospective, intended-use study with routine manual practice. *Acta Cytol* 42:214–220, 1998.)

AutoPap System–assisted analysis also indicated improved diagnostic specificity (Fig 1).

Conclusions.—AutoPap System–assisted analysis is more sensitive and specific than routine analysis. Its clinical use as a primary screening device should improve overall practice of cervical cytology and provide potential enhancement in overall laboratory productivity.

▶ Most of us are convinced that the way in which we do gynecologic cytology will be very different in the not too distant future, but are unsure in what ways the differences will be manifest. When the dust settles, the methods are adopted, and the review articles with their obligatory historical preambles are written, this article will be an oft-cited classic. It is this paper on which Food and Drug Administration approval of automated primary screening by this device—albeit with limitations—is predicated. (We shoud remember that automated primary screening means that some slides will never be microscopically examined by a human being.)

M.W. Stanley, M.D.

Suggested Reading

Automated primary screening for gynecologic cytology: An idea whose time has not yet come (editorial). *Am J Clin Pathol* 109:6–9, 1998.

Proposed guidelines for primary screening instruments for gynecologic cytology: Intersociety Working Group for Cytology Technologies. *Am J Clin Pathol* 109:10–15, 1998.

Cerebrospinal Fluid Cytology in Patients With Cancer: Minimizing False-Negative Results

Glantz MJ, Cole BF, Glantz LK, et al (Brown Univ, Providence, RI; Univ of Massachusetts, Worcester)

Cancer 82:733–739, 1998 2–7

Background.—The diagnostic gold standard for leptomeningeal carcinomatosis is detection of malignant cells on cytologic assessment of the

TABLE 3.—Percent of Positive Body Fluid Cytologies With Serial Taps: Review of the Literature

No. of patients	Type of fluid	Percent cytologically positive per sample: First	Second	Third	>Three (no.)	Authors
126	CSF	75%	92%	94%	95% (10)	Balm and Hammack[43] (1996)
68	CSF	57%	69%	76%	90% (?)	Fizazi et al.[45] (1996)
35	CSF	91%	97%			Jayson et al.[46] (1994)
34	CSF	94%			100% (?)	Nakagawa et al.[44] (1992)
44	CSF	91%	98%	100%		Boogerd et al.[39] (1991)
63	CSF	71%	92%	100%		Kaplan et al.[42] (1990)
90	CSF	54%	84%	86%	87% (7)	Wasserstrom et al.[2] (1982)
25	CSF	92%	100%			Yap et al.[5] (1978)
47	CSF	45%	64%	72%	74% (6)	Olson et al.[3] (1974)
532	All CSF studies	71%	86%	90%	93%	
55	Pleural	60%	92%	97%	100% (5)	Garcia et al.[47] (1994)
472	Pleural*	91%	93%	93%		Johnston[50] (1985)
64	Pleural	59%	65%	70%		Winkelmann and Pfizer[49] (1981)
95	Pleural	53%	64%	69%	73% (≥ 4)	Salver et al.[48] (1975)
282	Blood	92%	99%	100%		Weinstein et al.[51] (1983)
80	Blood	80%	89%	99%		Washington[52] (1975)

*Includes some pericardial and ascitic fluid specimens.

(Courtesy of Glantz MJ, Cole BF, Glantz LK, et al: Cerebrospinal fluid cytology in patients with cancer: Minimizing false-negative results. *Cancer* 82[4]:733–739. Copyright © 1998, American Cancer Society. Reprinted by permission of Wiley-Liss, Inc., a subsidiary of John Wiley & Sons, Inc.)

CSF. In most therapeutic trials, the absence of such cells is a primary end point. However, false-negative findings are common. In an attempt to minimize false-negative results, the contributions of 4 physician-dependent variables to the false-negative rate of CSF cytology were assessed.

Methods.—Thirty-nine patients with leptomeningeal carcinomatosis were enrolled in the prospective study. The 4 variables assessed were CSF sample volume, site of CSF sampling, processing time, and frequency of CSF sampling. Retrospective data were analyzed to determine the importance of these factors in daily practice.

Findings.—False-negative CSF cytologic findings were associated with small CSF volume, delayed processing, not obtaining CSF from a site of symptomatic or radiographically evident disease, and fewer than 2 samplings. During 1 year, 97% of CSF specimens were of inadequate volume, and more than 25% were processed too slowly (Table 3).

Conclusions.—False-negative CSF cytologic results can be minimized by withdrawing at least 10.5 mL of CSF for cytologic analysis, processing the CSF specimens immediately, and obtaining CSF from a site of known leptomeningeal disease. If initial cytology is negative, the procedure may be repeated.

▶ This is an important clinical and methodological review of a difficult subject. Furthermore, by evaluating a series of patients with known leptomeningeal carcinomatosis, the authors circumvent the usual situation in which the false-negative rate in CSF cytology is impossible to evaluate because of a lack of biopsy or autopsy documentation of disease. The findings have bearing on the fact that many CSF specimens are difficult to examine because of poor cellular preservation. Also, the authors effectively address the issue of repeated sampling in body fluid cytology.

M.W. Stanley, M.D.

Suggested Reading

Andrews JM, Schumann GB: Laboratory processing of cerebrospinal fluid specimens. *Diagn Cytopathol* 6:139–143, 1990.

Garcia LW, Ducatman BS, Wang HH: The value of multiple fluid specimens in the cytological diagnosis of malignancy. *Mod Pathol* 7:665–668, 1994.

A Comparison of the Effectiveness of Malignancy Detection in Body Fluid Examination by the Cytopathology and Hematology Laboratories

Kendall B, Dunn C, Solanki P (Wilford Hall Med Ctr, Lackland Air Force Base, Tex)

Arch Pathol Lab Med 121:976–979, 1997 2–8

Background.—At many centers, body fluid samples are submitted for cytologic examination as well as for assessment in a clinical microscopy or hematology laboratory. Cytologic assessment is generally considered the

TABLE 1.—All Cases Reviewed by Location and Diagnosis for Both Cytopathology and Hematology Laboratories

	Benign		Inconclusive		Malignant		
Specimen	Cytopathology	Hematology	Cytopathology	Hematology	Cytopathology	Hematology	Total
CSF	222	222	10	5	5	10	237
PC	3	3	0	0	1	1	4
PT	39	38	0	2	4	3	43
PL	93	89	3	4	17	20	113
Total	357	352	13	11	27	34	397

Abbreviations: PC, pericardial fluid; *PT*, peritoneal fluid; *PL*, pleural fluid.

(Courtesy of Kendall B, Dunn C, Solanki P: A comparison of the effectiveness of malignancy detection in body fluid examination by the cytopathology and hematology laboratories. *Arch Pathol Lab Med* 121:976–979, 1997.)

TABLE 2.—Clinical Diagnosis in 13 Cases With Discordant Results Between the 2 Methods of Evaluation

Case No.	Specimen	Cytopathology Diagnosis	Hematology Diagnosis	Primary Malignancy
1	CSF	Benign	Malignant	Squamous cell carcinoma
2	CSF	Benign	Malignant, lymphoma	Lymphoma (unspecified type)
3	CSF	Benign	Malignant, lymphoma	Large cell lymphoma
4	CSF	Inconclusive, consistent with blasts	Malignant, blasts present	Acute myelogenous leukemia
5	CSF	Inconclusive	Malignant	Transitional cell carcinoma with hydrocephalus
6	PL	Benign, scant cellularity	Malignant, few lymphomatous cells present	Burkitt's lymphoma
7	PL	Benign	Malignant lymphoma	Mantle cell lymphoma
8	PL	Benign	Malignant lymphoma	Mantle cell lymphoma
9	PL	Benign	Malignant	Suspected lung carcinoma
10	PL	Malignant, adenocarcinoma	Benign	Metastatic breast carcinoma
11	PL	Malignant, lymphoma	Atypical, suggestive of lymphoma	Unknown
12	PL	Inconclusive, suspicious for adenocarcinoma	Malignant	Metastatic abdominal tumor of unknown primary
13	PT	Malignant, lymphoma	Atypical	High-grade lymphoma (not further specified)

Abbreviations: PL, pleural fluid; *PT*, peritoneal fluid.

(Courtesy of Kendall B, Dunn C, Solanki P: A comparison of the effectiveness of malignancy detection in body fluid examination by the cytopathology and hematology laboratories. *Arch Pathol Lab Med* 121:976–979, 1997.)

standard for detecting malignancy, whereas the clinical microscopy laboratory is used mainly for cell counting and categorization. The efficacy of the hematology laboratory in detecting malignant fluids was investigated.

Methods.—Three hundred ninety-seven reports on body fluid specimens were reviewed. The cerebrospinal, pericardial, peritoneal, and pleural fluid samples had been submitted concurrently during a 1-year period to the cytopathology and hematology laboratories.

Findings.—In one or both examinations, 9.3% of the cases were diagnosed as malignant. Cytopathology assessment demonstrated that 73% of the 37 malignant cases were malignant and that 81.1% were at least atypical. Hematology reports indicated that 91.9% of the malignant cases were malignant and that 97.3% were at least atypical. In 64.9% of the malignant cases, the laboratories reported concordant malignant diagnoses (Tables 1 and 2).

Conclusions.—Hematology laboratory assessment of body fluid specimens can provide a very sensitive diagnostic assessment. Although such assessment is not advocated as a replacement for standard cytologic evaluation, it can serve as a useful complement.

► Should large laboratories combine the cytology and the clinical laboratories' interpretation of body fluid samples submitted for evaluation of possible malignancy? If we did this, would we improve efficiency or lower costs? What would be the impact on diagnostic accuracy? There is probably no universally applicable answer to this line of questioning. The impact of dual vs. single analysis might depend to some extent on the case mix. Referral centers that care for a relatively large number of leukemia/lymphoma patients are likely to have in-house experts in hematopathology and cytopathology. (Seven of 13 discordant cases in this article involved hematologic malignancies.) The fixed smears used in most cytology laboratories are regarded by many as suboptimal for recognition and classification of hematologic malignancies. Other factors include the possible improved diagnostic yield by use of cell blocks in cytology. Another difference in this study involves the details of cytocentrifuge operation; albumin was used in the clinical laboratory but not in cytology. This could explain some discordant cases, because albumin improves cell adhesion to slides and can increase the diagnostic yield with sparely celluar fluids. My reading of this literature suggests that we do not know enough to confidently alter current practices. Finally, these authors remind us that the results generated by 2 laboratories must be compared, and this comparison should be documented.

M.W. Stanley, M.D.

Suggested Reading

Ben-Ezra J, Stastny JF, Harris AC, et al: Comparison of the clinical microscopy laboratory with the cytopathology laboratory in the detection of malignant cells in body fluids. *Am J Clin Pathol* 102:439–442, 1994.

Clare N, Rone R: Detection of malignancy in body fluids. *Lab Med* 17:147–150, 1986.

Sulak LE: Comparison of the clinical microscopy laboratory with the cytopathology laboratory in the detection of malignant cells in body fluids (letter). *Am J Pathol* 103:533, 1995.

Significance of Intraperitoneal Cytology in Patients Undergoing Radical Hysterectomy
Estape R, Angioli R, Wagman F, et al (Univ of Miami, Fla)
Gynecol Oncol 68:169–171, 1998 2–9

Introduction.—Peritoneal washings are used in surgical staging for endometrial and ovarian cancer to improve prognostic assignment and to plan therapeutic modalities. The benefit of peritoneal washings in patients with cervical cancer is unknown. The incidence of positive peritoneal cytology in patients with early cervical cancer undergoing radical hysterectomy was prospectively assessed and compared with other surgical-pathological factors.

Methods.—Four hundred patients with early-stage cervical cancer underwent peritoneal washings before radical hysterectomy with pelvic and para-aortic lymphadenectomy. Cytologic and histologic specimens were used to determine stage and assign adjuvant therapy.

Results.—Seven of 400 patients (1.8%) had positive peritoneal washings. Of these, 4 had squamous cell carcinoma (compared with an overall rate of 94.7% for 400 patients), and 3 had adenocarcinoma (compared with an overall rate of 5.3% for 400 patients). Five of 7 patients had stage IB cervical cancer and 2 had stage IIA disease. Six of 7 patients had tumors greater than or equal to 3 cm; 2 had tumors 4 cm or greater. Three of 7 patients had positive pelvic nodes and 2 had lymphovascular space involvement. Four of 7 patients had greater than 50% stromal invasion; 61 of 400 had deep invasion. The overall 3-year survival for 400 patients was 88%, compared with 28.6% for 7 patients with positive peritoneal washings. Five of 7 had adjuvant therapy; 1 was still living at final follow-up.

Conclusions.—Yield for peritoneal cytology is very low for patients with cervical cancer. It does not add information to help patients in the decision-making process and should not be undertaken routinely.

▶ This study, which reviewed the outcomes of 400 patients with radical hysterectomies with concurrent peritoneal cytology, is an important step to understanding the importance of peritoneal cytology in patients with cervical cancer. Of importance is that less than 2% of the patients demonstrated positive peritoneal cytology, and all of these patients had well-defined risk factors obtained from surgical pathology material. In other words, the results of the peritoneal cytology did not add anything to the prognostic index for the patient. Unfortunately, a detailed cost analysis is not provided in this study, but it seems intuitive that the elimination of 400 peritoneal cytology wash specimens will result in a substantial savings for any cytology department, not only in materials but also in technologists' and pathologists' labor. It would have been nice to see a more detailed cost analysis in this paper.

D.J. Dabbs, M.D.

Telecytology: Diagnostic Accuracy Compared With Light Microscopy in the Bronchial Brush Specimen

Zaleski MS, Thomas PA, Lenel JC, et al (Univ of Iowa, Iowa City)
J Surg Pathol 3:67–72, 1998 2–10

Objective.—Telecytology, cytologic examination using a video monitor instead of a light microscope, has not been thoroughly evaluated for exfoliative specimens. The diagnostic accuracy of telecytology in the exfoliative specimen of the bronchial brush (BB) was assessed retrospectively using the receiver operating characteristic (ROC) curve analysis and the likelihood ratio (LR).

Methods.—Ten blinded observers reviewed 33 BBs for 12 seconds using a video monitor and, 1 month later, a light microscope and classified each as definitely benign, probably benign, possibly malignant, probably malignant, or definitely malignant. Diagnostic accuracy was calculated using ROC analysis and LRs.

Results.—Although the diagnostic accuracy of telecytology in the BB specimen is high, telecytology was significantly less accurate than light microscopy. Three observers had higher accuracy ratings using the video monitor than using the light microscope. LR values for both methods were similar.

Conclusion.—Although the diagnostic accuracy of telecytology is high, it is significantly less accurate than light microscopy for BB specimens. The reasons for the accuracy differences need to be investigated.

▶ Telepathology and telecytology are becoming frequent topics of conversation. It is easy to envision instantaneous consultations or practice extensions, should our profession agree that this is a technically acceptable mode of slide examination. Most previous work in telecytology has centered on cervicovaginal smears, but this paper attempts to extend the interpretive accuracy to bronchial brushings. These authors have been careful to describe their equipment in ways that help the reader and future investigators to make meaningful statements about video image quality. Not all such writings on this subject are so clear. The observation that some individuals do better with a light microscope, while others achieve improved accuracy with video images is fascinating and requires further study. The authors raise questions that are important for subsequent investigators, and for those wishing to employ this technology. Control over image selection would do much to improve some observers' comfort with this method of viewing slides. Binary diagnostic categories (cancer, yes; vs. cancer, no) probably led to more optimistic assessments of diagnostic accuracy than semiquantitative lists of possible diagnoses such as that used in this study.

M.W. Stanley, M.D.

Suggested Reading

Jensen CS, Zaleski MS, Thomas PA, et al: Telecytology: Diagnostic accuracy in cervical-vaginal smears with comparison to conventional light microscopy. *Mod Pathol* 8:41A, 1995.

Raab SS, Zaleski MS, Thomas PA, et al: Telecytology: Diagnostic accuracy in cervical vaginal smears. *Am J Clin Pathol* 105:599–603, 1996.

Ziol M, Vacher-Lavenu M, Ferrand J, et al: Telepathology and cervical Papanicolaou smears: Is teletransmission of selected fields available for interpretation of squamous cell abnormalities? *Acta Cytol* 39:376, 1995.

Diagnostic Pitfalls of Aspiration Cytology of Salivary Duct Carcinoma

Khurana KK, Pitman MB, Powers CN, et al (State Univ of New York, Syracuse; Harvard Med School, Boston; John L McClellan Mem Veterans Hosp, Little Rock, Ark; et al)

Cancer 81:373–378, 1997 2–11

Background.—Salivary duct carcinoma (SDC), a very aggressive primary salivary gland tumor, is histologically similar to intraductal and infiltrating breast carcinoma. The cytologic features of histologically

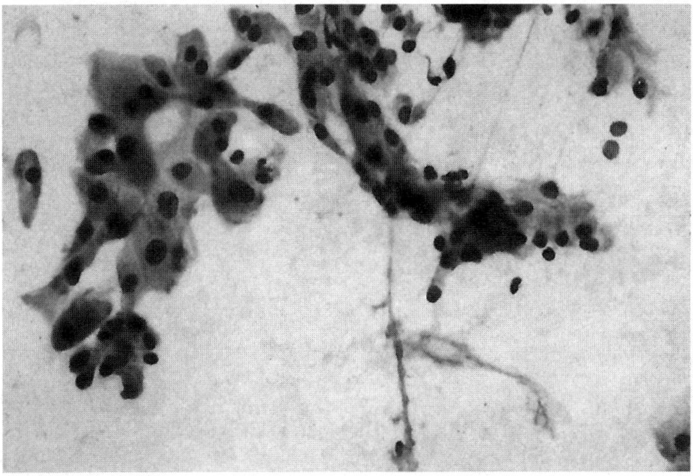

FIGURE 1.—Case 1. Bland tumor cells comprised of uniform round to oval nuclei and moderate amounts of cytoplasm. Isolated sheets of tumor cells also display a cribriform architecture (Papanicolaou stain, ×200). (Courtesy of Khurana KK, Pitman MB, Powers CN, et al: Diagnostic pitfalls of aspiration cytology of salivary duct carcinoma. *Cancer* 81[6]:373–378. Copyright © 1997, American Cancer Society. Reprinted by permission of Wiley-Liss, Inc., a subsidiary of John Wiley & Sons, Inc.)

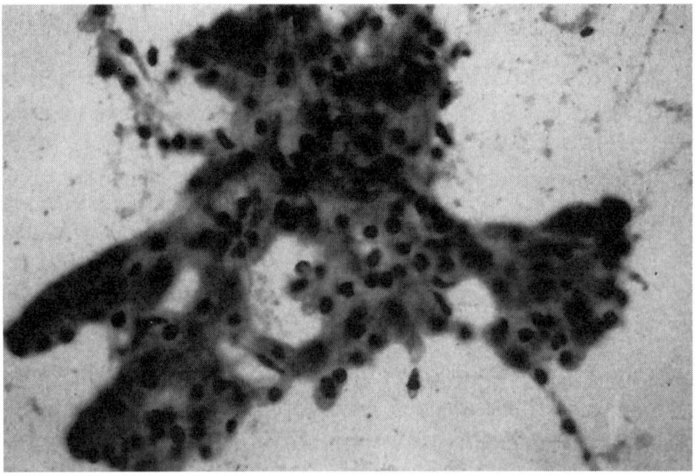

FIGURE 3.—Case 4. Tumor cells with abundant granular cytoplasm and moderate nuclear atypia. A prominent papillary configuration also is noted. (Papanicolaou stain, ×200). (Courtesy of Khurana KK, Pitman MB, Powers CN, et al: Diagnostic pitfalls of aspiration cytology of salivary duct carcinoma. *Cancer* 81[6]:373–378. Copyright © 1997, American Cancer Society. Reprinted by permission of Wiley-Liss, Inc., a subsidiary of John Wiley & Sons, Inc.)

proved SDC were reviewed, and possible pitfalls in cytologic diagnosis were identified.

Methods and Findings.—Nine patients aged 62–89 years were included in the review. Fine-needle aspiration cytology was performed in all. Cytologic diagnoses were pleomorphic adenoma in 3 patients; high-grade car-

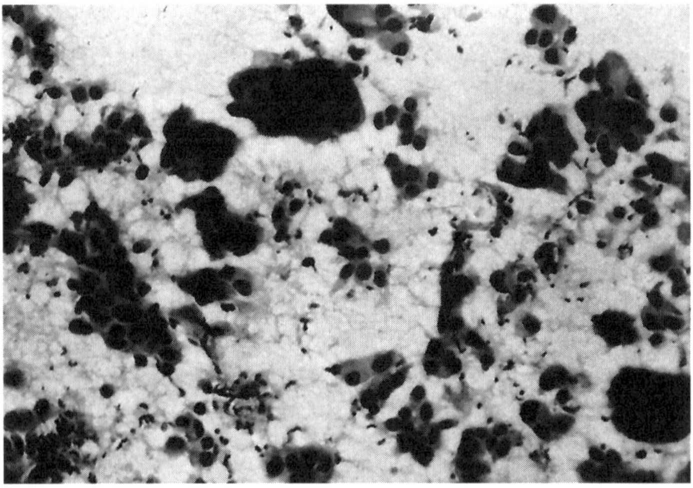

FIGURE 5.—A, Case 7. Poorly cohesive clusters of tumor cells exhibiting marked pleomorphism and irregular nuclear contours (Papanicolaou stain, ×200). (Courtesy of Khurana KK, Pitman MB, Powers CN, et al: Diagnostic pitfalls of aspiration cytology of salivary duct carcinoma. *Cancer* 81[6]:373–378. Copyright © 1997, American Cancer Society. Reprinted by permission of Wiley-Liss, Inc., a subsidiary of John Wiley & Sons, Inc.)

TABLE 1.—Clinical Findings and Initial Cytologic Diagnoses in Histologically Proven Cases of Salivary Duct Carcinoma of the Parotid Gland

Case no.	Age (yrs)	Gender	Initial cytologic diagnosis
1	75	M	Pleomorphic adenoma
2	69	M	Pleomorphic adenoma
3	81	M	Pleomorphic adenoma
4	71	M	Atypical cytology. Differential diagnosis includes oncocytoma, acinic cell carcinoma and mucoepidermoid carcinoma
5	69	M	Positive for malignancy. Consistent with high grade mucoepidermoid carcinoma
6	62	M	Positive for malignancy. Consistent with intermediate grade mucoepidermoid carcinoma
7	68	M	High grade carcinoma (NOS)
8	89	F	High grade carcinoma (NOS)
9	68	M	High grade carcinoma (NOS)

Abbreviations: M, male; *F*, female, *NOS*, not otherwise specified.

(Courtesy of Khurana KK, Pitman MB, Powers CN, et al: Diagnostic pitfalls of aspiration cytology of salivary duct carcinoma. *Cancer* 81[6]:373–378. Copyright © 1997, American Cancer Society. Reprinted by permission of Wiley-Liss, Inc., a subsidiary of John Wiley & Sons, Inc.)

cinoma not otherwise specified in 3; mucoepidermoid carcinoma in 2; and atypical cytology with differential diagnosis including mucoepidermoid carcinoma, oncocytoma, and acinic cell carcinoma in 1. Cytologic findings included broad flat sheets and 3-dimensional clusters. Mild-to-severe cellular pleomorphism and nuclear atypia were noted. In some specimens, papillary clusters and cribriforming were observed. In 3 patients, bland cytologic features and prominent hyaline stroma, representing the dense fibrosis on histologic sections, were interpreted cytologically as pleomorphic adenoma (Figs 1, 3, and 5; Table 1).

Conclusions.—Accurate interpretation of fine-needle aspiration of SDC may be difficult. In some patients, bland cytomorphologic features may result in a false-negative interpretation. This series demonstrates several clinically important pitfalls.

▶ This paper seems initially to be merely a report of a salivary gland neoplasm that is so rare, 4 large institutions were required to find 9 causes. In that light, it seems to be of relatively little utility except as an enhancement to the authors' CVs. However, it makes 2 points that deserve highlighting. The first, and less important, is that some SDCs are of lower grade than previously emphasized. This sets the stage for the second and more ominous problem. Our literature has emphasized the importance of fibrillar extracellular matrix material in the fine-needle aspiration diagnosis of benign mixed tumors (pleomorphic adenomas). In fact, identifying and characterizing this material is so important that it is one of the major reasons many of us prefer to approach salivary gland cytology with air-dried rather than fixed smears. Unfortunately, our literature is almost silent regarding the fact that the desmoplastic stroma accompanying many carcinomas can closely mimic this mixed tumor matrix; hence the false-negative cytologic diagnosis of 3 low-grade ductal carcinomas in this series as benign mixed tumors. This type of stroma has the same smear appearance when aspirated during study of invasive carcinomas in other body sites. However, in those areas, there is usually less danger of a false negative diagnosis.

M.W. Stanley, M.D.

Suggested Reading

Delgado R, Klimstra D, Albores-Saavedra J: Low grade salivary duct carcinoma: A distinctive variant with a low grade histology and a predominant intraductal growth pattern. *Cancer* 78:958–967, 1996.

Desai S, Krishnamurthy S: Stromal fragments in invasive carcinoma: Source of diagnostic difficulty in aspiration cytology. *Acta Cytol* 41:1747–1750, 1997.

Elsheikh TM, Bernacki EG Jr, Pisharodi L: Fine-needle aspiration cytology of salivary duct carcinoma. *Diagn Cytopathol* 11:47–51, 1994.

Fýrat P, Cramer H, Feczko JD, et al: Fine needle aspiration biopsy of salivary duct carcinoma: Report of five cases. *Diagn Cytopathol* 16:526–530, 1997.

Stanley MW, Bardales RH, Farmer CE, et al: Primary and metastatic high grade carcinoma of the salivary glands: A cytologic-histologic correlation study of twenty cases. *Diagn Cytopathol* 13:37–43, 1995.

Routine Addition of an Automated Biopsy Device to Fine-needle Aspiration of the Lung: A Prospective Assessment

Boiselle PM, Shepard J-AO, Mark EJ, et al (Massachusetts Gen Hosp, Boston)

AJR 169:661–666, 1997 2–12

Background.—Although percutaneous needle biopsy (PNB) of the lung using fine-needle aspiration (FNA) is very accurate in diagnosing malignant thoracic lesions, its role in assessing focal thoracic lesions is limited by its low diagnostic yield in benign lesions. The safety and value of the routine addition of an automated biopsy device (ABD) to FNA of the lung were determined.

Methods.—Fifty biopsies were performed in 49 patients under CT guidance using a coaxial method. A 19-gauge introducer needle and a 22-gauge aspirating needle were used, followed by a 20-gauge ABD. A mean of 3.5

TABLE 1.—Final Diagnosis and Diagnostic Accuracy of 50 Cases

Diagnosis	*n*	FNA Result No. (%)	ABD Result No. (%)
Malignant thoracic lesions	34	32 (94)	20 (59)
Bronchogenic carcinoma	27	25 (93)	14 (52)
Non–small cell lung cancer	25		
Adenocarcinoma	10		
Adenosquamous	3		
Squamous cell	2		
Large cell, undifferentiated	10		
Small cell carcinoma	2		
Metastatic disease	6	6 (100)	5 (83)
Thymic carcinoma	1	1 (100)	1 (100)
Benign conditions	16	5 (31)	11 (69)
Acute infections	8	4 (50)	5 (63)
Tuberculosis	3		
Fungal	2		
Bacterial	2		
Pneumocystis carinii pneumonia	1		
Other benign diagnoses	8	1 (12)	6 (75)
Chronic organizing pneumonia	3		
Acute fibrinous pneumonitis	1		
Organizing fibrinous pneumonitis	1		
Acute and chronic rejection*	1		
Hamartoma	1		
Fibrosis	1		

*Lung transplant patient.
Abbreviations: FNA, fine-needle aspiration; *ABD*, automated biopsy device.
(Courtesy of Boiselle PM, Shepard J-AO, Mark EJ, et al: Routine addition of an automated biopsy device to fine-needle aspiration of the lung: A prospective assessment. *AJR* 169:661–666, 1997.)

FNA specimens and 2.5 core specimens were acquired. Two experienced pathologists independently evaluated the specimens.

Findings.—For the 34 malignancies, FNA and core biopsy had diagnostic accuracies of 94% and 59%, respectively. The combined accuracy was 94%. For 16 benign lesions, accurate definitive diagnosis was established by FNA and core biopsy in 31% and 69%, respectively, with a combined accuracy of 69%. For 8 benign lesions that were not acute infections, FNA provided an accurate definitive benign diagnosis in 12%, and core biopsy in 75% (Table 1). There were no false-positive diagnoses of malignancies. Complications included pneumothorax in 18% of the patients, chest tube in 2%, minor pulmonary hemorrhage in 14%, and minor hemoptysis in 4%.

Conclusions.—Adding an ABD significantly enhances the diagnostic accuracy only for a subset of benign lesions that are not acute infections. The complication rates of FNA plus ABD are similar to those reported for FNA alone.

▶ There seems to be a rush among radiologists to embrace core biopsy and to replace FNA with the newer ABDs. In some institutions, this has already taken place and has been encouraged by some in the pathology community. This paper indicates that this is a good idea for benign lesions which do not represent acute infections. However, it provides no advantage when pulmonary malignancies are sampled with radiographic guidance. In our experience, many lung cancers can be diagnosed and reported (at least in a preliminary fashion) on FNA within a few minutes during the procedure. Thus, for the subset of lesions likely to represent malignancies, FNA, is, in my opinion, still the best place to start, because it will be rapid and inexpensive. As noted by other authors, the utility of FNA is maximized by having an individual experienced with preparation and evaluation of aspirate samples on site during the procedure. The current paper notwithstanding, others have found a higher complication rate for core biopsy than for FNA. The radiologists with whom I work have stated a preference for FNA over core biopsy in the majority of cases; the most often cited reasons are rapidity and the very low complication rate.

M.W. Stanley, M.D.

Suggested Reading

Austin JHM, Cohen MB: Value of having a cytopathologist present during percutaneous fine-needle aspiration biopsy of lung: Report of 55 cancer patients and metaanalysis of the literature. *AJR* 160:175–177, 1993.

Haramiti LB: CT-guided automated needle biopsy of the chest. *AJR* 165:53–55, 1995.

Klein JS, Salomon G, Stewart EA: Transthoracic needle biopsy with a coaxially placed 20–gauge automated cutting needle: Results in 122 patients. *Radiology* 198:715–720, 1996.

The Value of Immediate Cytologic Evaluation for Needle Aspiration Lung Biopsy

Padhani AR, Scott WW Jr, Cheema M, et al (Johns Hopkins Med Institutions, Baltimore, Md)

Invest Radiol 32:453–458, 1997 2–13

Background.—Although fine-needle aspiration biopsy (FNAB) is an effective method for acquiring material for cytologic study, it is limited by inadequate sampling resulting from small needle diameter. The value of immediate cytologic evaluation (ICE) with FNAB for lung lesions in patients at the greatest risk of pneumothorax was determined.

Methods.—Eighty patients with lung lesions surrounded by aerated parenchyma were included in the prospective, randomized study. All underwent FNAB with or without ICE.

Findings.—An increased number of needle passes was associated with immediate cytologic evaluation. In addition, fluoroscopic procedures required more time with ICE. Complication rates did not differ. Specimens were adequate in 74% and 64% of the samples in the ICE group and control group, respectively. The procedure was diagnostic in 79% and

TABLE 1.—Analysis of Lesions, Procedure, and Complications

	ICE Present (47)	No ICE (33)	Statistical test
Size of lesions (cm)			
0–1	5	1	χ^2 test: P = 0.15
1.1–2	12	7	
2.1–3	14	15	
>3	16	10	
Size <2 cm	17 (36%)	8 (24%)	χ^2 test: P = 0.18
Median size and range (cms)	2.5 (0.9–6.0)	2.0 (0.8–8.0)	
Pleural puncture time (minutes) for fluoroscopy procedures (median)	15 (4–49)	9 (4–30)	MW test: P = 0.002
Needle passes			
1	21 (45%)	19 (58%)	
2	15 (32%)	13 (39%)	
3	10 (21%)	1 (3%)	
4	0	0	
5	1 (2%)	0	
≥ 3 passes	23%	3%	χ^2 test: P = 0.01
Complications			
Pneumothorax	9 (19%)	6 (18%)	χ^2 test: P = NS
Chest drainage	2 (4%)	1 (3%)	
Hemoptysis	7 (15%)	8 (24%)	χ^2 test: P = NS

Abbreviations: ICE, immediate cytologic evaluation; *MW test,* Mann Whitney test; *NS,* not significant at 95% confidence level.

(Courtesy of Padhani AR, Scott WW Jr, Cheema M, et al: The value of immediate cytologic evaluation for needle aspiration lung biopsy. *Invest Radiol* 32:453–458, 1997.)

70%, respectively. Biopsy sensitivity, specificity, and accuracy did not differ significantly between groups (Tables 1 and 2).

Conclusions.—ICE marginally improved FNAB results in this patient population, with increased procedure time and needle passes. ICE may be most beneficial in patients at the lowest risk of complications to obviate the need for a second procedure.

▶ I was drawn to this paper because its findings seem so contrary to our cherished beliefs about the utility of ICE during guided lung aspiration (FNA). The ideas that ICE improves the procedure "marginally," that it makes the procedure several minutes longer, and that it results in more needle passes are the opposite of my own experiences. Table 1 causes us to ask why a majority of cases done without ICE were terminated after 1 pass. Was this a local institutional protocol? If so, it seems to differ from other centers and will inevitably result in an artifactually increased number of needle passes when ICE is used to evaluate the adequacy of the first pass. The fact that nearly half of all procedures were terminated because of patient or technical factors makes this a fairly small study and is another experience that differs strikingly from my own. Were these cases excluded for purposes of calculating pleural puncture time, complication rate, and the total number of needle passes? Finally, what is a cytotechnician?

M.W. Stanley, M.D.

TABLE 2.—Specimen Analysis, Diagnostic Yield and Accuracy

	ICE present (47)	No ICE (33)	Statistical test
Specimen Analysis			
Radiologist opinion (gross examination)			
Adequate specimen	38 (81%)	28 (85%)	
Cytopathologist's opinion (instant slide preparation)			
Adequate specimen	26 (55%)	—	
Cytopathology after laboratory processing of all specimens			
Adequate specimen	35 (74%)	21 (64%)	χ^2test: P = 0.21
Diagnostic group and final diagnosis			
Diagnostic biopsy	37 (79%)	23 (70%)	χ^2 test: P = NS
Primary lung cancer	19	16	
Secondary lung cancer	11	6	
Benign	7*	1†	
Suspicious for malignancy (insufficient sample for definite diagnosis)	3(6%)	4(12%)	
Primary lung cancer	2	1	
Secondary lung cancer	1	3	
Benign	0	0	
Nondiagnostic biopsy	7 (15%)	6 (18%)	
Primary lung cancer	1	4	
Secondary lung cancer	5	1	
Benign	1†	1‡	
Bayesian analysis			
Sensitivity	77%	71%	
Specificity	100%	100%	
Positive predictive value	100%	100%	
Negative predictive value	44%	10%	
Accuracy	80%	72%	

*Hamartoma 2, *Aspergillus* 1, lung abscess 1, tuberculosis 2.
†Tuberculosis.
‡Presumed inflammatory.
Abbreviations: ICE, immediate cytologic evaluation; *NS*, not significant at 95% confidence level.
(Courtesy of Padhani AR, Scott WW Jr, Cheema M, et al: The value of immediate cytologic evaluation for needle aspiration lung biopsy. *Invest Radiol* 32:453–458, 1997.)

Suggested Reading

Austin JH, Cohen MB: Value of having a cytopathologist present during percutaneous fine-needle aspiration biopsy of lung: Report of 55 cancer patients and metaanalysis of the literature. *AJR* 160:175–177, 1993.

Khouri NF, Stitik FP, Erozan YS, et al: Transthoracic needle aspiration biopsy of benign and malignant lung lesions. *AJR* 144:281–288, 1995.

Miller DA, Carrasco CH, Katz RL, et al: Fine needle aspiration biopsy: The role of immediate cytologic assessment. *AJR* 147:155–158, 1986.

Silverman JF, Finley JL, O'Brien KF, et al: Diagnostic accuracy and role of immediate interpretation of fine-needle aspiration biopsy from various sites. *Acta Cytol* 33:791–796, 1989.

Cytology of "Significant" Breast Ductal Proliferations

Gangopadhyay M, Nijhawan R, Joshi K, et al (Postgraduate Inst of Med Education and Research, Chandigarh, India)

Acta Cytol 41:1112–1120, 1997 2–14

Objective.—Whether atypical ductal hyperplasia can be distinguished from ductal carcinoma in situ and from infiltrating carcinoma using fine-needle aspiration (FNA) was evaluated.

Methods.—FNA cytology was performed at multiple sites in 30 patients, aged 20–65, with palpable breast lesions. Cytologic results were compared with histopathologic results on the excised lesions.

Results.—Cytologic and histopathologic results were correlated (Table 1). Cytoarchitecture, which was diagnosed histopathologically as ductal carcinoma in situ, varied from mild hyperplasia to marked atypia in 3 patients (Figs 1, 2, and 3).

Conclusion.—FNA cytologists should evaluate specimens based on the probability of their progressing to invasive cancer instead of attempting to classify lesions specifically. Significant breast ductal proliferations are characterized by the following features: 3-dimensional cell clusters, a swirling pattern of growth, sublumens, cell dyscohesion, conspicuous nuclear overlap, anisonucleosis, irregular nuclear membranes, clumped chromatin, and eosinophilic macronucleoli.

► I just don't get it. I keep thinking that the idea of classifying proliferative breast disease based on FNA will stop appearing in the literature, and then, it returns. My best reading of the experts' literature is that we cannot do this in most cases.

M.W. Stanley, M.D.

TABLE 1.—Cytohistologic Correlation (30 Cases)

Cytologic diagnosis	No. of cases	Histopathologic diagnosis	No. of cases
Mild hyperplasia	6	Mild hyperplasia 5, normal	1
Moderate to florid hyperplasia	14	Moderate to florid hyperplasia	12
		Fibroadenoma	2
ADH	7	ADH	3
		Moderate to florid hyperplasia	4
Marked atypia/? malignancy	3	DCIS	3

(Courtesy of Gangopadhyay M, Nijhawan R, Joshi K, et al: Cytology of "significant" breast ductal proliferations. *Acta Cytol* 41:1112–1120, 1997.)

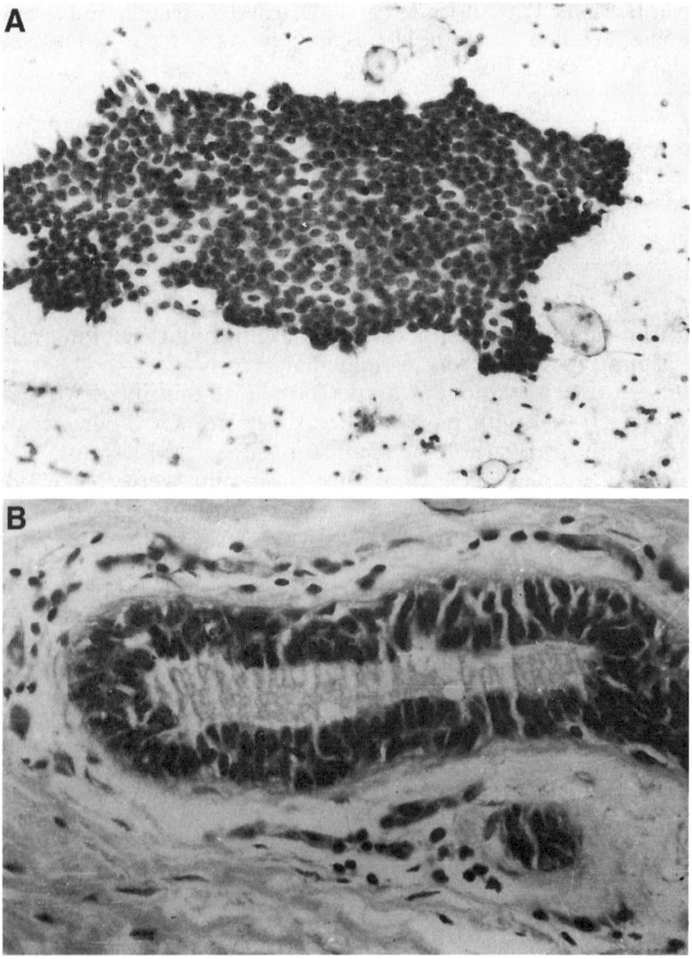

FIGURE 1.—A, FNA. Monolayered cell clusters (Papanicolaou stain, ×275). B, histopathology. Duct lined with two layers of cells; hematoxylin-eosin, original magnification, ×550. (Courtesy of Gangopadhyay M, Nijhawan R, Joshi K, et al: Cytology of "significant" breast ductal proliferations. *Acta Cytol* 41:1112–1120, 1997.)

Suggested Reading

Sidaway MK, Stoler MH, Frable WJ, et al: Interobserver variability in the classification of proliferative breast lesions by fine-needle aspiration: Results of the Papanicolaou Society of Cytopathology Study. *Diagn Cytopathol* 18:150–165, 1998.

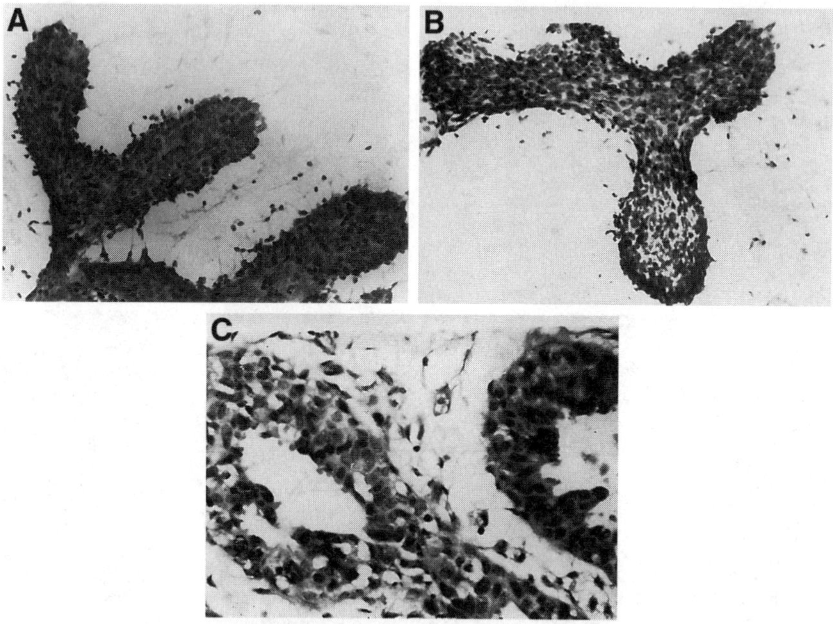

FIGURE 2.—Mild hyperplasia (A), FNA. Cell clusters with antler horn projections; Papanicolaou stain, ×275. (B), FNA. Clusters with well-outlined cell outgrowths; Papanicolaou stain, original magnification, ×275. C, histopathology. Ducts lined with two to four cell layers; (hematoxylin-eosin, original magnification, ×550. (Courtesy of Gangopadhyay M, Nijhawan R, Joshi K, et al: Cytology of "significant" breast ductal proliferations. *Acta Cytol* 41:1112–1120, 1997.)

Silverman JF, Masood S, Ducatman BS, et al: Can FNA biopsy separate atypical hyperplasia, carcinoma in situ, and invasive carcinoma of the breast? Cytomorphologic criteria and limitations in diagnosis. *Diagn Cytopathol* 9:713–728, 1993.

Stanley MW: Cytology of proliferative breast disease, in Schmidt W (ed): *Cytopathology Annual*, vol 7. Chicago, American Society of Clinical Pathologists Press, in press.

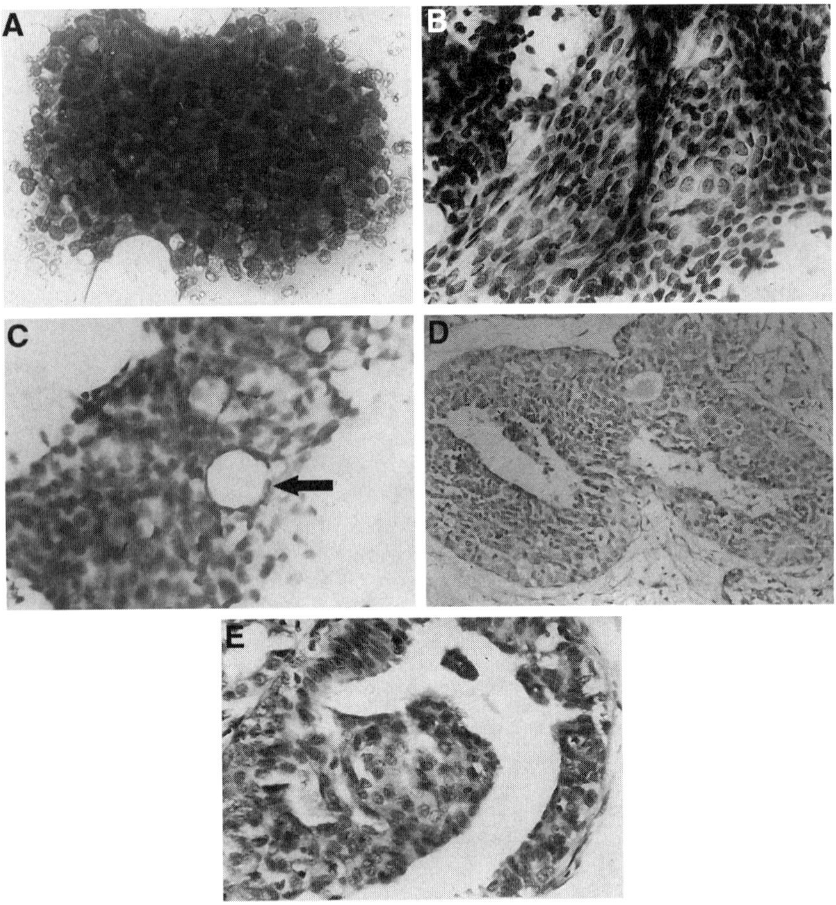

FIGURE 3.—Moderate hyperplasia. **A**, FNA. Three-dimensional, ball-like cell cluster; May-Grúnwald-Giemsa stain, original magnification, ×550. **B**, FNA. Swirling pattern of growth; hematoxylin-eosin; original magnification, ×550. **C**, FNA. Sublumen formation (hematoxylin-eosin, original magnification, ×550). **D**, histopathology. Ducts lined with more than four cell layers; hematoxylin-eosin; original magnification, ×275. **E**, histopathology. Duct with heaped-up epithelium; hematoxylin-eosin, original magnification, ×550). (Courtesy of Gangopadhyay M, Nijhawan R, Joshi K, et al: Cytology of "significant" breast ductal proliferations. *Acta Cytol* 41:1112–1120, 1997.)

Diagnostic Accuracy of Conventional Versus Sonography-guided Fine-Needle Aspiration Biopsy of Thyroid Nodules

Danese D, Sciacchitano S, Farsetti A, et al ("La Sapienza" Univ, Rome; Italian Air Force Med Inst, Rome; Inst of Experimental Med, Rome; et al)
Thyroid 8:15–21, 1998 2–15

Objective.—Fine-needle aspiration biopsy (FNAB) has improved the preoperative clinical evaluation of thyroid nodules. In patients where access to the thyroid is hampered, ultrasonic guidance has been suggested

TABLE 2.—Comparison Between Cytological and Histological Diagnosis in Thyroid Nodules Explored by C-FNAB

Cytologic diagnosis *Histologic diagnosis*

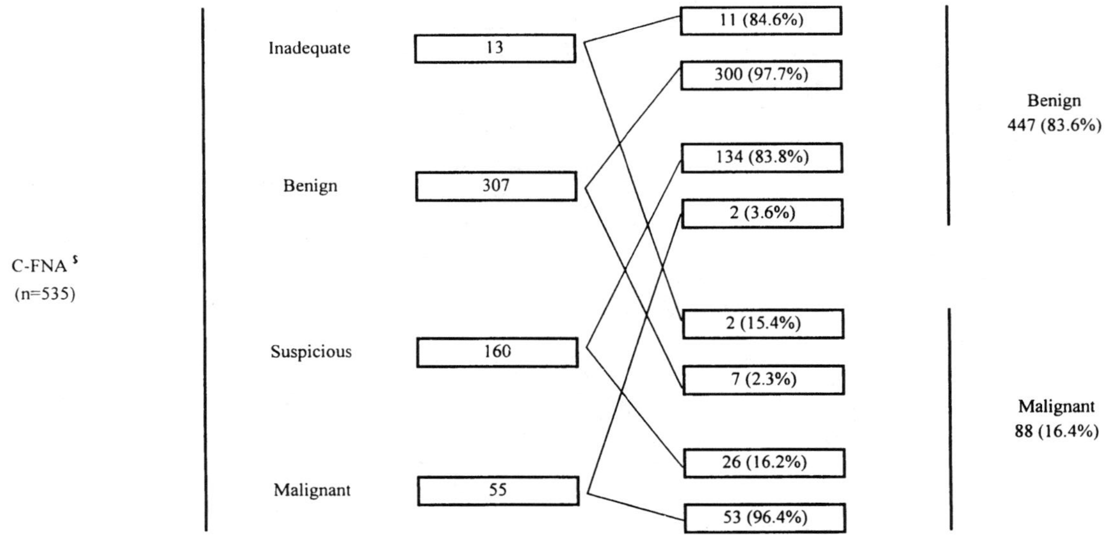

Abbreviation: C-FNAB, conventional fine-needle aspiration biopsy.
(Courtesy of Danese D, Sciacchitano S, Farsetti A, et al: Diagnostic accuracy of conventional versus sonography-guided fine-needle aspiration biopsy of thyroid nodules. *Thyroid* 8:15–21, 1998.)

TABLE 3.—Comparison Between Cytological and Histological Diagnosis in Thyroid Nodules Explored by SG-FNAB

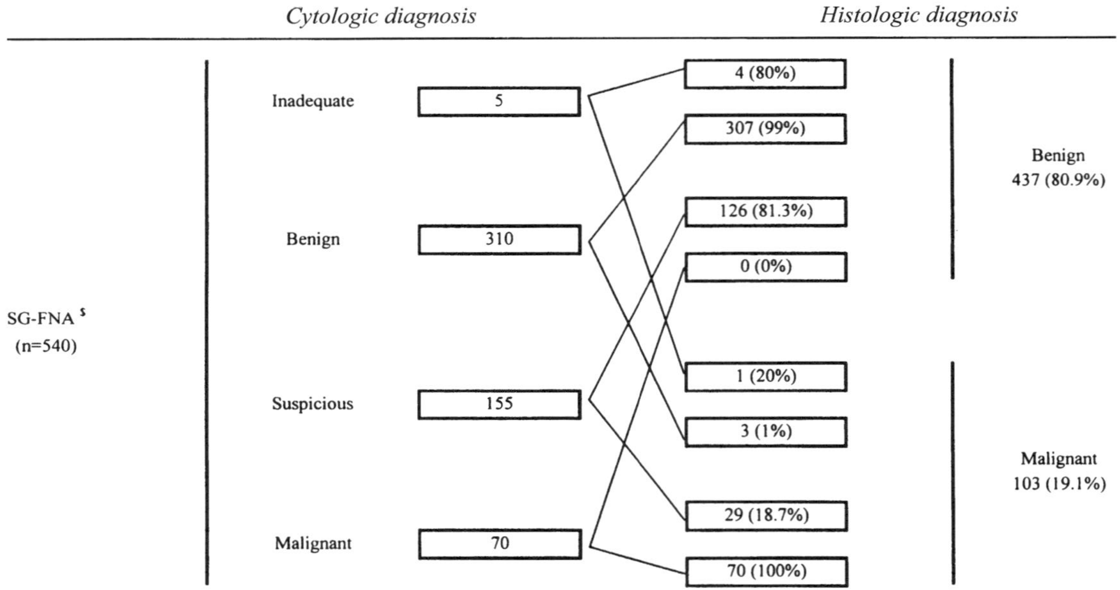

Abbreviation: SG-FNAB, sonography-guided fine-needle aspiration biopsy.
(Courtesy of Danese D, Sciacchitano S, Farsetti A, et al: Diagnostic accuracy of conventional versus sonography-guided fine-needle aspiration biopsy of thyroid nodules. *Thyroid* 8:15–21, 1998.)

TABLE 4.—Diagnostic Accuracy of C-FNAB vs. SG-FNAB

	*C-FNAB** (n = *522**)	*SG-FNAB** (n = *535**)
False-negative cases	7 (2.3%)	3 (1%)
Sensitivity	91.8%	97.1%
Specificity	68.8%	70.9%
Accuracy	72.6%	75.9%
Positive predictive value	36.7%	44%
Negative predictive value	97.7%	99%

*Inadequate specimens were not included in the calculation of indices of diagnostic accuracy.
Abbreviations: C-FNAB, conventional fine-needle aspiration biopsy; *SG-FNAB*, sonography-guided fine-needle aspiration biopsy.
(Courtesy of Danese D, Sciacchitano S, Farsetti A, et al: Diagnostic accuracy of conventional versus sonography-guided fine-needle aspiration biopsy of thyroid nodules. *Thyroid* 8:15–21, 1998.)

to improve diagnostic performance. The diagnostic accuracy of sonography-guided FNAB (SG-FNAB) was compared retrospectively with that of conventional FNAB (C-FNAB) in a large population of patients.

Methods.—Between 1982 and 1996, C-FNAB was performed on 4,986 patients (674 males), aged 2–87, and SG-FNAB was performed on 4,697 patients (681 males), aged 2–98. A minimum of 3 aspirations was performed on most nodules. Sensitivity, positive predictive value, negative predictive value, and accuracy were determined for both methods.

Results.—Insufficient material was obtained in 8.7% of C-FNAB specimens and in 3.5% of SG-FNAB specimens. Cytology identified benign lesions in 84.3% of C-FNAB specimens and in 89.4% of SG-FNAB specimens. C-FNAB detected a malignant lesion in 80 patients or a prevalence of 1.6%. SG-FNAB detected a malignant lesion in 100 patients or a prevalence of 2.1%. Of 160 lesions classified by cytology as potentially malignant by C-FNAB, 134 (81.2%) were found to be benign and 26 malignant by histology (Table 2). Of the 155 potentially malignant lesions identified by SG-FNAB, 126 were found to be benign and 29 malignant by histology (Table 3). The difference in cytologic results was significant. Suspicious lesions were found in 5.4% of C-FNAB specimens and in 5% of SG-FNAB specimens. The diagnostic accuracies of the 2 methods were similar (Table 4).

Conclusion.—SG-FNAB is an accurate, sensitive, and specific method for diagnosing thyroid nodules, particularly for lesions difficult to access. At earlier proliferative stages, SG-FNAB results in superior detection of thyroid malignancy.

► In my own practice, there is a marked trend for endocrinologists to send more thyroid aspirates that have been obtained with ultrasound guidance, even in cases where the mass is clearly palpable. Indeed, most of these patients arrive at the endocrinologist's office after another physician identifies a thyroid nodule on physical examination. Most are colloid nodules, and most aspirates are completely satisfactory. One improvement we have been able to bring about is teaching our clinical colleagues to use 25-gauge (0.5

mm) needles for the vast majority of these procedures. This has reduced the amount of blood on the smears and has decreased the unsatisfactory rates for all of our clinicians to very low levels. Another point that has nothing to do with this article, but has proven useful for maximizing specimen quality is that our clinicians (all of whom work off site) have been instructed to air dry all slides. In our experience, most doctors have difficulty getting slides fixed adequately, but air drying all slides and using a Romanowsky stain will solve this problem for those comfortable with interpreting this type of material.

M.W. Stanley, M.D.

Suggested Reading

Gharib H, Goellner JR, Johnson DA: Fine-needle aspiration cytology of the thyroid: A 12-year experience with 11,000 biopsies. *Clin Lab Med* 13:699–709, 1993.

Sanchez RB, van Sonnenberg E, D'Agostino HB: Ultrasound-guided biopsy of nonpalpable and difficult to palpate thyroid masses. *J Am Coll Surg* 178:33–37, 1994.

Cytologic Diagnosis of Anaplastic Large Cell Lymphoma

Sgrignoli A, Abati A (NIH, Bethesda, Md)
Acta Cytol 41:1048–1052, 1997 2–16

Objective.—Anaplastic large cell lymphoma (ALCL) is a rare malignancy and is sometimes difficult to recognize as a lymphoma. All cytologic material diagnosed as ALCL with histologic confirmation at the National Cancer Institute was reviewed retrospectively to identify morphologic and immunocytochemical staining patterns.

Methods.—Since 1990, 21 specimens from 7 patients (3 females), aged 2–83, were identified as ALCL. Immunochemical staining pattern and presence of CD30, CD3, L26, CD15, leukocyte common antigen, and epithelial membrane antigen (EMA) were investigated.

Results.—Two patients were HIV positive (Table 1). A smear pattern of cells that were largely dispersed with focal perivascular aggregates was common (Fig 2). Immunocytochemical studies were positive for CD30 in 4 patients and for EMA in 3 patients (Table 2).

Conclusion.—ALCL can be diagnosed in cytologic material on the basis of 9 characteristic features: (1) smear pattern of largely dispersed cells with focal aggregates; (2) variability in cell size; (3) deeply basophilic, variability vacuolated cytoplasm; (4) eccentric, round-to-oval nuclei with prominent nucleol; (5) ropy chromatin pattern; (6) proteinaceous background, particularly in cellular samples; (7) prominent necrosis; (8) lymphoglandular bodies and lymphoid tangles not prominent; and (9) expression of CD30 and one or more of EMA, LCA, T- or B-cell markers.

TABLE 1.—Clinicopathologic Data on Patients With Anaplastic Large Cell Lymphoma

Patient	Age (yr)	Sex	HIV status	Case no.	Specimen
1	3	F	+	1	FNA neck
				2	FNA lung
2	2	M	+	3	CSF
3	43	M		4	FNA pelvis Soft tissue
4	41	F		5	FNA Mediastinum
5	34	M		6	Pleural fluid
				7	Pleural fluid
				8	CSF
				9	CSF
				10	CSF
				11	CSF
				12	CSF
				13	CSF
				14	CSF
				15	CSF
				16	CSF
				17	CSF
				18	CSF
6	83	F		19	FNA lymph node
7	46	M		20	FNA groin
				21	FNA lymph node

Abbreviation: CSF, cerebrospinal fluid.
(Courtesy of Sgrignoli A, Abati A: Cytologic diagnosis of anaplastic large cell lymphoma. *Acta Cytol* 41:1048–1052, 1997.)

▶ ALCL causes diagnostic problems because of clinical and pathologic findings that require its distinction from Hodgkin's disease, metastatic carcinoma, malignant melanoma, or even a sarcoma. These authors warn that lymphoglandular bodies and lymphoid tangles may not be prominent, and this can add to diagnostic uncertainty. Immunohistochemical findings are very helpful, but only if one thinks of the diagnosis. Furthermore, even those who do not endorse primary diagnosis of malignant lymphoma by FNA occasionally "bump into" these neoplasms, and from time to time may encounter ALCL; we have certainly had this experience in our own laboratory. These authors also highlight the cytologic findings in exfoliative specimens.

M.W. Stanley, M.D.

Suggested Reading

Akhtar M, Ali MA, Haider A, et al: Fine-needle aspiration biopsy of Ki-1-positive anaplastic large-cell lymphoma. *Diagn Cytopathol* 8:242–247, 1992.

Tani E, Löwhagen T, Nasiell K, et al: Fine-needle aspiration cytology and immunocytochemistry of large-cell lymphomas expressing the Ki-1 antigen. *Acta Cytol* 33:359–362, 1989.

Zakowski MF, Feiner-H, Finfer M; et al: Cytology of extranodal Ki-1 anaplastic large-cell lymphoma. *Diagn Cytopathol* 14:155–160, 1996.

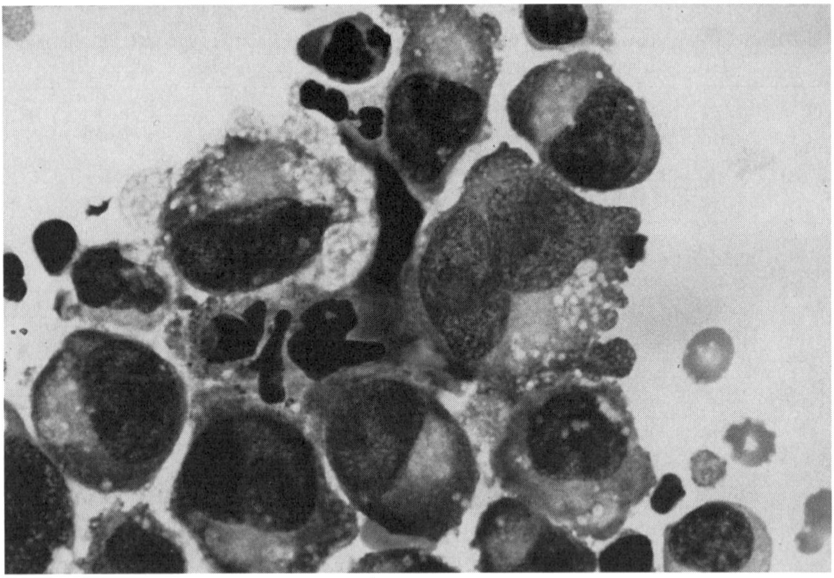

FIGURE 2.—ALCL in pleural fluid. Note the very large cell size (six to seven times the diameter of a RBC), variability in cell size, eccentrically placed nuclei, prominent nucleoli, deeply basophilic cytoplasm, cytoplasmic vacuoles and ropy chromatin pattern. Scattered binucleated or multinucleated cells are present. In this case, pallor in a perinuclear Golgi distribution was prominent; Diff-Quik, original magnification, ×1,000. (Courtesy of Sgrignoli A, Abati A: Cytologic diagnosis of anaplastic large cell lymphoma. *Acta Cytol* 41:1048–1052, 1997.)

TABLE 2.—Immunocytochemical Staining Pattern in Six Cases of ALCL

Patient no.	CD30	EMA	LCA	L26	CD3	CD15
1	+	–	Weakly +	–	–	–
	+	+	Unsatisfactory	–	+	–
2	+					
	+	+	Weakly +	–	Weakly +	Weakly +
3	+					
4	+	Weakly +		+	+	–

(Courtesy of Sgrignoli A, Abati A: Cytologic diagnosis of anaplastic large cell lymphoma. *Acta Cytol* 41:1048–1052, 1997.)

Rate of Insufficient Samples for Fine-needle Aspiration for Nonpalpable Breast Lesions in a Multicenter Clinical Trial: The Radiologic Diagnostic Oncology Group 5 Study

Pisano ED, Fajardo LL, Tsimikas J, et al (Univ of North Carolina, Chapel Hill; Univ of Virginia, Charlottesville; Harvard Univ, Boston; et al)

Cancer 82:679–688, 1988 2–17

Background.—Fine-needle aspiration (FNA) of nonpalpable breast lesions has variable results. Whether variations are caused by technical limitations, use of different methods, or the experience of the operator is not clear. The Radiologic Diagnostic Oncology Group 5 (RDOG5) multicenter clinical trial evaluated FNA of nonpalpable breast lesions by multiple operators using the same protocol.

Methods.—Eighteen institutions enrolled 419 women with nonpalpable lesions detected by mammography. Criteria for inclusion and exclusion are indicated in (Table 1). The women were randomly assigned to group A, which received stereotactically guided FNA (SFNA) followed by stereotactically guided core needle biopsy (SCNB) or SCNB alone, or to group B,

TABLE 1.—Mammographic Criteria for Inclusion and Exclusion From the Protocol

Mammographic lesions eligible for entry onto protocol
Any circumscribed solid mass over 1 cm in size
Any circumscribed, solid mass under 1 cm in size that has grown since a prior mammogram
Area of architectural distortion with a lucent center (probably a radial scar)
Area of architectural distortion, unless in a known prior biopsy site
Microlobulated noncystic mass, regardless of size
Spiculated noncystic mass, regardless of size
Noncystic mass with indistinct borders
Noncystic mass associated with suspicious calcifications, architectural distortion, focal skin thickening, or a focal solitary dilated duct
Clustered calcifications that are pleomorphic, linear, branching, variable in size, and/or very small and granular
Asymmetry associated with a noncystic mass, suspicious calcifications, architectural distortion, a solitary dilated duct and/or focal skin thickening
Mammographic lesions specifically excluded from entry onto protocol
Single dilated duct not associated with spontaneous nipple discharge
Localized center of tiny round or oval uniform calcifications
Circumscribed, low density mass <1 cm in size unless changed since prior mammogram
Mass containing intralesional fat density that is pathognomonic for lymph node, lipid (oil) cyst, or hamartoma
Localized focal asymmetric area of fibroglandular density
Subtle area of architectural distortion without central increased fibroglandular density in an area of prior biopsy
Discrete cluster or clusters of calcifications suggestive of milk of calcium, secretory disease, or sclerosing adenosis
Diffuse nonclustered calcifications suggestive of milk of calcium (a mammographically pathognomonic type of fibrocystic change), secretory disease, or sclerosing adenosis
Multiple noncalcified, well defined mass
Any lesion found to be a cyst at ultrasound

(Courtesy of Pisano ED, Fajardo LL, Tsimikas J, et al: Rate of insufficient samples for fine-needle aspiration for nonpalpable breast lesions in a multicenter clinical trial: The Radiologic Diagnostic Oncology Group 5 Study. *Cancer* 82[4]:679–688, 1988.

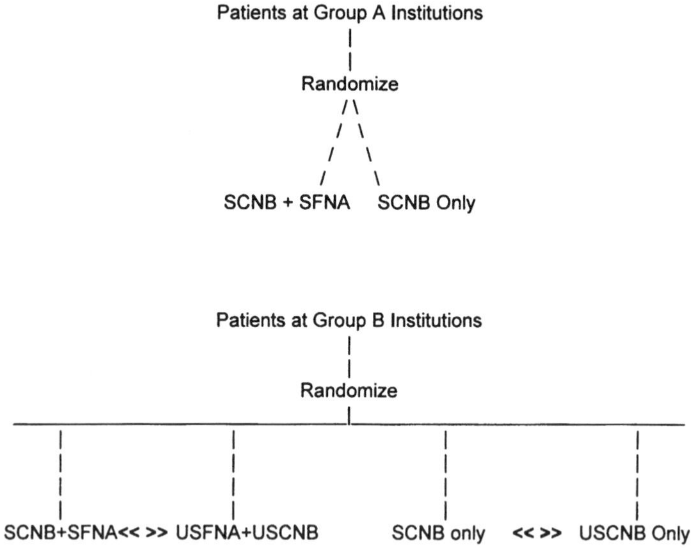

FIGURE 1.—Radiologic Diagnostic Oncology Group 5 study scheme. *Abbreviations: SCNB*, stereotactically guided core needle biopsy; *SNFA*, stereotactically guided fine-needle biopsy; *USFNA*, ultrasonographically guided fine-needle aspiration biopsy; *USCNB*, ultrasonographically guided core needle biopsy. Brackets indicate crossover allowed in both directions. (Courtesy of Pisano ED, Fajardo LL, Tsimikas J, et al: Rate of insufficient samples for fine-needle aspiration for nonpalpable breast lesions in a multicenter clinical trial: The Radiologic Diagnostic Oncology Group 5 Study. *Cancer* 82[4]:679–688, 1988. © 1988 American Cancer Society. Reprinted by permission of Wiley-Liss, Inc., a subsidiary of John Wiley & Sons, Inc.)

which received SFNA and SCNB, SCNB alone, ultrasonographically guided FNA followed by ultrasonographically guided core needle biopsy (USCNB), or USCNB alone (Fig 1). The insufficient sampling rates overall and according to the mammographic characteristics of the lesion were analyzed. Pathologic diagnosis by FNA was compared with diagnosis by SCNB or surgery.

Results.—Of the 377 women (236 with mass lesions and 141 with calcified lesions) whose results were eligible for analysis, 128 (34%) had insufficient FNA samples. Calcified lesions had a significantly higher rate of insufficient sampling than mass lesions (46.1% vs. 29.2%; $P < 0.001$). The radiologist's level of suspicion was a significant predictor of insufficient sampling for calcified lesions but not for mass lesions. Of the 336 lesions for which histologic data were available, insufficient samples were significantly more common for benign than malignant masses (34.2% vs. 12.5%) and for benign than malignant calcified lesions (55.9% vs. 33.3%) (Table 3). The insufficient sampling rates for malignant masses were 34.3% using stereotactic guidance and 8.6% using ultrasound guidance. The insufficient sampling rates for calcified lesions were 46.4% using stereotactic guidance and 0% using ultrasound guidance. The presence of an on-site cytopathologist significantly improved the sufficiency of FNA sampling for both mass lesions and calcifications (Table 4).

TABLE 3.—FNA Sample Sufficiency According to Histopathology and Lesion Type

Lesion type	Histologic results	FNA results No. (% of histologic type) Sufficient	Insufficient	Total
Mass	Benign	106 (65.8)	55 (34.2)*	161
	ALH/LCIS/ ADH	2 (100.0)	0	2
	DCIS/ invasive carcinoma	35 (87.5)	5 12.5)*	40
	Total	143 (70.4)	60 (29.6)	203
Calcifications	Benign	45 (41.1)	57 (55.9)†	102
	ALH/LCIS/ ADH	6 (85.7)	1 (14.3)	7
	DCIS/ invasive carcinoma	14 (66.7)	7 (33.3)†	21
	Total	65 (50.0)	65 (50.0)	133
Total		208 (62.5)	125 (37.5)	336

*$P = 0.007$.
†$P = 0.06$.
Abbreviations: FNA, fine-needle aspiration; *ALH*, atypical lobular hyperplasia; *LCIS*, lobular carcinoma in situ; *ADH*, atypical ductal hyperplasia; *DCIS*, ductal carcinoma in situ.
(Courtesy of Pisano ED, Fajardo LL, Tsimikas J, et al: Rate of insufficient samples for fine-needle aspiration for nonpalpable breast lesions in a multicenter clinical trial: The Radiologic Diagnostic Oncology Group 5 Study. Cancer 82[4]:679–688, 1998. © 1988 American Cancer Society. Reprinted by permission of Wiley-Liss, Inc., a subsidiary of John Wiley & Sons, Inc.)

Conclusion.—Fine-needle aspiration of nonpalpable breast lesions—both malignant masses and calcified lesions—resulted in such a high rate of insufficient samples that the study was terminated early.

► This paper has implications that go beyond application of FNA to nonpalpable breast lesions. Perhaps the most interesting is the statement that "No special training for FNA or specimen preparation was provided to the clinicians as part of this study." The benefits of FNA in many clinical settings are

TABLE 4.—FNA Sample Sufficiency by Cytopathologist and Lesion Type

Lesion type	On-site cytopathologist	FNA results No. (% of category) Sufficient	Insufficient	Total
Mass	No	119 (68.8)	54 (31.2)	173
	Yes	53 (85.5)	9 (14.5)	62
Calcifications	No	55 (50.0)	55 (50.0)	110
	Yes	20 (74.1)	7 (25.9)	27

Abbreviation: FNA, fine-needle aspiration.
(Courtesy of Pisano ED, Fajardo LL, Tsimikas L, et al: Rate of insufficient samples for fine-needle aspiration for nonpalpable breast lesions in a multicenter clinical trial: The Radiologic Diagnostic Oncology Group 5 Study. Cancer 82[4]:679–688, 1998. © 1988 American Cancer Society. Reprinted by permission of Wiley-Liss, Inc., a subsidiary of John Wiley & Sons, Inc.)

obvious to all. However, in my opinion, the main reason for our failure to disseminate the method to the majority of practitioners and patients who might benefit from it is the fact that it does not work very well (and can even be diagnostically dangerous) in untrained or inexperienced hands. It's just not as easy as it looks. The only way to learn this method is to work side by side with an expert and compare your samples with his or hers. For this reason, I would suggest that RDOG5 was fatally flawed from its conception and does not constitute a meaningful evaluation of FNA. In contrast, I would offer the very successful integration of FNA into breast evaluation by Dr. Sanchez and coworkers.[1] They have been so successful that the Swedes have asked them to visit and instruct them in the technique. This maturation of American FNA practice contrasts sharply with the failure of RDOG5.

M.W. Stanley, M.D.

Reference

1. Sanchez M, Stahl R, Goldfischer M: The use of fine needle aspiration and core biopsies in the diagnosis of nonpalpable breast lesions, in Schmidt W (ed): *Cytopathology Annual*, vol 6. American Society of Clinical Pathologists Press, in press.

Suggested Reading

Hayes MK, DeBruhl ND, Hirschowitz S, et al: Mammographically-guided fine-needle aspiration cytology of the breast: Reducing the rate of insufficient specimens. *AJR* 167:381–384, 1996.

Sneige N, Fornage BD, Saleh G: Ultrasound-guided fine-needle aspiration of non-palpable breast lesions. Cytologic and histologic findings. *Am J Clin Pathol* 102(1):98–101, 1994.

3 Female Genital Tract

Fine-needle Aspiration Cytology Versus Core Biopsies in the Evaluation of Recurrent Gynecologic Malignancies

Malmström H (Univ Hosp, Linköping, Sweden)
Gynecol Oncol 65:69–73, 1997 3–1

Introduction.—In all women with possible gynecologic tumors, there is a need for definitive cytologic or histologic diagnosis before additional treatment can be given. The standard method for verification of various primary or recurrent tumors has been the use of the fine-needle aspiration, but there is a problem with false-negative results, because the small dimensions of the needle obtain insufficient tissue material. To obtain a tissue specimen for histologic evaluation, automatic biopsy needle devices can be used. The accuracies of fine-needle aspiration and core biopsies were evaluated in gynecologic cancer.

Methods.—There were 85 patients with gynecologic cancer in a 9-year period. An automatic biopsy instrument with a specially designed needle guide, called Biopty, was used to investigate the histology and cytology of gynecologic lesions. All women also had fine-needle aspiration for cytology. The patients had persistent, recurrent, or metastatic disease. Three hundred thirty-nine fine-needle aspirations and 141 biopsies using the core instrument were obtained.

Results.—Fine-needle aspiration cytology resulted in correct diagnoses in 67 of 85 patients (79%) and Biopty core instrument biopsies resulted in correct diagnoses in 62 of 85 patients (73%) (Table 2). In 12 of 85 patients who had aspiration cytology, there was insufficient material for evaluation (14%), and in biopsies, there was insufficient material in 10 of 85 patients (12%). In 5% of the patients with fine-needle aspiration cytology, false-negative diagnoses occurred, compared to 15% of the patients with the biopsies. The sensitivity of the biopsies was 73% and the specificity

TABLE 2.—Results of Find-needle Aspiration and Biopty Core Instrument Samples

	Malignant *n* (%)	Benign *n* (%)	Inadequate material *n* (%)	False neg. *n* (%)	False pos. *n* (%)	Correct *n* (%)
FNA	45 (53)	22 (26)	12 (14)	4 (5)	2 (2)	67 (79)
BCI	35 (41)	27 (32)	10 (12)	13 (15)	0 (0)	62 (73)

(Courtesy of Malmström H: Fine-needle aspiration cytology versus core biopsies in the evaluation of recurrent gynecologic malignancies. *Gynecol Oncol* 65:69–73, 1997.)

TABLE 3.—Sensitivity, Specificity, and Predictive Value for the Biopty Core Instrument and Fine-needle Aspiration Methods

	FNA	BCI	*P*
Sensitivity	45/(45 + 4) = 92%	35/(35 + 13) = 73%	0.01
Specificity	22/(22 + 2) = 92%	27/(27 + 0) = 100%	0.14
Predictive value of positive results	45/(45 + 2) = 96%	35/(35 + 0) = 100%	

(Courtesy of Malmström H: Fine-needle aspiration cytology versus core biopsies in the evaluation of recurrent gynecologic malignancies. *Gynecol Oncol* 65:69–73, 1997.)

was 100%, whereas with the fine-needle aspiration, the sensitivity was 92% and the specificity was 92% (Table 3). The predictive value of positive results for fine-needle aspiration was 96% and for biopsies, it was 100%. There was a negligible complication rate.

Conclusion.—Fine-needle aspiration in combination with Biopty core instrument in gynecologic lesions is a simple and safe operation using needle guides. The sensitivity for Biopty core instrument is lower than for fine-needle aspiration cytology, but the specificity is higher. Between the 2 methods, no significant differences were found in accuracy. In the subset of patients in whom additional information about the tumor is desired for planning the treatment of recurrent disease, Biopty core instrument biopsy should be considered.

▶ The abstract of this article results speaks for itself. Surprisingly, there are no prior studies comparing these 2 methods in patients with gynecologic malignancies. In this patient series, 72% of the specimens were obtained transvaginally, 15% transrectally, and 13% percutaneously. The importance of using a needle guide for transvaginal/transrectal approach is critical. One particular advantage of using the biopsy core is in situations in which tumors are difficult to keep in a fixed position. The high-speed bore of the biopsy tool aids the harvesting of the tissue.

D.J. Dabbs, M.D.

Angiomyofibroblastoma of the Female Genital Tract: Analysis of 17 Cases Including a Lipomatous Variant

Laskin WB, Fetsch JF, Tavassoli FA (Northwestern Univ, Chicago; Armed Forces Inst of Pathology, Washington, DC)

Hum Pathol 28:1046–1055, 1997 3–2

Objective.—Angiomyofibroblastoma (AMF) is a rare, indolent mesenchymal tumor characterized by a well-circumscribed, subcutaneous vulvovaginal tumor. Only 38 cases have been reported. The clinicopathologic and immunohistochemical features of 17 cases were reviewed.

Findings.—The 17 cases involved women, aged 38–60 years, with 15 tumors in the vulva, 1 in the inguinal region, and 1 in the perineum.

Tumors ranged in size from 2 to 8 cm, were well circumscribed, round to ovoid, had a soft-to-rubbery consistency, and were pinkish. Cells were plump, spindled, and epithelioid, with numerous, focally clustered, patent vessels in a collagenous stroma. Mitotic activity ranged from 1 to 7 mitoses in 9 cases. There was little cytologic atypia. There were 12 fatty tumors, and 2 were composed mainly of fatty tissue (a variant of AMF). Five tumors tested for vimentin expressed it strongly. Six of 8 tumors showed desmin activity, 5 of 6 progesterone receptor protein, 1 of 6 CD34, and 1 of 7 smooth muscle actin. None of 8 patients followed up for 1–25 years had a recurrence or metastases after simple excision.

Conclusions.—The benign nature of AMF tumors is confirmed, and a histogenetic link to lipomatous tumors is suggested.

► The important differential diagnosis of AMF includes the aggressive angiomyxoma, cutaneous myxoma, fibroepithelial polyps with cellular stroma, smooth muscle and glomus tumors, neurofibromas, Schwannoma, and solitary fibrous tumor. The aggressive angiomyxoma presents without the typical clustered vascular patterns seen in AMF, and thus is relatively hypovascular with a predominance of myxoid-edematous stroma. The short spindle and stellate cells are also unlike the plump epithelioid collections cuffed around the vessels in AMF. The superficial or cutaneous myxoma is a nodular mass that is superficial, lobular, and contains abundant mucin again without the cell population or vascularity. Although the presence of intralesional fat is common in AMF, an abundant content is referred to as the lipomatous variant and should not be confused with angiolipoma.

D.J. Dabbs, M.D.

Expression of Vascular Endothelial Growth Factor (VEGF) in Epithelial Ovarian Neoplasms: Correlation With Clinicopathology and Patient Survival, and Analysis of Serum VEGF Levels

Yamamoto S, Konishi I, Mandai M, et al (Kyoto Univ, Japan)

Br J Cancer 76:1221–1227, 1997 3–3

Introduction.—Vascular endothelial growth factor (VEGF) is generated by various solid tumors and may be involved in microvascular permeability and/or angiogenesis. The expression of VEGF was analyzed immunohistochemically in 110 epithelial ovarian tumors to determine the relationship between VEGF expression in ovarian neoplasms and clinicopathological factors or patient survival.

Methods.—The VEGF levels in the tumor fluid in 17 patients, ascites in 12 patients, and sera in 38 patients were analyzed via enzyme immunoassay. Patient survival curves and the correlations between immunoreactivity and the clinicopathological factors of patients with ovarian tumors were calculated.

Results.—Positive immunostaining for VEGF was seen in 97% of ovarian carcinomas, a significantly higher percentage than in tumors of low malignant potential and in benign cystadenomas. Strong VEGF immunostaining was also seen more frequently in tumors of clear cell type in advanced stage of disease and with positive peritoneal cytology. Patients with strong VEGF staining had significantly lower survival rates than did patients with weak or no immunostaining for VEGF.

Conclusion.—Strong VEGF expression was important in the tumor progression of ovarian carcinoma. The enzyme immunoassay showed higher serum VEGF levels in patients with carcinoma than in patients with tumors of low malignant potential or with benign tumors. Serum VEGF levels did decrease after successful removal of tumors in patients with ovarian cancer. Serum VEGF was re-elevated in 1 patient during relapse. Serum VEGF may be used as a marker for managing the clinical course in patients with ovarian cancer.

► VEGF has been reported to be synthesized or secreted by a variety of cultured tumor cells and solid human tumors, such as tumors of the brain, lung, breast, gastrointestinal tract, kidney, and urinary bladder, as well as by epithelial ovarian carcinomas. In most studies, as in this one, prognostic information was obtained from examining the distribution of VEGF immunostaining in tumor tissues. Certainly the presence of strong VEGF staining of tumor cells implies a survival advantage for the tumor cells, as the VEGF supplies the stimulus for nutrient vessels and capillaries to appear. Even if the tumor is not capable of metastasizing, its life can be prolonged by the presence of new vessels, so VEGF may well play a critical role in the progression of the tumor. The longer the neoplasm lives, the more genetic abnormalities pile up, which can ultimately lead to a more aggressive behavior. The intriguing aspect of this article is the enzyme immunoassay used to examine serum VEGF in carcinoma patients. Further work needs to be done, but the basic premise is that any VEGF detectable in peripheral blood would be suspect for neoplasm.

D.J. Dabbs, M.D.

Carcinosarcomas (Malignant Mixed Mullerian Tumors) of the Female Genital Tract: Comparative Molecular Analysis of Epithelial and Mesenchymal Components

Kounelis S, Jones MW, Papadaki H, et al (Magee-Women's Hosp, Pittsburgh, Pa; Univ of Pittsburgh, Pa)

Hum Pathol 29:82–87, 1998 3–4

Background.—Female genital tract carcinosarcomas (FGTCS), or malignant mixed mullerian tumors, are highly aggressive, biphasic neoplasms made up of carcinomatous and sarcomatous components. The histogenesis of these tumors may involve simultaneous formation of 2 independent tumors or multidirectional differentiation of a single tumor. Previous p53-immunobased studies of FGTCS have supported the monoclonal theory.

Topographic genotyping (TG) was used to establish the biclonal vs. monoclonal origin of FGTCS.

Methods.—Immunostaining for p53 protein was performed in 43 cases of FGTCS, 32 uterine and 11 ovarian. Thirty-five of these tumors showed strong immunopositivity for p53. Nine of these tumors had distinct carcinomatous and sarcomatous components for effective sampling. These were subjected to TG to determine the presence of specific genotype and timing of p53 mutational change.

Results.—The 9 p53-immunopositive tumors all showed point mutations on p53 exons 5 through 8. Both components of all 9 tumors showed the same point mutational genotype. In each case, loss of the wild-type allele appeared to have occurred before separation into biphasic tumor.

Conclusions.—The findings support the monoclonal theory of FGTCS histogenesis. In FGTCS, p53 immunopositivity is a very common finding, suggesting that p53 gene mutation is a frequent event in the progression of FGTCS. The results are consistent with the classification of FGTCS as a separate histologic entity with an unfavorable prognosis. Specialized techniques such as TG have an important role to play in dealing with selected investigations unresolved by other techniques.

▶ The limitations of pure ultrastructural morphology in the study of these neoplasms is evident with this molecular study. Whereas prior ultrastructural studies demonstrated distinct, independent epithelial and stromal differentiation with no transition between the two, this analysis of p53 mutations provides evidence that in fact these tumors demonstrate multidirectional differentiation from an initial single malignant clone. Unfortunate is the small number of cases that were available for this topographic genotyping study. A sample of only 9 cases is small indeed, and larger numbers would be of further interest to ascertain the spectrum of possible p53 mutations. In addition, further studies using microsatellite instability as clonality markers would be most interesting and perhaps, more definitive.

D.J. Dabbs, M.D.

Mucinous Tumors of the Vermiform Appendix and Ovary, and Pseudomyxoma Peritonei: Histogenetic Implications of Cytokeratin 7 Expression

Guerrieri C, Frånlund B, Fristedt S, et al (Univ Hosp, Linköping, Sweden; St Vincent's Hosp, New York)

Hum Pathol 28:1039–1045, 1997 3–5

Introduction.—Pseudomyxoma peritonei and simultaneous mucinous tumors involving the veriform appendix and ovaries are 2 entities that have come under increasing scrutiny by pathologists. Knowing the site of origin of these tumors would help increase understanding of the disease process. Cytokeratin 7 is expressed in all ovarian epithelial tumors, and this expression has not been adequately studied in appendiceal epithelial tumors. The expression of cytokeratin 7 in a series of primary appendiceal mucinous tumors, primary ovarian mucinous borderline tumors, simultaneous mucinous tumors of the appendix and ovary, and pseudomyxoma peritonei was investigated.

Methods.—There were 17 appendiceal cystadenomas and carcinomas, 20 mucinous borderline tumors of the ovary, 10 simultaneous mucinous tumors of the appendix and ovary, 3 high-stage mucinous borderline tumors of the ovary, and 3 pseudomyxoma peritonei of unknown origin that were investigated for their expression of cytokeratin 7.

Results.—Cytokeratin 7 was negative in 9 appendiceal cystadenomas, 2 of which were associated with pseudomyxoma peritonei, with the peritoneal lesions being Cytokeratin negative as well. More negative cytokeratin 7 findings occurred in 3 appendiceal carcinomas, 1 of which had metastases also found to be negative, 6 simultaneous mucinous tumors of the ovary and appendix and their peritoneal mucinous deposits, and 2 of 3 high-stage ovarian borderline tumors. Three cystadenomas, 2 appendiceal carcinomas, all 20 ovarian borderline tumors, 4 simultaneous mucinous tumors at the appendiceal and ovarian sites, and all 3 pseudomyxoma peritonei of unknown origin were cytokeratin 7 positive.

Conclusion.—Ovarian mucinous borderline tumors are always cytokeratin 7 positive, and appendiceal cystadenomas are often cytokeratin 7 negative. An appendiceal origin is suspected for simultaneous mucinous tumors involving the appendix and ovary, because the concordant staining pattern shows that 60% of these tumors were cytokeratin negative. For any cytokeratin 7 negative mucinous tumor involving the ovary or the peritoneum, an appendiceal or colonic source is supported. Mucinous borderline tumors in the ovary associated with pseudomyxoma peritonei are often metastatic from an appendiceal or other mucinous tumor, rather than being ovarian in origin.

► The findings of this article are most compatible with the conclusion that mucinous borderline tumors of the ovary associated with pseudomyxoma peritonei are not ovarian in origin, but are almost always metastatic from the appendix or other gastrointestinal based mucinous tumors. The study, based on the expression of cytokeratin 7, relies on the faithful uniform expression of cytokeratin 7 in all ovarian mucinous neoplasms, but in only approximately 12% of gastrointestinal mucinous tumors that originate in the appendix. Thus, the finding of cytokeratin negative pseudomyxoma peritonei is most compatible with origin in the gastrointestinal tract, particularly the appendix. The same holds true for so-called mucinous borderline tumors in the ovary associated with pseudomyxoma peritonei, because they are almost invariably cytokeratin negative, again indicative of an appendiceal origin. The current study is corroborated by other molecular studies, including 1 in which the loss of heterozygosity showed that some synchronous mucinous tumors of the ovary and appendix were appendiceal in origin. Another study demonstrated C-Ki-RAS mutation patterns, suggesting that the tumors were appendiceal in origin. In my experience with examining ovarian mucin tumors approximately 10 years ago, another useful antibody would be carcinoembryonic antigen (CEA), because ovarian mucinous epithelium is negative for CEA. In contrast, the mucinous epithelial cells and strips of epithelial cells seen in pseudomyxoma peritonei with appendiceal origin are invariably positive. Carcinoembryonic antigen, particularly the antibody that recognizes the epitope CEA-D14, is most useful.

D.J. Dabbs, M.D.

Suggested Reading

Chuaqui RF, Zhuang Z, Emmert-Buck BR, et al: Genetic analysis of synchronous mucinous tumors of the ovary and appendix. *Hum Pathol* 27:165–171, 1996.

Cuatrecasas M, Matias-Guiu X, Prat J: Synchronous mucinous tumors of the appendix and the ovary associated with pseudomyxoma peritonei: A clinicopathologic study of six cases with comparative analysis of c-Ci-*ras* mutations. *Am J Surg Pathol* 20:739–746, 1996.

Loy T, Calaluce R, Keeney G: Cytokeratin immunostaining in differentiating primary ovarian carcinoma from metastatic colonic adenocarcinoma. *Mod Pathol* 9:1040–1045, 1996.

Ronnett BM, Shmookler BM, Diener-West M, et al: Immunohistochemical evidence supporting the appendiceal origin of pseudomyxoma peritonei in women. *Int J Gynecol Pathol* 16:1–9, 1997.

Wang NP, Zee S, Zarbo RJ, et al: Coordinate expression of cytokeratins 7 and 20 defines unique subsets of carcinomas. *Appl Immunohistochem* 3:99–107, 1995.

Immunohistochemical Staining of Ovarian Granulosa Cell Tumors With Monoclonal Antibody Against Inhibin

McCluggage WG, Maxwell P, Sloan JM (Royal Group of Hosps Trust, Belfast, Ireland; Queen's Univ of Belfast, Ireland)
Hum Pathol 28:1034–1038, 1997 3–6

Introduction.—Classified within the sex cord–stroma group of ovarian neoplasms, adult granulosa cell tumor accounts for 1.5% of all ovarian neoplasms and for 6% of all malignant ovarian tumors. On occasion, it may be difficult to separate from other ovarian neoplasms. Because no marker has been proven to be specific for adult granulosa cell tumor, immunohistochemistry has generally been of limited value. Inhibin, a peptide hormone normally produced by ovarian granulosa cells, inhibits the release of follicle-stimulating hormone from the pituitary gland, and its detection in serum has been used for early diagnosis of tumor growth or metastasis before clinical disease is apparent. It was determined whether positive immunohistochemical staining with antibodies against inhibitor were specific for ovarian adult granulosa cell tumor.

Methods.—There were 16 patients with ovarian adult granulosa cell tumors, 15 patients with other ovarian sex cord-stromal tumors, and 51 patients with a range of ovarian and extraovarian neoplasms, many of which may mimic granulosa cell tumor. All cases were stained by an antibody against the alpha-subunit of human inhibin.

Results.—In all patients with adult granulosa cell tumor, there was diffuse strong cytoplasmic staining. In all Leydig cell tumors, diffuse positive staining was observed. In a proportion of fibrothecomas, there was focal staining. In 1 patient with ovarian clear cell carcinoma, there was focal weak staining, but no staining was seen of other ovarian and extraovarian neoplasms.

Conclusion.—In the diagnosis of granulosa cell tumor and in the distinction of this neoplasm from others that may mimic it, immunohistochemical staining with antibodies against inhibin is of value. The antibody also may be useful in the confirmation of late metastasis of granulosa cell tumor, especially when the previous history is not known.

► Granulosa cell tumors of the ovary can be difficult to differentiate from small cell carcinoma of the ovary or metastatic small cell carcinoma of the ovary. Normally produced by ovarian granulosa cells, this peptide is recapitulated in the adult granulosa cell tumor, being faithfully expressed strongly in virtually all cases. In a similar fashion, metastatic ovarian granulosa cell tumors may mimic small cell neoplasms in another site, and thus the expression of inhibin could be quite valuable in making this differential diagnosis in metastatic sites. In addition, Chivite et al. recently described the distribution of inhibin expression in the adrenal gland and its neoplasms.[1] In the normal adrenal gland, inhibin is expressed with increasing density from the glomerulosa level through the reticularis level. Adrenal cortical adenomas and carcinomas are almost uniformly diffusely positive for inhibin, whereas pheochromocytomas are almost all negative. In addition, a large number of metastatic neoplasms to the adrenal gland have been negative for inhibin. Even in high-grade adrenal cortical carcinomas vs. poorly differentiated chromocytomas and metastatic carcinomas, the expression of inhibin in adrenal cortical tumors has been faithful. The list of cells and tumors that express inhibin is widening, and includes granulosa cells, theca cells, Sertoli cells, Leydig cells, and adrenal cortical tumors. Clear cell renal cell carcinomas are universally negative for inhibin, a key to useful diagnostic differentiation from primary adrenal cortical tumors.

D.J. Dabbs, M.D.

Reference

1. Chivite A, Matias-Guiu X, Pons C, et al: Inhibin A expression in adrenal neoplasms, a new histochemical marker for adrenal cortical tumors. *Appl Immunohistochem* 6:42–49, 1998.

Telomerase Activity in Human Gynaecological Malignancies
Gorham H, Yoshida K, Sugino T, et al (Univ of Oxford, England)
J Clin Pathol 50:501–504, 1997 3–7

Introduction.—Maintenance of telomere length, which can be achieved by activating telomerase, a ribonucleoprotein RNA dependent DNA polymerase that adds telomeric hexanucleotide repeats to the ends of replicating chromosomes, is considered necessary for continued cell division and immortalization. In the vast majority of human cancer cell lines and tumors tested, telomerase activity has been demonstrated, but it was absent or present at very low levels in somatic cells. The telomeric repeat amplification protocol has been used, to detect the presence of telomerase activity in carcinomas from a number of organs, but few studies have assessed the value of this assay in detecting carcinoma in samples from the female reproductive tract.

Methods.—Telomerase activity was examined in frozen tissue samples of histologically confirmed lesions of the endometrium, ovary, and cervix. There were 6 endometrial carcinomas, 8 normal endometria, 13 ovarian carcinomas, 5 benign ovarian tumors, 6 cervical carcinomas, and 5 normal cervices. The exfoliated cells in cervical smears from patients with premalignant and malignant lesions, and the ascitic fluid obtained from patients with malignant or non-malignant ovarian tumors, were also examined for telomerase activity.

Results.—In all specimens of endometrial (6 of 6) and cervical (6 of 6) origin, and in almost all from the ovary (12 of 13), solid tissues from carcinomas were telomerase positive. The result was telomerase negative in the normal tissues from the cervix (0 of 5) and the ovary (0 of 5). Telomerase activity was seen in samples from normal endometrium, possibly because of the cyclical regenerative nature of this tissue. Detectable telomerase activity was rarely seen in dissociated cells in cervical smears from preneoplastic and frankly neoplastic lesions. In 1 of 2 patients, smears from malignant tumors were positive, but smears from cervical intraepithelial neoplasia-22 (0 of 5) and cervical intraepithelial neoplasia-3 (1 of 17) lesions and from normal samples (0 of 10) were almost all negative. In cells obtained from ascitic fluid from patients with ovarian tumors, telomerase activity was scarcely detectable.

Conclusion.—Malignant tumors of the female reproductive tract have increased telomerase activity, as do tumors in many other organs, but such activity is still not a reliable indicator of the exfoliated cancerous or precancerous cells in clinical specimens. Until more extensive studies have been conducted, interpretation should be guarded. Activation of this enzyme is a major hallmark of the neoplastic process.

► Using the telomeric repeat amplification protocol assay, the authors investigated whether exfoliated cellular material or fluid specimens could demonstrate the presence of telomerase activity to confirm the presence of malignant cells. The solid neoplasms examined from the ovary, cervix, and endometrium all clearly showed prominent telomerase activity. However, cellular material from cysts, ascitic fluid, and cervical vaginal specimens showed no appreciable telomerase activity in cervical intraepithelial neoplasia cells, and no activity in the fluid specimens. The overall number of specimens examined in this article is small, and perhaps is the largest limitation of the study. Nevertheless, it certainly would be ideal to be able to detect such enzymatic activity readily as a marker for malignant cells, as we can for bladder washings, colonic washings, and fine needle aspirates of breast carcinomas. The nature of the clinical specimens in this study, for example, the age of the exfoliated cells in secretions and the possible dilutional effects of cells basking in fluid, may impede the detection of telomerase activity, A larger, more comprehensive study is needed to confirm these findings.

D.J. Dabbs, M.D.

Distribution of Epithelial-specific Antigen in Uterine Cervix With Endocervical Glandular Dysplasia

Umezaki K, Sanezumi M, Okada H, et al (Kansai Med Univ, Moriguchi, Osaka, Japan)

Gynecol Oncol 66:393–398, 1997 3–8

Introduction.—Up to 10% of primary malignant tumors of the uterine cervix are cervical adenocarcinomas, but they are difficult to diagnose by means of Pap smear because the lesions are located higher in the endocervical canal. The natural history of cervical adenocarcinomas is also unknown, as is whether endocervical glandular dysplasia is a precursor lesion to malignant tumor formation. The relationship of endocervical glandular dysplasia to the uterine endocervical adenocarcinoma was clarified.

Methods.—There were 31 patients with glandular abnormalities of the uterine cervix identified in an 8-year period, including 11 patients with endocervical glandular dysplasia, 5 with adenocarcinoma in situ, 4 with microinvasive adenocarcinoma, and 11 with invasive adenocarcinoma. Ten normal endocervical specimens were compared with the immunohistochemical localization of epithelial-specific antigen in the patients with endocervical glandular dysplasia and related lesions.

Results.—In the basolateral membrane of endocervical cells in the normal endocervix, the epithelial-specific antigen immunoreactivities were usually present. In 6 of 11 patients with glandular dysplasia, in 9 of 9 patients with in situ and microinvasive adenocarcinomas, and in 11 of 11 patients with invasive adenocarcinomas, the expressions of epithelial-specific antigens were increasing from the basolateral membrane to the diffuse cytoplasmic membrane, along with the malignant transformation of the endocervical cells.

Conclusion.—For endocervical glandular dysplasia and related lesions with malignant transformation, epithelial-specific antigen is a useful marker, and it also suggests that endocervical glandular dysplasia may be a precursor lesion to uterine cervical adenocarcinomas.

▶ This article deserves scrutiny because it addresses the usefulness of epithelial-specific antigen antibody in detecting endocervical glandular dysplasia/in situ adenocarcinoma. Indeed, this detection is an age-old problem and 1 area where we can use all the help we can get diagnostically. In addition, such immunocytochemical techniques would be more than welcome on Papanicolaou smears in the quagmire of atypical glandular cells of undetermined significance. Other avenues that have been examined to detect endocervical dysplasias include differential mucin staining and carcinoembryonic antigen antibody reactivity, but neither of these is consistent. The epithelial-specific antigen antibody recognizes a 40-kd cell surface glycoprotein and it decorates a variety of epithelial cells. In this case, it is a matter of distribution of the antibody staining, predominantly basolateral in normal endocervix and apical/cytoplasmic in dysplasias. This pilot is in need of a larger study to corroborate these findings.

D.J. Dabbs, M.D.

Suggested Reading

Hurlimann J, Gloor E: Adenocarcinoma in situ and invasive adenocarcinoma of the uterine cervix: An immunohistologic study with antibodies specific for several epithelial markers. *Cancer* 54:103–109, 1984.

Nanbu Y, Fujii S, Konihi I, et al: Immunohistochemical localization of CA125, carcinoembryonic antigen, and CA19-9 in normal and neoplastic glandular cells of the uterine cervix. *Cancer* 62:2580–2588, 1988.

Rollason TP, Byrne P, Williams A, et al: Expression of epithelial membrane and 3-fucosyl-N-acetyllactosamine antigen in cervix uteri with particular reference to adenocarcinoma in situ. *J Clin Pathol* 41:547–552, 1988.

Inhibin Immunohistochemistry Applied to Ovarian Neoplasms: A Novel, Effective, Diagnostic Tool

Costa MJ, Ames PF, Walls J, et al (Univ of California, Sacramento; Indiana Univ, Indianapolis)

Hum Pathol 28:1247–1254, 1997 3–9

Introduction.—Sex cord–stromal tumors (SCSTs) account for only 8% of ovarian tumors, and half of these are benign fibromas. Diagnostic recognition of granulosa cell tumors (GCTs) or Sertoli–stromal cell tumors (SSCTs) is essential, because the neoplasms they may be confused with have completely different treatment and follow-up. Human inhibin is a peptide hormone produced by ovarian granulosa cells to inhibit follicle-stimulating hormone. Immunohistochemical studies using monoclonal antibodies against inhibin have recently come into use. Inhibin immunohistochemistry was evaluated for its ability to distinguish between SCSTs and other primary ovarian neoplasms.

Methods.—A total of 186 primary ovarian tumors were retrospectively studied. Hematoxylin-and-eosin–stained slides and clinical data from these tumors were reviewed to verify the diagnosis. Immunostaining with antiinhibin was performed in representative paraffin sections. Each specimen was graded as showing weak (W) vs. strong (S) immunoreactivity. In addition, the percentage of strongly staining cells was graded as S1, less than 10%; S2, 10% to 50%; and S3, greater than 50%.

Results.—Of 66 GCTs, 100% showed inhibin immunoreactivity: S3 in 80% and S2 in 20%. Immunoreactivity rate was also 100% in 17 SSCTs (90% S3 and 10% S2), 13 hyperplastic follicular/stromal lesions (90% S3 and 10% S2), and 6 steroid cell tumors (all S3). Ninety percent of 18 thecomas also showed inhibin immunoreactivity (40% S3, 10% S2, and 30% S1). Inhibin immunoreactivity was not observed in any of 12 fibromas, 3 myxomas, or 2 sclerosing stromal tumors. None of 49 other ovarian neoplasms showed immunoreactivity, including 22 carcinomas, 12 carcinosarcomas, 7 small-cell carcinomas, 6 germ cell tumors, and 2 lymphomas.

Conclusions.—Inhibin immunohistochemistry may be useful in distinguishing SCSTs and GCTs from other ovarian neoplasms, when this distinction cannot be made by routine pathologic examination. Study findings demonstrate that SCSTs and GCTs are positive on inhibin immunohistochemistry, whereas other ovarian tumors that could be confused with these entities have been negative so far. The findings must be independently confirmed before this test is adopted into general clinical practice.

► In general, the vast majority of SCSTs can be differentiated from other common epithelial tumors of the ovary and germ cell tumors. However, the subsets of SCSTs that can be confused with other, primary ovarian tumors principally include the GCT and small cell carcinoma of the ovary. In addition, lymphomas can be included in this small cell group of potentially undifferentiated ovarian carcinomas that are difficult to distinguish from each other. Inhibin, the glycoprotein hormone that inhibits the production and secretion of pituitary gonadotropins (principally follicle-stimulating hormone, is produced by ovarian granulosa cells. The literature contains 17 small cell carcinomas of the ovary that have been tested immunohistochemically with inhibin. All have been negative for inhibin. This study did address the diagnostic problems in which SCSTs and GCTs can be confused with other ovarian neoplasms. Thus, inhibin is a valuable marker in making these diagnostic distinctions, particularly in concert with established immunohistochemical algorithms for this group of tumors, which includes cytokeratins, vimentin, and epithelial membrane antigen.

D.J. Dabbs, M.D.

Value of Inhibin in the Identification of Granulosa Cell Tumors of the Ovary

Hildebrandt RH, Rouse RV, Longacre TA (Stanford Univ, Calif; Veterans Affairs Med Ctr, Palo Alto, Calif)

Hum Pathol 28:1387–1395, 1997 3–10

Objective.—Although diagnosis of adult granulosa cell tumors is usually straightforward, it can be difficult to differentiate these tumors from various primary and metastatic ovarian neoplasms. This distinction cannot always be made by immunohistochemistry. Cells of sex cord–stromal derivation selectively express inhibins, which are peptide hormones that take part in regulation of the pituitary-gonadal feedback system. Inhibin was evaluated as an immunohistochemical marker to detect adult and juvenile granulosa cell tumors.

Methods.—The study included formalin-fixed, paraffin-embedded specimens of 134 primary and metastatic ovarian lesions. The specimens included various sex cord–stromal tumors (SCSTs), including 35 adult and juvenile granulosa cell tumors, 14 fibroma-thecomas, and 18 other sex cord–stromal proliferations. Non–granulosa cell neoplasms included 33 surface epithelial neoplasms, 12 germ cell tumors, 11 metastatic lesions, and 11 miscellaneous ovarian neoplasms. Each specimen was studied by immunohistochemistry using a monoclonal antibody reactive with the α-subunit of inhibin.

Results.—Inhibin immunoreactivity was observed in 94% of granulosa cell tumors, compared with 17% of primary ovarian endometrioid tumors, 11% of primary ovarian transitional cell proliferations, and 18% of other primary and metastatic poorly differentiated carcinomas. Eighty-nine percent of granulosa cell tumors showed moderate-to-strong inhibin staining, or staining in at least half of cells. This was so for only 6% of primary surface epithelial neoplasms, with weak staining in 70% to 80% of cells. Inhibin positivity was noted in 71% of ovarian fibroma-thecomas and 94% of other sex cord–stromal proliferations. In about one third of evaluable cases, nonneoplastic luteinized stromal cells showed positive staining for inhibin.

Conclusions.—Inhibin immunohistochemistry is not a specific or reliable test for distinguishing between granulosa cell tumors vs. fibroma-thecomas or other ovarian sex cord–stromal proliferations. However, this test may be of value in differentiating SCSTs from most primary and metastatic non-SCSTs. Various primary and metastatic ovarian tumors may include luteinizing cells that stain positively for inhibin, underscoring the need for caution in the interpretation of inhibin-positive cells.

► In comparison with the paper by Costa et al. (Abstract 3–9), this study also includes a substantial number of extraovarian tumors that may mimic some SCSTs. Importantly, the antibody to the α-subunit of inhibin was found to stain focally and weakly in a substantial number of other primary and metastatic poorly differentiated carcinomas, including primary ovarian endometrioid tumors, primary ovarian transitional cell carcinoma, and metastatic adenoid cystic carcinoma.

This emphasizes the importance of performance of immunohistochemical patterns in the study of these SCSTs, for while granulosa cell tumors may be focally positive with low molecular cytokeratins, they are invariably negative for epithelial membrane antigen (EMA), whereas other primary ovarian carcinomas are strongly positive for EMA. Thus, panels that include low–molecular weight cytokeratins, along with vimentin, EMA, and other appropriate antibody studies (depending on the diagnostic dilemma), should discriminate SCSTs from other tumors.

D.J. Dabbs, M.D.

Telomerase Activity in the Female Reproductive Tract and Neoplasms

Yokoyama Y, Takahashi Y, Shinohara A, et al (Gifu Univ, Japan)

Gynecol Oncol 68:145–149, 1998 3–11

Introduction.—Telomerase synthesizes telomeric DNA onto chromosomal ends by using a segment of its RNA component as a template. It counteracts the mitotic clock of telomere shortening. Telomerase activity has been measured in several tissues and cells. Most cancer cells, immortal cells, and germ line cells demonstrate telomerase activity, whereas normal somatic cells do not have this activity. It is possible that determination of telomerase activity could be useful in diagnosis of cancer. Telomerase activity of female reproductive tissues was evaluated to determine its significance in the diagnosis of gynecologic neoplasms.

Methods.—Of 227 tissue samples evaluated for telomerase activity, 114 were normal tissue samples of reproductive age, 10 were fallopian tubes of postmenopausal age, and 103 were neoplastic tissues from female reproductive tracts (Table 1). Telomerase activity was compared in normal and

TABLE 1.—Number of Samples Examined and Age Distribution

Tissue	Sample number (age)
Ovari	
Normal ovary	10 (24–49)
Cystadenoma	15 (34–57)
Epithelial carcinoma	25 (45–78)
Oviduct	
Epithelium	28 (35–78)
Uterus	
Endometrium	44 (35–49)
Endometrial carcinoma	28 (36–78)
Epithelium of endocervix	12 (34–49)
Epithelium of exocervix	12 (34–50)
Epidermoid carcinoma of the cervix	20 (35–68)
Myometrium	18 (35–49)
Leiomyoma	15 (35–50)

(Courtesy of Yokoyama Y, Takahashi Y, Shinohara A, et al: Telomerase activity in the female reproductive tract and neoplasms. *Gynecol Oncol* 68:145–149, 1998.)

TABLE 2.—Positivity of Telomerase Activity

Tissue	Telomerase positive (%)
Ovari	
Normal ovary	3/10 (30)
Cystadenoma	6/15 (40)
Epithelial carcinoma	24/25 (96)
Oviduct	
Epithelium of menstruating patient	16/18 (89)
Epithelium of post-menopausal patient	3/10 (30)
Uterus	
Endometrium	39/44 (89)
Endometrial carcinoma	28/28 (100)
Epithelium of endocervix	11/12 (92)
Epithelium of exocervix	11/12 (92)
Epidermoid carcinoma of the cervix	19/20 (95)
Myometrium	2/18 (11)
Leiomyoma	4/15 (27)

(Courtesy of Yokoyama Y, Takahashi Y, Shinohara A, et al: Telomerase activity in the female reproductive tract and neoplasms. *Gynecol Oncol* 68:145–149, 1998.)

carcinoma tissues.

Results.—Telomerase activity was detected in 71 (97.3%) of 73 tissue samples of ovarian carcinoma, endometrial carcinoma, and epidermoid carcinoma of the cervix, and 77 (89.5%) of 86 of the epithelia of the reproductive-aged uterus and fallopian tube. The frequency of positivity was significantly higher for epithelia of the fallopian tube of reproductive age, compared with postmenopausal epithelia (16 of 18 vs. 3 of 10). Telomerase activity was similar for endometrial carcinomas and normal proliferative endometria. Ovarian epithelial carcinoma and epidermoid carcinoma of the cervix had significantly higher activity, compared with normal tissues. Telomerase activity was detected in 11 (92%) of 12 of normal exocervix and 3 (30%) of 10 of the normal ovary (Table 2).

Conclusions.—Telomerase activity is maintained by most epithelia of the female reproductive tract during reproductive ages. Detection of malignancies by telomerase may be possible in ovarian and epidermoid carcinoma of the cervix, but quantification of activity would be necessary.

▶ The presence of telomerase activity in tissues has been associated with prolonged or continued proliferative activity. In the normal state, certain tissues retain telomerase activity; such tissues as germ cells and gastrointestinal epithelium are prime examples of tissues that retain telomerase activity. In this study, telomerase activity was also found in virtually all of the female reproductive tract, including the normal ovary, fallopian tube, endometrium, exocervical epithelium, endocervical epithelium and myometrium. The implication in a practical sense is that the identification of telomerase activity in the female genital tract would not be a reliable marker of neoplastic transformation. Interestingly, some other normal tissues that retain telomerase activity are also under endocrine manipulation, namely, the epithelial cells in the proliferating zones of hair bulbs. Perhaps this is why the endocrine system evolved, to orchestrate selective tissues for coordinating specific sites of continued telomerase activity.

In somatic tissues in which telomerase activity is not normally present, the appearance of such telomerase activity may be useful in substantiating a cancer diagnosis. However, this does not appear to be a reliable method in the female genital tract. Accurate quantification of differences of baseline telomerase activity compared with neoplastic transformation may be a potential useful distinction between normal tissues and neoplastic tissues.

D.J. Dabbs, M.D.

Ovarian Serous Borderline Tumors With Invasive Peritoneal Implants

Gershenson DM, Silva EG, Levy L, et al (Univ of Texas MD Anderson Cancer Ctr, Houston)

Cancer 82:1096–1103, 1998 3–12

Background.—There is no accepted standard postoperative treatment for women with serous borderline tumors (SBTs) with peritoneal implants. The prognostic factors and the effects of postoperative treatment were retrospectively determined in a large series of these patients.

Study Design.—The study group consisted of 39 women, aged 17–60 years, with diagnosed primary ovarian SBT with invasive peritoneal implants. The women were seen at the M.D. Anderson Cancer Center between 1956 and mid-1996. Invasive implants were subdivided into early and frankly invasive types. All patients had surgery as the initial treatment. For those who had second-look surgery, surgicopathologic response was evaluated. There was a median follow-up of 111 months. The Cox proportional hazards model was used for identification of prognostic factors.

Findings.—Of these 39 patients, 30 had both noninvasive and invasive peritoneal implants. Early invasive implants were detected in 35 and frankly invasive implants were detected in 9, with 5 patients having both types. Postoperative chemotherapy was used in 31 patients, of whom 22 received platinum-based and 9 received melphalan chemotherapy. At second-look surgery in 18 patients, 11 had no macroscopic disease and findings were either negative in 9 or demonstrated involvement of only the residual ovary in 2 patients. Of the remaining 7 patients, 1 had a complete surgicopathologic response to chemotherapy, 3 had a partial response, and 3 had no response to chemotherapy. During follow-up, 12 patients had progression or recurrence, with a median time from diagnosis of 24 months. Time to progression was significantly longer for those patients with no macroscopic residual disease after initial surgery or for those with early invasive peritoneal implants. Platinum-based chemotherapy was associated with significantly shorter progression-free survival.

Conclusions.—This largest retrospective study of women with ovarian SBTs with invasive peritoneal implants revealed that more than 30% of these women will have progressive or recurrent tumor. The most important prognostic factor was the presence of macroscopic residual tumor after initial surgery. In this study, the role of postoperative therapy could not be defined. Further study is necessary to determine appropriate postoperative treatment for women with ovarian SBTs with invasive peritoneal implants.

▶ Currently, patients with stage 1 SBTs have a disease-free survival rate approaching 100% with surgery alone. Patients with SBTs and peritoneal implants may carry a different prognosis depending on the rate of recurrence and nature of recurrence. Currently, there is a large Gynecologic Oncology Group (GOG) study attempting to address these questions. No clear picture emerges regarding the prognostic significance of the type of peritoneal implant. In this study, there was no appreciable difference in overall survival between the groups of patients who had noninvasive and invasive peritoneal implants. Only the presence of macroscopic tumor at the initial surgery influenced the time to recurrence or progression and survival.

While awaiting the results of a prospective GOG trial in these groups of patients, the authors recommend continued use of platinum-based chemotherapy for patients with SBTs and invasive peritoneal implants.

D.J. Dabbs, M.D.

4 Breast

Premalignant and Malignant Disease of the Breast: The Roles of the Pathologist

Page DL, Jensen RA, Simpson JF (Vanderbilt Univ, Nashville, Tenn)

Mod Pathol 11:120–128, 1998 4–1

Background.—The role of the pathologist in the diagnosis and management of breast disease has evolved with the increasing complexity of the approach to breast cancer. The practical evaluation of breast biopsy specimens was reviewed.

Premalignancy and Atypical Hyperplasias.—It is now widely accepted that most women undergoing benign breast biopsy do not have an increased risk of subsequent breast cancer. Only a minority will have some measurable risk of later breast cancer, based on histologic patterns of disease (Tables 1 and 2). Higher risk groups of women have been identified using specific definitions of atypical hyperplasias. Atypical hyperplasias indicate a subsequent increase in risk anywhere in either breast and thus may be considered markers of generalized increased risk. The criteria for atypical ductal hyperplasia (ADH) include certain cytologic features, histologic patterns, and some indication of size or extent. Thus a tissue biopsy is needed to identify any changes that indicate increased risk. The uniform cytologic appearance and even placement of cells extending over 5–8 mm are indicative of ductal carcinoma in situ (DCIS). Typically, ADH lesions are less than 3 mm overall and are limited to an individual lobular unit.

Prognostication in Invasive Breast Carcinoma.—In the current era of mammography, overdiagnosis of malignancy is the greatest concern. In addition to guarding against this, pathologists are responsible for reporting specific information in an orderly fashion to clinicians to use in decision-making. Assigning prognoses of very good or very poor can be done without special studies of biological indicators (Table 4).

Conclusions.—Pathologists will continue to face the challenge of identifying the best categorization of breast cancer and its putative precursors. This article reviewed the major areas of the pathologist's responsibility in the diagnosis of breast disease, covering premalignancy and the stratification and prognosis of invasive carcinomas.

▶ Diagnosis of breast disease—particularly premalignant lesions and the carcinomas in situ—has changed drastically during many of our careers.

TABLE 1.—Categories of Benign Breast Disease and Risk and Location of Subsequent Carcinoma Development

General category	Risk implications*	Specific lesion	Locality of risk
Benign	No increased risk of later invasive cancer	Cysts, fibrosis, apocrine change, most fibroadenomas	None
	Slightly increased cancer risk, reliably approaching double that of comparable women	Well-developed patterns of usual hyperplasia; sclerosing adenosis, subsets of fibroadenoma; possibly many large and recurring cysts	Either breast
Benign, elevated cancer concern in some age groups	Moderate magnitude and generalized increased risk	Specific patterns of atypia, cytologic and histologic criteria; atypical ductal hyperplasia; atypical lobular hyperplasia; lobular carcinoma *in situ*	Either breast
Carcinoma *in situ*	Prolonged evolution to invasive carcinoma	Low grade DCIS, < 1 cm in extent	Local area from which DCIS was diagnosed
	Evolution to invasion, − 50% in 3 yr for large lesions incompletely removed	High grade DCIS	Region from which DCIS was diagnosed

*Risk is relative to women of comparable age without specific lesion.
Abbreviation: DCIS, ductal carcinoma in situ.
(Courtesy of Page DL, Jensen RA, Simpson JF: Premalignant and malignant disease of the breast: The roles of the pathologist. *Mod Pathol* 11[2]:120–128, 1998.)

TABLE 2.—Features Associated With Fibroadenoma That Elevate Breast Cancer Risk*

Complex histologic characteristics (any combination of apocrine change, cysts, sclerosing adenoisis, and/or epithelial-related calcification within fibroadenoma)
Usual patterns of hyperplasia, moderate and florid in surrounding parenchyma (similar to that of women without fibroadenoma)
History of breast cancer in a first-degree relative (slightly higher than the history of cancer in a relative alone)

*Most of the risk is operative after 10–15 years following diagnosis.
(Courtesy of Page DL, Jensen RA, Simpson JF: Premalignant and malignant disease of the breast: The roles of the pathologist. *Mod Pathol* 11[2]:120–128, 1998.)

Furthermore, change continues and involves not only terminology, but criteria, concepts, and our notions of clinical relevance. This article offers a thorough, up to date, and careful look at the impact and limitations of various breast diagnoses. The impact of various prognostic assessments and the importance of grading are noted. The discussion of who should and who should not receive chemotherapy highlights both the importance of our tasks and the quandary in which our clinical colleagues often find themselves. We will need periodic reviews of this type in the foreseeable future.

M.W. Stanley, M.D.

Suggested Reading

Mansour EG, Ravdin PM, Dressler L: Prognostic factors in early breast carcinoma. *Cancer* 74:381–400, 1994.

Simpson JF, Page DL: Status of breast cancer prognostication based on histopathologic data. *Am J Clin Pathol* 102:35–85, 1994.

Wold LE, Ingle JN, Pisansky TM, et al: Prognostic factors for patients with carcinoma of the breast. *Mayo Clin Proc* 70:678–679, 1995.

TABLE 4.—Predictors of Good and Bad Prognosis in Invasive Breast Cancer

Lower grade and most special type invasive carcinomas	Especially good prognosis in low stage: good prognosis even in high stage: prolonged disease-free interval and reduced metastatic events	Tubular, cribriform, mucinous, pure invasive lobular, and any low combined histologic grade cancer
High grade carcinomas	Stage (size and nodal status) is critical to prognosis	High and intermediate grade "no special type" (ductal) carcinomas

(Courtesy of Page DL, Jensen RA, Simpson JF: Premalignant and malignant disease of the breast: The roles of the pathologist. *Mod Pathol* 11[2]:120–128, 1998.)

Consensus Conference on the Classification of Ductal Carcinoma In Situ
Schwartz GF, for the Consensus Conference Committee (Jefferson Med College, Philadelphia; et al)
Cancer 80:1798–1802, 1997 4–2

Objective.—Because invasive cancer develops in only a minority of patients with ductal carcinoma in situ (DCIS), some physicians have opted to treat the disease by local incision or local incision and radiation. Because there is no general agreement on the optimum treatment for these patients, an international consensus conference was convened in Philadelphia in April of 1997 to discuss the pathologic classification of DCIS, the identification of prognostic features, methods of sizing and determining the extent of DCIS, margin assessment, and appropriate processing of surgical specimens.

Classification.—The panel recommended documenting nuclear grade, necrosis, polarization, and architectural pattern in the pathology report. Also included would be information about margins; size (extent and distribution of DCIS); microcalcifications; and correlation of tissue specimens, x-ray specimens, and mammographic findings. A synoptic report for DCIS was also suggested. Attendees recommended establishing a grading system to include probability of local recurrence, risk of subsequent mastectomy, probability of invasive disease, and specific mortality. Definitions of nuclear grade, necrosis, cell polarization and architectural pattern were provided. Optimal tissue processing recommendations were included.

Invasion.—Any report of invasion should also include microinvasion.

Biological Markers.—Biological markers for guiding management of DCIS should be evaluated as they become available.

Future Directions.—A standard classification system for DCIS must be established. Biological and molecular markers of progression, recurrence, and response to therapy need to be identified. Attendees recommended using the term "mammary intraepithelial neoplasia" to include DCIS in the general category of proliferative breast lesions.

▶ The classification, optimal treatment and prognostic significance (in terms of recurrence or development of infiltrating carcinoma) of DCIS represent important but controversial topics. This international consensus conference report describes a major effort to ameliorate this situation by standardizing the classification of DCIS. Furthermore, problems related to determining the extent of a lesion, evaluating margins, and specimen handling were addressed. The classification is based on nuclear grade, necrosis, cell polarization (lumen formation), and architectural pattern (comedo, cribriform, papillary, micropapillary or solid). The uncoupling of necrosis and architectural pattern led the panel to consider all centrally necrotic proliferations to be "comedo," regardless of nuclear grade. Thus, low nuclear grade, centrally necrotic examples of DCIS have been removed from the limbo that was their most recent residence. Most of the tissue handling suggestions are now fairly standard for most of us. It is comforting to have these practices concisely described by this panel. It was noted that biologic marker studies (including hormone receptor analyses) have no "uniquely definitive role in management." However, the paper goes on to note that because they may be useful in the future, and because most are evaluated in paraffin sections, we should not discard these blocks after any length of time.

M.W. Stanley, M.D.

Suggested Reading

Cheng L, Al-Kaisi NK, Gordon NH, et al: Relationship between the size and margin status of ductal carcinoma in situ of the breast and residual disease. *J Natl Cancer Inst* 89:1356–1360, 1997.

Tavassoli FA: Ductal carcinoma in situ: Introduction of the concept of ductal intraepithelial neoplasia. *Mod Pathol* 11:140–154, 1998.

Winchester DP, Strom EA: Standards for diagnosis and management of ductal carcinoma in situ (DCIS) of the breast. *CA Cancer J Clin* 48:108–128, 1998.

Statewide Study of Diagnostic Agreement in Breast Pathology

Wells WA, Carney PA, Eliassen MS, et al (Dartmouth Med School, Hanover, NH)

J Natl Cancer Inst 90:142–145, 1998 4–3

Background.—Previous researchers have reported relatively poor agreement among pathologists in their diagnostic assessments of breast disease. However, these studies mostly involved academic centers with a special interest in breast pathology and slides of tumors with challenging histologic features. The degree of diagnostic agreement among community-based general pathologists reading slides of a representative mixture of breast tissue specimens was determined.

Methods.—Twenty-six New Hampshire pathologists assessed slides of breast tissue from 30 patients selected randomly from a state breast pathology database (Table 1). Diagnostic categories included benign, benign with atypia, noninvasive malignant, and invasive malignant.

TABLE 1.—Characteristics of Eligible Participating and Nonparticipating Pathologists

Characteristic *	Eligible nonparticipants (n = 17)	Participants (n = 26)
Median age in y (range)	53 (35–65)	47 (36–65)
Median time in practice in y (range)	15 (4–20)	16 (2–37)
% Male	100	69

*One pathologist (W.A. Wells) is excluded from this table (ineligible to participate in slide read, but contributed reports to the database).

(Reprinted by permission of Oxford University Press, from Wells WA, Carney PA, Eliassen MS, et al: Statewide study of diagnostic agreement in breast pathology. *J Natl Cancer Inst* 90:142–145, 1998.)

TABLE 2.—Distribution of Diagnoses (n) by Slide for the 30 Representative Cases

Slide	Benign (n)	Benign with atypia (n)	Noninvasive malignant (n)	Invasive malignant (n)
A	26	0	0	0
B	26	0	0	0
C	26	0	0	0
D	26	0	0	0
E	26	0	0	0
F	26	0	0	0
G	24	0	0	0
H	25	1	0	0
I	25	1	0	0
J	25	1	0	0
K	25	1	0	0
L	25	1	0	0
M	25	1	0	0
N	24	1	0	1
O	23	1	1	0
P	23	1	0	1
Q	22	3	1	0
R	22	4	0	0
S	19	6	1	0
T	13	12	1	0
U	13	12	1	0
V	0	1	25	0
W	0	0	1	25
X	0	0	6	20
Y	0	0	13	12
Z	0	0	16	10
AA	0	0	0	26
BB	0	0	0	26
CC	0	0	0	26
DD	0	0	0	26

(Reprinted by permission of Oxford University Press, from Wells WA, Carney PA, Eliassen MS, et al: Statewide study of diagnostic agreement in breast pathology. *J Natl Cancer Inst* 90:142–145, 1998.)

Results.—Agreement among pathologists was high for assignment of the diagnostic category; the kappa coefficient was 0.71 (Table 2). Agreement was also high for the pathologists' selection of benign vs. malignant categories (kappa coefficient, 0.95). Agreement was lower in comparison with all other categories for the noninvasive malignant (kappa coefficient, 0.59) and benign with atypia (kappa coefficient, 0.22) categories. Levels of agreement were apparently unrelated to specimen type and perceived slide quality.

Conclusions.—Overall, diagnostic agreement among community-based pathologists in the diagnosis of breast tissue specimens is high. However, clinically important disagreement may occur in the evaluation of noninvasive malignant diagnoses. Policies for rereading slides of lesions in certain diagnostic categories may decrease the possibility of overtreatment or undertreatment resulting from misdiagnosis.

▶ This interesting study begins with some findings that are not too surprising. They center largely on disagreements between immediately adjacent categories in Table 1. Each of us can probably recall any number of intradepartmental consultations in each of these situations. Furthermore, there is good literature showing that when one considers the categories of "benign with atypia," and "noninvasive malignant," similar problems may haunt groups of experts. Although the sample is fairly small, I was surprised to learn that only 30% of the participating pathologists are seeing breast core biopsy samples on a routine basis. It might be interesting to perform a larger study of this type with a focus on core vs. excisional biopsy.

M.W. Stanley, M.D.

Suggested Reading

Fisher ER, Costantino J: Quality assurance of pathology in clinical trials: The National Surgical Adjuvant Breast and Bowel Project experience. *Cancer* 74 (Suppl 9):2638–2641, 1994.

Robbins P, Pinder S, de Klerk N, et al: Histological grading of breast carcinomas: A study of interobserver agreement. *Hum Pathol* 26:873–879, 1995.

Rosai J: Borderline epithelial lesions of breast. *Am J Surg Pathol* 15:209–221, 1991.

Schnitt SJ, Connolly JL, Tavrssoli FA, et al: Interobserver reproducibility in the diagnosis of ductal proliferative breast lesions using standardized criteria. *Am J Surg Pathol* 16:1133–1143, 1992.

The Role of Histologic Grading in the Prognosis of Patients With Carcinoma of the Breast: Is This a Neglected Opportunity?

Roberti NE (Oceanside, Calif)

Cancer 80:1708–1716, 1997 4–4

Background.—Although quantified grading of breast carcinoma through histologic analysis has been done for many years, it is generally not used in treatment decision making. The role of histologic grading in determining the prognosis of breast carcinoma was investigated.

Methods and Findings.—The literature was reviewed to explore this issue. The analysis indicated that, at all disease stages, histologic features suitable for grading provide important prognostic information. However, there is no agreement on the methodology for the application of this information. Because of the persisting disagreement about its validity, this information is frequently ignored.

Conclusions.—Serious attempts should be made to overcome the perceived problems with the grading of breast carcinoma. Authorities should come to a consensus about a methodology for quantifying this well-established index of the virulence of disease comparable to that attained in the American Joint Committee on Cancer staging of the extent of disease. Such information could then be used in clinical trials.

► This review incorporates an historical overview of breast cancer grading and its clinical utility to illuminate how we arrived at our current situation. The core issue is that before the concept of disseminated at diagnosis and the advent of systemic therapy, a contiguous spread model led to some surgically mediated therapeutic successes. Currently, however, the goal is identification of patients most likely to have occult metastases and to benefit from adjuvant therapy. (With wider application of these therapies, the object has actually become identification of those who are not likely to benefit. This concept is further developed by Page and coworkers, as reviewed in Abstract 4–1.) I found it surprising that the author was able to cite numerous recent breast cancer studies in which grading information was not available.

M.W. Stanley, M.D.

Suggested Reading

Dalton LW, Page DL, DuPont WD: Histologic grading of breast cancer: A reproducibility study. *Cancer* 73:2765–2770, 1994.

Report of the Council of Scientific Affairs AMA: Management of patients with node-negative breast cancer. *Arch Intern Med* 153:58–67, 1993.

Evidence of Effectiveness of Clinical Audit in Improving Histopathology Reporting Standards of Mastectomy Specimens

Appleton MAC, Douglas-Jones AG, Morgan JM (Univ of Wales College of Medicine, Cardiff)

J Clin Pathol 51:30–33, 1998 4–5

Background.—In the past 5 years, clinical audit has been introduced into the routine practice of medicine. The efficacy of clinical audit in improving standards in the histopathologic reporting of mastectomy specimens was investigated.

Methods.—Ten reports each from 1990, 1992, 1994, and 1996 were scored for informative content. All reports were on mastectomy specimens containing tumor and were issued by nonspecialist histopathologists. The 1992 and 1994 audits were performed after the establishment of written guidelines, specifying 6 essential pieces of information. In 1996 the reports were issued using a proforma.

Findings.—After the written guidelines were introduced, the amount of information increased significantly. However, over time the amount of information declined. In 1990, none of the reports included all 6 pieces of mandatory information, compared with 4 in 1992 and only 1 in 1994. The introduction of the proforma resulted in improvements, with all ten 1996 reports containing all mandatory information.

Conclusions.—Successive rounds of audit appear to increase the standard of histopathologic reporting. Continued monitoring is needed because standards may deteriorate over time. The use of a proforma for reporting on complex specimens significantly enhances information content.

▶ Iterative, cyclical auditing of adherence to clinical practice standards has become a routine quality improvement device. These authors perform a similar audit of breast cancer reporting. The message of this article is that our adherence to even fairly straightforward and obviously important guidelines can deteriorate over time. Periodic report audits and some use of "proforma" documents are techniques that will increasingly characterize the practice of diagnostic pathology.

M.W. Stanley, M.D.

Suggested Reading

Leslie KO, Rosai J: Standardization of the surgical pathology report: Formats, templates and synoptic reports. *Semin Diagn Pathol* 11:253–257, 1994.

Parham DM: The hidden increase in histopathologists' workload. *J Clin Pathol* 49:689–690, 1996.

The Pathological and Biological Nature of Screen-detected Breast Carcinomas: A Morphological and Immunohistochemical Study

Cowan WK, Kelly P, Sawan A, et al (Queen Elizabeth, Gateshead, England; Royal Victoria Infirmary, Newcastle upon Tyne, England; Univ of Teesside, England)

J Pathol 182:29–35, 1997 4–6

Introduction.—It has been suggested that breast cancers detected by screening differ in several ways from those detected clinically. The biological characteristics of screening-detected tumors may have important implications for the rationale of breast cancer screening programs. The characteristics of screening-detected versus clinically detected tumors were compared.

Methods.—The study included 3 groups of women with breast cancers: (1) 356 detected as a result of screening under the U.K. National Health Service Breast Screening Programme; (2) 60 detected in other screening programs; and (3) 267 detected clinically, usually with a breast lump or symptoms. The screen-detected and clinically detected tumors were compared for their characteristics. The comparison included not only conventional prognostic indicators, but also various immunohistochemical markers thought to be related to tumor behavior. These included epidermal growth factor receptor, c-*erb*B-2 protein, estrogen and progesterone receptors, cathepsin D, p53, and retinoblastoma protein.

Results.—There were no significant differences between the tumors detected by population screening or other screening programs. The screening-detected cancers were more likely to be in situ cancers than those detected clinically (Table 2). When invasive, the screening-detected cancers

TABLE 2.—Comparison of Invasion Status and Histopathological Features of Invasive Cancers According to Detection Mode

		Screen-detected No. (%)	'Clinical' No. (%)	Odds ratio* (95% confidence interval)	Significance
In situ		92 (20)	13 (5)	5·1 (2·8–9·4)	*P*<0·0001
Invasive		363 (80)	264 (95)		
Size (invasive)	3–10 mm	82 (23)	16 (6·0)		
	11–20 mm	200 (55)	104 (39·5)		
	21–30 mm	56 (15)	77 (29·0)		*P*<0·0001
	>30 mm	25 (7)	67 (25·5)		
Grade	I	150 (41·3)	44 (17)	4·7 (2·8–7·9)†	*P*<0·0001
	II	150 (41·3)	93 (35)	1·6 (1·0–2·7)‡	*P*=0·04
	III	63 (17·4)	127 (48)	2·5 (1·6–3·8)§	*P*<0·0001
Vascular invasion	Absent	304 (84)	106 (40)		
	Present	59 (16)	158 (60)	5·0 (3·3–7·7)	*P*<0·0001
Definite BV invasion	Absent	353 (97)	226 (86)		
	Present	10 (3)	38 (14)	3·3 (1·6–7·1)	*P*<0·0001
Perineural invasion	Absent	286 (79)	163 (62)		
	Present	77 (21)	101 (38)	2·15 (1·5–3·1)	*P*<0·0001
Lymph node	Positive	81 (26·5)	97 (50)		
(invasive tumours)	Negative	225 (73·5)	96 (50)	2·81 (1·9–4·1)	*P*<0·001
Lymph node	Positive (4 or more)	19 (6·2)	38 (19·7)	3·7 (2·1–6·6)	*P*<0·0001
	Negative (plus pos: 1,2,3)	287 (93·8)	155 (80·3)		

*Adjusted for age and tumor size.
†Odds ratio for grade III vs. grade I.
‡Odds ratio for grade II vs. grade I.
§Odds ratio for grade II + III vs. grade I.
(Reprinted by permission of John Wiley & Sons, Ltd., from Cowan WK, Kelly P, Sawan A, et al: The pathological and biological nature of screen-detected breast carcinomas: A morphological and immunohistochemical study. *J Pathol* 182:29–35. Copyright 1997, John Wiley & Sons, Ltd.)

were more likely to be smaller, of lower grade, and less likely to have invaded vessels, perineural spaces, and lymph nodes. Patients in the screening groups were more likely to have tubular- and cribriform-type tumors. None of the immunohistochemical markers were significantly different between the screening-detected and clinically detected tumors (Table 7).

Conclusions.—No biological differences were found between breast cancers detected at screening and those detected clinically. Instead, the screening-detected tumors apparently were the same lesions recognized at an earlier stage in their natural history. Although immunohistochemical markers tend to remain the same, some breast cancers at least dedifferentiate as they enlarge. The implications of these findings require long-term follow-up.

► The thrust of this article is to disagree with those who feel that small mammographically detected breast cancers may fundamentally differ biologically and prognostically from palpable tumors. To explore this question, the authors contrast the pathologic and immunohistochemical tumor characteristics in 2 large patient groups. As presented, the data seem compelling. However, some concerns come to mind. The screen-detected group is substantially enriched for tubular carcinoma (7.7% vs. 1.1%), which clearly

TABLE 7.—Immunohistochemical Examination for Epidermal Growth Factor Receptor (EGFR), c-*erb*B-2 Protein, Estrogen Receptor (ER), Progesterone Receptor (PgR), Cathepsin D, Retinoblastoma Gene Protein (Rb), and p53 Protein in Relation to Detection Mode

Marker		Screen detected No. (%)	'Clinical' No. (%)	Odds ratio* (95% confidence interval)	Significance
EGFR	+ ve	104 (40)	70 (40)	0·91	NS *P*=0·65
	− ve	155 (60)	105 (60)	(0·59−1·38)	
c-*erb*B-2	+ ve	74 (21)	42 (20)	0·90	NS *P*=0·86
	− ve	273 (79)	171 (80)	(0·27−2·95)	
ER	+ ve	102 (77)	64 (75)	1·07	NS *P*=0·87
	− ve	30 (23)	21 (25)	(0·50−2·29)	
PgR	+ ve	119 (68)	76 (65)	0·88	NS *P*=0·63
	− ve	55 (32)	40 (35)	(0·51−1·51)	
Cathepsin D	+ ve	147 (62)	105 (61)	0·95	NS *P*=0·83
	− ve	89 (38)	67 (39)	(0·62−1·47)	
Rb	+ ve	59 (84)	48 (92)	2·35	NS *P*=0·23
	− ve	11 (16)	4 (8)	(0·59−9·40)	
P53	+ ve	55 (26)	46 (33)	1·19	NS *P*=0·53
	− ve	153 (74)	93 (67)	(0·69−2·02)	

*Adjusted for age and tumor size.
Abbreviation: NS, not significant.
(Reprinted by permission of John Wiley & Sons, Ltd., from Cowan WK, Kelly P, Sawan A, et al: The pathological and biological nature of screen-detected breast carcinomas: A morphological and immunohistochemical study. *J Pathol* 182:29–35. Copyright 1997, John Wiley & Sons, Ltd.)

differs biologically from garden variety infiltrating ductal carcinoma. Furthermore, as discussed elsewhere in this section, different investigators employ different criteria for the diagnosis of tubular carcinoma, but no criteria are described in this study. Methods and criteria for identification of vascular invasion have been reviewed previously (see references), but are not discussed by these authors. It is unclear what is meant by "cribriform carcinoma," even though it is said to be more common in the screen-detected group. Infiltrating cribriform carcinoma is a rare lesion, so more details would be interesting. It is unclear what subsets of these heterogeneous neoplasm collections were subjected to immunohistochemical analysis, so these data are impossible to interpret.

M.W. Stanley, M.D.

Suggested Reading

Klemi, PJ, Joensuu H, Toikkannen S, et al: Aggressiveness of breast cancers found with and without screening. *BMJ* 304:467–469, 1992.

Lee AKC, DeLellis RA, Silverman ML, et al: Lymphatic and blood vessel invasion in breast carcinoma: A useful prognostic indicator? *Hum Pathol* 17:984–987, 1986.

Moezzi M, Melamed J, Vamvakas, et al: Morphological and biological characteristics of mammogram-detected invasive breast cancer. *Hum Pathol* 27:944–948, 1996.

Axillary Staging Utilizing Selective Sentinel Lymphadenectomy for Patients With Invasive Breast Carcinoma

Dale PS, Williams JT IV (Mercer Univ, Macon, Ga)

Am Surg 64:28–32, 1998 4–7

Objective.—Although breast conservation with axillary dissection is the treatment of choice for small primary breast cancers, less invasive axillary sampling or partial axillary dissections have been reported to understage the axilla in 10% to 45% of patients. The feasibility and accuracy of selective sentinel lymphadenectomy for patients with invasive breast cancer are reported.

Methods.—Between July 1995 and January 1997, 20 patients, aged 27–80 years, underwent 21 selective sentinel lymphadenectomy. Three to 5 mL of 1% Isosulfan Blue dye were injected into the 4 quadrants surrounding the primary tumor or biopsy site. Sentinel nodes were identified and removed during axillary dissection with level I, level II, and partial level III dissections. Mastectomies were subsequently performed.

Results.—There were 13 modified radical mastectomies and 8 breast-conserving operations. One sentinel lymph node was found in 11 patients, and 2 sentinel lymph nodes were identified in 3 patients. There were no level III lymph nodes. Five patients had 15 (8.9%) positive sentinel nodes and 10 (5.9%) positive nonsentinel nodes out of 169 nodes harvested. The sentinel node was the only positive node in 3 patients, and 2 had microscopic disease only. Nine patients had no positive nodes.

Conclusion.—Identification of sentinel lymph nodes using Isosulfan Blue is an accurate method for staging patients with primary breast cancer.

► This paper describes a relatively small experience, but it is a very up-to-date investigation and offers reflections on the idea of sentinel node biopsy for cancer staging. Both noninvasive assessment of the axilla and partial dissections lead to frequent understaging of breast cancer patients. Sentinel node sampling involves injection of a mobile, node-marking substance (methylene blue, other dyes, or a radioactive isotope) into the region of a tumor or a previous excision site. In these authors experience with 20 patients, 66% had an identifiable sentinel node in Level I or Level II of the axilla; there was no example of a skip directly to Level III. In 3 of 5 patients with a positive sentinel node, this was their only positive axillary lymph node, and in 2 of these, the metastases were microscopic. Sentinel node labeling has improved the staging of patients with malignant melanoma and appears to be advancing as a standard method in breast cancer staging.

M.W. Stanley, M.D.

Suggested Reading

Albertini JJ, Lyman GH, Reintgen DS, et al: Lymphatic mapping and sentinel node biopsy in the patient with breast cancer. *JAMA* 276:1818–1822, 1996.

Morton D, Wen DR, Wong J, et al: Technical details of intraoperative lymphatic mapping for early stage melanoma. *Arch Surg* 127:392–399, 1992.

Pathology of Familial Breast Cancer: Differences Between Breast Cancers in Carriers of *BRCA1* or *BRCA2* Mutations and Sporadic Cases

Stratton MR, and the Breast Cancer Linkage Consortium (Inst of Cancer Research, Sutton, Surrey, England; et al)

Lancet 349:1505–1510, 1997 4–8

Introduction.—Some breast cancers, particularly those in young patients, can be attributed to a hereditary predisposition. This is a highly penetrant autosomal dominant trait for which some causative genes have been identified, mainly mutations of the *BRCA1* and *BRCA2* genes. It is unclear whether any particular type of breast cancer is more common in patients with a family history of the disease. The histologic features of breast cancers in women with *BRCA1* or *BRCA2* mutations were analyzed.

Methods.—The study included specimens of breast cancers from 440 women with familial breast cancer. Of these patients, 118 (27%) were carriers of *BRCA1* mutations and 78 (18%) were carriers of *BRCA2* mutations (Table 3). The morphologic characteristics of these familial cases were compared with those of 547 age-matched control subjects unselected for a history of breast cancer.

Results.—The cancers from patients with *BRCA1* and *BRCA2* mutations had a higher average grade than cancers from patients in the control groups. Sixty-six percent of cancers from carriers of *BRCA1* genes and 41% of cancers from patients with *BRCA2* mutations were grade 2, compared with 36% of control specimens. Compared with the control group, the cancers of patients with *BRCA1* mutations had more pleomorphism, a higher mitotic count, and less tubule formation. The cancers of patients with *BRCA2* mutations also had less tubule formation, but were similar to control cancers in the other 2 indices (Table 4). No differences in the incidence of invasive lobular carcinoma or invasive ductal carcinoma were noted. Medullary or atypical medullary carcinoma was found in 13% of patients with *BRCA1* mutations, compared with 3% of patients with *BRCA2* mutations and 2% of control subjects. Patients with *BRCA2* mutations were less likely to have tubular carcinomas. All cases of mucoid carcinoma occurred in patients with familial breast cancer. Ductal carcinoma in situ was found around the invasive lesion in 41% of carriers of *BRCA1* mutations, compared with 56% of controls. Though lobular carcinoma in situ was less frequent in patients with familial breast cancer, this difference was not significant for patients with *BRCA1* or *BRCA2* mutations.

Conclusions.—The histologic findings are different for women with a family history of breast cancer than for those with sporadic disease. Some differences are noted in patients with *BRCA1* and *BRCA2* mutations as

TABLE 3.—Histological Type/Subtype Diagnosis According to Familial Disposition

Characteristics	Control observations	Familial patients			
		BRCA1 observations	Odds ratio (95% CI)	*BRCA2* observations	Odds ratio (95%) CI)
Invasive ductal no special type	810 (74%)	171 (74%)	1·00	119 (76)	1·00
Invasive lobular	113 (10%)	8 (3%)	0·36 (0·15–0·86)	16 (10%)	1·04 (0·50–2·13)
Tubular	51 (5%)	5 (2%)	0·50 (0·16–1·50)	0 (0%)	..
Mucoid	0 (0%)	3 (1%)	..	2 (1%)	..
Medullary/atypical medullary	19 (2%)	30 (13%)	5·16 (2·42–11·03)	4 (3%)	1·60 (0·49–5·29)
Ductal lobular	33 (3%)	2 (1%)	0·32 (0·07–1·34)	4 (3%)	0·81 (0·28–2·32)
Others	67 (6%)	13 (6%)	0·92 (0·41–2·03)	11 (7%)	1·08 (0·44–2·65)
Ductal carcinoma in situ absent	486 (44%)	138 (59%)	1·00	75 (48%)	1·00
Ductal carcinoma in situ present	607 (56%)	94 (41%)	0·51 (0·35–0·75)	81 (52%)	0·81 (0·52–1·26)
Lobular carcinoma in situ absent	1030 (94%)	228 (98%)	1·00	152 (97%)	1·00
Lobular carcinoma in situ present	63 (6%)	4 (2%)	0·31 (0·09–1·09)	4 (3%)	0·38 (0·12–1·26)

(Courtesy of Stratton MR, and the Breast Cancer Linkage Consortium: Pathology of familial breast cancer: Differences between breast cancers in carriers of *BRCA1* or *BRCA2* mutations and sporadic cases. *Lancet* 349:1505–1510. Copyright 1997 by The Lancet Ltd.)

TABLE 4.—Grading According to Familial Predisposition

Characteristics	Control observations	Familial patients			
		BRCA1 observations	Odds ratio (95% CI)	*BRCA2* observations	Odds ratio (95% CI)
Overall grade					
1	247 (24%)	19 (9%)	1·00	15 (11%)	1·00
2	405 (40%)	52 (25%)	1·65 (0·87–3·14)	68 (48%)	2·72 (1·47–5·04)
3	368 (36%)	139 (66%)	4·43 (2·34–8·38)	58 (41%)	2·55 (1·26–5·13)
Tubule formation					
1	78 (8%)	9 (4%)	1·00	1 (1%)	1·00
2	267 (26%)	28 (13%)	1·01 (0·36–2·79)	18 (12%)	5·38 (0·97–29·75)
3	685 (66%)	177 (83%)	2·22 (0·85–5·80)	124 (87%)	14·60 (2·50–85·35)
Pleomorphism					
1	106 (10%)	9 (4%)	1·00	8 (5%)	1·00
2	393 (38%)	49 (23%)	1·43 (0·67–3·04)	57 (40%)	1·78 (0·78–4·06)
3	532 (52%)	156 (73%)	2·96 (1·32–6·63)	78 (55%)	1·76 (0·73–4·21)
Mitoses					
1	537 (53%)	55 (26%)	1·00	66 (47%)	1·00
2	180 (17%)	32 (15%)	1·66 (0·99–2·78)	37 (26%)	1·63 (1·05–2·53)
3	303 (30%)	123 (59%)	3·71 (2·37–5·81)	38 (27%)	1·00 (0·58–1·73)
Mitotic count					
0–4	586 (56%)	51 (23%)	1·00	70 (50%)	1·00
5–9	141 (13%)	27 (12%)	2·16 (1·22–3·69)	26 (19%)	1·58 (0·91–2·67)
10–19	153 (15%)	52 (24%)	3·87 (2·29–6·60)	27 (19%)	1·50 (0·83–2·67)
20–39	96 (9%)	61 (28%)	6·90 (3·95–11·67)	16 (11%)	1·48 (0·69–2·97)
>40	70 (7%)	28 (13%)	4·16 (2·09–8·14)	2 (1%)	0·24 (0·06–1·01)

(Courtesy of Stratton MR, and the Breast Cancer Linkage Consortium: Pathology of familial breast cancer: Differences between breast cancers in carriers of *BRCA1* or *BRCA2* mutations and sporadic cases. *Lancet* 349:1505–1510. Copyright 1997 by The Lancet Ltd.)

well. The natural history of breast cancer in carriers of *BRCA1* mutations may be different from that of patients with *BRCA2* mutations or nonfamilial disease. These histologic differences could have research, screening, and treatment implications.

▶ This is a fascinating paper, and the authors state clearly the implications of their findings for breast cancer detection and management. Is medullary carcinoma really so common in *BRCA1* patients (13%)? If strict criteria are used for this diagnosis, many of us find it to be a very uncommon entity. The idea of "atypical" medullary carcinoma seems very fuzzy in the context of *BRCA1* cases of which 73% were noted to have grade 3 nuclear pleomorphism. These are relatively minor points of curiosity that detract only slightly.

M.W. Stanley, M.D.

Suggested Reading

Eisinger F, Stoppa Lyonnet D, Longy M, et al: Germ line mutation at *BRCA1* affects the histoprognostic grade in hereditary breast cancer. *Cancer Res* 56:471–474, 1996.

Marcus JN, Watson P, Page DL, et al: Hereditary breast cancer: Pathobiology, prognosis, and *BRCA1* and *BRCA2* linkage. *Cancer* 77:697–709, 1996.

Prognostic Value of DNA Ploidy Using Flow Cytometry in 1301 Breast Cancer Patients: Results of the Prospective Multicenter Morphometric Mammary Carcinoma Project

Bergers E, Baak JPA, van Diest PJ, et al (Free Univ, Amsterdam; St Jans Gasthuis, Weert, The Netherlands; Ignatius Hosp, Breda, The Netherlands; et al)

Mod Pathol 10:762–768, 1997 4–9

Background.—The prognostic value of DNA ploidy determined on the basis of flow cytometric DNA histograms is unclear. Previous conflicting findings may be the result of different DNA ploidy classification methods.

TABLE 1.—DNA Ploidy Classification into Subgroups on the Basis of the DNA Index

DNA ploidy	Definition	*n*
Diploid	one cell cycle, DNA index = 1.00	510
Hyperdiploid	two cell cycles, 1.00 < DNA index < 1.90	516
Tetraploid	two cell cycles, 1.90 ≤ DNA index ≤ 2.10	192
Hypertetraploid	two cell cycles, DNA index > 2.10	42
Multiploid	three or more cell cycles	41

(Courtesy of Bergers E, Baak JPA, van Diest PJ, et al: Prognostic value of DNA ploidy using flow cytometry in 1301 breast cancer patients: Results of the prospective multicenter morphometric mammary carcinoma project. *Mod Pathol* 10:[8]762–768, 1997.)

TABLE 6.—Overview of the Results in the Literature as to the Prognostic Value of Cell Cycle Variables. The P-Value 0.05 Was Regarded as Significant

Author (ref.)	*n*	Tissue	Diploid *vs* nondiploid Overall survival	Diploid *vs* nondiploid Disease-free survival
Aasmundstad and Haugen (11)	84	Paraffin	NS	NS
Arnerlöv *et al.* (38)	158	Paraffin	NS	SG
Baildam *et al.* (12)	136	Paraffin	NS	NS
Beerman *et al.* (1)	690	Paraffin, fresh	SG	SG
Bosari *et al.* (13)	147	Paraffin	–	NS
Clark *et al.* (37)	395	Frozen	NS	SG
Cornelisse *et al.* (40)	565	Paraffin, frozen	SG	NS
Dressler *et al.* (14)	565	Paraffin	–	NS
Eskelinen *et al.* (2, 3)	117	Paraffin	SG	–
Fisher *et al.* (15)	398	Paraffin	NS	NS
Joensuu *et al.* (4)	222	Paraffin	SG	–
Johnson *et al.* (5)	100	Paraffin	SG	–
Kallioniemi *et al.* (6)	93	Paraffin	NS	SG
Kallioniemi *et al.* (38)	308	Paraffin	SG	–
Keyhani-Rofagha *et al.* (16)	165	Paraffin	NS	NS
Klintenberg *et al.* (17)	191	Frozen	NS	NS
Kute *et al.* (18)	197	Paraffin	NS	NS
Kute *et al.* (19)	400	Paraffin	NS	NS
Lewis (7)	155	Paraffin	SG	SG
Merkel *et al.* (20)	280	Paraffin	NS	NS
Muss *et al.* (21)	101	Frozen	NS	NS
Noguchi *et al.* (8)	207	Paraffin	SG	–
O'Reilly *et al.* (22)	140	Paraffin	NS	NS
Owainati *et al.* (23)	280	Paraffin, Frozen	NS	NS
Pfisterer *et al.* (24)	139	Paraffin	–	NS
Sigurdsson *et al.* (25)	367	Frozen	NS	NS
Stål *et al.* (9)	472	Frozen	SG	SG
Stuart-Harris *et al.* (26)	42	Paraffin	NS	–
Toikkanen *et al.* (27)	351	Paraffin	NS	–
Toikkanen *et al.* (28)	95	Paraffin	NS	–
Uyterlinde *et al.* (29)	63	Paraffin	NS	–
Uyterlinde *et al.* (10)	225	Paraffin	SG	–
Witzig *et al.* (30)	265	Paraffin	NS	NS

Abbreviations: SG, significant; *NS*, not significant.

(Courtesy of Bergers E, Baak JPA, van Diest PJ, et al: Prognostic value of DNA ploidy using flow cytometry in 1301 breast cancer patients: Results of the prospective multicenter morphometric mammary carcinoma project. *Mod Pathol* 10:[8]762–768, 1997.)

The prognostic power of DNA ploidy was investigated using different classification methods.

Methods.—A total of 1,301 patients with breast cancer were studied prospectively. Flow cytometric DNA histograms were obtained from fresh-frozen material and interpreted using a commercially available computer program. The DNA ploidy was classified by different methods on the basis of the number of stemlines and the DNA index (Table 1).

Results.—Classification of DNA as diploid or nondiploid provided the best prognostic significance for overall survival (OS) and disease-free survival (DFS). This was also true for OS in the lymph node-positive subgroup but not in the node-negative subgroup. In subgroups classified according to tumor size, DNA ploidy had prognostic significance for DFS only in tumors smaller than 2 cm or larger than 5 cm. In a multivariate analysis, DNA ploidy did not contribute additional prognostic power to the prognostic significance of lymph node status and tumor size (Table 6).

Conclusions.—Compared with other prognostic parameters, DNA ploidy appears to be of little clinical importance in breast cancer. Past disagreement in the literature may have been a result of the need for large study groups to achieve statistical significance.

► The goal of this study is to sort out some of the conflicting reports on the prognostic usefulness of ploidy analysis in breast cancer. Importantly, this study was larger than most, used a single processing method and looked at several operational ploidy classifications. The authors' conclusion that this type of analysis has little clinical usefulness seems justified.

M.W. Stanley, M.D.

Comparative Study of Computer-assisted Image Analysis and Light-Microscopically Determined Estrogen Receptor Status of Breast Carcinomas

Bejar J, Sabo E, Misselevich I, et al (Technion–Israel Inst of Technology, Haifa)

Arch Pathol Lab Med 122:346–352, 1998 4–10

Objective.—Because semiquantification of estrogen receptor (ER) status in patients with breast cancer is a tedious and subjective task, a "quick-score" method has been developed to differentiate between negative and low-grade positive ER scores. The ability of pathologists to provide a correct reading of ER status was compared with results from the histomorphometrically measured contents of the ERs of breast carcinomas.

Methods.—ER status of hematoxylin-eosin-stained lumpectomy specimens was determined by 2 pathologists using immunohistologic staining and light microscopic evaluation. Histomorphometric assessments were performed using a computer-supported analysis of sections stained with ER antibody by the immunoperoxidase method. Pathologists' assessments were compared with histomorphometric results.

Results.—On a case-by-case basis of 3 grades of positivity, the kappa coefficient of agreement was only 0.28. When carcinomas were allocated to binary categories (positively vs. negatively-stained cell nuclei), the kappa coefficient increased to 0.52. When a weighted score of 1.2 was applied as the cut-off value for ER-negativity, and tumors were grouped into binary categories with negative scores adjusted by including all cases with a weighted score of 1.2 or less to ER negativity, the kappa coefficient between pathologists findings and histomorphometric results was 0.89 (Fig 3).

Conclusion.—The optimum rating of ER status is accomplished when breast tumors with a weighted score of 1.2 or less are placed in the

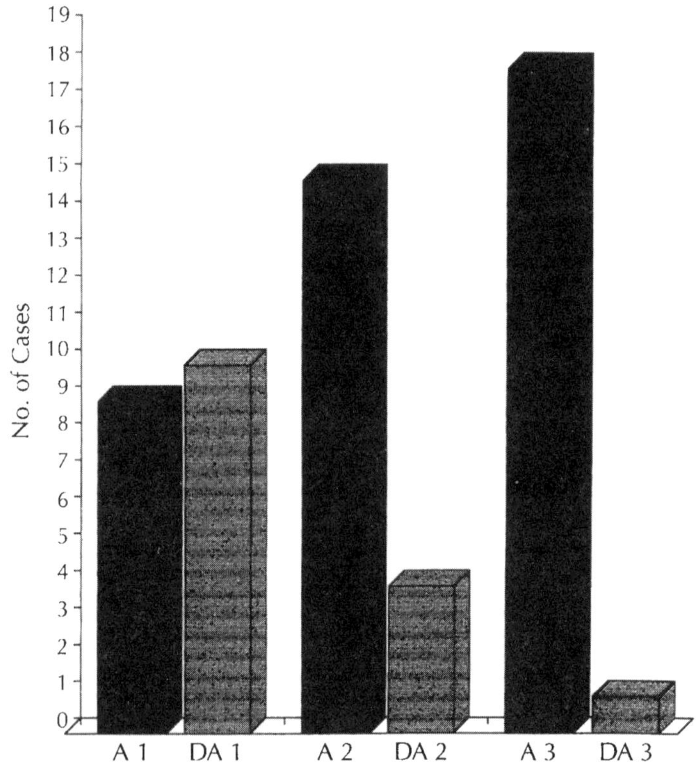

FIGURE 3.—Bar graph showing the number of breast carcinoma cases in which there was agreement and disagreement in the grades of estrogen receptor status assigned by the pathologists and the grades of estrogen receptor contents measured by the computer-assisted image analysis. *A1* indicates agreement based on case-by-case evaluation; *DA1*, disagreement based on case-by-case evaluation; *A2*, agreement based on the binary categories of tumor cells that were positive (grades 1+, 2+, or 3+) for estrogen receptor; *DA2*, disagreement based on the binary categories of tumor cells that were positive (grades 1+, 2+, or 3+) for estrogen receptor; *A3*, agreement based on binary categories using a weighted score of 1.2 as the cut-off value to discriminate between ER-positive and ER-negative carcinomas; and *DA3*, disagreement based on binary categories using a weighted score of 1.2 as the cut-off value to discriminate between ER-positive and ER-negative carcinomas. (Courtesy of Bejar J, Sabo E, Misselevich I, et al: Comparative study of computer-assisted image analysis and light-microscopically determined estrogen receptor status of breast carcinomas. *Arch Pathol Lab Med* 122:346–352, 1998.)

ER-negative category and those with a weighted score of 1.3 or more are placed into the ER-positive category.

▶ This paper looks at pathologists' ability to semiquantitatively evaluate ER immunostains and compares their performance with computer-assisted image analysis. The primary focus was on the ability to distinguish between ER-negative and low-grade positive cases. The pathologists' readings are analyzed in various ways, but calculation of a score [(staining intensity graded as 0, 1+, 2+, or 3+) × (percent of 200 cells with staining)] and setting the lowest score for ER-positive at 1.3 was effective. Problems with reproducibility of 4-grade systems are emphasized, and the biologically relevant distinction between ER-positive and ER-negative results emerges as a factor favoring the type of system suggested by the authors. The danger they wish to avoid is that some patients with minimally positive ER results may be denied appropriate therapy. The actual problem with semiquantitation by inspection is the human eye's inability to distinguish small differences in staining intensity. Image analysis computers, on the other hand, excel in this task. This study probably has relevance to other semiquantitative methods in pathology.

M.W. Stanley, M.D.

Suggested Reading

Andersen J: Determination of oestrogen receptors in paraffin-embedded tissue. *Acta Oncol* 31:611–627, 1992.

Detre S, Saccani Jotti G, Dowsett M: A "quickscore" method for immunohistochemical semiquantitation: Validation for oestrogen receptor in breast carcinomas. *J Clin Pathol* 48:876–878, 1995.

A Comparative Study of Pure Tubular and Tubulolobular Carcinoma of the Breast

Green I, McCormick B, Cranor M, et al (Mem Sloan–Kettering Cancer Ctr, New York)

Am J Surg Pathol 21:653–657, 1997 4–11

Objective.—Although pure tubular carcinoma (PTC) can be treated successfully by modified radical mastectomy, less is known about the treatment for tubulolobular carcinoma (TLC). PTC and TLC were compared with respect to tumor size, multifocality, axillary lymph node metastases, and likelihood of lymph node metastases.

Methods.—Pathology records and specimens of 90 cases of PTC and 17 cases of TLC were reviewed to compare the frequency of prognostic factors (Table 1). The average patient age was 42.

Results.—PTC tumors contained more than 75% neoplastic growth with amphophilic cytoplasm and cells with apical apocrine snouts at the luminal border (Fig 2). TLC tumors had both tubular and infiltrating growth patterns. Intraductal carcinoma was found in 42% of the cases; of

TABLE 1.—Prognostic Indicators in PTC and TLC

Prognostic indicators	PTC	TLC
Total no. of cases	90	17
Tumor size mean (cm)	1.2	1.3
% MF cases	20	29
% Cases with pos ALN	12	43
Recurrences	1 (1%)	2 (12%)
No. of local recurrences	1	1
No. of systemic recurrences	0	1

Abbreviations: MF, multifocal; *pos ALN,* positive axillary lymph node.

(Courtesy of Green I, McCormick B, Cranor M, et al: A comparative study of pure tubular and tubulolobular carcinoma of the breast. *Am J Surg Pathol* 21:653–657, 1997.)

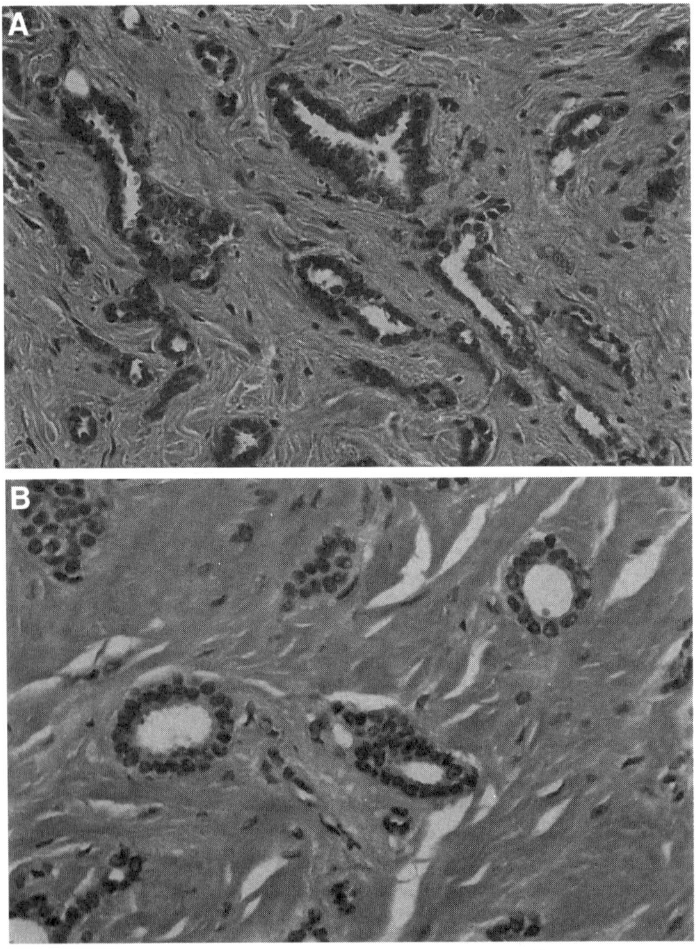

FIGURE 2.—Pure tubular carcinoma at high power. **A,** angulated tubular glands. **B,** round glands. (Courtesy of Green I, McCormick B, Cranor M, et al: A comparative study of pure tubular and tubulolobular carcinoma of the breast. *Am J Surg Pathol* 21:653–657, 1997.)

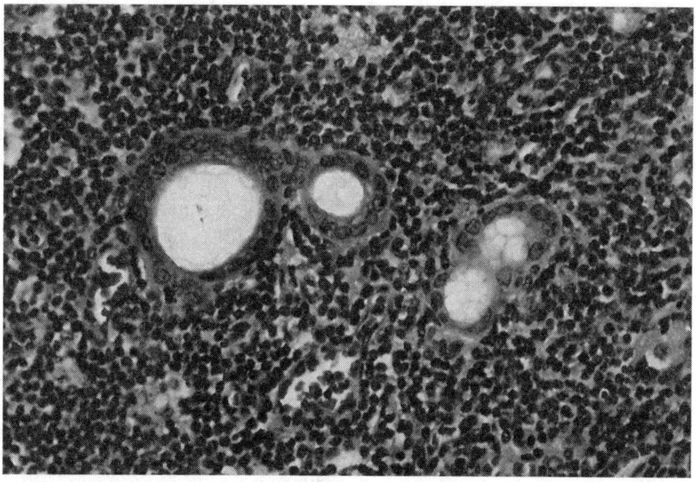

FIGURE 3.—Metastatic tubular carcinoma in a lymph node demonstrating preservation of tubule formation. (Courtesy of Green I, McCormick B, Cranor M, et al: A comparative study of pure tubular and tubulolobular carcinoma of the breast. *Am J Surg Pathol* 21:653–657, 1997.)

these, coexisting foci of lobular carcinoma were found in 10%. Although some breasts contained multiple foci of tubular carcinoma, no examples of bilateral tubular carcinoma were detected. Forty percent of tumors exhibited calcification. Axillary lymph nodes were positive in 6 (11.8%) of 51 PTC patients and 6 (42.8%) of 14 TLC patients. Tubular metastases were seen in the axillary lymph nodes (Fig 3). One PLC and 2 TLC patients had a local recurrence. In PTC patients with multifocal disease, 33% of lymph nodes were positive. In TLC patients with multifocal disease, 60% of lymph nodes were positive. In nonmultifocal cases, 7% of lymph nodes were positive in PTC patients, and 33% of lymph nodes were positive in TLC patients.

Conclusion.—TLC contained features of both tubular and lobular carcinoma and was significantly more frequently associated with lobular carcinoma. TLC had higher rates of multifocality, axillary lymph node metastases, and recurrences, suggesting that it might be a higher-grade lesion than PLC.

▶ Many of us now encounter PTC of the breast more frequently than in previous years, presumably owing to mammographic detection of small lesions. It is inevitable that the apparent incidence of uncommon PTC variants also increases. The importance of this problem lies in the fact that these adulterated neoplasms do not have the excellent prognosis that attends PTC. The best known variant is the mixed PTC in which less than 75% of the tumor shows tubular differentiation. The TLC variant is infrequently encountered, and questions about the clinical significance of this diagnosis always arise. This study will be the one to cite in trying to address these questions. By comparing 17 examples of TLC with 90 cases of PTC, these authors found higher risks for multicentricity, axillary nodal metastases and recurrence in TLC. The suggestion that TLC represents a distinct clinicopathologic entity that should be separated from other types of breast carcinoma seems completely justified. Matters to be addressed more completely in the future include the clinical significance of multifocality in both tumor types, the prognosis of TLC, and the best treatment for this uncommon PTC variant. When this diagnosis is made, and the questions arise, we can now give more answers than in the past, but some questions obviously remain.

M.W. Stanley, M.D.

Suggested Reading

Deos PH, Norris HJ: Well-differentiated (tubular) carcinoma of the breast: A clinicopathologic study of 145 pure and mixed cases. *Am J Clin Pathol* 78:1–7, 1982.

Fisher ER, Gregorio RM, Redmond C, et al: Tubulolobular invasive breast carcinoma: A variant of lobular invasive cancer. *Hum Pathol* 8:679–683, 1977.

McDiritt RW, Boyce W, Gersell D: Tubular carcinoma of the breast. *Am J Surg Pathol* 6:401–411, 1982.

Tubular Carcinoma of the Breast: An Institutional Review

McBoyle MF, Razek HA, Carter JL, et al (Univ of Kansas, Wichita; Via Christi Regional Med Ctr, Wichita, Kan)
Am Surg 63:639–645, 1997 4–12

Background.—Tubular carcinoma (TC) of the breast is a rare, differentiated variant of infiltrating ductal carcinoma. It can be recognized by its distinct histologic appearance and is known to have a favorable prognosis. However, many unanswered questions exist concerning its frequency, mammographic appearance, incidence of metastases, and the need for axillary lymph node dissection. Concern has been expressed that this

TABLE 1.—Combined Results for Those Studies That Defined Tubular Carcinoma as Breast Lesions With the Tubular Component >90% and Concurrent Axillary Lymph Node Involvement

First author (Year)	Positive Axillary Dissections/ Total Axillary Dissections (%)
Cooper (1978)[7]	1/12 (8.3)
Peters (1981)[8]	0/16 (0)
Deos (1982)[5]	4/65 (6.2)
Leibman (1993)[4]	0/9 (0)
Winchester (1996)[1]	6/40 (15)
McBoyle (current study)	1/22 (4.5)
Total	12/164 (7.3)

(Courtesy of McBoyle MF, Razek HA, Carter JL, et al: Tubular carcinoma of the breast: An institutional review. *Am Surg* 63:639–645, 1997.)

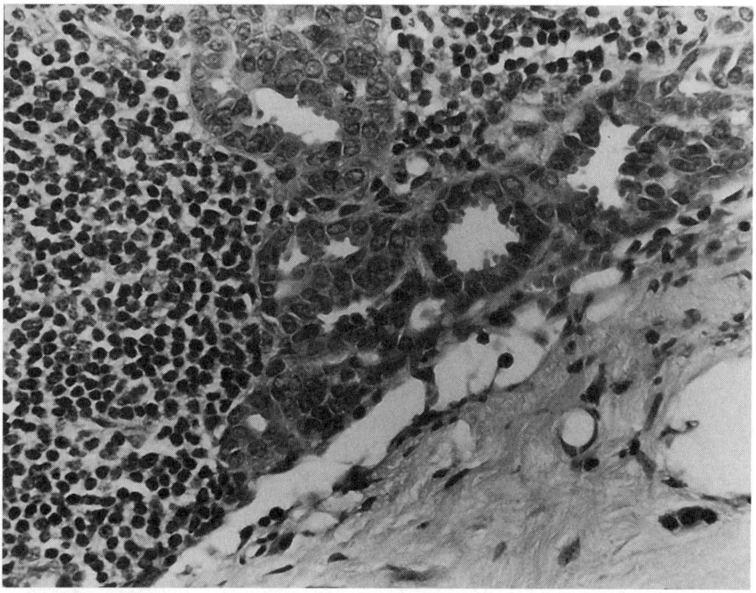

FIGURE 4.—High power microscopic image of a low axillary lymph node with microscopic focus of metastatic tubular carcinoma. (Courtesy of McBoyle MF, Razek HA, Carter JL, et al: Tubular carcinoma of the breast: An institutional review. *Am Surg* 63:639–645, 1997.)

tumor may be surgically overtreated. One institution's retrospective experience with tubular carcinoma of the breast from January 1984 to September 1995 was reviewed.

Methods.—The 12-year review identified 22 cases of pure TC among 1,483 patients with invasive breast carcinoma, representing an incidence of 1.5%. Pure TC was defined as having a tubular component of more than 90%. The patients' mean age was 58 years. In 14 (63.6%) patients, the cancers were detected solely by mammography; in this group, the mean tumor size was 1.0 cm. After biopsy, usually open biopsy, 14 patients underwent modified radical mastectomies, and 8 patients had breast-preserving therapy. Six patients received adjuvant therapy (chemotherapy in 2 and tamoxifen in 4).

Results.—On pathologic examination, the mean tumor size was 1.2 cm. All patients underwent axillary dissection, which recovered a mean of 19 nodes (Table 1). Of the 22 patients, one (4.5%) patient had tubular metastasis to a single lymph node (Fig 4). At a mean follow-up of 3.5 years, 18 (81.8%) patients were alive and disease free. The other 4 patients were disease free when they died or died of unknown causes.

Conclusions.—This review suggests that pure TC is a rare disease, with small lesions. No mammographic characteristics distinguish it from other invasive carcinomas. TC has an excellent prognosis, and patients with this diagnosis are ideal candidates for breast-preserving therapy. Although the rate of lymph node metastases is low, they can occur.

▶ As noted elsewhere in this section, many of us now encounter TC more frequently than in the past; most cases are nonpalpable and mammographically detected. This article does not contain any great surprises, but it does afford us an opportunity to reflect on the definition of tubular carcinoma (and perhaps other uncommon cancer variants, as well). Most investigators require at least 75% tubular morphology, while these authors require 90%. It is clear that as this type of quantitative criterion is made more stringent, the frequency of TC decreases, while its prognosis improves and the incidence of nodal metastases decreases. Pure TC constitutes less than 2% of infiltrating breast malignancies, but authors permitting as little as 50% tubular morphology find it to be much more common and to more frequently metastasize or recur. The message seems to be that we must read the literature critically, and that we must communicate our histologic findings in a clear fashion, if patients are to be optimally managed.

M.W. Stanley, M.D.

Suggested Reading

McDivitt RW, Boyce W, Gersell D: Tubular carcinoma of the breast: Clinical and pathological observations concerning 135 cases. *Am J Surg Pathol* 6:401–411, 1982.

Oberman H, Fidler W: Tubular carcinoma of the breast. *Am J Surg Pathol* 3:387–395, 1979.

Page D, Anderson T: *Diagnostic Histopathology of the Breast*. New York, Churchill Livingstone, 1987, pp 211, 213, 214.

Cytogenetic Findings in Phyllodes Tumors of the Breast: Karyotypic Complexity Differentiates Between Malignant and Benign Tumors

Dietrich CU, Pandis N, Rizou H, et al (Norwegian Radium Hosp, Oslo, Norway; Saint Savas Anticancer Hosp, Athens, Greece; Univ Hosp, Odense, Denmark; et al)

Hum Pathol 28:1379–1382, 1997 4–13

Background.—Cytogenetic assessment of phyllodes tumors of the breast may be of clinical value, suggesting why some tumors transform malignantly, as well as providing important pathogenetic information. To date, karyotypic abnormalities have been reported in only 8 primary tumors and 2 cell lines. The cytogenetic findings in short-term cultures from 5 benign and 1 malignant phyllodes tumor of the breast were reported.

Methods and Findings.—Clonal karyotypic abnormalities were identified in short-term cell cultures from 6 phyllodes breast tumors. The 5 benign tumors had simple chromosomal changes. By contrast, the highly malignant tumor had a near-triploid stemline, showing that karyotypic complexity is a marker of malignancy in these lesions. In 2 benign tumors, the only aberrations were interstitial deletions of the short arm of chromosome 3, del(3)(p12p14) and del(3)(p21p23). Three benign tumors showed cytogenetic polyclonality, 2 of which had cytogenetically unrelated clones. The third had 3 different, karyotypically related cell populations as evidence of clonal evolution.

Conclusions.—The finding of clonal chromosome abnormalities in the epithelial and connective tissue components of the phyllodes tumors shows that they are biphasic, both components being part of the neoplastic parenchyma. The 5 benign phyllodes tumors studied all carried simple chromosomal changes and were markedly different from the complex cytogenetic profile of the malignant tumor.

▶ This is one of those neoplasms to which we have difficulty assigning a prognosis; we are usually confident about only the most banal and the most flamboyantly malignant examples. It would be very nice if cytogenetic analysis could facilitate identification of those neoplasms that would go on to behave badly. However, the authors' case material does not allow testing of this idea. We have no histologic illustrations to review, but descriptions of the cases clearly give us the impression that the most karyotypically deranged tumor was histologically malignant, whereas those with less severe abnormalities were much more bland. The histogenetic implications of the observation that epithelial and mesenchymal tumor compartments share clonal chromosomal abnormalities are fascinating.

M.W. Stanley, M.D.

Suggested Reading

Norris HJ, Taylor HN: Relationship of histologic features to behavior of cystosarcoma phyllodes: Analysis of ninety-four cases. *Cancer* 20:2090–2099, 1967.

Pandis N, Heim S, Bardi G, et al: Improved technique for short-term culture and cytogenetic analysis of human breast cancer. *Genes Chromosom Cancer* 5:14–20, 1992.

Stephenson CF, Davis RI, Moore GE, et al: Cytogenetic and fluorescence in situ hybridization analysis of breast fibroadenomas. *Cancer Genet Cytogenet* 63:32–36, 1992.

Myofibroblastoma of the Breast: Cytologic, Histologic, Immunohistochemical, and Ultrastructural Findings in Two Cases With Differing Cellularity

Deligeorgi-Politi H, Kontozoglou T, Joseph M, et al (Univ of Athens, Greece; St Joseph's Health Centre, London, Ont)

Breast J 3:365–371, 1997 4–14

Background.—The widespread use of fine-needle aspiration (FNA) has led to an increased recognition of new pathologic entities. The cytologic,

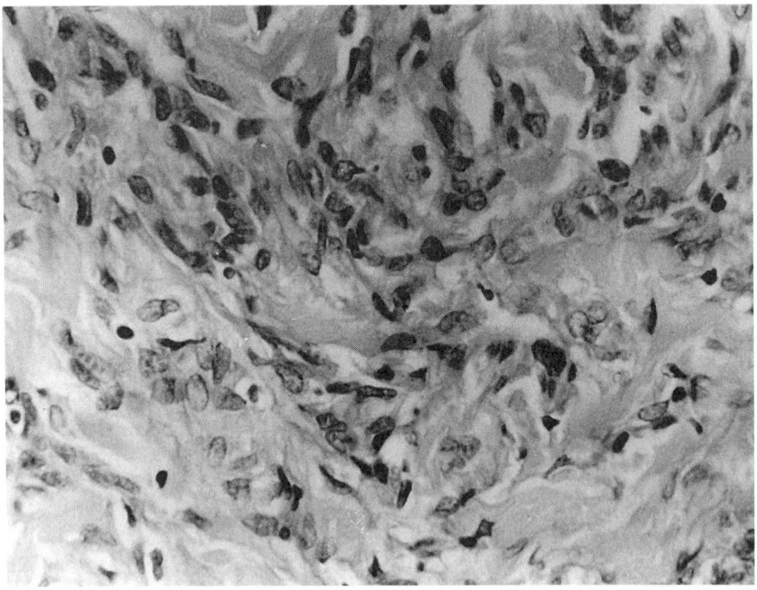

FIGURE 5.—Case 1. A paucicellular area with dense collagen globules in close apposition to rather plump, elongated cells; hematoxylin and eosin, ×250. (Courtesy of Deligeorgi-Politi H, Kontozoglou T, Joseph M, et al: Myofibroblastoma of the breast: Cytologic, histologic, immunohistochemical, and ultrastructural findings in two cases with differing cellularity. *Breast J* 3:365–371, 1997.)

histologic, immunohistochemical, and ultrastructural features of 2 patients with myofibroblastomas with different cellularity were reported.

Case Reports.—The 2 patients were a 31-year-old woman and a 78-year-old man. In the first patient, FNA revealed a benign paucicellular tumor of the breast. In the second case, FNA suggested hypercellular tumor of the breast. In both patients, immunohistochemistry demonstrated smooth muscle–specific actin, vimentin, and desmin positivity consistent with myofibroblastic differentiation. Both tumors showed positivity to CD34, suggesting that they may be associated with the so-called solitary fibrous tumor. In the patient with hypercellular disease, there was strong progesterone- and weak estrogen-receptor positivity ion, a novel finding with possible histogenetic implications. In the first patient, ultrastructural findings were consistent with the myofibroblastic tumor origin (Figs 5 and 6).

Conclusions.—Myofibroblastomas of the breast are rare, benign neoplasms. The 2 case reports show that myofibroblastomas may include a spectrum of variable features, ranging from the bland, paucicellular, mostly collagenous, fibrotic, benign tumor to a hypercellular, atypical soft-tissue tumor with increased mitotic activity.

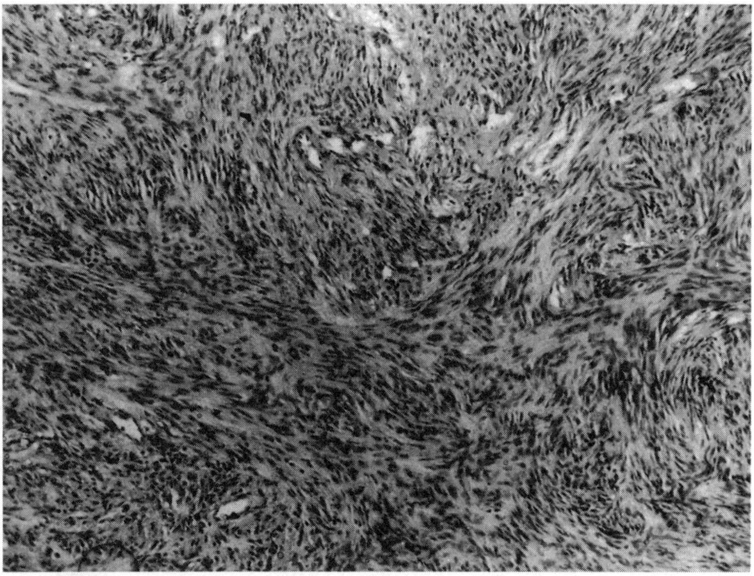

FIGURE 6.—Case 2. Interlacing fascicles of spindle cells with relatively little amount of intervening stroma; hematoxylin and eosin, ×100. (Courtesy of Deligeorgi-Politi H, Kontozoglou T, Joseph M, et al: Myofibroblastoma of the breast: Cytologic, histologic, immunohistochemical, and ultrastructural findings in two cases with differing cellularity. *Breast J* 3:365–371, 1997.)

► Spindle cell lesions that appear clinically as breast masses can actually arise from the breast, the overlying skin, or the chest wall. They comprise a wide array of pathologic entities, and diagnosis is complicated by the fact that none are common. Thus, we can be presented with difficulties resulting from the complexity of the differential diagnosis, as well as our relative paucity of experience with each entity. Myofibroblastoma is a good example of this situation. In this article, the situation is further complicated by the fact that each case was initially investigated by FNA. The equivocal interpretations of the cytology studies were probably unavoidable. The authors provide a useful reminder of the histologic variations in this tumor, as well as a caution that not all examples occur in the male breast.

M.W. Stanley, M.D.

Suggested Reading

Bardales RH, Stanley MW: Benign spindle and inflammatory lesions of the breast: Diagnosis by fine-needle aspiration. *Diagn Cytopathol* 12:126–130, 1995.

Silverman JF, Geisinger KR, Frable WJ: Fine needle aspiration cytology of mesenchymal tumors of the breast. *Diagn Cytopathol* 4:50–58, 1988.

Wargotz ES, Weiss SW, Norris HJ: Myofibroblastoma of the breast. Sixteen cases of a distinctive benign mesenchymal tumor. *Am J Surg Pathol* 11:493–502, 1987.

5 Gastrointestinal System

Squamous Islands in Barrett's Esophagus: What Lies Underneath?

Sharma P, Morales TG, Bhattacharyya A, et al (Tucson VA Med Ctr, Ariz)
Am J Gastroenterol 93:332–335, 1998 5–1

Background.—Patients with Barrett's esophagus have a distal esophagus with columnar-lined epithelium, intestinal metaplasia, instead of normal squamous cell epithelium. This condition often occurs in patients with gastroesophageal reflux disease. These patients are prone to developing adenocarcinoma of the esophagus. Endoscopic examination of Barrett's esophagus frequently reveals macroscopic islands of squamous epithelium.

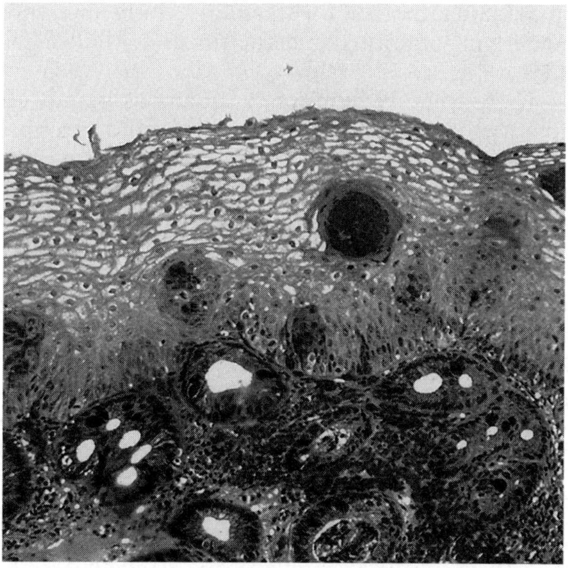

FIGURE 2.—Intestinal metaplasia underlying squamous epithelium; hematoxylin and eosin with alcian blue stain at pH 2.5; original magnification ×246. Biopsy of squamous island obtained from an 80-year-old patient with Barrett's esophagus who was treated with lansoprazole (60 mg/day) for 2.5 years. (Courtesy of Sharma P, Morales TG, Bhattacharyya A, et al: Squamous islands in Barrett's esophagus: What lies underneath? *Am J Gastroenterol* 93:332–335, 1998.)

TABLE 1.—Patient Characteristics According to Squamous Island Histology

	Squamous Epithelium	Squamous Epithelium With Underlying IM
Number of patients	12	10
Mean age (yr)	65.4	65.3
Mean Barrett's length (cm)	5.7	5.5
Mean PPI dose (mg/day)		
Omeprazole	25.7	35
Lansoprazole	60	60
Mean duration of PPI therapy (months)	23.5	30.1

Abbreviations: IM, intestinal metaplasia; *PPI*, proton pump inhibitor.
(Courtesy of Sharma P, Morales TG, Bhattacharyya A, et al: Squamous islands in Barrett's esophagus: What lies underneath? *Am J Gastroenterol* 93:332–335, 1998.)

This has been taken as a sign of regression, but its significance is not known. Macroscopic squamous islands from patients with Barrett's esophagus were systematically biopsied to define their histologic characteristics.

Study Design.—The study group consisted of 22 patients, 20 men and 2 women, with documented Barrett's esophagus, who had macroscopic squamous islands detected at endoscopy. Each squamous island was individually biopsied and examined for squamous epithelium, squamous basal layer, and underlying intestinal metaplasia in a blinded fashion by an independent pathologist.

Findings.—There were 39 biopsies of squamous islands obtained from the 22 patients with Barrett's esophagus in this study group. The average length of Barrett's mucosa was 5.6 cm. Of the 22 patients, 18 (82%) were on proton pump inhibitor therapy for a mean of 2.3 years. Of the remaining 4 (18%) patients, 3 were on H_2-blocker therapy, and 1 had no acid suppression therapy. Histologic analysis revealed that 61.5% of the specimens were exclusively squamous, and 38.5% of specimens had intestinal metaplasia underlying the squamous epithelium (Fig 2). There was no significant difference in age, length of Barrett's mucosa, and dose or duration of proton pump inhibitor therapy between those patients with and without underlying intestinal metaplasia in their biopsies (Table 1).

Conclusions.—Many patients with Barrett's esophagus have macroscopic islands of squamous mucosa that can be detected endoscopically. Systematic biopsy and histologic assessment of these squamous islands indicated that many of these islands have underlying intestinal metaplasia. The presence of these islands cannot be considered evidence of regression or of reduced risk of adenocarcinoma of the esophagus.

► As pathologists looking at "esophagus" biopsies and evaluating the presence or absence of Barrett's metaplasia (to say nothing about the presence or absence of dysplasia), we sometimes find ourselves wondering about the endoscope's precise location. The presence of macroscopic, and thus endoscopically visible squamous islands may further increase our confusion regarding relationships between clinical and histologic findings, unless communication from the endoscopist is clear. These authors have tried to address the question of whether or not these islands represent regression of Barrett's metaplasia. After detecting glandular foci deep to the surface squamous island in 38.5% of biopsies, they conclude that they do not. Lacking sequential studies, we could wonder whether this change might actually represent incomplete (early?) regression that will proceed to more complete resolution in some fraction of cases. Perhaps it is regression that has been halted for some reason and is now reverting to a fully metaplastic surface. The caution that squamous islands may not be taken as an indication of reduced cancer risk seems very reasonable, given our current knowledge of whatever process they represent.

M.W. Stanley, M.D.

Suggested Reading

Malesci A, Savarino V, Zentilin P, et al: Partial regression of Barrett's esophagus by long-term therapy with high-dose omeprazole. *Gastrointest Endosc* 44:700–705, 1996.

Pera M, Cameron AJ, Trastek VF, et al: Increasing incidence of adenocarcinoma of the esophagus and esophagogastric junction. *Gastroenterology* 104:510–513, 1993.

Sampliner RE, Garewal HS, Fennerty MB, et al: Lack of impact of therapy on extent of Barrett's esophagus in 67 patients. *Dig Dis Sci* 35:93–96, 1990.

Inflammation and Intestinal Metaplasia of the Gastric Cardia: The Role of Gastroesophageal Reflux and *H. pylori* Infection

Goldblum JR, Vicari JJ, Falk GW, et al (Cleveland Clinic Found, Ohio; Nashville VA Hosp, Tenn)
Gastroenterology 114:633–639, 1998 5–2

Background.—The gastric cardia is the portion of the stomach immediately distal to the esophagogastric junction. Inflammation of this area is referred to as carditis. The relationship of carditis to gastroesophageal reflux disease (GERD) and *Helicobacter pylori* infection was investigated.

Study Design.—The study group consisted of 58 patients with GERD and 27 control group patients undergoing endoscopy at the Cleveland Clinic Foundation or the Nashville Department of Veterans Affairs Medical Center from September 1995 to January 1997. Two biopsy specimens were obtained from the distal esophagus, the pyloric antrum, the fundus and the cardia from each patient. All specimens were analyzed histologically and for evidence of *H. pylori* infection. Serologic tests for infection were also performed.

TABLE 1.—Prevalence of *H. pylori* Infection and Carditis in Patients With GERD and Controls

Condition	Control group n/n (%)	GERD group n/n (%)
H. pylori infection	13/27 (48)	24/58 (41)
Carditis	11/27 (41)	23/58 (40)
H. pylori+ carditis	11/11 (100)	22/23 (96)

(Courtesy of Goldblum JR, Vicari JJ, Falk GW, et al: Inflammation and intestinal metaplasia of the gastric cardia: The role of gastroesophageal reflux and *H. pylori* infection. *Gastroenterology* 114:633–639, 1998.)

Findings.—The prevalence of *H. pylori* infection and carditis was not significantly different between GERD patients and control (Table 1). There was no significant difference in inflammation intensity or degree of colonization in different parts of the stomach of patients with infection-related pangastritis (Table 2). All 11 control patients with carditis and 22 of the 23 GERD patients with carditis had *H. pylori* infections (Fig 2). Esophagitis was significantly more common among the GERD patients than among the control patients. Cardia intestinal metaplasia was significantly more common among the control patients than the GERD patients. All of the control group patients with intestinal metaplasia had cardia inflammation,

TABLE 2.—Intensity of Acute and Chronic Inflammation and Degree of *H. pylori* Colonization in Different Parts of the Stomach in Patients With *H. pylori*–related Pangastritis

	Site					
	Antrum		Fundus		Cardia	
	Frequency	%	Frequency	%	Frequency	%
Mononuclear cells						
None	5	13.5	7	18.9	5	13.5
Mild	14	37.8	18	48.6	16	43.2
Moderate	10	27.0	6	16.2	10	27.0
Severe	8	21.6	6	16.2	6	16.2
Neutrophil-mediated gland injury (activity)						
None	21	56.8	25	67.6	23	62.2
Mild	10	27.0	9	24.3	10	27.0
Moderate	5	13.5	1	5.4	4	10.8
Severe	1	2.7	1	2.7	0	0.0
H. pylori colonization						
None	5	13.5	5	13.5	5	13.5
Mild	13	35.1	17	45.9	19	51.4
Moderate	8	21.6	4	10.8	5	13.5
Severe	11	29.7	11	29.7	8	21.6

(Courtesy of Goldblum JR, Vicari JJ, Falk GW, et al: Inflammation and intestinal metaplasia of the gastric cardia: The role of gastroesophageal reflux and *H. pylori* infection. *Gastroenterology* 114:633–639, 1998.)

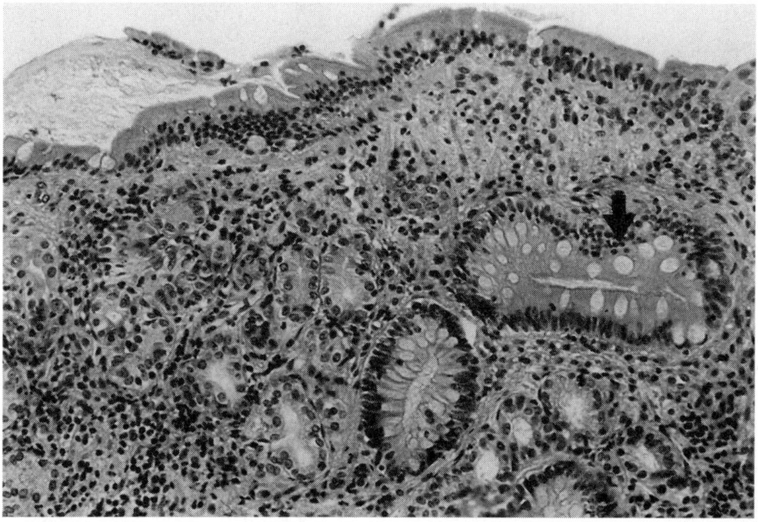

FIGURE 2.—Intestinal metaplasia of the cardia in a background of carditis. There is focal replacement of the gastric glands by intestinal metaplasia, characterized by the presence of goblet cells (*arrow*). The surrounding lamina propria is expanded predominantly by lymphocytes and plasma cells, indicative of carditis. Hematoxylin and eosin stain; original magnification x20. (Courtesy of Goldblum JR, Vicari JJ, Falk GW, et al: Inflammation and intestinal metaplasia of the gastric cardia: The role of gastroesophageal reflux and *H. pylori* infection. *Gastroenterology* 114:633–639, 1998.)

88% were infected with *H. pylori* and 75% had intestinal metaplasia in other parts of the stomach (Table 4).

Conclusions.—The prevalence of carditis was similar in patients undergoing endoscopy, with or without GERD. An association was seen between carditis and infection with *H. pylori* in both the control group and GERD patients. Intestinal metaplasia of the cardia was associated with infection-related carditis and with intestinal metaplasia in other parts of

TABLE 4.—Prevalence of Intestinal Metaplasia of the Gastric Cardia in Patients With GERD and Controls

Condition	Control group n/n (%)	GERD group n/n (%)
IM of the cardia	6/27 (22)	2/58 (3)*
Carditis in patients with IM of the cardia	6/6 (100)	2/2 (100)
H. pylori+ in patients with IM of the cardia	6/6 (100)	1/2 (50)
IM of antrum/fundus in patients with IM of the cardia	5/6 (83)	1/2 (50)

$^*P = 0.01$, Fisher's Exact Test.

Abbreviation: IM, intestinal metaplasia.

(Courtesy of Goldblum JR, Vicari JJ, Falk GW, et al: Inflammation and intestinal metaplasia of the gastric cardia: The role of gastroesophageal reflux and *H. pylori* infection. *Gastroenterology* 114:633–639, 1998.)

the stomach. The role of *H. pylori* infection and intestinal metaplasia of the cardia in the development of adenocarcinoma remains to be determined.

▶ These authors have investigated the degree to which inflammation of the gastric cardia is associated with either the pangastritis of *H. pylori* infection or gastroesophageal reflux disease. This is of great interest, because adenocarcinomas of the upper stomach and lower esophagus appear to be increasingly common, in contrast with other types of gastric carcinoma. The data indicate that intestinal metaplasia in the gastric cardia is associated with similar alterations elsewhere in the stomach mucosa and is related to *Helicobacter* rather than representing a part of gastroesophageal reflux disease. This is in contrast to some previous work in which inflammation of the gastric cardia appeared to be a reasonable marker of reflux. These authors make the important point that some earlier work did not adequately address the issue of *Helicobacter* and its role in gastritis and intestinal metaplasia. Another important contribution is that these authors emphasize the need to carefully evaluate studies based on upper gastrointestinal tract endoscopy; precise identification of the gastroesophageal junction remains difficult. Also, different studies vary widely in their assessment of *Helicobacter* infection and may employ variable combinations of routine microscopy, special stains, and serology. Furthermore, the number of biopsies varies widely.

M.W. Stanley, M.D.

Suggested Reading

Morale TG, Sampliner RE, Bhattacharyya A: Intestinal metaplasia of the gastric cardia. *Am J Gastroenterol* 92:414–418, 1997.

Spechler SJ, Wang HH, Chen YY, et al: Inflammation of the gastric cardia and *H. pylori* infection are not risk factors for intestinal metaplasia at the esophagogastric junction. *Gastroenterology* 112:297A, 1997.

Helicobacter pylori **Gastritis, Peptic Ulcer, and Gastric Cancer: Clinical and Molecular Aspects**

Goodwin CS (St George's Hosp Med School, London)
Clin Infect Dis 25:1017–1019, 1997 5–3

Introduction.—Infection with *Helicobacter pylori* is associated with specific ultrastructural changes to gastric mucosa and increased risk for duodenal ulcer and gastric cancer. This brief review describes the epidemiology, molecular biology, and clinical aspects of infection with *H. pylori.*

Epidemiology and Clinical Aspects.—In developing countries infection is common at a young age. When infection occurs in children aged 5 years or less, inflammation takes place throughout the stomach causing damage to acid-producing cells and permanently reducing acid output. These infected children do not acquire duodenal ulcers, but the chronic inflammation, in association with other factors, may lead to gastric cancer. Infection is also associated with persistent diarrhea and malnutrition, as well as short stature. When the age of occurrence is greater than 5 years, the acid-producing cells of the stomach are not damaged, duodenitis can then occur, and a duodenal ulcer may form.

Molecular Biology.—*H. pylori* secretes chaperonins, such as *hp*cpn60, which induce macrophages to secrete cytokines and stimulate T cells. The expression of this chaperonin increases after either exposure to 42°C or acidic conditions. This protein binds to sulfoglycolipid, which is present in the stomach. Exposure of *H. pylori* to the conditions in the stomach increases expression of the chaperonin/adhesin *HP*cpn60 to alter the binding specificity to sulfoglycolipid. *H. pylori* type I strains have the *cagA* gene, express vacuolating cytotoxin, and are associated with more severe gastritis, peptic ulcer, and gastric cancer. Strains with the *picB* gene induce cytokine IL-8, which causes inflammation and mucosal injury.

▶ This article provides a quick review of epidemiologic and clinical aspects of *H. pylori* infection. Also interesting is the brief discussion of its molecular biology.

M.W. Stanley, M.D.

Suggested Reading

Moayyedi P, Axon ATR: *Helicobacter pylori*: The research explosion. *Curr Opin Infect Dis* 8:374–379, 1995.

McCarthy C, Patchett S, Collins RM, et al: Long-term prospective study of *Helicobacter pylori* in nonulcer dyspepsia. *Dig Dis Sci* 40:114–119, 1995.

Histologic Assessment of *Helicobacter pylori* Status After Therapy: Comparison of Giemsa, Diff-Quik, and Genta Stains

El-Zimaity HMT, Segura AM, Genta RM, et al (VA Med Ctr, Houston; Baylor College of Medicine, Houston)
Mod Pathol 11:288–291, 1998 5–4

Background.—It is frequently difficult to determine whether a patient has been cured of *Helicobacter pylori* infection. To assess the efficacy of commonly used stains, positive and negative biopsy specimens were stained with Diff-Quik, Giemsa, and Genta and examined for the presence of *H. pylori.*

Study Design.—A series of 100 large-cup forceps biopsy specimens were chosen retrospectively. Of these 100 specimens, 64 were from patients with active infections and 36 were from cured patients 4–6 weeks after treatment, but with a background of chronic inflammation. Three tissue sections were cut from each block, and 1 section was stained with each of the 3 stains. The slides were independently examined in a blinded fashion by 2 pathologists and a trainee. The time required was also recorded.

Findings.—Of 72 *H. pylori*–negative slides there were 1.3% false positives with Diff-Quik, 3% with Genta and 4% with Giemsa. Of 128 *H. pylori*–positive slides there were 4% false negatives with Diff-Quik, 6% with Genta and 11% with Giemsa. Although no grade 2 slides were missed by Genta or Diff-Quik stains, three (15%) of 20 grade 2 slides were missed with Giemsa. Diff-Quik was cheaper and more available than Genta but required more time.

Conclusions.—The sensitivity and specificity of several special stains were compared for the detection of *H. pylori* infection. Our data indicated that the Genta stain is the best of the 3 stains studied. Genta stain had a specificity of 97% and a sensitivity of 94% but had a high cost and lower availability than other stains. Giemsa was not accurate for the assessment of infection status. Inexpensive Diff-Quik had excellent sensitivity and specificity, although it required more time than the Genta stain. The combination of hematoxylin and eosin (H&E) and Diff-Quik stains can provide accuracy similar to that of Genta stain but will increase processing time. The ^{13}C-urea breath test is another accurate method of evaluating *H. pylori* status.

▶ Morphologic evaluation of antibiotic treatment response after a diagnosis of *H. pylori* gastritis remains difficult; inflammation persists, and organisms may be very rare. The usual response to this dilemma is use of a special stain to highlight any remaining organisms. In these authors' experience, a combination of H&E and Diff-Quik brand stains gave the best overall results, especially when the time and difficulty of both staining and microscopy were considered. They also point out that the urea breath test is often the preferred method for evaluation of treatment response and that its accuracy for *Helicobacter* detection rivals that of multiple biopsies with histology.

M.W. Stanley, M.D.

Suggested Reading

Ashton-Key M, Diss TC, Isaacson PG: Detection of *Helicobacter pylori* in gastric biopsy and resection specimens. *J Clin Pathol* 49:107–111, 1996.

El-Zimaity HM, Graham DY, Al-Assi MT, et al: Interobserver variation in the histopathological assessment of *Helicobacter pylori* gastritis. *Hum Pathol* 27:35–41, 1996.

Kawanishi M, Fukuda S, Kawaguchi H, et al: Significance of rapid urease test for identification of *Helicobacter pylori* in comparison with histological and culture studies. *J Gastroenterol* 30:16–20, 1995.

Anti–*Helicobacter pylori* Specific Antibody Immunohistochemistry Improves the Diagnostic Accuracy of *Helicobacter pylori* in Biopsy Specimen From Patients Treated With Triple Therapy

Marzio L, Angelucci D, Grossi L, et al (Università G D'Annunzio, Chieti, Italy)

Am J Gastroenterol 93:223–226, 1998 5–5

Background.—Infection with *Helicobacter pylori* is associated with gastritis, peptic ulcers, gastric cancer, and lymphoma of mucosa-associated lymphoid tissue type (MALT). After therapy, *H. pylori* infection may remain in a cryptic coccoid form that does not produce urea and is not culturable in vitro, but may still trigger relapses. An immunohistochemical detection method involving rabbit anti–*H. pylori* polyclonal antibody (anti-HPAb) was assessed to determine its effectiveness in detecting cryptic forms of infection in gastric biopsy specimens.

Study Design.—The study group consisted of 40 adult patients with active gastritis and *H. pylori* infection. Six biopsies were obtained: 3 from the antrum and 3 from the corpus. One from each location was for urease test, 1 for culture and 1 for routine histopathological assessment. All patients then had triple therapy with omeprazole, amoxicillin, and metronidazole for 1 week. Two months after therapy, histology and culture tests were repeated to determine evidence of infection. Those patients who were considered cured had specimens assayed with the anti-HPAb test by 2 blinded pathologists.

Findings.—In 37.5% of the patients considered cured by culture, urease, and histology, persistent bacteria were recognized by the anti-HPAb test.

Conclusions.—This study indicates that the anti-HPAb immunohistochemical test is more sensitive than histology, culture or urease test for the detection of the persistence of *H. pylori* organisms after therapy. In more than one third of the patients considered cured by histology, urease, and culture methods, persistent infection was detected by the anti-HPAb. Whether the bacteria detected by this test are capable of reactivating infection to produce gastritis, ulcer, and MALT lesions remains to be determined.

► These authors emphasize the difficulty in identifying *H. pylori* after antibiotic therapy for gastritis. They note the existence of coccoid forms that are impossible to morphologically identify as *Helicobacter*. Furthermore, these altered organisms are urea negative and cannot be cultured. This report describes preliminary experience with a commercially available polyclonal anti-*Helicobacter* antibody. Using this method, they found persistent organisms in more than one third of treated individuals. If confirmed by others, this could explain recurrent infections, as well as persistence or progression of MALT proliferative lesions.

M.W. Stanley, M.D.

Suggested Reading

Ashton-Key M, Diss TC, Isaacson PG: Detection of *Helicobacter pylori* in gastric biopsy and resection specimens. *J Clin Pathol* 49:107–111, 1996.

Cammarota G, Tursi A, Montalto M, et al: Prevention and treatment of low-grade B-cell primary gastric lymphoma by anti–*H. pylori* therapy. *J Clin Gastroenterol* 21:118–122, 1995.

Chan WY, Hui PK, Leung KM, et al: Coccoid forms of *Helicobacter pylori* in the human stomach. *Am J Clin Pathol* 102:503–507, 1994.

Classification of Primary Gastric Lymphomas According to Histologic Features

Hsi ED, Eisbruch A, Greenson JK, et al (Univ of Michigan, Ann Arbor)
Am J Surg Pathol 22:17–27, 1998 5–6

Background.—Low-grade gastric lymphomas of mucosa-associated lymphoid tissue (MALT) can transform to a large-cell, or high-grade, lymphoma. High-grade gastric lymphomas were characterized histologically to distinguish between MALT-type and non–MALT-type lesions.

Methods.—Sixty gastric lymphomas were characterized clinically, histopathologically, and immunophenotypically. Based on the presence or absence of a low-grade component and lymphoepithelial lesions (LELs), high-grade lymphomas were classified as high-grade MALT lymphomas appearing in low-grade MALT lymphomas (LG/HG MALT lymphoma); large cell lymphoma with LELs composed of large cells (high-grade LELs) but without a low-grade component (HG MALT lymphoma); or diffuse large cell lymphoma without a low-grade MALT lymphoma component or LELs (DLCL).

Findings.—Twenty-two lymphomas were classified as low-grade MALT lymphomas; 16, LG/HG MALT lymphomas; 10, HG MALT lymphomas; and 12, DLCL. In all 55 cases undergoing immunophenotyping, B-cell immunophenotype was confirmed. Low-grade LELs were observed in all low-grade MALT lymphomas. In all 20 cases, CD20(L26) expression confirmed B-cell phenotype in the LELs. Mean clinical follow-up of 56 patients was 57 months. Clinical stage was highly significant in actuarial disease-specific and relapse-free survival. Histologic type and grade approached statistical significance. In a multivariate analysis, clinical stage was the only significant variable in relapse-free and disease-specific survival (Fig 6).

Conclusions.—Most of the primary gastric lymphomas in this series had features of MALT. In this retrospective analysis, clinical stage and histologic grade were the only significant prognostic indicators in a univariate analysis. Although only clinical stage remained significant in a multivariate analysis, histologic type showed a trend toward significance.

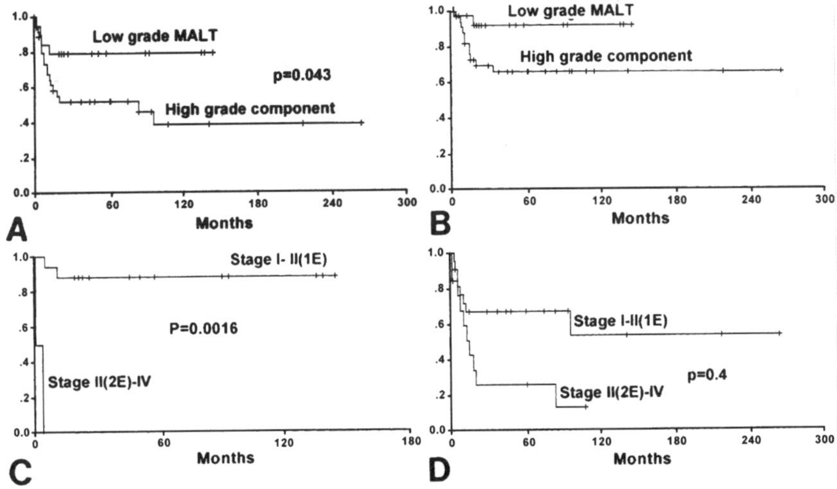

FIGURE 6.—A, actuarial relapse-free survival by histologic grade; low-grade = low-grade mucosa-associated lymphoid tissue (MALT); high-grade = other types. B, actuarial disease-specific survival by histologic grade. C, actuarial relapse-free survival of patients with low-grade MALT lymphoma. A highly significant difference exists between patients with low stages (I–II[1E]) and high stages (II[2E]–IV). D, actuarial relapse-free survival of the patients with high-grade lymphoma (low-grade/high-grade, high-grade MALT and diffuse large cell lymphoma). A trend toward a better outcome of patients with lower stages does not reach statistical significance. (Courtesy of Hsi ED, Eisbruch A, Greenson JK, et al: Classification of primary gastric lymphomas according to histologic features. *Am J Surg Pathol* 22:17–27, 1998.)

▶ The authors of this study did not show statistical significance regarding histologic types or grades; however, they did reveal prognostic trends according to histologic subclassification. Several studies that have analyzed a larger population,[1, 2] only resection specimens,[1–3] or extensively endoscopically biopsied patients[4] have shown statistical significance regarding the prognosis of histologic classification. In general, these other studies have demonstrated that with increasing large cells, the prognosis becomes worse. In the cases with focal large cell transformation (sheets or large aggregates of large transformed cells in a small portion of the specimen), there is an intermediate prognosis between low-grade MALT lymphoma and high-grade MALT lymphoma (predominantly diffuse large cells) at 5 years' follow-up.[1, 2] At 10 years' follow-up, the prognosis of cases with focal large cell transformation appears more similar to the cases of high-grade MALT lymphoma.[1]

Hsi et al. segregated the large cell lymphomas into high-grade MALT lymphomas or diffuse large cell lymphomas based on the presence of lymphoepithelial lesions composed of large cells. Interestingly, they show a trend for better disease-specific survival for patients with high-grade MALT lymphoma than for those with diffuse large cell lymphoma. In addition, they demonstrate that the relapse-free survival for patients with low-stage diffuse large cell lymphoma is significantly worse than for patients with high-grade MALT lymphoma. Other studies have not evaluated the clinical significance of lymphoepithelial lesions composed of large cells.

This study as well as others have demonstrated the importance of clinical staging of gastric lymphomas using the Musshoff modification of the Ann Arbor system that divides stage II into either II_{1E} or II_{2E}. Involvement of perigastric lymph nodes, stage II_{1E}, has a much better prognosis than involvement of nonregional lymph nodes on the same side of the diaphragm, stage II_{2E}.

J.F. Turner, Jr., M.D.

References

1. Akaza K, Motoori T, Nakamura S, et al: Clinicopathologic study of primary gastric lymphoma of B-cell phenotype with special reference to low-grade B-cell lymphoma of mucosa-associated lymphoid tissue among the Japanese. *Pathol Int* 45:832–845, 1995.
2. Nakamura S, Akazawa K, Yao T, et al: Primary gastric lymphoma: A clinicopathologic study of 233 cases with special reference to evaluation with the MIB-1 index. *Cancer* 76:1313–1324, 1995.
3. Hoshida Y, Kusakabe H, Furukawa H, et al: Reassessment of gastric lymphoma in light of the concept of mucosa-associated lymphoid tissue lymphoma: Analysis of 53 patients. *Cancer* 80:1151–1159, 1997.
4. De Jong D, Boot H, Van Heerde P, et al: Histological grading in gastric lymphoma: Pretreatment criteria and clinical relevance. *Gastroenterology* 112:1466–1474, 1997.

Suggested Reading

Chan JKC: Gastrointestinal lymphomas: An overview with emphasis on new findings and diagnostic problems. *Semin Diagn Pathol* 13:260–296, 1996.

Histology of the Stomach and Duodenum in Crohn's Disease

Wright CL, Riddell RH (McMaster Univ, Hamilton, Ont)

Am J Surg Pathol 22:383–390, 1998 5–7

Background.—Although Crohn's disease (CD) can affect the stomach and duodenum, its histologic appearance beyond the identification of granulomas has not been well described. A pattern of focal acute *Helicobacter pylori*–negative gastritis or duodenitis appears sometimes in CD. This occurrence was further examined.

Methods.—Two hundred nine upper gastrointestinal biopsy specimens from 80 sets of biopsies obtained from 49 patients with CD were studied retrospectively. For comparison, biopsy specimens were selected from age- and sex-matched patients with *H. pylori* gastritis, with a known history of nonsteroidal anti-inflammatory drug use, and with ulcerative colitis (Table 2).

Findings.—More than three fourths of the patients with CD had abnormal biopsy findings. Fifty-six percent of the patients with CD had acute inflammation, but only 10% of the patients had *H. pylori* infection. *Helicobacter pylori*–negative CD was characterized by focal acute inflammation, which was much less common in the patients who did not have CD (Tables 3 and 4). Surface intraepithelial neutrophils of the duodenum

TABLE 2.—Distribution of Patients (n), Diagnoses, Biopsy Sites, and Number of Biopsies

	Stomach (n = 70)	Duodenum (n = 73)
Crohn's (n = 80)		
209 biopsies	102 biopsies	107 biopsies
Non-Crohn's (n = 49)		
99 biopsies		
H. pylori (n = 34)		
73 biopsies	53 biopsies	20 biopsies
NSAIDs (n = 12)		
18 biopsies	12 biopsies	6 biopsies
Ulcerative colitis (n = 3)		
8 biopsies	4 biopsies	4 biopsies

Abbreviation: NSAID, nonsteroidal anti-inflammatory drug.
(Courtesy of Wright CL, Riddell RH: Histology of the stomach and duodenum in Crohn's disease. *Am J Surg Pathol* 22:383–390, 1998.)

occurred in 25% of those with CD and only 4% of those without CD. In addition, deep acute inflammation of the duodenum was more likely to occur in *H. pylori*–negative patients with CD. Granulomas occurred in only 9% of the patients with CD.

Conclusions.—In this series, more than three fourths of the patients with CD had abnormal histologic findings in the stomach or duodenum. Focal acute inflammation of the gastroduodenum, especially in the presence of uninflamed mucosa, is strong evidence for CD in the appropriate clinical context (Table 6). However, the stomach and duodenum must be sampled properly and examined carefully for evidence of *H. pylori*.

▶ This careful study does much to answer questions about the histology and frequency of CD in the upper gastrointestinal tract. The message seems to be that it is more common than previously thought, and that in the correct clinical setting (a very important requirement), acute mucosal inflammation is the typical findings in *H. pylori*–negative individuals. Traditionally, diagnosis of upper tract involvement has been reserved for those uncommon patients with granulomatous inflammation in histologic samples. The current investigation highlights how rare this finding is in biopsy material. The authors also remind us that only half of granulomatous gastritis cases represent CD. They also underscore the importance, and methods of completely eliminating *H. pylori* as a cause of the patient's problems, before considering a *de novo* upper gastrointestinal presentation of CD.

M.W. Stanley, M.D.

Suggested Reading

Alcantara M, Rodriquez R, Potenciano JLM, et al: Endoscopic and bioptic findings in the upper gastrointestinal tract in patients with Crohn's disease. *Endoscopy* 25:282–286, 1993.

TABLE 3.—Gastric Biopsies: Crohn's vs. non-Crohn's

	Crohn's Disease (CD)						
Histologic feature	All Crohn's (n = 70) no. (%)	p*	HP-pos (n = 8) no. (%)	p†	HP-negative (n = 62) no. (%)	p‡	Non-CD (n = 49) no. (%)
Gland atrophy	9 (12.9)	ns	2 (25)	ns	7 (11.3)	ns	7 (14.3)
Erosions	3 (4.3)	ns	0	ns	3 (4.8)	ns	2 (4.1)
Mucin depletion	38 (54.3)	ns	8 (100)	<0.01	30 (48.4)	ns	31 (63.3)
Foveolar hyperplasia	25 (35.7)	0.04	2 (25)	ns	23 (37.1)	0.02	8 (16.3)
Intestinal metaplasia	2 (2.9)	ns	1 (12.5)	ns	1 (1.6)	ns	0
Regenerative nuclei	18 (25.7)	ns	4 (50)	ns	14 (22.6)	ns	7 (14.3)
Fibrosis	17 (24.3)	<0.01	1 (12.5)	ns	16 (25.8)	ns	8 (16.3)
Smooth muscle	3 (4.3)	ns	0	ns	3 (4.8)	ns	2 (4.1)
Edema	8 (11.4)	ns	1 (12.5)	ns	7 (11.3)	ns	8 (16.3)
Helicobacter pylori	8 (11.4)	<0.01	8 (100)	ns	n/a	ns	35 (71.4)
Granuloma	6 (8.6)	ns	0	ns	6 (9.7)	ns	0
Focal inflammation	19 (27.1)	<0.01	0	ns	19 (30.6)	<0.01	1 (2.0)
Neutrophils							
surface	11 (15.7)	ns	1 (12.5)	ns	10 (16.1)	ns	6 (12.2)
pit	18 (25.7)	0.01	7 (87.5)	<0.01	11 (17.7)	<0.01	24 (49.0)
gland	16 (22.9)	ns	4 (50)	ns	12 (19.4)	ns	6 (12.2)
superficial l.p.	19 (27.1)	0.03	6 (75)	<0.01	13 (21.0)	<0.01	23 (46.9)
deep l.p.	11 (15.7)	ns	2 (25)	ns	9 (14.5)	ns	4 (8.2)
Eosinophils							
surface	3 (4.3)	ns	0	ns	3 (4.8)	ns	1 (2.0)
pit	2 (2.9)	ns	0	ns	2 (3.2)	ns	5 (10.2)
gland	1 (1.4)	ns	0	ns	1 (1.6)	ns	1 (2.0)
superficial l.p.	35 (50.0)	ns	6 (75)	ns	29 (46.8)	ns	30 (60.2)
deep l.p.	39 (55.7)	ns	7 (87.5)	ns	32 (51.6)	ns	33 (67.3)
Plasma cells							
superficial	63 (90.0)	ns	8 (100)	ns	55 (88.7)	ns	42 (85.7)
Plasma cells							
deep l.p.	49 (70.0)	ns	6 (75)	ns	43 (69.4)	ns	39 (79.6)
IELs	4 (5.7)	ns	0	ns	4 (5.7)	ns	3 (6.1)
Lymphoid aggregates	18 (25.7)	<0.01	8 (100)	<0.01	10 (16.1)	<0.01	29 (59.2)
Lymphoid follicles	0	0.01	0	ns	0	<0.01	5 (10.2)

**P* values, CD vs. non-CD.
†*P* values, HP-pos vs. HP-neg CD.
‡*P* values, HP-neg CD vs. non-CD.
Abbreviations: CD, Crohn's disease; *HP-pos, H. pylori* positive; *IEL*, intraepithelial lymphocytes; *l.p.*, lamina propia; *ns*, no significant difference.
(Courtesy of Wright CL, Riddell RH: Histology of the stomach and duodenum in Crohn's disease. *Am J Surg Pathol* 22:383–390, 1998.)

TABLE 4.—Duodenal Biopsies: Crohn's vs. non-Crohn's

			CD				
Histologic feature	All CD (n = 73) no. (%)	p*	HP-positive (n = 8) no. (%)	p†	HP-negative (n = 65) no. (%)	p‡	non-CD (n = 24) no. (%)
Villous atrophy	17 (23.3)	ns	4 (50)	ns	13 (20.0)	ns	4 (16.7)
Erosions	2 (2.7)	ns	0	ns	2 (3.1)	ns	0
Gastric metaplasia	13 (17.8)	ns	1 (12.5)	ns	12 (18.5)	ns	3 (12.5)
Edema	2 (2.7)	ns	0	ns	2 (3.1)	ns	0
Helicobacter pylori	0	ns	0	ns	n/a	ns	1 (4.2)
Granulomas	1 (1.4)	ns	0	ns	1 (1.5)	ns	0
Focal inflammation	29 (39.7)	<0.01	3 (37.5)	ns	26 (40.0)	<0.01	2 (8.3)
Neutrophils							
surface	16 (21.9)	ns	0	ns	16 (24.6)	0.03	1 (4.2)
gland	10 (13.7)	ns	1 (12.5)	ns	9 (13.8)	ns	1 (4.2)
superficial l.p.	23 (31.5)	ns	1 (12.5)	ns	22 (33.8)	ns	5 (20.8)
deep l.p.	14 (19.2)	0.04	2 (25)	ns	12 (18.5)	0.03	0
eosinophils							
surface	8 (11)	ns	0	ns	8 (12.3)	ns	2 (8.3)
gland	6 (8.2)	ns	0	ns	6 (9.2)	ns	4 (16.7)
superficial l.p.	59 (80.8)	ns	6 (75)	ns	53 (81.5)	ns	16 (66.7)
deep l.p.	63 (86.3)	ns	6 (75)	ns	57 (87.7)	ns	18 (75.0)
Plasma cells							
superficial l.p.	50 (68.5)	ns	6 (75)	ns	44 (67.7)	ns	13 (54.2)
Plasma cells							
deep l.p.	15 (20.5)	ns	2 (25)	ns	13 (20)	ns	4 (16.7)
IELs	16 (21.9)	ns	2 (25)	ns	14 (21.5)	ns	4 (16.7)

**P* values, CD vs. non-CD.
†*P* values, HP-pos vs. HP-neg CD.
‡*P* values, HP-neg CD vs. non-CD.
Abbreviations: CD, Crohn's disease, *HP-pos, H. pylori* positive; *IEL*, intraepithelial lymphocytes; *l.p.*, lamina propia; *ns*, no significant difference.
(Courtesy of Wright CL, Riddell RH: Histology of the stomach and duodenum in Crohn's disease. *Am J Surg Pathol* 22:383–390, 1998.)

TABLE 6.—Sites of Acute Inflammation in Crohn's Group*

Site of acute inflammation	All Crohn's (n = 57) no. (%)	*H. pylori* negative Crohn's (n = 49) no. (%)
Duodenum only	9 (15.8)	9 (18.4)
Stomach only	10 (17.5)	5 (10.2)
Duodenum and stomach	11 (19.3)	9 (18.4)
None	27 (47.4)	26 (53.1)

*Biopsy sets that included duodenum and stomach both.

(Courtesy of Wright CL, Riddell RH: Histology of the stomach and duodenum in Crohn's disease. *Am J Surg Pathol* 22:383–390, 1998.)

Ectors NL, Dixon MF, Geboes KJ, et al: Granulomatous gastritis: A morphological and diagnostic approach. *Histopathology* 23:55–61, 1993.

Shapiro JL, Goldblum JR, Petras RE, et al: A clinicopathologic study of 42 patients with granulomatous gastritis: Is there really an "idiopathic" granulomatous gastritis? *Am J Surg Pathol* 20:462–470, 1996.

Whipple Disease: Clinical Review of 52 Cases

Durand DV, and the SNFMI Research Group on Whipple Disease (Centre Hospitalier Lyon Sud, Pierre-Bénite, France; et al)
Medicine 76:170–184, 1997 5–8

Background.—Whipple disease is a rare disorder that affects multiple organs and has prominent intestinal manifestations. A clinical review of 52 patients was presented.

Patients and Findings.—The patients were recruited in various parts of France between 1967 and 1994. Seventy-three percent were male. Before diagnosis, clinical symptoms and signs were articular in 67%, digestive in 15%, general in 14%, and neurologic in 4%. At a later disease stage, 85% of the patients had diarrhea, weight loss, and malabsorption. The remaining 15% had no gastrointestinal symptoms throughout their disease course. Eighty-three percent of the patients had arthralgia or arthritis, and 21% had prominent neurologic symptoms. In addition, 17% had cardiovascular symptoms; 17%, mucocutaneous symptoms; 13%, pleuropulmonary symptoms; and 10%, ophthalmologic symptoms. Diagnosis was based on histopathologic criteria in all but 1 patient. With treatment, the disease course was favorable in 90% of the patients. Of the 5 with an unfavorable course, 2 patients had digestive symptoms unresponsive to antimicrobial treatment, 1 patient had chronic dementia, and 2 patients died from neurologic involvement. No relapses occurred in any of the patients treated with trimethoprim-sulfamethoxazole, alone or after combination treatment with penicillin and streptomycin or penicillin and streptomycin.

Conclusions.—Diagnosing Whipple disease in an early stage or in the absence of digestive symptoms continues to be difficult. Proximal enteroscopy as well as a normal erythrocyte sedimentation rate can be misleading. The key to diagnosis is histopathology, sometimes requiring repeated biopsies. Trimethoprim-sulfamethoxazole should be the antimicrobial agent of choice.

► Whipple disease has in common with Wilson's disease and a number of other conditions the fact that it enters our differential diagnostic thinking much more often than it emerges as the correct answer for a difficult bowel, lymph node, CNS, or other biopsy. The most often considered differential diagnoses include systemic histoplasmosis and a disseminated mycobacterial infection. This review article provides a periodically necessary update of clinical, pathologic, therapeutic, and prognostic factors in this condition. Of particular interest is the wide range of articular and CNS problems that may exist for years before a diagnosis. The relapsing and occasionally fatal or chronically debilitating (dementia) nature of Whipple disease are not often discussed, but come through clearly in this article. The utility of the polymerase chain reaction for diagnosis is briefly mentioned as a "note added in proof."

M.W. Stanley, M.D.

Suggested Reading

Ramzan NN, Loftus E, Burgart LJ, et al: Diagnosis and monitoring of Whipple disease by polymerase chain reaction. *Ann Intern Med* 126:520–527, 1997.

Von Herbay A, Ditton H-J, Schuhmacher F, et al: Whipple's disease: Staging and monitoring cytology and polymerase chain reaction analysis of cerebrospinal fluid. *Gastroenterology* 113:434–441, 1997.

Small Intestinal Stromal Tumors: A Clinicopathologic Study of 20 Cases With Immunohistochemical Assessment of Cell Differentiation and the Prognostic Role of Proliferation Antigens

Ma CK, De Peralta MN, Amin MB, et al (Henry Ford Hosp, Detroit)
Am J Clin Pathol 108:641–651, 1997 5–9

Background.—Small intestinal stromal tumors (SISTs) are less common than gastric stromal tumors, and even less well understood. A series of 22 SISTs from 20 patients were examined to identify potential prognostic features.

Study Design.—The 22 tumors were divided into 3 categories based on mitotic count (MC) per 50 high-power fields (Table 2) and tumor size: 6 were benign, 6 were borderline and 10 were malignant (Figs 3, 4, and 5). Tissue sections were analyzed histologically and immunohistochemically and a tumor proliferation index was calculated. Each tumor was

TABLE 2.—Clinicopathologic Data for 22 Small Intestinal Stromal Tumors

Case No.	Age(y)	Sex	Site	Size (cm)	Cell Type	Necrosis (%)	Cellularity*	Atypia*	Mitoses per 50 HPF	TPI PCNA (%)	TPI MIB-1 (%)	Outcome, Follow-Up (mo)
Benign tumors												
1	54	M	Unknown	2.0	Spindle	0	2+	1+	0.5	1.6	NI	Alive, no evidence of disease, 108
2	54	M	Jejunum	2.5	Spindle	0	2+	2+	0.0	1.2	0.6	Alive, no evidence of disease, 108
3	72	F	Jejunum	3.5	Spindle	10	2+	1+	1.0	1.7	1.2	Alive, no evidence of disease, 96
4	84	F	Unknown	3.5	Spindle	5	2+	1+	1.0	1.6	2.0	Alive, no evidence of disease, 84
5	75	F	Duodenum	1.5	Spindle	5	2+	1+	0.0	0.0	0.0	Incidental finding at autopsy
6	72	M	Ileum	3.5	Spindle and focal epithelioid	5	2+	3+	0.0	1.4	1.4	Died of other disease, no evidence of disease, 24
Borderline tumors												
7	70	M	Ileum	15.0	Spindle	0	2+	2+	1.0	2.4	NI	Alive, no evidence of disease, 276
8	64	M	Jejunum	14.0	Spindle	20	2+	1+	2.5	1.6	1.4	Died of disease, 36
9	75	M	Ileum	12.0	Spindle and focal epithelioid	5	3+	2+	4.5	1.6	3.2	Died of disease, 20
10	46	F	Jejunum	7.0	Spindle	10	2+	2+	0.5	NI	0.8	Died of disease, 96

11	35	F	Ileum	5.5	Spindle	5	2+	1+	4.0	17.6	0.8	Alive, no evidence of disease, 40
12	45	M	Ileum	5.0	Spindle	5	2+	2+	0.5	0.2	2.4	Alive, no evidence of disease, 24
Malignant tumors												
13	47	M	Jejuhum	2.0	Spindle	< 5	3+	3+	26.0	41.2	8.0	Died of disease, 22
14	68	M	Jejunum	> 10	Spindle	10	3+	3+, P	7.0	13.4	5.6	Died of disease, 10
15	66	M	Jejunum	7.5	Spindle	0	3+	3+	10.5	14.0	9.2	Died of disease, 36
16	63	M	Ileum	3.5	Spindle	5	2+	3+, P	109.0	39.6	11.4	Died of other disease, no evidence of disease, 108
17	76	M	Ileum	6.0	Spindle	0	3+	2+, P	60.5	49.2	NI	Died of disease, 8
18	82	F	Ileum	8.5	Epithelioid, 75%; spindle, 25%	0	2+	3+, P	10.5	23.2	5.2	Died of disease, 48
19	54	F	Duodenum	14.0	Spindle	5	3+	3+, P	154.0	66.0	2.4	Died of disease, 48
20	60	F	Unknown	34.0	Epithelioid	0	2+	2+, P	8.5	12.4	NI	Died of disease, 17
21	50	M	Duodenum	4.8	Spindle, 70%; epithelioid, 30%	0	2+	2+	12.5	10.4	2.6	Died of disease, 31
22	57	M	Ileum	12.0	Spindle	20	3+	3+, P	14.0	24.8	5.2	Died of disease, 13

*Cellularity and atypia were judged from 1+ to 3+.

Abbreviations: HPF, high-power field; *PI*, tumor proliferation index; *PCNA*, proliferating cell nuclear antigen; *MIB-1*, Ki-67 antigen; *NI*, not interpretable, *P*, pleomorphism present.

(Courtesy of Ma CK, De Peralta MN, Amin MB, et al: Small intestinal stromal tumors: A clinicopathologic study of 20 cases with immunohistochemical assessment of cell differentiation and the prognostic role of proliferation antigens. *Am J Clin Pathol* 108:641–651. Copyright 1997, by the American Society of Clinical Pathologists. Reprinted with permission.)

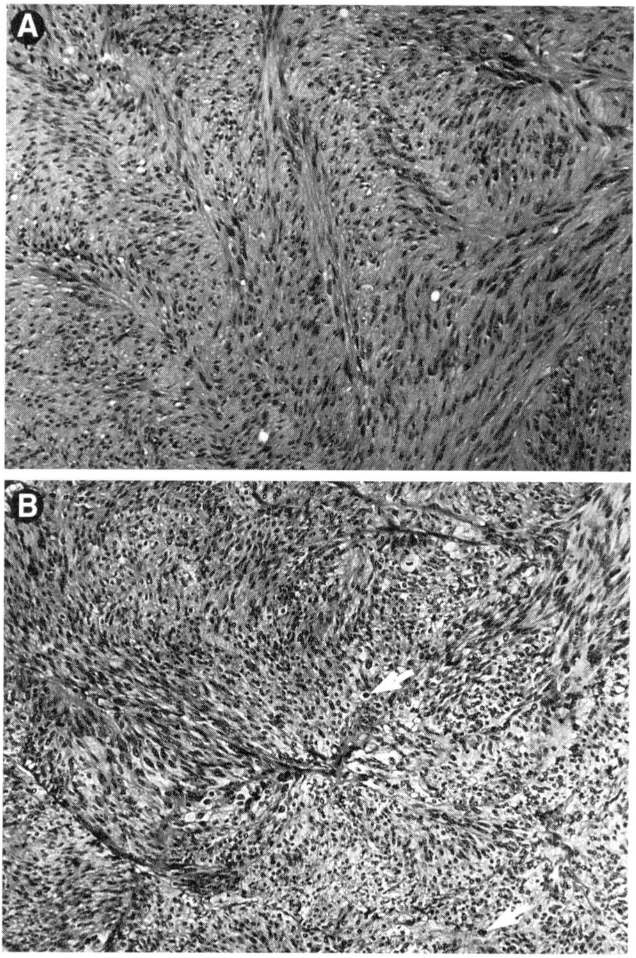

FIGURE 3.—Stromal tumors composed of fascicles uniform spindle cells. Panel **A**, benign; hematoxylin-eosin; original magnification ×33. **B**, malignant, note the mitotic figures in **B** (*arrows*); hematoxylin-eosin; original magnification ×80. (Courtesy of Ma CK, De Peralta MN, Amin MB, et al: Small intestinal stromal tumors: A clinicopathologic study of 20 cases with immunohistochemical assessment of cell differentiation and the prognostic role of proliferation antigens. *Am J Clin Pathol* 108:641–651. Copyright 1997, by the American Society of Clinical Pathologists. Reprinted with permission.)

assessed for cellularity, degree of anaplasia, pleomorphism, necrosis, MC, and predominant cell type (epithelioid or spindle).

Findings.—After an average of 96 months of follow-up, none of the patients with benign SISTs progressed, but half of the patients with borderline tumors and almost 90% of the patients with malignant tumors died of their disease. Cox Proportional Hazard regression analysis demonstrated that MC, tumor size, and cellularity were significant prognostic factors. Proliferating cell nuclear antigen, Ki-67 (MIB-1), tumor necrosis, and atypia were not significant predictors of survival. All tumors

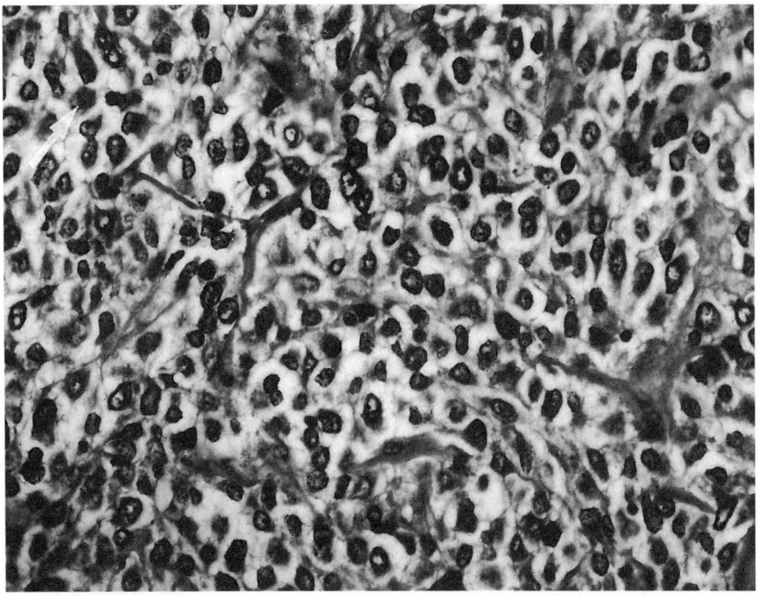

FIGURE 4.—Malignant stromal tumor composed of epithelioid cells with occasional mitotic figures (*arrows*); hematoxylin-eosin; original magnification ×80. (Courtesy of Ma CK, De Peralta MN, Amin MB, et al: Small intestinal stromal tumors: A clinicopathologic study of 20 cases with immunohistochemical assessment of cell differentiation and the prognostic role of proliferation antigens. *Am J Clin Pathol* 108:641–651. Copyright 1997, by the American Society of Clinical Pathologists. Reprinted with permission.)

were stained with vimentin; 77% immunoreacted with muscle-specific actin markers and 59% immunoreacted with alpha smooth muscle actin. One tumor stained with desmin, whereas none of the tumors stained with S-100 protein, neurofilament, or glial fibrillary acidic protein. Immunoreactions were not significantly different for benign, borderline, or malignant tumors. The tumor proliferation index was significantly different between benign or borderline and malignant tumors, but not between benign and borderline tumors.

Conclusion.—In this series of 22 small intestinal stromal tumors, the best predictors of clinical outcome were mitotic count, size, and cellularity (Table 5). The majority of SISTs demonstrated smooth muscle differentiation. The tumor proliferative index correlated with MC, but could not be used to predict survival. The SISTs were morphologically and immunologically similar to gastric stromal tumors, but appeared to have more potential for malignancy.

► SISTs represent another one of those entities that cause problems whenever they occur. These stem from the fact that almost none of us has enough experience to make reliable statements about prognosis. Cellularity, MC, and tumor size emerge from this study as important outcome indicators. (Note that the mitoses are counted per 50 high-magnification fields.) Ultimately, these authors conclude that any mitotic activity in a SIST larger than

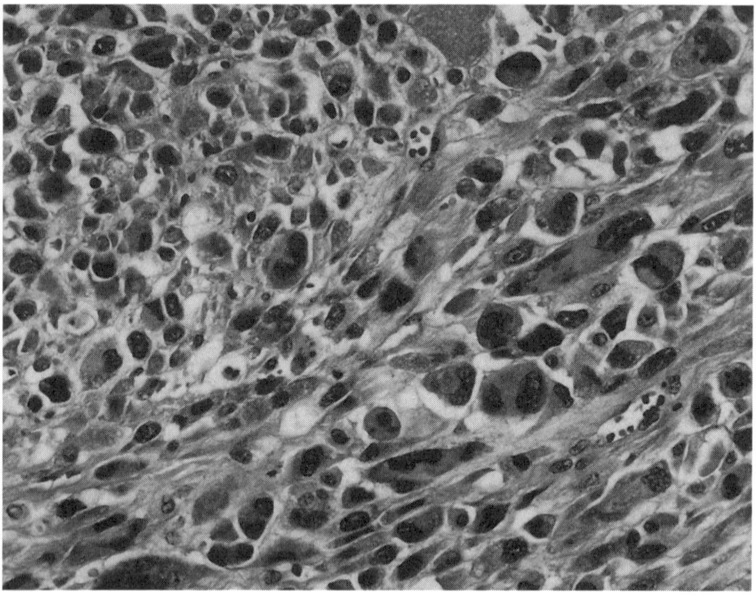

FIGURE 5.—Malignant spindle cell stromal tumor with pleomorphism and numerous mitoses; hematoxylin-eosin; original magnification ×66. (Courtesy of Ma CK, De Peralta MN, Amin MB, et al: Small intestinal stromal tumors: A clinicopathologic study of 20 cases with immunohistochemical assessment of cell differentiation and the prognostic role of proliferation antigens. *Am J Clin Pathol* 108:641–651. Copyright 1997, by the American Society of Clinical Pathologists. Reprinted with permission.)

1 cm indicates that it is "potentially malignant." These results support the idea that SISTs behave more aggressively than their morphologically similar gastric counterparts. Other schemes for denoting a tumor as benign, borderline, or malignant are similar, as summarized in Table 5.

M.W. Stanley, M.D.

Suggested Reading

Frangnemont DW, Frierson HF Jr: Proliferating cell nuclear antigen immuno-reactivity and prognosis of gastrointestinal stromal tumors. *Mod Pathol* 8:473–477, 1995.

Goldblum JR, Appelman HD: Stromal tumors of the duodenum: A histologic and immunochemical study of 20 cases. *Am J Surg Pathol* 19:71–80, 1995.

TABLE 5.—Histologic Grading of Small Intestinal Stromal Tumors Based on Tumor Size and Mitotic Count

Author	No. of Cases	Benign		Borderline		Malignant	
		Size (cm)	Mitoses	Size (cm)	Mitoses	Size (cm)	Mitoses
Goldblum and Appelman[27]	20 (duodenal)	< 4.5	< 2/50 HPF	—	—	≥ 4.5	≥ 2/50HPF
Franquemont and Frierson[29]	16	< 5.0	< 2/10 HPF	≥ 5.0 or	≥ 2/10 HPF	≥ 5.0 and	≥ 2/10HPF
Current study	22	< 5.0	< 5/50 HPF	≥ 5.0	< 5/50 HPF	Any	≥ 5/50HPF

Abbreviation: HPF, high-power field.

(Courtesy of Ma CK, De Peralta MN, Amin MB, et al: Small intestinal stromal tumors: A clinicopathologic study of 20 cases with immunohistochemical assessment of cell differentiation and the prognostic role of proliferation antigens. *Am J Clin Pathol* 108:641–651. Copyright 1997, by the American Society of Clinical Pathologists. Reprinted with permission.)

The Spectrum of Mucosa-associated Lymphoid Tissue Lesions in Pediatric Patients Infected With HIV: A Clinicopathologic Study of Six Cases

Joshi VV, Gagnon GA, Chadwick EG, et al (East Carolina Univ, Greenville, NC; Northwestern Univ, Chicago; St Jude Children's Research Hosp, Memphis, Tenn; et al)

Am J Clin Pathol 107:592–600, 1997 5–10

Introduction.—This retrospective case study describes a series of 6 pediatric AIDS patients with extrapulmonary mucosa-associated lymphoid tissue (MALT) lesions.

Study Design.—The study group consisted of 6 pediatric AIDS patients with MALT lesions. Half of these patients acquired HIV infection perinatally and half acquired HIV infection through transfusion (Table 1). Clinical data were collected through reviews of patient records.

Findings.—Mucosal sites of involvement (Table 3) included: salivary gland in 4 patients, bronchiolar mucosa in 2 patients and oropharyngeal mucosa in 1 patient. Histologic diagnoses (Table 4) included: myoepithelial sialadenitis (MESA), MESA with low-grade MALT lymphoma (Fig 6), diffuse large cell lymphoma (DLCL) (Fig 1), and atypical pulmonary lymphoid hyperplasia and lymphoid interstitial pneumonitis complex (Figs 2 and 7). Epstein-Barr virus (EBV) genome quantitation by polymerase chain reaction in 2 of these patients revealed high copy number in peripheral blood mononuclear cells, but low copy number in MALT lesions suggesting that MALT lesions and EBV infection may not be directly associated. The 2 patients with high-grade DLCL tumors, were successfully treated with chemotherapy and radiation therapy. MALT lesions had an indolent course in all patients.

Conclusions.—This case review describes mucosa-associated lymphoid tissue lesions in 6 pediatric AIDS patients. Clinicians should be aware that MALT lesions are not uncommon in pediatric AIDS patients. These lesions appear to follow an indolent course.

► This interesting study of six patients who acquired HIV infection during the pediatric age period encompasses the entire spectrum of MALT proliferative processes from hyperplasias to high grade malignant lymphomas. The rarity of gastrointestinal involvement among these cases is striking. Considerable attention has been given to searching for an infectious agent that leads to MALT lesions in these patients in a manner analogous to that in which *Helicobacter* is related to gastric lesions in non-HIV infected individuals; none has been identified to date. Candidates include HIV itself. Results regarding EBV have been somewhat confusing, and this small series provides relatively little opportunity for elucidation of this area. The authors note that although salivary gland enlargements are relatively common in pediatric HIV patients, biopsy of these swellings is rarely performed. This seems to be an excellent place for fine-needle aspiration. We would use 25-gauge needles (0.5 mm), and in most instances this procedure would yield tissue sufficient for morphologic evaluation, cell marker studies, and investigation of viral DNA. Furthermore, this procedure is essentially free of

TABLE 1.—Clinical Features of Patients With Proliferative Lesions of Mucosa-associated Lymphoid Tissue

Case	Age (yr) Sex	Mode of HIV Transmission	$CD4/mm^3$ at Diagnosis	Clinical Classification*	Clinical Presentation	Treatment/Outcome
1	8 10/12, female	Perinatal	1,562	A1	5-cm mass in parotid gland; cervical lymphadenopathy (3 cm)	α-Interferon; partial (75%) response
2	23, male	Transfusion (during childhood)	10	C3	Firm, nontender mass in parotid gland enlarging over 5 months to 10 × 9 cm	Unresponsive to combination cytoxan, Adriamycin, vincristine, prednisone; resolved with radiation therapy for 1 month; no recurrence after 1 year follow-up
3	11 1/2, female	Perinatal	150	A3	Respiratory distress, tonsillar mass, extensive lymphadenopathy	Vincristine, Adriamycin, prednisone, methotrexate, and cytosine arabinoside; complete remission of disease
4	17, female	Transfusion	212	B2	Right ear pain; parotid and submandibular gland swelling	No specific therapy, 6 months follow-up
5	2 4/12, male	Perinatal	Not done	B	Progressive pulmonary infiltrates	No treatment acutely/ required corticosteroid therapy for hypoxemia 3 years later
6	16, male	Transfusion	140	A3	Recurrent painful parotid gland swelling	No specific therapy, 10-year follow up

*Centers for Disease Control and Prevention classification system for HIV infection.

(Courtesy of Joshi VV, Gagnon GA, Chadwick EG, et al: The spectrum of mucosa-associated lymphoid tissue lesions in pediatric patients infected with HIV: A clinicopathologic study of six cases. *Am J Clin Pathol* 107:592–600. Copyright 1997, by the American Society of Clinical Pathologists. Reprinted with permission.)

TABLE 3.—Mucosa-associated Lymphoid Tissue (MALT) Lesions in Pediatric AIDS: Morphologic Features

	Case 1			Case 3				
	A	B	Case 2	A	B	Case 4	Case 5	Case 6
Mucosal site	Parotid	Parotid and adjacent LN	Parotid	Bronchial	Tonsil oropharynx	Parotid	Bronchial	Parotid
Reactive follicles	+++	++	–	++	–	+	++	++
Follicular colonization	++	++	–	+	–	+	++	–
Clusters of CCL/ monocytoid cells	+++	+++	+/–	++	–	+++	+++	+
Lymphoepithelial lesions	+++	++	–	++	–	++	++	++
Plasma cells	++	++	–	++	–	+	+	–
Immunoblasts	+	+	+++	++	+++	+	++	++
Other	Microcysts	Microcysts	Necrosis ++	Necrosis+	Necrosis+++			Microcysts
Diagnosis	MESA with focal lymphoma	Low-grade MALT lymphoma	Diffuse LCL	Atypical PLH/LIP complex	Diffuse LCL	Low-grade MALT Lymphoma	Atypical PLH/LIP complex	MESA

*(–), not present; (+), few; (++), moderate; (+++), marked.

Abbreviations: CCL, centrocyte-like; *MESA*, myoepithelial sialadenitis; *LN*, lymph node; *LCL*, large cell lymphoma; *PLH/LIP*, pulmonary lymphoid hyperplasia/lymphoid interstitial pneumonitis complex.

(Courtesy of Joshi VV, Gagnon GA, Chadwick EG, et al: The spectrum of mucosa-associated lymphoid tissue lesions in pediatric patients infected with HIV: A clinicopathologic study of six cases. *Am J Clin Pathol* 107:592–600. Copyright 1997, by the American Society of Clinical Pathologists. Reprinted with permission.)

TABLE 4.—Mucosa-associated Lymphoid Tissue (MALT) and Non-MALT Lesions Belonging to the Spectrum of Systemic Lymphoproliferation in Children With AIDS

- Follicular hyperplasia (lymph node, gastrointestinal tract)
- Lymphoid follicles/nodules (liver, thymus)
- Thymitis and multilocular thymic cyst
- Pulmonary lymphoid hyperplasia/lymphoid interstitial pneumonitis complex, typical and atypical
- Polyclonal, polymorphic B-cell lymphoproliferative disorder
- Myoepithelial sialadenitis
- MALT lymphoma (involving lungs, tonsils, and salivary glands)
- Non-MALT lymphoma (involving nodal and extranodal sites)

(Courtesy of Joshi VV, Gagnon GA, Chadwick EG, et al: The spectrum of mucosa-associated lymphoid tissue lesions in pediatric patients infected with HIV: A clinicopathologic study of six cases. *Am J Clin Pathol* 107:592–600. Copyright 1997, by the American Society of Clinical Pathologists. Reprinted with permission.)

complications and is well tolerated. This opens the possibility of sequential studies over a period of time.

M.W. Stanley, M.D.

Suggested Reading

Pelstring RJ, Essell JH, Kurtin PJ, et al: Diversity of organ site involvement among malignant lymphomas of mucosa-associated lymphoid tissue. *Am J Clin Pathol* 96:738–745, 1991.

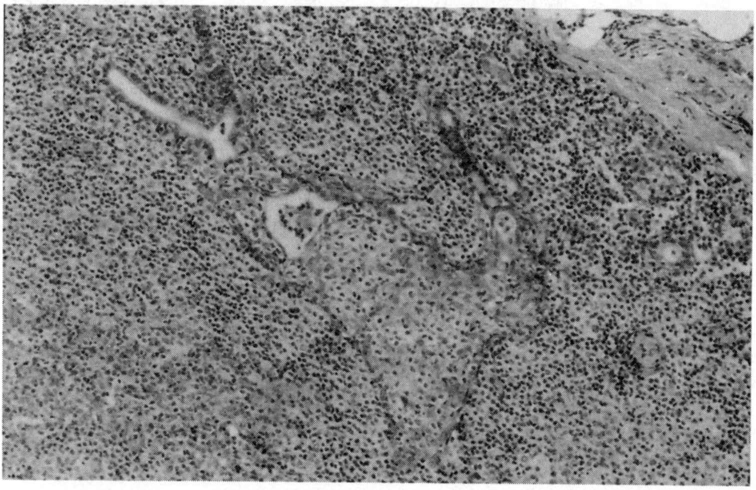

FIGURE 6.—Case 1. Salivary gland lymphoepithelial lesions in a patient who had myoepithelial sialadenitis and low-grade mucosa-associated lymphoid tissue lymphoma. (Courtesy of Joshi VV, Gagnon GA, Chadwick EG, et al: The spectrum of mucosa-associated lymphoid tissue lesions in pediatric patients infected with HIV: A clinicopathologic study of six cases. *Am J Clin Pathol* 107:592–600. Copyright 1997, by the American Society of Clinical Pathologists. Reprinted with permission.)

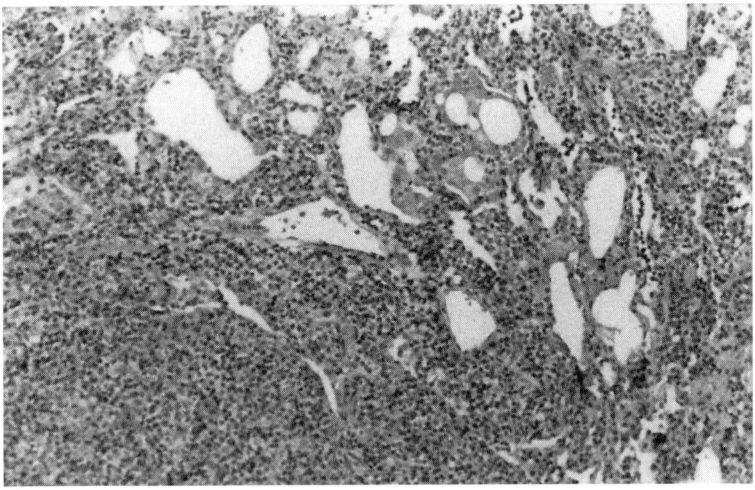

FIGURE 1.—Case 3. Nodular lymphoid aggregate in the lung with extension of lymphoid infiltrate into the septa of the surrounding alveoli. (Courtesy of Joshi VV, Gagnon GA, Chadwick EG, et al: The spectrum of mucosa-associated lymphoid tissue lesions in pediatric patients infected with HIV: A clinicopathologic study of six cases. *Am J Clin Pathol* 107:592–600. Copyright 1997, by the American Society of Clinical Pathologists. Reprinted with permission.)

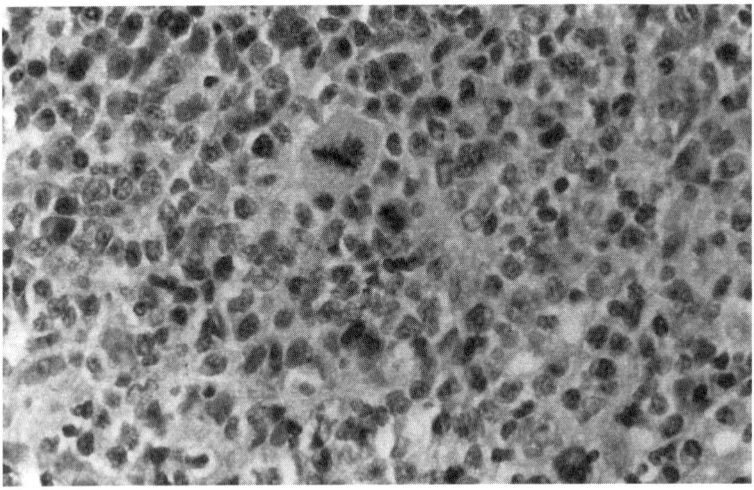

FIGURE 2.—Case 5. Admixture of centrocyte-like cells and immunoblasts in larger numbers than usually seen in pulmonary lymphoid hyperplasia and lymphoid interstitial pneumonitis complex. Note the prominent mitotic figure. (Courtesy of Joshi VV, Gagnon GA, Chadwick EG, et al: The spectrum of mucosa-associated lymphoid tissue lesions in pediatric patients infected with HIV: A clinicopathologic study of six cases. *Am J Clin Pathol* 107:592–600. Copyright 1997, by the American Society of Clinical Pathologists. Reprinted with permission.)

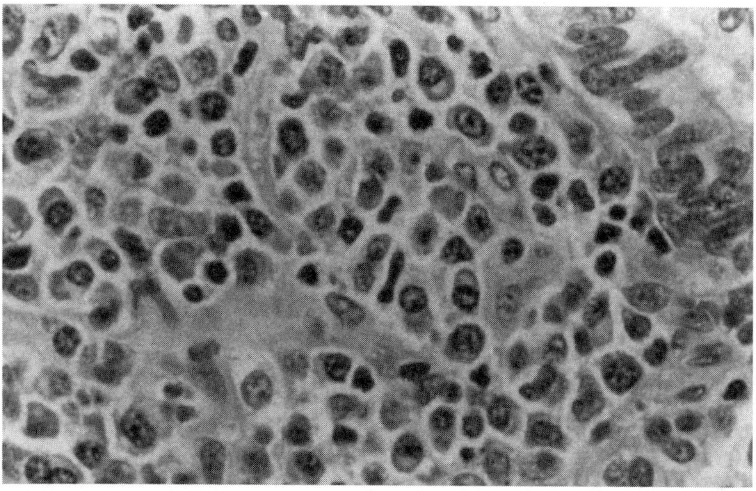

FIGURE 7.—Case 5. Plasma cells and plasmacytoid lymphocytes in the lymphoepithelial lesion. (Courtesy of Joshi VV, Gagnon GA, Chadwick EG, et al: The spectrum of mucosa-associated lymphoid tissue lesions in pediatric patients infected with HIV: A clinicopathologic study of six cases. *Am J Clin Pathol* 107:592–600. Copyright 1997, by the American Society of Clinical Pathologists. Reprinted with permission.)

Teruya-Feldstein J, Teemeck BL, Sloas MM, et al: Pulmonary malignant lymphoma of mucosa-associated lymphoid tissue (MALT) arising in a pediatric HIV-positive patient. *Am J Surg Pathol* 19:357–363, 1995.

Polypoid Dysplasia and Adenomas in Inflammatory Bowel Disease: A Clinical, Pathologic, and Follow-up Study of 89 Polyps From 59 Patients

Torres C, Antonioli D, Odze RD (Harvard Med School, Boston)

Am J Surg Pathol 22:275–284, 1998 5–11

Introduction.—Patients with inflammatory bowel disease (IBD) are at increased risk for developing adenocarcinoma of the colon. The marker with the highest prognostic significance for malignancy in these patients is epithelial dysplasia, which can be flat or raised (dysplasia-associated lesion or mass, DALM). Some DALMs present as discrete polyps that are difficult to distinguish from sporadic adenomas (SAs). This distinction is important as IBD-associated polypoid dysplastic (IPD) lesions are an indication for colectomy, whereas sporadic adenomas can be treated with polypectomy. A retrospective case study was performed to determine whether there are clinical, endoscopic, or pathologic findings that can be used to differentiate IPD from SA.

Study Design.—The study group consisted of 51 chronic ulcerative colitis and 8 Crohn's colitis patients with at least 1 IPD or SA, selected from records obtained from 1985 to 1995 files in Beth Israel Hospital or Brigham and Women's Hospital. Included were 35 men and 24 women, aged 27–85 years. Patient charts and endoscopic reports were reviewed.

TABLE 1.—Summary of Clinical Data and Comparison of Clinical and Endoscopic Features Between IBD Patients With Polyps Considered Probable SA, Probable IPD, or IND (N = 59)

Clinical feature	Total	SA (n = 16)	IND (n = 30)	IPD (n = 13)	P_1	P_2
		No. of patients/(%)				
Male/Female Ratio	35/24	10/6	16/14	9/4	0.5	0.507
Median age (years)	57 (27–85)	63.5	62.5	48	0.39	0.0913
IBD type					0.729	0.606
Ulcerative colitis	51 (86.5%)	13 (81.3%)	26 (86.7%)	12 (92.3%)		
Crohn's disease	8 (13.5%)	3 (18.7%)	4 (13.3%)	1 (7.7%)		
Mean duration of disease (years)	10 (1–45)	5	10	11	0.05*	0.0047*
Disease activity					0.101	0.058
Active	39 (66.1%)	8 (50.0%)	20 (66.7%)	11 (84.6%)		
Inactive	20 (33.9%)	8 (50.0%)	10 (33.3%)	2 (15.4%)		
Pancolitis					N/A	N/A
Present	29 (49.2%)	0 (0%)	18 (60.0%)	11 (84.6%)		
Absent	30 (50.8%)	16 (100%)	12 (40.0%)	2 (15.4%)		
No. of polyps					0.192	0.223
1	41 (69.5%)	13 (81.2%)	20 (66.7%)	8 (61.5%)		
≥2	18 (30.5%)	3 (18.7%)	10 (33.3%)	5 (38.5%)		
Polyp location					N/A	N/A
Right and transverse colon	33 (37%)	16 (64.0%)	10 (23.0%)	7 (35.0%)		
Left colon and rectum	56 (63%)	9 (36.0%)	34 (77.0%)	13 (65.0%)		

*Statistically significant.

Abbreviations: P_1, SA vs. Other (IND + IPD); P_2, SA vs. IPD only; *IBD*, inflammatory bowel disease; *IND*, indeterminate; *IPD*, polypoid dysplastic lesion; *N/A*, not applicable (SA defined in this study as a polyp occurring in nondiseased colon; therefore, all patients with SA had subtotal colitis); *SA*, sporadic adenomas.

(Courtesy of Torres C, Antonioli D, Odze RD: Polypoid dysplasia and adenomas in inflammatory bowel disease: A clinical, pathologic, and follow-up study of 89 polyps from 59 patients. *Am J Surg Pathol* 22:275–284, 1998.)

TABLE 2.—Summary and Comparison of Pathologic Features Between Patients With IBD With Polyps Considered Probable SA, Probable IPD, or IND (n = 89)

Clinical feature	Total	SA (n = 25)	IND (n = 44) No. of polyps (%)	IPD (n = 20)	p_1	p_2
Median polyp size (mm)	5.0 (2–50)	4.0	6.0	5.0	0.253	0.5091
Tubulovillous or villous architecture					0.013*	0.033*
Present	14 (15.7%)	0 (0%)	10 (22.7%)	4 (20.0%)		
Absent	75 (84.3%)	25 (100%)	34 (77.3%)	16 (80.0%)		
High grade dysplasia					0.237	0.570
Present	32 (36.0%)	7 (28.0%)	19 (43.0%)	6 (30.0%)		
Absent	57 (64.0%)	18 (72.0%)	25 (57.0%)	14 (70.0%)		
Admixture†					0.101	0.003*
Present	27 (30.3%)	4 (16.0%)	11 (25.0%)	12 (60.0%)		
Absent	62 (69.7%)	21 (84.0%)	33 (75.0%)	8 (40.0%)		
Metaplasia					0.575	0.460
Present	29 (32.6%)	9 (36.0%)	14 (31.8%)	6 (30.0%)		
Absent	60 (67.6%)	16 (64.0%)	30 (68.2%)	14 (70.0%)		
Lamina propria inflam (mono)					0.016*	0.003*
Normal	54 (60.7%)	21 (84.0%)	25 (56.8%)	8 (40.0%)		
Increase (1+ and 2+)	35 (39.3%)	4 (16.0%)	19 (43.2%)	12 (60.0%)		
Lamina propria inflam (poly)					0.062	0.096
Normal	42 (47.1%)	16 (64.0%)	18 (40.9%)	8 (40.0%)		
Increase (1+ and 2+)	47 (52.9%)	9 (36.0%)	26 (39.1%)	12 (60.0%)		
Intraepithelial inflam (mono)					0.455	0.231
Normal	78 (87.6%)	23 (92.0%)	39 (88.6%)	16 (80.0%)		
Increase (1+ and 2+)	11 (12.4%)	2 (8.0%)	5 (11.4%)	4 (20.0%)		
Intraepithelial inflam (poly)					0.098	0.165
Normal	44 (49.4%)	16 (64.0%)	19 (43.2%)	9 (45.0%)		
Increase (1+ and 2+)	45 (50.6%)	9 (36.0%)	25 (56.8%)	11 (55.0%)		

*Statistically significant.

†Admixture = admixture of normal and dysplastic crypts at polyp surface.

Abbreviations: p_1 = SA vs. Other (IND + IPD); p_2 = SA vs. IPD only; *IBD*, inflammatory bowel disease; *IND*, indeterminate; *IPD*, polypoid dysplastic lesion; *SA*, sporadic adenoma.

(Courtesy of Torres C, Antonioli D, Odze RD: Polypoid dysplasia and adenomas in inflammatory bowel disease: A clinical, pathologic, and follow-up study of 89 polyps from 59 patients. *Am J Surg Pathol* 22:275–284, 1998.)

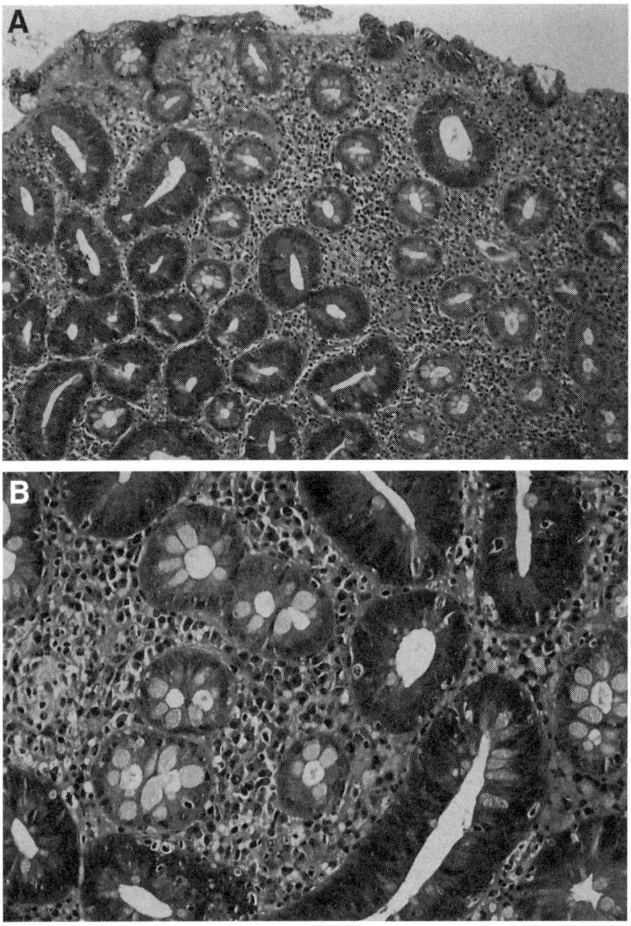

FIGURE 1.—A, Medium power view of a probable inflammatory bowel disease-associated polypoid-dysplastic lesion that shows a mixture of dysplastic and normal crypts at the surface of the polyp and increased inflammation in the lamina propria. B, High-power view of another area of the same polyp that highlights these features. (Courtesy of Torres C, Antonioli D, Odze RD: Polypoid dysplasia and adenomas in inflammatory bowel disease: A clinical, pathologic, and follow-up study of 89 polyps from 59 patients. *Am J Surg Pathol* 22:275–284, 1998.)

Tissue sections from 89 specimens of these 59 patients were evaluated for polyp size, architecture, dysplasia, surface crypts or villi, metaplasia, and infiltration of lamina propria or intraepithelial mono- or polymorphonuclear cell. The polyps were subclassified as probable SA, IPD, or indeterminate (IND). Pathologic, clinical, and endoscopic features were correlated.

Findings.—The average disease duration of the 59 patients in the study group was 10 years. Of these 59 patients, 49 (83%) had pancolitis. Histologically active disease was present in 39 (66%). The majority of these patients had only 1 polyp (Table 1). Only 8% of the polyps were

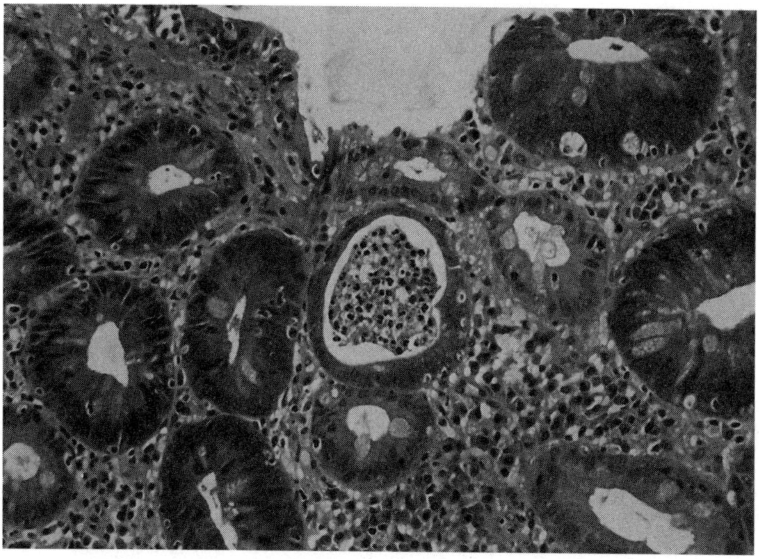

FIGURE 2.—High-power view of the surface of another probable inflammatory bowel disease-associated polypoid-dysplastic lesion that shows a dysplastic crypt abscess and increased lamina propria and intraepithelial mononuclear inflammation. (Courtesy of Torres C, Antonioli D, Odze RD: Polypoid dysplasia and adenomas in inflammatory bowel disease: A clinical, pathologic, and follow-up study of 89 polyps from 59 patients. *Am J Surg Pathol* 22:275–284, 1998.)

pedunculated. Size of the polyps ranged from 2 to 50 mm, with a median of 5 mm. Most of the polyps had tubular architecture and contained low-grade dysplasia (Table 2). The majority of these polyps had increased lamina propria inflammation and intraepithelial neutrophilic and mononuclear inflammation (Figs 1 and 2). After a median follow-up period of 13 months, an additional neoplastic lesion developed in 20% of the patients low-grade flat dysplasia was detected in 12.5%, additional benign polypoid epithelial neoplasms developed in 37.5%, and adenocarcinoma developed in 7.5%. Dysplasia and adenocarcinoma did not develop in any patients with lesions outside areas of colitis. Patients with probable IPD had significantly longer disease duration, as well as patients with polyps with tubulovillous or villous architecture, a mixture of normal and dysplastic surface epithelium, and increased lamina propria mononuclear inflammation, compared with patients with probable SA (Table 3).

Conclusions.—Patients with probable IPD were younger, had active colitis and longer disease duration. Histologically, IPD lesions differed from SA lesions in that IPD lesions exhibited more mononuclear inflammation in the lamina propria, tubulovillous or villous architecture, and had a mixture of normal and adenomatous crypts at the polyp surface. These distinguishing features may be useful for clinicians trying to differentiate these lesions.

▶ This paper addresses a very important and vexing problem in surgical pathology. Even in IBD, a sporadically occurring neoplastic polyp of the

TABLE 3.—Summary of Distinguishing Clinical, Endoscopic and Pathologic Features Between Patients With Probable SA or Probable IPD

Feature	SA	IPD
Patient age	Older (median age = 63.5 yrs)	Younger (median age = 48.0 yrs)
Disease activity	Inactive (50%)	Active (85%)
Duration of disease*	Shorter (median: 5 yrs)	Longer (median: 11 yrs)
Increased lamina propria inflammation* (mononuclear)	Uncommon (16%)	Common (60%)
Increased lamina propria inflammation (polymorphonuclear)	Less Common (36%)	Common (60%)
Tubullovillous/Villous architecture*	Absent (0%)	Occasional (20%)
Admixture*†	Uncommon (16%)	Common (60%)

*SA versus IPD; $P < 0.05$

†Admixture = admixture of normal and dysplastic crypts at polyp surface.

Abbreviations: IPD, polypoid dysplastic lesion; *SA*, sporadic adenoma.

(Courtesy of Torres C, Antonioli D, Odze RD: Polypoid dysplasia and adenomas in inflammatory bowel disease: A clinical, pathologic, and follow-up study of 89 polyps from 59 patients. *Am J Surg Pathol* 22:275–284, 1998.)

large bowel can often be treated with polypectomy, although many would consider polypoid dysplasia an indication for colectomy. Some have suggested that sporadic polyps occur more often in older colitis, and that polypoid lesions with neoplastic epithelium are more likely to represent dysplasia in younger patients. However, overlap occurs and age is not a sufficiently discriminating diagnostic criterion. These authors have attempted to develop a set of clinicopathologic criteria that can be used to distinguish sporadic polyps that occur by chance in an individual with preexisting IBD from polypoid dysplasia. It seems clear that this distinction cannot be made solely on the basis of histologic findings, as the "adenomatous" epithelium in neoplastic polyps closely resembles the dysplastic epithelial alterations of IBD. The clinicopathologic criteria that they propose include whether the polypoid lesion under investigation has arisen in a site of documented colitis, and whether dysplasia is present or absent in adjacent or distant mucosal foci. These authors suggest that the significance of dysplasia in the polyp's stalk is difficult to evaluate, because the finding of a pedunculated lesion that has been completely removed is relatively rare in this setting. This is the first study of such lesions in Crohn's disease as well as in chronic ulcerative colitis, but only a few examples were available for evaluation. These criteria seem sensible and useful. Their ultimate usefulness in guiding therapy will probably require additional testing.

M.W. Stanley, M.D.

Suggested Reading

Schneider A, Stolte M: Differential diagnosis of adenomas and dysplastic lesions in patients with ulcerative colitis. *Z Gastroenterol* 31:653–656, 1993.

Adenocarcinoma of the Ampulla of Vater: A 28-Year Experience

Talamini MA, Moesinger RC, Pitt HA, et al (Johns Hopkins Med Insts, Baltimore, Md)

Ann Surg 225:590–600, 1997 5–12

Introduction.—Adenocarcinoma of the ampulla of Vater is considered to be the most curable of all carcinomas of the upper gastrointestinal tract. Reported series are small and treatment of periampullary cancer has changed significantly in recent years. The experience with treatment of patients with adenocarcinoma of the ampulla of Vater was retrospectively assessed during a 28-year period to determine the factors that influence patient outcome.

Methods.—Medical records from 1969 to 1996 of 120 patients with adenocarcinoma of the ampulla of Vater were reviewed for demographics, history, physical findings, laboratory data, radiologic evaluation, procedures, pathologic evaluation, complications, and treatment. Morbidity and long-term survival were calculated.

Results.—One hundred six (88%) of 120 patients underwent resection. Of these, 105 (99%) underwent pancreaticoduodenal resection (103) or total pancreatectomy (2). The number of patients who underwent resection increased from 62% in the 1970s to 82% in the 1980s, and increased to 96% in the 1990s. The median survival period over 5 years for patients who could not undergo resection was 5 months, and the mean survival rate was 0%. For patients who underwent resection, these numbers were 46 months over the 5-year period and 38% for the mean survival rate. The number of transfusions significantly decreased from 1.5 in the 1980s to 0.82 in the 1990s. The 5-year survival rate of patients with blood transfusions was 30% and the survival rate of patients without transfusions was 53%, which indicated a significant adverse effect of transfusions on survival. There was a significant decrease in morbidity from 70% before to 38% after December 1992. Factors influencing long-term outcome were resection, no perioperative blood transfusions, negative lymph node status, and moderately or well-differentiated tumors. The best predictor of prolonged survival was the absence of perioperative blood transfusions.

Conclusion.—This is the first time that the use of perioperative transfusions has been shown to be a significant factor affecting the long-term survival in patients with adenocarcinomas of the ampulla of Vater. Survival rates were also better in patients with resectable tumors, negative lymph nodes, and moderately or well-differentiated histologic features.

▶ This article is an interesting and useful description of ampullary carcinoma, primarily because of the large number of patients described. The discussions of clinical management for various patients and pathologies will be helpful when we encounter these uncommon lesions.

M.W. Stanley, M.D.

Suggested Reading

Branum GD, Pappas TN, Meyers WC: The management of tumors of the ampulla of Vater by local resection. *Ann Surg* 224:621–627, 1996.

6 Hepatobiliary System and Pancreas

Protocol for the Examination of Specimens Removed From Patients With Carcinoma of the Exocrine Pancreas: A Basis for Checklists

Compton CC, for Members of the Cancer Committee (Massachusetts Gen Hosp, Boston; et al)

Arch Pathol Lab Med 121:1129–1136, 1997 6–1

Background.—The Cancer Committee of the College of American Pathologists develops protocols for the pathologic examination of surgical specimens from patients with cancer. Previous protocols have addressed Hodgkin's disease and cancers of the breast, bladder, colon and rectum, and lung. The protocols are based on synoptic reporting, in which checklists or other descriptive formats are used to ensure a uniform system of reporting. The Committee presents its protocol for data to be included in surgical pathology reports on patients with carcinoma of the exocrine pancreas.

Protocol for Carcinomas of the Exocrine Pancreas.—The protocol is divided into 4 segments, reflecting the surgical procedures typically used in patients with carcinoma of the pancreas: acquisition of cytologic material; incisional biopsy; partial pancreatectomy; and the Whipple procedure, i.e., partial or complete pancreaticoduodenectomy, with or without partial gastrectomy. Items to be included in the report under each category include clinical information and the results of macroscopic and microscopic examination. Extensive notes, which apply across categories, are included. The notes regard the presence of tumor; their histologic type and grade; tumor location, configuration, and staging; the presence of blood/lymphatic vessel or perineural invasion; tumor margins; and other issues.

Conclusions.—A protocol for surgical pathologic examination of specimens from patients with carcinoma of the exocrine pancreas is reported. The protocol can provide a basis for the development of checklists, an outline for full narrative reporting, or a guide for other types of synoptic or reporting formats. The protocol specifies important information regarding the surgical specimen and other data that will be used to select treatment, estimate prognosis, and analyze outcome.

► This is one of a series of articles from the College of American Pathologists Cancer Committee providing practical information on handling of oncologic resection specimens, including the reporting of results. Whipple, or lesser, procedures are relatively uncommon, so standardization of handling of specimens is critical. This article should well serve that purpose. Another proposal was recently published by the Association of Directors of Anatomic and Surgical Pathology.[1]

M.B. Cohen, M.D.

Reference

1. Association of Directors of Anatomic and Surgical Pathology: Recommendations for reporting resected pancreatic neoplasms. *Mod Pathol* 11:500–504, 1998.

Intraductal Papillary Tumors and Mucinous Cystic Tumors of the Pancreas: Clinicopathologic Study of 38 Cases

Fukushima N, Mukai K, Kanai Y, et al (Natl Cancer Ctr Research Inst, East, Kashiwa, Japan; Natl Cancer Ctr Research Inst, Tokyo; Natl Cancer Ctr Hosp, Tokyo; et al)

Hum Pathol 28:1010–1017, 1997 6–2

Background.—Intraductal papillary tumor (IDPT) of the pancreas is a specific entity of pancreatic ductal tumors that shows diffuse or segmental dilatation of the pancreatic ducts and intraductal papillary growth. In mucinous cystic tumor (MCT) of the pancreas, the formation of large multilocular or unilocular cells lined by tall or flattened mucus-producing cells is typically seen, often associated with papillary projections. The differences between IDPT and MCT have not been well characterized. The clinicopathologic features of 28 patients with IDPT and 10 with MCT were investigated.

Methods and Findings.—Both entities showed papillary projections of the epithelium, with abundant mucus secretion in the ectatic ducts or cystic spaces. Three fourths of the IDPTs were in the pancreatic head. Mean tumor size was 3.5 cm. One patient had a local recurrence but none died of IDPT. None of the MCTs arose in the pancreatic head. Mean tumor size in this group was 7.1 cm. One patient died of MCT, and the remainder survived with no recurrence. Eight IDPTs and 3 MCTs invaded the surrounding pancreatic tissue. Muconodular infiltration was found primarily in 5 IDPTs and 1 MCT. Tubular infiltration occurred in 3 IDPTs and 2 MCTs. In IDPT, a characteristic histologic finding associated with the muconodular infiltration was subepithelial "mucin droplets," which seemed to represent a change in polarity of mucus secretion. The forma-

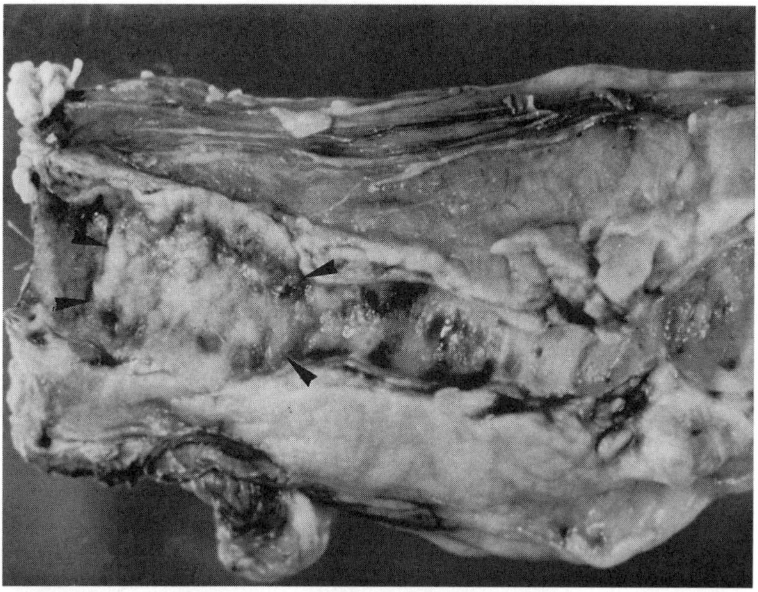

FIGURE 1, A.—Gross features and panoramic view of intraductal papillary tumor (IDPT). Intraductal papillary adenoma, main duct type (IDPT, case 3). Marked dilatation of the main pancreatic duct is seen. Part of the mucosal surface of the main pancreatic duct is granular (*arrow*). (Courtesy of Fukushima N, Mukai K, Kanai Y, et al: Intraductal papillary tumors and mucinous cystic tumors of the pancreas: Clinicopathologic study of 38 cases. *Hum Pathol* 28:1010–1017, 1997.)

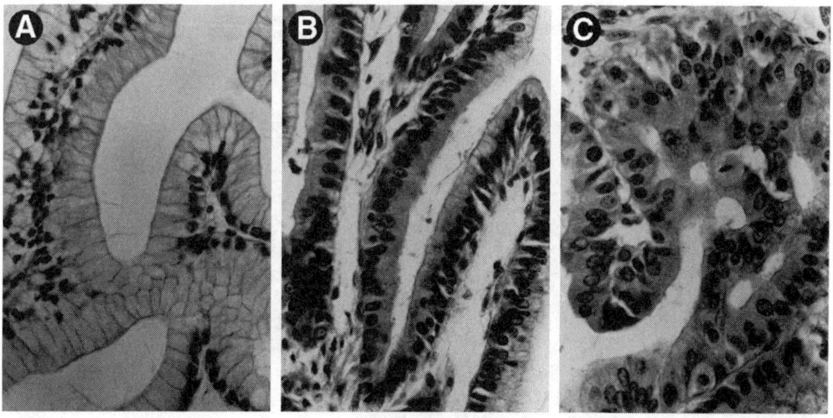

FIGURE 3.—Microscopic features of intraductal papillary tumor (IDPT, case 25). Epithelium with various grades of atypia is evident in this tumor. **A**, hyperplastic epithelium: tall columnar cells with abundant mucin in the cytoplasm. Nuclear atypia is not apparent. **B**, moderately dysplastic epithelium with slight nuclear atypia and focal nuclear pseudostratification. **C**, carcinomatous epithelium increased nuclear atypia and mitotic figures. Glandular structures without a fibrovascular stroma are observed. (Hematoxylin-eosin, original magnifications, **A–C**, ×305.) (Courtesy of Fukushima N, Mukai K, Kanai Y, et al: Intraductal papillary tumors and mucinous cystic tumors of the pancreas: Clinicopathologic study of 38 cases. *Hum Pathol* 28:1010–1017, 1997.)

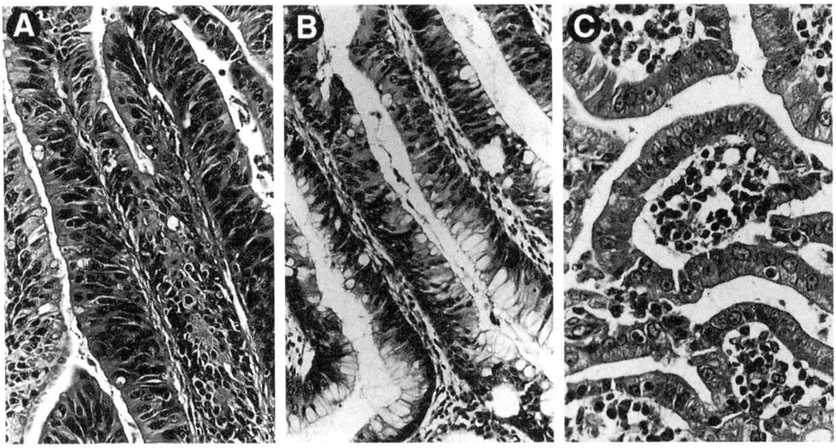

FIGURE 4.—Three types of carcinomatous cells in intraductal papillary tumor (IDPT). **A**, tall columnar cells with slightly basophilic dense cytoplasm. **B**, tall columnar cells with clear cytoplasm. **C**, round to cuboidal cells with eosinophilic dense cytoplasm. (Hematoxylin-eosin, original magnification ×153.) (Courtesy of Fukushima N, Mukai K, Kanai Y, et al: Intraductal papillary tumors and mucinous cystic tumors of the pancreas: Clinicopathologic study of 38 cases. *Hum Pathol* 28:1010–1017, 1997.)

tion of such droplets may be the first step of muconodular infiltration in IDPT (Figs 1, A; 3; 4; 5; 6, A; and 7).

Conclusions.—Although IDPT and MCT are similar morphologically, they have obvious clinicopathologic differences. These tumors should be

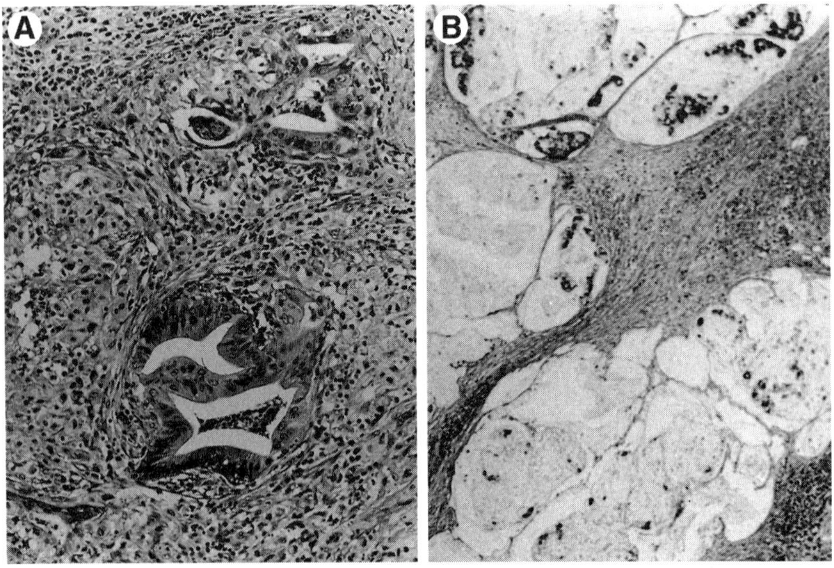

FIGURE 5.—Tubular infiltration (**A**) and muconodular infiltration (**B**) associated with intraductal papillary tumor (IDPT). (Hematoxylin-eosin, original magnification ×76.) (Courtesy of Fukushima N, Mukai K, Kanai Y, et al: Intraductal papillary tumors and mucinous cystic tumors of the pancreas: Clinicopathologic study of 38 cases. *Hum Pathol* 28:1010–1017, 1997.)

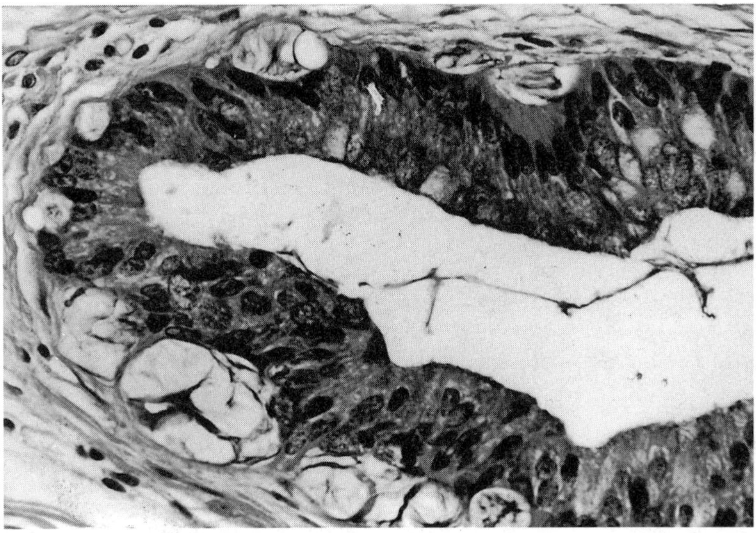

FIGURE 6, A.—Proposed sequence in the development of a mucus lake in intraductal papillary tumor (IDPT). "Mucin droplets" are seen in the subepithelial space. This feature is called "mucin droplets" in this article. The epithelium is markedly dysplastic. (Hematoxylin-eosin, original magnification ×305.) (Courtesy of Fukushima N, Mukai K, Kanai Y, et al: Intraductal papillary tumors and mucinous cystic tumors of the pancreas: Clinicopathologic study of 38 cases. *Hum Pathol* 28:1010–1017, 1997.)

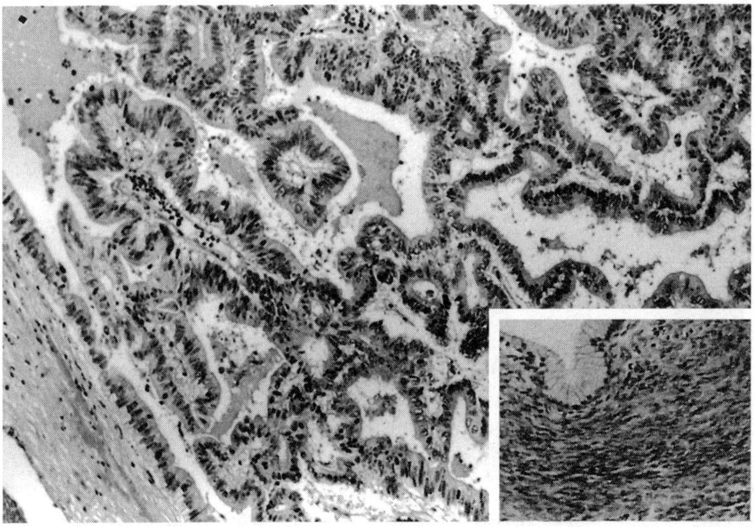

FIGURE 7.—Histologic features of mucinous cystic tumor (MCT). Marked papillary growth in the cystic space. The wall of the MCT is composed of cellular connective tissue that resembles ovarian stroma (**inset**). (Hematoxylin-eosin, original magnification ×76; **inset**, ×153.) (Courtesy of Fukushima N, Mukai K, Kanai Y, et al: Intraductal papillary tumors and mucinous cystic tumors of the pancreas: Clinicopathologic study of 38 cases. *Hum Pathol* 28:1010–1017, 1997.)

divided and recorded in different categories. Subepithelial "mucin droplets" may be the initial step in muconodular infiltration in IDPT.

▶ This recently described entity (1982) has received several names, most incorporating some form of the words mucin and cyst. They are sometimes detected in older patients with unexplained bouts of recurrent pancreatitis. Endoscopy shows pancreatic duct dilatation with mucin accumulation and discharge of mucin through the ampulla of Vater. This article compares these IDPTs and MCTs. Noting differences in tumor location and patient gender, the authors encourage continued separate classification of these 2 neoplasm groups. They proposed the interesting idea that subepithelial mucin droplets herald invasion and represent morphological evidence of a breakdown in the polarized cell phenotype.

M.W. Stanley, M.D.

Suggested Reading

Compagno J, Oertel JE: Mucinous cystic neoplasms of the pancreas with overt and latent malignancy (cystoadenocarcinoma and cystadenoma): A clinicopathologic study of 41 cases. *Am J Clin Pathol* 69:573–580, 1978.

Madura JA, Wiebke EA, Howard TJ, et al: Mucin-hypersecreting intraductal neoplasms of the pancreas: A precursor to cystic pancreatic malignancies. *Surgery* 122:786–793, 1997.

Ohhashi K, Murakami Y, Maruyama M, et al: Four cases of mucous secreting pancreatic cancer. *Prog Digest Endosc* 20:348–351, 1982.

Undifferentiated Carcinoma With Osteoclast-like Giant Cells of the Pancreas and Periampullary Region

Molberg KH, Heffess C, Delgado R, et al (Univ of Texas, Dallas; Armed Forces Inst of Pathology, Washington, DC)

Cancer 82:1279–1287, 1998 6–3

Background.—Undifferentiated carcinomas with osteoclast-like giant cells are rare pancreatic and periampullary neoplasms that are morphologically similar to giant cell tumor of the bone. The histogenesis, terminology, and biological behavior associated with these tumors are still debated.

Methods.—Nine pancreatic neoplasms and 1 periampullary lesion of this type were studied. Immunohistochemistry was done in 9 cases. For 8, clinical follow-up data were available.

Findings.—The mean size of the lesions was 9 cm. The lesions were partially or completely multicystic, and hemorrhagic. Histologic examination showed that they consisted mainly of ovoid or spindle-shaped bland mononuclear cells and evenly spaced osteoclast-like giant cells (Fig 1). However, in the foci of 3 neoplasms, the nuclear pleomorphism of the

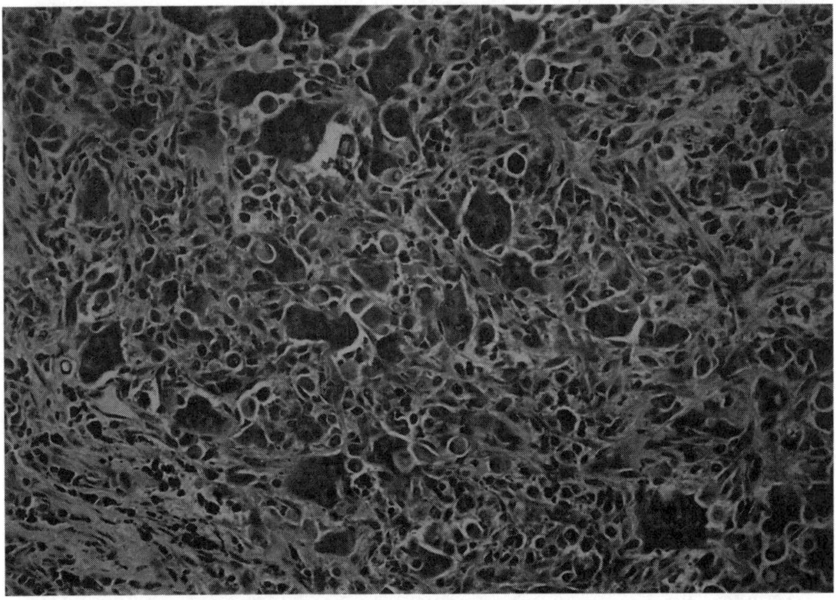

FIGURE 1.—Mononuclear and osteoclast-like giant cells closely resembing giant cell tumor of bone (hematoxylin and eosin, ×100). (Courtesy of Molberg KH, Heffess C, Delgado R, et al: Undifferentiated carcinoma with osteoclast-like giant cells of the pancreas and periampullary region. *Cancer* 82[7]:1279–1287. Copyright 1998, American Cancer Society. Reprinted by permission of Wiley-Liss, Inc., a subsidiary of John Wiley & Sons, Inc.)

mononuclear cells approached that seen in anaplastic spindle and giant cell carcinomas. Other histologic features were phagocytosis of the mononuclear cells by the osteoclast-like giant cells in 7 of 10 cases (Fig 2), osteoid or bone formation in 3 of 10, and chondroid differentiation in 1 of 10. Four neoplasms had foci of conventional adenocarcinoma. Two arose in preexisting mucinous cystic neoplasms of the pancreas. In 6 of 9 tumors tested, the mononuclear cells were positive for epithelial markers and negative for histiocytic markers. By contrast, the osteoclast-like giant cells in all 9 were positive for CD-68 and negative for cytokeratins; in 4, they were positive for lysozyme. In 3 cases, p53 stained the mononuclear tumor cells, and in 4, MIB-1 stained the mononuclear tumor cells. However, the osteoclast-like giant cells did not stain with either antibody in any of the 9 cases tested. Most patients died of disease within 1 year of diagnosis. Only 1 was alive and free of disease 14 years after surgery (Table 1).

Conclusions.—These data suggest an epithelial phenotype for the mononuclear cells and a reactive histiocytic lineage for the nonneoplastic osteoclast-like giant cells. These neoplasms follow an aggressive course, resulting in the death of most patients within 1 year. Such lesions should be classified as undifferentiated carcinoma.

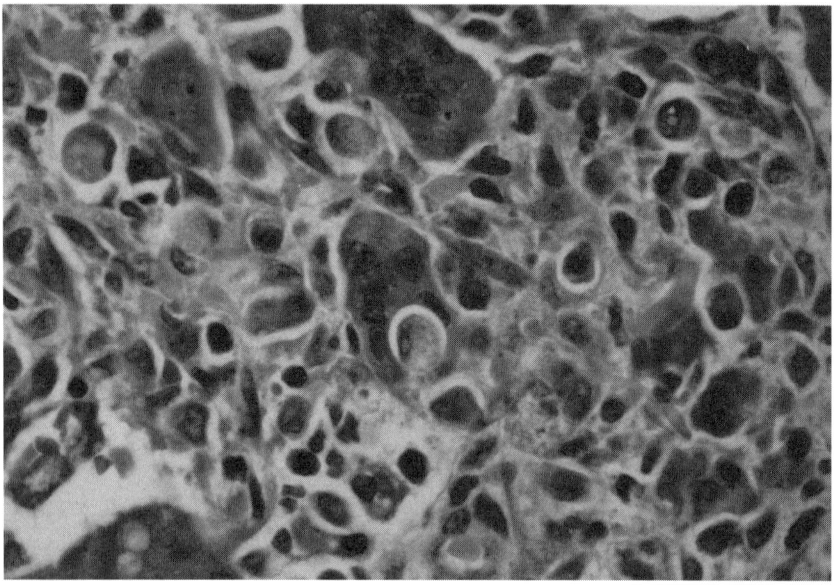

FIGURE 2.—Detail of mononuclear and osteoclast-like giant cells. Note the phagocytosis of mononuclear cells by osteoclast-like giant cells (hematoxylin and eosin, ×400). (Courtesy of Molberg KH, Heffess C, Delgado R, et al: Undifferentiated carcinoma with osteoclast-like giant cells of the pancreas and periampullary region. *Cancer* 82[7]:1279–1287. Copyright 1998, American Cancer Society. Reprinted by permission of Wiley-Liss, Inc., a subsidiary of John Wiley & Sons, Inc.)

► This relatively large series of undifferentiated pancreatic carcinomas with osteoclast-like giant cells is probably the best source for detailed study of this entity.

M.W. Stanley, M.D.

TABLE 1.—Clinical and Pathological Features of 9 Patients With Undifferentiated Carcinoma With Osteoclast-like Giant Cells

Case	Age (yrs)	Sex	Location	Size (cm)	Therapy	Follow up
1	70	F	Head of pancreas	11	Whipple procedure	LFU
2	62	F	Head of pancreas	6	Whipple procedure	DOD 10 months
3	33	M	Not stated	NA	Biopsy	DOC 1 month
4	58	F	Head of pancreas	13	Whipple procedure	NED 14 years
5	43	F	Tail of pancreas	7	Distal pancreatectomy	DOD 8 months
6	88	F	Tail of pancreas	14	Distal pancreatectomy	DOD 2 months
7	85	F	Periampullary region	3.5	Local resection of periampullary tumor	DOD 6 months
8	75	M	Not stated	12	Biopsy	AWD 7 months
9	88	M	Tail of pancreas	11	Distal pancreatectomy	LFU
10	63	M	Head of pancreas	5	Whipple procedure	DOD 11 months

Abbreviations: LFU, lost to follow-up; *DOD,* dead of disease; *DOC,* dead of other causes; *NED,* no evidence of disease; *AWD,* alive with disease; *NA,* not available.

(Courtesy of Molberg KH, Heffess C, Delgado R, et al: Undifferentiated carcinoma with osteoclast-like giant cells of the pancreas and periampullary region. *Cancer* 82[7]:1279–1287. Copyright 1988, American Cancer Society. Reprinted by permission of Wiley-Liss, Inc., a subsidiary of John Wiley & Sons, Inc.)

Suggested Reading

Goldberg RO, Michelassi F, Montag AG: Osteoclast-like giant cell tumor of the pancreas: Immunophenotypic similarity to giant cell tumor of bone. *Hum Pathol* 22:618–622, 1991.

Martin A, Texier P, Bahnini JM, et al: An unusual epithelial pleomorphic giant cell tumour of the pancreas with osteoclast-type cells. *J Clin Pathol* 47:372–374, 1994.

Liver Hemangioma: US-guided 18-Gauge Core-Needle Biopsy
Heilo A, Stenwig AE (Norwegian Radium Hosp, Oslo, Norway)
Radiology 204:719–722, 1997 6–4

Background.—An absolute histologic diagnosis of a liver lesion is sometimes necessary, especially in patients with a known malignancy. The clinical utility of US-guided, 18-gauge core-needle biopsy of liver hemangiomas done with a 1-hand automatic-sampling technique was determined.

Methods and Findings.—Of 491 US-guided core-needle liver biopsies, hemangioma was suspected at US in 51 and confirmed histologically in 29. Eighteen lesions that appeared malignant on US were diagnosed as hemangiomas. Mean diameter was 45 mm, with a range of 7–114 mm. On histologic assessment, 47 biopsy specimens were diagnosed unequivocally as hemangiomas. In all but 1 procedure, a cuff of normal hepatic parenchyma could be interposed between the capsule and margin of the heman-

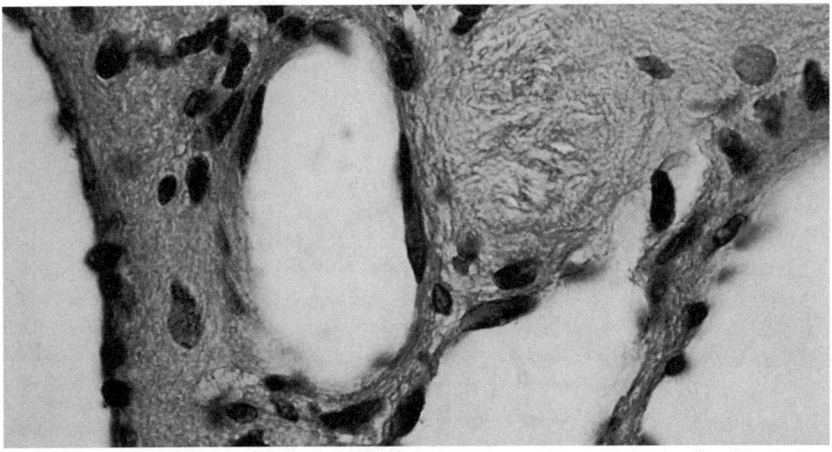

FIGURE D.—Photomicrograph of a liver hemangioma shows flattened endothelium lines the dilated vessels. (Hematoxylin-eosin stain; original magnification, ×576). (Courtesy of Heilo A, Stenwig AE: Liver hemangioma: US-guided 18-gauge core-needle biopsy. *Radiology* 204:719–722. Copyright 1997, Radiological Society of North America.)

gioma. The mean number of punctures done at each biopsy session was 1.4. None of the findings were false positive, and 15 or 16 were false negative. No serious complications occurred (Fig D).

Conclusions.—When the diagnosis of hemangioma must be established, US-guided core-needle biopsy appears to be safe. Conclusive biopsy findings may shorten the diagnostic workup, to the benefit of both patient and hospital.

▶ Hepatic hemangiomas are very common and must be investigated in some patients, particularly those with prior history of malignancy. However, radiographic studies are not always definitive. I have made this diagnosis by fine-needle aspiration, when a paraffin-embedded cell block preparation of solid tissue particles was available. These authors present a sizable series based on 18-gauge core biopsies; importantly, there were no complications. The article makes the point that even if one plans to avoid biopsy of hemangiomas, their puncture among a series of liver masses in cancer patients will occur periodically by chance alone and is thus unavoidable. For this reason, documentation of the procedure's safety and the laboratory's diagnostic accuracy is important. This is analogous to those individuals who do not wish to study malignant lymphoma by fine-needle aspiration. If you look at enough aspirates, you will inevitably "bump into" a lymphoma once in a while.

M.W. Stanley, M.D.

Suggested Reading

Kaw YT, Esparza AR: Cytologic diagnosis of cavernous hemangioma of the liver with fine-needle biopsy. *Diagn Cytopathol* 7:628–630, 1991.

Takayasu K, Uesaka K: Is fine needle biopsy of liver hemangioma hazardous (reply). *AJR* 148:231–232, 1987.

Turlington BS, Charboneau JW, Reading CC, et al: Percutaneous needle biopsy of hepatic cavernous hemangiomas. *Radiology* 181(P):224, 1991.

Choledochal Cyst and Neoplasm: A Comprehensive Review of 106 Cases and Presentation of Two Original Cases

Fieber SS, Nance FC (Saint Barnabas Med Ctr, Livingston, NJ; Univ of Medicine and Dentistry of New Jersey, Newark)

Am Surg 63:982–987, 1997 6–5

Objective.—Over 3,000 cases of cystic dilation of the biliary tree have been reported in the literature. Complications of choledochal cysts include cholangitis, biliary cirrhosis, portal hypertension, lithiasis, rupture, and carcinoma. One hundred six cases of choledochal cysts associated with neoplasms have been identified. This report analyzes the relationship be-

TABLE 3.—Age Associated With Choledochal Cysts With Neoplasm

Age (Years)	106 Cases Listed in Collated Series
0–10	4%
11–20	18%
21–30	20%
31–40	18%
41–50	14%
51–60	13%
61–70	9%
71–80	2%

(Courtesy of Fieber SS, Nance FC: Choledochal cyst and neoplasm: A comprehensive review of 106 cases and presentation of two original cases. *Am Surg* 63:982–987, 1997.)

tween choledochal cyst and primary neoplasm in situ or in the biliary tract, gallbladder, or pancreas.

Findings.—The review included the 106 cases from the literature and 2 new cases. The estimated incidence of choledochal cysts was 1 per 13,000 U.S. hospital admissions. Neoplasm with choledochal cyst was most likely to occur in the second to fourth decades of life (Table 3). Of the reported cases, the choledochal cyst was the primary site of adenocarcinoma in 31% of cases (Table 4). Of the extracystic sites, 43% involved cholangiocarcinoma and 7% anaplastic carcinoma. In 68 cases, neoplasms were identified at the initial laparotomy. Resection was performed in 20 patients; 20 of these patients survived for longer than 1 year, including 7 patients who underwent biliary pancreaticoduodenostomy. Elective surgery was performed in 38 patients with "pristine" choledochal cysts, and 28 underwent internal drainage. In 3 patients, carcinoma of the biliary tract developed decades after choledochocystoduodenostomy.

TABLE 4.—Pathology in 106 Choledochal Cysts With Neoplasia

Pathology	Percentage
Cholangiocarcinoma	43%
Choledochal cyst (*in situ*; primary adenocarcinoma and a squamous cell carcinoma)	31%
Anaplastic carcinoma (pleomorphic giant cell, poorly differentiated, carcinomatosis)	7%
Primary carcinoma of the gallbladder	9%
Primary carcinoma gallbladder and choledochal cyst	3%
Carcinoma of pancreas	3%
Miscellaneous	5%
Botryoides sarcoma	
Squamous cell carcinoma	
Intrahepatic bile duct sarcoma	
Adenoacanthoma of cyst	
Papilloma in choledochal cyst	

(Courtesy of Fieber SS, Nance FC: Choledochal cyst and neoplasm: A comprehensive review of 106 cases and presentation of two original cases. *Am Surg* 63:982–987, 1997.)

Conclusions.—A comprehensive review of the literature suggests that patients with choledochal cysts may develop neoplasia at any time along the biliary tract or in the gallbladder or pancreas. Patients with choledochal cysts and neoplasia have a high incidence of anomalous relation at the pancreaticobiliary duct junction. The malignancy is noted at the initial laparotomy in nearly two thirds of cases.

▶ Most references on the topic of choledochal cyst are in the surgery literature, and most are pediatric. This article shifts the focus to those patients (106 total) with choledochal cyst-related malignancy, and with this shift comes a range of older individuals. The cysts are uncommon, and only a minority of affected patients develop a related neoplasm. It is important to note, however, that the neoplasm may be in any portion of the biliary tract or be in the pancreas. A high percentage are cholangiocarcinomas. As noted in the authors' Case 1 and in their literature review, a lengthy interval may separate a pediatric presentation of choledochal cyst from development of a lethal malignancy in adulthood. Interesting factors of potential pathogenetic significance merit further investigation and include associated anatomic variations in the pancreaticobiliary junction and K-*ras* oncogene mutations.

M.W. Stanley, M.D.

Suggested Reading

Albores-Saavedra J, Defortuna SM, Smothermon WE: Primary papillary hyperplasia of the gallbladder and cystic and common bile ducts. *Hum Pathol* 21:228–231, 1990.

Reliability of Frozen Section Diagnosis of Gallbladder Tumor for Detecting Carcinoma and Depth of Its Invasion

Yamaguchi K, Chijiiwa K, Saiki S, et al (Kyushu Univ, Fukuoka, Japan)
J Surg Oncol 65:132–136, 1997 6–6

Background.—Deciding the most appropriate treatment strategy during surgery for gallbladder tumor relies on accurate frozen section diagnosis. However, the accuracy of frozen section diagnosis of the gallbladder has not been well documented.

Methods.—Eighty-six consecutive patients with gallbladder tumors were studied to determine the reliability of frozen section diagnosis. Thirty-two patients had polypoid lesions and 54 had nonpolypoid tumors.

Findings.—Frozen tissue and final diagnoses were concordant in 82 patients, being benign in 65 and malignant in 17. Frozen diagnosis had an overall accuracy of 95.3%. The accuracy of frozen section diagnosis was 91% in 32 polypoid lesions and 98% in 54 nonpolypoid lesions. Diagnoses of depth of invasion were concordant in 70% of the 10 carcinomas examined. Frozen section diagnoses were changed in 7 patients, 5 of whom had a polypoid tumor (Tables 1, 2, and 3).

TABLE 1.—Total Accuracy of Frozen Section Diagnosis and Accuracy of Frozen Section Diagnosis of Benign Disease and Malignant Disease

	Total accuracy (%)	Benign disease (%)	Malignant disease (%)
Polypoid lesion	90.6	92.6	80.0
Nonpolypoid tumor-like lesion	98.1	100	92.9
Total	95.3	97.0	94.7

(Courtesy of Yamaguchi K, Chijiiwa K, Saiki S, et al: Reliability of frozen section diagnosis of gallbladder tumor for detecting carcinoma and depth of its invasion. *J Surg Oncol* 65:132–136. Copyright 1997, John Wiley & Sons, Inc. Reprinted by permission of Wiley-Liss, Inc., a subsidiary of John Wiley & Sons, Inc.)

Conclusions.—Intraoperative frozen tissue diagnosis is fairly reliable in patients with gallbladder lesions, although its accuracy is low in those with polypoid tumors. In addition, frozen section diagnosis is not a reliable indicator of the depth of invasion of gallbladder carcinoma.

► This article from the surgical literature is useful to us in that it adjusts our expectations regarding these very difficult frozen section diagnoses. The authors devote considerable energy to discussing the implications of laparoscopic techniques for cholecystectomy. Various approaches have been advocated when an unclassified mass lesion is under investigation. In most cases frozen section evaluation will be requested. In those instances where the extent of surgery is determined in part by the depth of tumor invasion, frozen section and its attendant sampling error may not be fully reliable. Another interesting note about this article is the discussion of port site tumor recurrences after laparoscopy. We have also seen this in colon cancer and ovarian carcinoma. In our experience, fine-needle aspiration of these masses provides rapid confirmation of the clinical impression.

M.W. Stanley, M.D.

TABLE 2.—Final Diagnosis of 86 Patients Who Underwent Frozen Section Examination of the Gallbladder

Polypoid lesion (32)		Nonpolypoid tumor-like lesion (54)	
Benign		Benign	
Cholesterol polyp	13	Chronic cholecystitis	33
Chronic cholecystitis	5	Xanthogranulomatous cholecystitis	2
Inflammatory polyp	1	Cholesterolosis	1
Hyperplastic polyp	1	Cholesterol polyp	1
Polyp (nonspecific)	1	Adenomyoma	3
Adenomyoma	1	Adenoma	1
Adenoma	4		
Malignant		Malignant	
Adenocarcinoma	6	Adenocarcinoma	13

(Courtesy of Yamaguchi K, Chijiiwa K, Saiki S, et al: Reliability of frozen section diagnosis of gallbladder tumor for detecting carcinoma and depth of its invasion. *J Surg Oncol* 65:132–136. Copyright 1997, John Wiley & Sons, Inc. Reprinted by permission of Wiley-Liss, Inc. a subsidiary of John Wiley & Sons, Inc.)

TABLE 3.—Alteration of Frozen Section Diagnosis of Benign or Malignant Gallbladder Disease

Frozen section diagnosis	Final diagnosis
Hyperplastic polyp	Adenocarcinoma (ss)
Adenoma	Adenocarcinoma (m)
Adenocarcinoma (m)	Adenoma
Adenocarcinoma (ss)	Chronic cholecystitis

Abbreviations: m, limited to the mucosa; *ss*, invading the subserosal layer.

(Courtesy of Yamaguchi K, Chijiiwa K, Saiki S, et al: Reliability of frozen section diagnosis of gallbladder tumor for detecting carcinoma and depth of its invasion. *J Surg Oncol* 65:132–136. Copyright 1997, John Wiley & Sons, Inc. Reprinted by permission of Wiley-Liss, Inc., a subsidiary of John Wiley & Sons, Inc.)

Suggested Reading

Ishibashi T, Nagai H, Yasuda T, et al: Two cases of early gallbladder cancer incidentally discovered by laparoscopic cholecystectomy. *Surg Laparosc Endosc* 5:21–26, 1995.

O'Rourke N, Price P, Kelly S, et al: Tumour inoculation during laparoscopy. *Lancet* 342:368–369, 1993.

7 Endocrine System

Vascularity in Human Adrenal Cortex

Susano H, Ohashi Y, Suzuki T, et al (Tohoku Univ, Sendai, Japan)

Mod Pathol 11:329–333, 1998 7–1

Background.—It has been hypothesized that angiogenesis is a major factor in tumor cell proliferation and hormonal secretion of endocrine tumors, including adrenocortical neoplasms. However, there are no detailed reports of vascularity in adrenocortical tumors.

Methods.—Vascular density, endothelial area of each vessel, and vascular area were analyzed in adrenocortical carcinoma, Cushing's adenoma, aldosterone-producing adenoma, nonfunctioning hormonally inactive adenoma, and normal adrenal gland. Immunohistochemical analysis of CD34 and the CAS 200 image analysis system were used.

Results.—Analysis showed that the endothelial area and the vascular area in adrenocortical carcinomas were significantly higher than in adenomas and normal adrenal tissues. No significant differences in vascular density were seen among normal specimens, adenomas, and carcinomas (Fig 2). No significant differences in vascularity were seen in the zona glomerulosa, zona fasciculata, and zona reticularis of aldosteronomas, Cushing's adenomas, and nonfunctioning hormonally inactive adenomas. There were no significant differences in vascularity between specimens from patients who died of the disease and patients who did not.

Discussion.—These findings indicate an association between adrenocortical carcinoma and increased endothelial cell proliferation, but not with an increased number of intratumoral microvessels. Further studies using a larger sample and factor VIII immunostain are needed to establish an association between vascularity and outcome in patients with adrenocortical carcinoma.

► Angiogenesis is thought to play a fundamental role in tumor progression. Recent attention in the scientific and lay literature to angiogenesis inhibitors as therapeutic agents is one such example. With respect to histopathology, attention has focused on the (mean) vascular density in tumors. In this report, the authors focus their studies on the adrenal, an intrinsically vascular organ. Using standard immunohistochemical techniques combined with image analysis, vascular density as well as endothelial area in each vessel and vascular area were assessed in a series on normal and neoplastic adrenals.

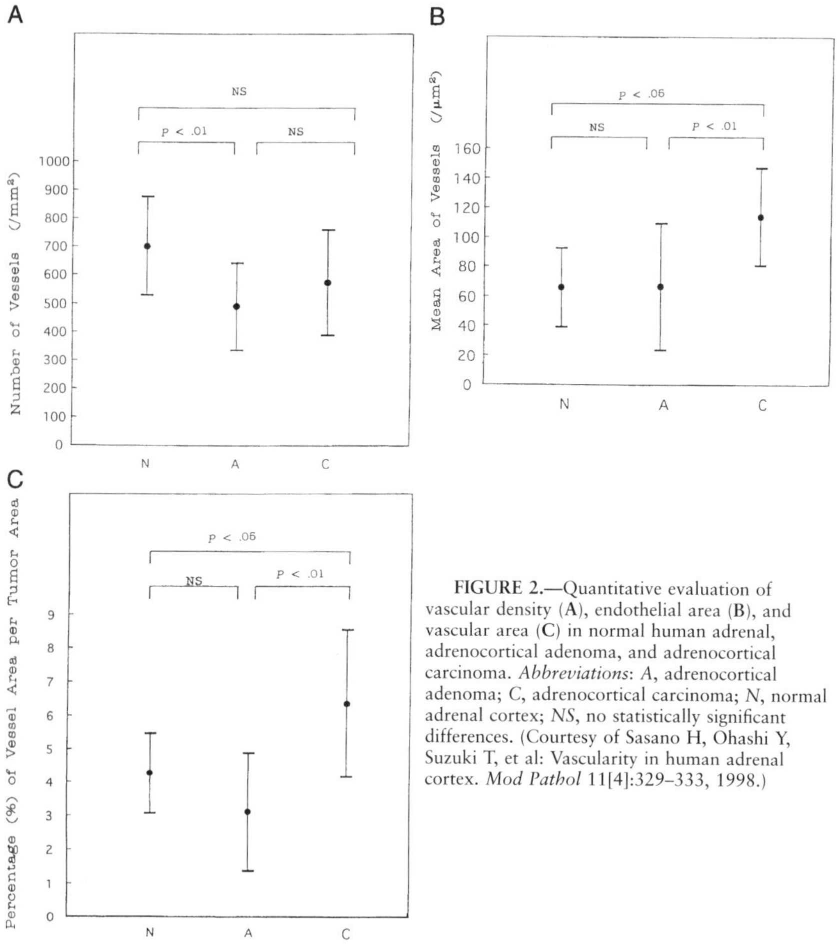

FIGURE 2.—Quantitative evaluation of vascular density (**A**), endothelial area (**B**), and vascular area (**C**) in normal human adrenal, adrenocortical adenoma, and adrenocortical carcinoma. *Abbreviations*: *A*, adrenocortical adenoma; *C*, adrenocortical carcinoma; *N*, normal adrenal cortex; *NS*, no statistically significant differences. (Courtesy of Sasano H, Ohashi Y, Suzuki T, et al: Vascularity in human adrenal cortex. *Mod Pathol* 11[4]:329–333, 1998.)

The results indicate that only the vascular area was statistically significant between normal glands and adenomas when compared with carcinomas. However, given the error bars, there was overlap between all three entities. Consequently, it would appear that assessment of vascular density or related parameters is difficult to apply prospectively to individual patients.

M.B. Cohen, M.D.

CD44 Expression in Normal Adrenal Tissue and Adrenal Tumours

Barshack I, Goldberg I, Nass D, et al (Tel-Aviv Univ, Israel)
J Clin Pathol 51:52–54, 1998 7–2

Objective.—CD44 is a cell surface glycoprotein that is expressed in standard form by normal cells and in variant forms (CD44-V) by malignant cells. The CD44 expression was examined in different layers of the cortical cortex, in adrenal medulla, and in adrenal tumors. Differences were characterized to determine if they were helpful in the diagnosis and differentiation of distinct adrenal tumors.

Methods.—Immunohistochemical staining was performed on 12 adrenal cortical adenomas, 3 adrenal cortical carcinomas, 10 pheochromocytomas, and 4 normal adrenal glands. CD44-V6 and CD44-S expression were determined.

Results.—Different zones of the adrenal cortex showed different cytoplasmic staining intensities for CD44-V6. CD44-V6 and CD44-S cytoplasmic expression was found in adrenal cortical adenomas and carcinomas. Pheochromocytoma cells expressed CD44-S and CD44-V6, but in 5 of 10 specimens CD44-V6 expression was sparse, focal, and primarily perinuclear. Among patients with cortical adenomas, 4 were cortisol secretors, 3 were aldosterone secretors, and the remainder were nonsecretors.

Conclusion.—Strong membranous CD44 expression may help to distinguish between pheochromocytomas and weaker staining adrenal cortical adenomas.

▶ CD44 is a glycoprotein (?proteoglycan) cellular adhesion molecule that has received a lot of attention as a "prognostic" marker. The gene contains 19 exons, which may be alternatively spliced, resulting in variant isoforms. The most prevalent form is the "standard" form (CD44-S), and the V6 isoform (CD44-V6), in particular, has received attention. In this study, the authors assessed CD44 expression in a relatively small panel of medullary and cortical tumors. The conclusion by the authors suggests a role for CD44-S in separating pheochromocytomas from cortical adenomas. Other approaches to this differential diagnosis are available, not the least of which is morphologic. Further, the significance of cytoplasmic staining of CD44-V6 is unclear. This observation has been noted in a number of other tumors. It is intriguing since CD44 is a transmembrane molecule, although a soluble form is known to exist. Further studies are clearly warranted. With respect to CD44 expression as a prognostic marker in adrenal tumors, this study is too small to answer the question.

M.B. Cohen, M.D.

Extracapsular Invasion of Lymph Node Metastasis Is an Indicator of Distant Metastasis and Poor Prognosis in Patients With Thyroid Papillary Carcinoma

Yamashita H, Noguchi S, Murakami N, et al (Oita Med Univ, Japan; Noguchi Thyroid Clinic and Hosp Found, Oita, Japan)

Cancer 80:2268–2272, 1997 7–3

Background.—Age and presence or absence of distant metastasis are important prognostic factors in patients with papillary carcinoma of the

TABLE 2.—Incidence of Histologic Findings in the Two Groups

Factors	Control	Metastatic	*P* values
Extranodal invasion	18	41	0.0000
Large lymph node deposit	11	30	0.0001
Bone at the periphery of the tumor	7	0	0.0014
Perithyroidal muscular invasion	0	5	0.0073
Pure papillary carcinoma	15	6	0.0252
Lymph node deposit	37	44	0.0716
Capsule invasion	21	26	0.3160
Tumor necrosis	4	7	0.3349
Poorly differentiated carcinoma	6	9	0.3995
Vascular invasion	4	6	0.5037

(Courtesy of Yamashita H, Noguchi S, Murakami N, et al: Extracapsular invasion of lymph node metastasis is an indicator of distant metastasis and poor prognosis in patients with thyroid papillary carcinoma. *Cancer* 80[12]:2268–2272. Copyright 1997, American Cancer Society. Reprinted by permission of Wiley-Liss, Inc. a subsidiary of John Wiley & Sons, Inc.)

thyroid. The histologic characteristics of papillary carcinoma that develops distant metastasis, however, have not been defined.

Methods.—There were 50 patients with papillary carcinoma of the thyroid in whom distant metastasis developed and 50 control patients without distant metastasis or local recurrence. The histologic findings and prognosis of the patients in these two groups were compared. The group with metastasis and the control group were matched for age, tumor size, and gender ratio. Univariate and multivariate analyses were performed. Mean follow-up was more than 13 years.

Results.—Univariate analysis showed a significantly higher incidence of nonpure papillary carcinoma, absence of bone at the periphery of the tumor, invasion of the perithyroidal muscle, large lymph node deposits, and extranodal invasion in patients who had metastasis (Table 2). Multivariate analysis showed that only extranodal invasion was significant. The odds ratio of extranodal invasion in cases of distant metastasis was 9. Patients with extranodal invasion had a higher risk of death from thyroid carcinoma than those without extranodal invasion.

Discussion.—These results suggest that the presence of extranodal invasion in patients with papillary carcinoma of the thyroid indicates distant metastasis and a poor prognosis.

► This study was based on an emerging theme: the importance of extracapsular lymph node extension (ECLNE) as a poor prognostic marker. In this instance, the tumor of focus is papillary carcinoma of the thyroid. The data (see, for example, the authors' Table 2), appear to be compelling. There are, however, some concerns about this study; three examples follow. This is a retrospective study of 100 patients who were identified on the basis of the absence or presence of distant metastases. The details of how the 50 patients in each group were selected are not fully provided. Further, having had some experience with this type of study, myself, it is difficult to understand how there were no equivocal cases of ECLNE. Finally, the impact of different methods of treatment on the analysis is not entirely clear. Nonetheless, the results are intriguing and worthy of further study by other groups to validate these findings.

M.B. Cohen, M.D.

Thyroid Papillary Carcinoma of Columnar Cell Type: A Clinicopathologic Study of 16 Cases

Wenig BM, Thompson LDR, Adair CF, et al (Armed Forces Inst of Pathology, Washington, DC; Washington Hosp Ctr, Washington, DC)

Cancer 82:740–753, 1998 7–4

Background.—Thyroid papillary carcinoma of columnar cell type is an uncommon histologic variant of papillary carcinoma. It is characterized by its morphologic and aggressive features.

Methods.—Sixteen cases of thyroid papillary carcinoma of columnar cell type were investigated. Clinical records and follow-up data were available for all 16 cases. Paraffin blocks from 15 patients were analyzed histochemically and immunohistochemically. Of the 16 patients, 13 were female and 3 were male. The patients were between 16 and 76 years old.

Results.—The most common clinical symptom was an asymptomatic neck mass. Macroscopically, the tumors ranged from 1.5 cm to 6.5 cm,

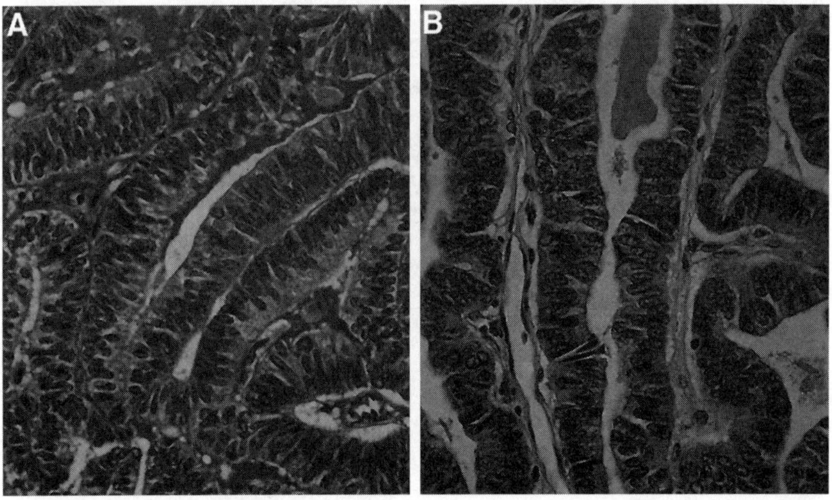

FIGURE 3.—The cytomorphologic characteristics of thyroid papillary carcinoma of columnar cell type include columnar-appearing cells with elongated nuclei showing nuclear stratification. In (**B**), there are hyperchromatic nuclei lying between the columnar cells. (Courtesy of Wenig BM, Thompson LDR, Adair CF, et al: Thyroid papillary carcinoma of columnar cell type: A clinicopathologic study of 16 cases. *Cancer* 82[4]:740–753. Copyright 1998, American Cancer Society. Reprinted by permission of Wiley-Liss, Inc., a subsidiary of John Wiley & Sons, Inc.)

and were circumscribed or encapsulated to infiltrative. Histologically, the growth patterns included papillary, solid, microfollicular, and cribriform. A common pattern consisted of markedly elongated follicles arranged in parallel cords. All patients had colloid-filled follicles. Histologically, the tumors were characterized by elongated cells with nuclear stratification (Fig 3). There were also cells that appeared vacuolated, spindle-shaped cells, and squamoid nests. Limited areas had morphologic features typical of papillary carcinoma of the thyroid. In 14 cases, the tumor was encapsulated, had limited invasive growth, or was microscopic. In 2 cases, extrathyroidal invasion was present. Immunohistochemical studies showed consistent reactivity with cytokeratin and vimentin; varied reactivity with thyroglobulin, epithelial membrane antigen, carcinoembryonic antigen, and LeuM1; and no reactivity with calcitonin or chromogranin. All patients underwent surgical resection, and 8 patients had adjunctive radioactive iodine treatment. Thirteen patients were alive and free of disease or had died of unrelated causes at 2–11 years; the tumor was completely confined to the thyroid gland in these 13 patients. One patient died 4 months after diagnosis secondary to a septic condition. Two patients had an aggressive biologic course; both had extrathyroidal invasion. One of these two patients died of metastatic disease to the lungs at 3 years, and the other was alive with bilateral pulmonary metastases at 9 years.

Discussion.—These results indicate that thyroid papillary carcinoma of columnar cell type is a distinct morphologic type of thyroid papillary carcinoma, but not a distinct clinical type. Its biologic behavior is based on clinical stage; the most important feature is presence or absence of extrathyroidal invasion. Treatment should be based on clinical stage, not morphologic appearance.

▶ This article represents a "victory" for the lumpers; the conclusion clearly states that this morphologically unique variant of papillary carcinoma (see Fig 3) has a biologic behavior similar to that of the usual papillary carcinoma of the thyroid. Consequently, the importance of this variant is of interest chiefly to pathologists. It should be pointed out, though, that the basis for this conclusion cannot necessarily be independently assessed by the reader because primary follow-up data from patients with the usual papillary carcinoma of the thyroid are not provided. The remainder of the study itself, however, including the ancillary staining results, is well done and includes a detailed discussion of the previous literature.

M.B. Cohen, M.D.

Metastatic Tumors of the Thyroid Gland: A Study of 79 Cases in Chinese Patients

Lam KY, Lo CY (Queen Mary Hosp, Hong Kong)

Arch Pathol Lab Med 122:37–41, 1998 7–5

Objective.—Because metastases to the thyroid gland are rare, there are few case reports of such occurrences. The incidence, histology, site of primary tumor, clinical presentation, and course of metastatic lesions in the thyroid gland in a Chinese population over a period of 26 years were studied retrospectively.

Methods.—When autopsy and biopsy reports between 1971 and 1997 from the Queen Mary Hospital in Hong Kong were reviewed for the presence of metastatic thyroid tumors, 79 patients (38 male), aged 12–94, with secondary thyroid tumors were identified.

Results.—About half of the patients were in their 50s and 60s. The incidence of metastatic tumors of the thyroid gland at autopsy was 0.5%, and the incidence at thyroidectomy was 1.2%. Eighteen patients (6 men) were symptomatic and had a mass in the thyroid. Primary tumors were found in the lung (n = 9), lymphoid tissue (n = 3), breast (n = 2), bone (n = 1), uterus (n = 1), nasopharynx (n = 1), and colon (n = 1). Tumors in 6 patients were correctly diagnosed, whereas the other patients were thought to have thyroid tumors (n = 8) or nodular hyperplasia (n = 4). Six patients died before their tumors were diagnosed. Whereas 4 of 5 fine-needle aspiration cytologic examinations demonstrated malignancy, only 2 were specific for metastatic disease. Thyroid metastases were detected either simultaneously (n = 48) or after (n = 24) diagnosis of the primary disease. In 4 patients, thyroid metastases appeared as goiter. Whereas the average time to appearance of thyroid metastases was 9 months, metastatic tumors were detected as long as 7 years after resection of the primary tumor. The 79 lesions were carcinomas in 81% of cases, lymphoid malignancies in 15%, and sarcomas in 4%. Primary sites included lung (n = 34), breast (n = 7), and stomach (n = 6), and more rarely kidney, pancreas, nasopharynx, bladder, liver, cervix, uterus, and placenta. Adenocarcinomas were the most common metastatic cancers, with almost half being moderately or poorly differentiated. Rare secondary cancers included choriocarcinoma, osteosarcoma, malignant phylloides, and nasopharyngeal carcinoma. There were 24 solitary lesions, 8 with diffuse infiltration of the thyroid gland, and 11 multiple lesions. All patients died soon after the metastatic lesions were detected.

Conclusion.—Metastasis to the thyroid gland can be difficult to diagnose. All patients in this study died shortly after metastases were detected.

▶ This retrospective study of both surgical-pathologic (n = 18) and autopsy (n = 61) material describes a single institution's 26-year experience with metastasis to the thyroid. The incidence varied somewhat based on the source, but given the low incidence rates it is hard to be sure if these are significant. Based on the authors' literature review, it is also difficult to compare the incidence with previous reports. In addition, although cytologic and clinical diagnoses of metastasis were apparently considered, it is unclear from the details how they may add (or subtract) from the denominator. By far the most common primary site was the lung (n = 34, including 6 small cell carcinomas), followed by hematopoietic neoplasms (n = 12). The literature would suggest that other common primary sites include breast, kidney, and stomach. Metastatic thyroid disease is uncommon, but the diagnosis should be entertained in the morphologic evaluation of any unusual tumor, especially cytologically.

M.B. Cohen, M.D.

Insular Carcinoma: A Distinct De Novo Entity Among Follicular Carcinomas of the Thyroid Gland

Pilotti S, Collini P, Mariani L, et al (Istituto Nazionale Tumori, Milan, Italy)

Am J Surg Pathol 21:1466–1473, 1997 7–6

Objective.—There appears to be a connection between insular carcinoma and the follicular type of thyroid gland tumors. To determine whether the insular carcinoma entity belonged to the papillary or follicular carcinoma category, a large series of thyroid gland carcinomas were reclassified. Clinicopathologic characteristics of insular carcinomas and widely invasive follicular carcinomas (WIFC) were compared.

Methods.—The clinicopathologic characteristics of 27 patients (8 men), aged 17–69, with insular carcinoma and 29 patients (13 men), aged 28–82 with WIFC, diagnosed and treated between 1975 and 1993, were compared statistically. Patients were followed up until June 1995 or until death. Kaplan-Meier survival curves were constructed and compared, and the association between patient survival and occurrence of visceral metastases was evaluated. Tumor DNA samples from 7 insular carcinoma and 7 WIFC tumors were analyzed for *ras* point mutations using polymerase chain reaction (PCR)–single-strand conformation polymorphism.

Results.—Of the 27 patients with insular carcinomas, 14 had multifocal disease. Sixteen (59%) lesions were pT4, 13 (48%) were pN1, and 12 (44%) were pM1/M1C2. Of the 29 patients with WIFC, 7 had multifocal disease. Two (7%) lesions were pT4, 2 (7%) were pN1, and 19 (66%) were pM1/M1C2. Whereas pT4 and pN1 categories were significantly more common in insular carcinomas than in WIFC, overall, relative, and metastasis-free survival rates were similar for both groups. Age and pathologic pM/MC2 stage were significantly associated with increased survival. Visceral metastases were significantly associated with decreased survival. Five of 8 insular carcinomas assessed by PCR-SSCP showed a *ras* gene family point mutation at codon 61. Three of 8 WIFCs assessed by PCR-SSCP showed an H-*ras* point mutation at codon 61 and 2 had an N-*ras* point mutation at codon 61.

Conclusion.—Insular carcinomas appear to be different from WIFC, although both share *ras* gene family point mutations. WIFC were more often poorly differentiated, whereas pT4 and pN1 categories were significantly more common in insular carcinomas. Survival data were similar for both carcinomas.

► Since the report by Carcangui et al.[1] in 1984, which reintroduced insular carcinoma of the thyroid, there has been particular interest in this relatively rare tumor. In this report, Pilotti et al. describe their experience with 27 such cases. Of particular interest was the molecular analysis of *ras* point mutations in 8 cases. Three of the *ras* genes were sequenced at the 2 common sites for mutations (codons 12/13 and 61). Of importance, mutations were assessed by PCR-SSCP and not direct sequencing. Five of the 8 cases showed a mutation at N61. However, 2 of 8 WIFCs studied also showed this pattern. The conclusion by the authors that insular carcinoma is distinct from WIFC is reasonable but not fully supported by their findings. Additional molecular-based studies into this unusual tumor are needed to help define its biology.

M.B. Cohen, M.D.

Reference

1. Carcangui ML, Zampi G, Rosai J: Poorly differentiated (insular) thyroid carcinoma. *Am J Surg Pathol* 8:655–668, 1984.

8 Head and Neck

Salivary Gland Lymphoid Infiltrates Associated With Lymphoepithelial Lesions: A Clinicopathologic, Immunophenotypic, and Genotypic Study
Quintana PG, Kapadia SB, Bahler DW, et al (Univ of Pittsburgh, Pa)
Hum Pathol 28:850–861, 1997 8–1

Background.—The significance of genotypically documented clonality in distinguishing benign lymphoepithelial lesions (BLEL) from low-grade B-cell lymphomas of mucosa-associated lymphoid tissue (MALT) type in salivary glands has not been established. The clinical implications of a neoplastic diagnosis are also uncertain.

Methods.—The histopathologic features of 68 specimens from 49 patients with at least 1 salivary gland biopsy with lymphoepithelial lesions (LEL) were studied, along with available clinical data. Assessments included paraffin section immunohistochemical stains for κ, λ, CD3, CD20, and CD43; in situ hybridization for κ and λ; and polymerase chain reaction for immunoglobulin HC rearrangement.

Findings.—The specimens included 13 BLEL, 8 BLEL with monocytoid B-cell halos, 24 low-grade B-cell lymphomas of MALT type with confluent zones of monocytoid B-cells or other atypical lymphocytes (ML-MALT), 12 low-grade B-cell lymphomas of MALT type with monoclonal plasma cells, and 4 high-grade B-cell lymphomas of MALT type (MALT-HC). Most often, CD43+ B cells were seen in ML-MALT, though they occurred in all but MALT-HC. Clonal B cells were detected in 5 of 12 BLEL, 5 of 8 BLEL with halos, 17 of 22 ML-MALT, 6 of 10 ML-MALT with plasma cells, and all 3 MALT-HC biopsies (Table 6).

Findings.—Two types of borderline lesions occur in the spectrum of lymphoid proliferations associated with salivary gland LEL. One type has clonal B cells without histologic characteristics of neoplasia, and the other has nonconfluent monocytoid B-cells extending beyond the limits of LEL. The best treatment for the borderline and low-grade lesions has yet to be determined. Why so many of the lymphoproliferative lesions associated with LEL remain localized in the neck is also unknown.

► The criteria are evolving for distinguishing benign LELs from low-grade B-cell lymphomas of MALT. Historically, the presence of an LEL was a histologic indicator of a benign lesion; however, this same morphologic feature is currently 1 criterion for diagnosing MALT-type lymphomas of the

TABLE 6.—Ancillary Studies

Diagnosis	No. of Specimens	Monoclonal by Immunostains (%)*	Monoclonal by In Situ Hybridization (%)*	CD43+ B-cells (%)	No. With Successful Paraffin IgHC PCR†	Monoclonal by Paraffin IgHC PCR (%)	Monoclonal by Any Method (%)‡
1. BLEL	13	0/13 (0)	0/12 (0)	5/12 (42)	12	42	42
2. BLEL-halo	8	0/8 (0)	0/13 (0)	4/8 (50)	8	63	63
3. ML-MALT	24	0/22 (0)	1/22 (5)	19/22 (86)	22	77	77
4. ML-MALT-PC	12	12/12 (100)	10/10 (100)	4/11 (36)	9	67	100
5. MALT-high grade	4	0/4 (0)	0/4 (0)	0/3 (0)	3	100	100

Note: Statistical comparisons showing significance (*P* less than .05): monoclonal by immunostains and ISH: 1 vs 4, 2 vs 4, 3 vs 4, and 4 vs 5; monoclonal by paraffin IgHC: 1 vs 3; monoclonal by any method: 1 vs 3, 1 vs 4, and 2 vs 4; CD43: 1 vs 3, 3 vs 4, and 3 vs 5.

*All monoclonal cases were κ positive. Cases with nonevaluable staining are not included in the denominator.

†No amplification was obtained in 1 ML-MALT-PC.

‡The denominator includes only cases with successful paraffin IgHC PCR, except the ML-MALT-PC category.

Abbreviations: IgHC PCR, immunoglobulin heavy-chain rearrangement by the polymerase chain reaction technique; *BLEL*, benign lymphoepithelial lesions; *ML-MALT*, low-grade B-cell lymphomas of MALT type; *ML-MALT-PC*, low-grade B-cell lymphoma of MALT type with monoclonal plasma cells; *MALT*, mucosa-associated lymphoid tissue; *ISH*, in situ hybridization.

(Courtesy of Quintana PG, Kapadia SB, Bahler DW, et al: Salivary gland lymphoid infiltrates associated with lymphoepithelial lesions: A clinicopathologic, immunophenotypic, and genotypic study. *Hum Pathol* 28:850–861, 1997.)

salivary glands. Additional histologic features in the context of LELs are required for a diagnosis of MALT-type lymphoma. Generally accepted criteria are a dense lymphoid infiltrate accompanied by confluent areas of monocytoid B-cells/centrocyte-like cells, and a dense lymphoid infiltrate accompanied by monoclonality of plasma cells. Polymerase chain reaction (PCR) analysis of immunoglobulin heavy chain gene rearrangements, $CD43^+$ B-cells, and expanded halos of monocytoid B-cells/centrocyte-like cells that surround epimyoepithelial islands are controversial observations that need clinical correlation for determination of their significance in detecting B-cell monoclonality.

This study is well suited for determining the clinical significance of these findings, because very few patients have received treatment. The authors have demonstrated 2 borderline lesions within the spectrum of salivary gland lymphoid infiltrates associated with LELs. One is an LEL with clonal B-cells that lacks atypical histopathologic features. Polymerase chain reaction-detected B-cell monoclonality and $CD43^+$ B-cells were evident in 42% of 12 benign LELs. These cases had no evidence of disseminated lymphoma after a follow-up ranging from 1 to 130 months. The significance of monoclonality detected in these histologically benign infiltrates remains uncertain and is similar to PCR-detected B-cell monoclonality in cases of chronic active gastritis.[1]

LEL with halos of monocytoid B-cells are another borderline entity. PCR-detected B-cell monoclonality was observed in 63% of 8 cases with these morphologic features. In addition, $CD43^+$ B-cells were detected in 50% of these cases. Clinical follow-up, ranging from 6 to 36 months, did not demonstrate dissemination or transformation of lymphoma. However, this follow-up is relatively short for justifying conclusions about the clinical significance of this morphologic feature.

Patients with low-grade MALT-type lymphomas had a higher rate of PCR-detected B-monoclonality (77% of 22 patients). Eighty-six percent of these patients also had $CD43^+$ positive B-cells. The clinical follow-up for these patients was longer (up to 128 months), with only 1 case transforming to a diffuse large-cell lymphoma. In addition, only 1 of the patients with plasmacytic differentiation developed disseminated disease.

By studying a previously untreated group of patients, the indolent natural history of most of these low-grade lesions becomes apparent. Given the indolent clinical course of the low-grade MALT lymphomas occurring in the salivary region, signing out the borderline lesions as an atypical lymphoproliferatives disorder of uncertain significance[2] is probably warranted. Because these low-grade lymphoproliferative lesions may transform to a higher-grade lymphoma or disseminate, clinical follow-up of the borderline lesions and biopsies of persistent or enlarging lesions are advisable.

J.F. Turner, Jr., M.D.

References

1. Hsi ED, Greenson JK, Singleton TP, et al: Detection of immunoglobulin heavy chain gene rearrangement by polymerase chain reaction in chronic active gastritis associated with *Helicobacter pylori*. *Hum Pathol* 27:290–296, 1996.
2. Collins RD: Is clonality equivalent to malignancy: Specifically, is immunoglobulin gene rearrangement diagnostic of malignant lymphoma? *Hum Pathol* 28:757–759, 1997.

Suggested Reading

Diss TC, Wotherspoon AC, Speight P, et al: B-cell monoclonality, Epstein-Barr virus, and t(14;18) in myoepithelial sialadenitis and low-grade B-cell MALT lymphoma of the parotid gland. *Am J Surg Pathol* 19:531–536, 1995.

Hsi ED, Zukerberg LR, Schnitzer B, et al: Development of extrasalivary gland lymphoma in myoepithelial sialadenitis. *Mod Pathol* 8:817–824, 1995.

Basal Cell Adenocarcinoma of the Salivary Glands: Comparison With Basal Cell Adenoma Through Assessment of Cell Proliferation, Apoptosis, and Expression of p53 and *bcl*-2

Nagao T, Sugano I, Ishida Y, et al (Teikyo Univ, Ichihara, Japan; Chiba Cancer Ctr Hosp, Japan)

Cancer 82:439–447, 1998 8–2

Purpose.—Basal cell adenocarcinoma (BCAC) is a newly categorized entity of the World Health Organization classification of salivary gland tumors. This is a rare tumor that is of low-grade malignancy; although it has a relatively high recurrence rate, the prognosis is good. It has some clinical and histologic characteristics in common with basal cell adenoma (BCA). BCAC and BCA were compared in terms of cell proliferative activity; apoptosis; and expression of p53, *bcl*-2, and epidermal growth factor receptor (EGFR).

Methods.—From a surgical series of 1,851 primary tumors of the major salivary gland, 11 cases of BCAC and 9 of BCA were identified. This represented a 0.6% incidence of BCAC. Formalin-fixed, paraffin-embedded specimens of these tumors were studied by immunostaining for Ki-67, p53, *bcl*-2, and EGFR. Terminal deoxynucleotidyl transferase–mediated dUTP-digoxigenin nick end labeling studies were performed to assess apoptosis.

Results.—Of the 11 cases of BCAC, 9 arose in the parotid gland and 2 in the submandibular gland. Recurrences developed in 5 of 10 patients for whom follow-up was available, but none had metastases or died of BCAC. Seventy-five percent of BCAC patients had vascular involvement, 36% had perineural invasion, and 45% had necrosis. Compared with BCAs, the BCACs showed significantly greater cell proliferative activity, Ki-67 labeling index, and apoptotic index. Only BCACs showed more than 4 mitotic figures per 10 high-power fields, or a Ki-67 labeling index of greater than

5%. Fifty-five percent of BCACs were positive for p53 and 27% were positive for EGFR—compared with 100% of BCAs—when 10% positive tumor cells was used as the cutoff point. Whereas all BCAs were strongly positive for *bcl*-2, 27% of BCACs were completely negative.

Conclusions.—Assessment of cell proliferation, apoptosis, and expression of p53, *bcl*-2, and EGFR may help in distinguishing between benign and malignant basal cell tumors of the salivary gland. The findings suggest greater biological activity of BCAC compared with BCA, consistent with the histologic aggressiveness of BCAC.

▶ The BCAC of the salivary gland is a newly recognized entity in the World Health Organization classification of salivary gland tumors. It is considered to be a low-grade malignancy, and morphologically consists of basals cells similar to those seen in BCAs. The diagnostic value of the information from this paper lies in the fact that we rarely see either of these tumor types because they represent such a small fraction of tumors of the salivary gland. Both tumors can assume morphological patterns of solid, trabecular, tubular, and membranous patterns. Thus, the immunohistochemical findings of high Ki-67 labeling index, and labeling for p53 or EGFR favor the more aggressive BCAC.

D.J. Dabbs, M.D.

Immunolocalization of Three Novel Smooth Muscle–specific Proteins in Salivary Gland Pleomorphic Adenoma: Assessment of the Morphogenetic Role of Myoepithelium

Savera AT, Gown AM, Zarbo RJ (Henry Ford Hosp, Detroit; Univ of Washington, Seattle)

Mod Pathol 10:1093–1100, 1997 8–3

Introduction.—Myoepithelial cells of salivary glands have an elaborate cytoskeletal immunophenotype. The immunohistochemical expression of 3 novel monoclonal antibodies (MAbs) to α smooth-muscle actin (α-SMA), smooth-muscle myosin heavy (SMMH) chains, and calponin in formalin-fixed tissues of 65 pleomorphic adenomas was assessed to determine the smooth-muscle phenotype of salivary gland myoepithelium and analyze its contribution to the histogenesis of pleomorphic adenomas.

Methods.—Slides of 65 pleomorphic adenomas were reviewed retrospectively. Fifty-one tumors contained additional surrounding normal salivary gland. Sections 4–5 μm thick were deparaffinized, rehydrated, and subjected to heat-induced epitope retrieval. Sections were incubated with primary antibodies before antibody localization and counterstaining with methyl green.

Results.—There were several varieties of cell types observed: inner-tubular epithelial cells, myoepithelium-like cells (juxtatubular, cuboidal, and spindle), modified myoepithelium (myxoid, chondroid, and hyaline), and transformed myoepithelium (solid epithelioid, squamous, and basaloid-cribriform). The periancinar and periductal myoepithelial cells of all 51 normal salivary glands were diffusely stained by all 3 MAbs; all ancinar/ductal epithelial cells tested negative. Sixty-one (94%) of pleomorphic adenomas reacted to all 3 MAbs. The inner-tubular epithelial cells were stained by any of the smooth muscle markers. The α-SMA and SMMH MAbs were primarily limited to the myoepithelium-like cells. The modified and transformed myoepithelia lacked these myofilaments. Calponin was observed in 64 tumors (98%) and reacted to nearly all of the myoepithelium-like cells, 60% of modified myoepithelium, and 30% of transformed myoepithelium.

Conclusion.—These findings extend the smooth muscle phenotype characterization of normal and neoplastic myoepithelium and broaden the role of myoepithelium in the histogenesis of pleomorphic adenomas. The 3 smooth muscle markers, especially calponin, might be helpful in various aspects of diagnostic surgical pathology of the breast and salivary gland.

▶ SMMH chain and calponin are new antibody names to remember because they will have far-reaching consequences for diagnostic surgical pathologists. More specific than α-SMA, these antibodies are very important for at least 2 reasons: (1) they allow us to visualize the amazing morphological arrays that myoepithelial cells can take, especially in salivary gland neoplasms, and (2) the absence of myoepithelial cells is associated with certain morphological malignant conditions, and the use of these antibodies can only help in increasing the sensitivity when looking for these cells. Important current uses could include the examination of breast lesions for myoepithelial cells.

D.J. Dabbs, M.D.

Suggested Reading

Wang NP, Wan BC, Skelly M, et al: Antibodies to novel myoepithelium associated proteins distinguish benign lesions and carcinoma in situ from invasive carcinoma of the breast. *Appl Immunohistochem* 5:141–151, 1997.

Lymphoepithelial Cysts of Salivary Glands: An Immunohistochemical Study of HIV-related and HIV-unrelated Lesions

Maiorano E, Favia G, Viale G (Univ of Bari, Italy; Univ of Milan, Italy)

Hum Pathol 29:260–265, 1998 8–4

Introduction.—Patients infected by the human immunodeficiency virus may be affected by different diseases of the secretory component or the intraparenchymal lymph nodes of the salivary glands. Some typical features include xerostomia and salivary gland lymphoid infiltration in these patients, who may be affected by a distinct clinicopathologic entity characterized by multiple cysts lined by epithelial and lymphoid cells arising in the parotid glands. Little is known about the pathogenesis of lymphoepithelial cysts. To assess the possible morphological and immunohistochemical similarities of cystic lesions in HIV-positive and HIV-negative patients, lymphoepithelial cysts from HIV-positive and HIV-negative patients were evaluated.

Methods.—There were 6 HIV-positive patients and 5 HIV-negative patients whose lymphoepithelial cysts were examined. The paraffin sections were immunostained. Macroscopic features, histologic features, and immunohistochemistry features were compared.

Results.—In HIV-positive and HIV-negative patients, the lymphoepithelial cysts have similar histological and immunohistochemical features, which may simultaneously affect the salivary gland parenchyma and the intrasalivary lymph nodes. A diffuse lymphoid infiltrate is invariably observed in the glandular tissue around lymphoepithelial cysts and is consistently associated with ectatic changes of the striated ducts. The proliferation fraction of the epithelial cells in lymphoepithelial cysts is comparable to that of epithelial cells in salivary retention cysts, indicating that the expansion of the epithelial compartment may be secondary to the accumulation of the lymphoid cell component, which may represent the initial trigger of lymphoepithelial cysts.

Conclusion.—Cyst formation is most likely secondary to the obstruction of salivary ducts by exuberant lymphoid infiltration, as evidenced by the finding of an equivalent proliferation fraction of the epithelial compartment in lymphoepithelial cysts and salivary retention cysts. Direct viral infection of salivary glands has been repeatedly postulated, but never definitely ascertained.

▶ Even though the histopathologic features of lymphoepithelial cysts in these groups of patients parallel each other, the lymphoepithelial cysts in HIV-positive patients were larger and more numerous. In the larger cysts of HIV-positive patients, lymphoid follicles had a spectrum of atrophy, with increasing numbers of T-suppressor cells compared to T-helper cells. Otherwise, the morphologic features are quite similar. It is hypothesized that whatever stimulates the lymphoid proliferation, the lymphoid proliferation causes ductal obstruction and cyst formation.

D.J. Dabbs, M.D.

Suggested Reading

Ihrler S, Zietz C, Riederer A, et al: HIV-related parotid lymphoepithelial cysts: Immunohistochemistry and 3-D reconstruction of surgical and autopsy material with special reference to formal pathogenesis. *Virchows Arch* 429:139–147, 1996.

Clonal Salivary Gland Infiltrates Associated With Myoepithelial Sialadenitis (Sjögren's Syndrome) Begin as Nonmalignant Antigen-selected Expansions

Bahler DW, Swerdlow SH (Univ of Pittsburgh, Pa)

Blood 91:1864–1872, 1998 8–5

Background.—Reactive myoepithelial sialadenitis (MESA) occurs in Sjögren's syndrome and is believed to be a precursor to mucosa-associated lymphoid tissue (MALT) lymphomas. Exogenous antigens or autoantigens have been implicated in the pathogenesis by causing B-cell proliferation and encouraging B-cell transformation. However, monoclonal B cells are also found in histologically benign tissues from MESA-associated salivary glands. This study examined VH genes from patients with MESA or MALT to determine whether monoclonal B cells in MESA-associated lesions represent early MALT lymphoma or are merely a benign expansion, and to determine any role of antigen stimulation in MESA-associated clones.

Methods.—Seven patients with MESA, MESA with halos of monocytoid cells, or low-grade MALT lymphoma provided biopsy specimens. Follow-up biopsy of contralateral sites was performed from 3 to 122 months after the initial procedure. VH genes were amplified from DNA by electrophoresis and were cloned and sequenced by polymerase chain reaction.

Findings.—In 3 cases, the polyclonal B cells present in the first specimen were also present in the subsequent specimen. In 3 cases, single clones in the follow-up specimen were different from those in the initial sample. And in 1 case, there were 2 clones in the second biopsy specimen, and 1 of these differed from the clone in the initial sample. Thus, 11 distinct clones were identified. Three of these clones were derived from a V3-7 VH gene segment and 8 were derived from a V1-69 VH gene segment (5 with homology to the 51p1 gene and 3 with homology to allelic variant 7M27, which differs from the 51p1 gene by 1 nucleotide). Gene restriction was evident, in that 10 of 11 VH gene segments used a J4 segment and 8 of 11 gene segments used D segments. Seven of 11 clones also conserved amino acids in the CDR3 sequences, with evidence of N nucleotides at the VH-D junction. VH mutations showed significant intraclonal heterogeneity, with many noncommon mutations and few replacement mutations. VH mutation rates in samples of MALT lymphoma were more than twice as high as mutation rates in benign MESA-associated lesions (1.8 vs. 074).

Conclusion.—The similarities in VH gene expression and in CDR3 sequences and the marked VH gene restriction make it likely that MESA-associated clones would bind the same or similar antigens. Thus, a possible pathogenetic scenario is that stimulation of appropriate VH gene structures by immunoglobulin binding to a common antigen causes B cell expansion. Early, nonmalignant clones appear to be more likely to be found in MESA-associated lesions that are histologically more benign.

► The lesions we recognize as MESA appear benign histologically. As a MALT lymphoma, the MESA is similar pathogenetically to the MALT lymphomas that occur in the stomach in association with *Helicobacter* infection. This current study of the clonality of lymphoid cells in the MESA is genetic evidence that a clonal dysplastic process has begun but is not recognizable morphologically. Indeed, the MALT lymphomas of the stomach, in their earliest stages, may represent a benign histomorphology with abundant benign-appearing lymphoid follicles.

This information adds to the knowledge of our understanding of the neoplastic progression in lymphoma genesis. Nevertheless, just as we now know the importance of eradicating *Helicobacter* to head off the process of lymphoma genesis, these findings tell us of the importance of treating and eradicating the immunoinflammatory reactions of this syndrome. This information also should alter the rules by which we identify malignancy. Traditionally, the identification of clonal cell lines, particularly on lymphoid lesions, has been heralded as a sign of malignancy. However, we now know that clonal cell lines can be generated via antigen selection, and, thus, probably represent a dysplastic step in the progression to malignant behavior and malignant histomorphology.

D.J. Dabbs, M.D.

Homologous Carcinomas of the Breasts, Skin, and Salivary Glands: A Histologic and Immunohistochemical Comparison of Ductal Mammary Carcinoma, Ductal Sweat Gland Carcinoma, and Salivary Duct Carcinoma

Wick MR, Ockner DM, Mills SE, et al (Washington Univ, St Louis; Univ of Virginia, Charlottesville)

Am J Clin Pathol 109:75–94, 1998 8–6

Introduction.—The morphologic mimicry among malignant neoplasms is a well-recognized phenomenon in surgical pathology. Both undifferentiated and committed neoplasms can demonstrate this trait. Adenocarcinomas of the breast, sweat glands, and salivary glands are almost identical under light microscopic analysis. The histological identity in this group of tumors is also mirrored in part by biochemical similarity. One hundred three homologous carcinomas of the breast, skin, and salivary glands underwent microscopic and immunohistochemical examination to codify points of potential pathologic similarity and difference.

Findings.—All lesions had characteristic, irregularly permeative clusters and cords of atypical polygonal cells with variable luminal differentiation. A proportion of primary neoplasms in each site revealed in situ ductal components. It was not possible to make topography-related morphologic distinctions among these neoplasms without these components. Immunostaining for gross cytic disease fluid protein-15, carcinoembryonic antigen, S100 protein, c-erb-B-2 oncoprotein, estrogen receptor protein, and progesterone receptor protein also revealed largely overlapping phenotypes in all 3 tumor categories, with some exceptions. These differences were clarified through paired x^2 analysis, and included a significant infrequency of gross cystic disease fluid protein-15 in eccrine sweat gland carcinomas, a paucity of carcinoembryonic antigen in breast cancers, and an absence of estrogen receptor protein in salivary duct carcinomas.

Conclusion.—These findings may be beneficial in predefined differential diagnostic settings involving the distinction between primary and metastatic ductal cancers of the breast, skin, and salivary glands. The striking homologies among such tumors at structural and protein-synthetic levels of comparison demand that all available clinicopathologic information be used in this context.

► Because of the minor immunohistochemical differences among these 3 groups of tumors, which may appear virtually identical in tissue, careful histologic examination with inclusion of an abundance of clinical information is critical to arriving at the correct diagnosis. Using antibodies to carcinoembryonic antigen, gross cystic disease fluid protein-15, and estrogen receptor protein, a few statistically significant differences among these 3 tumor types surface. One should not, however, rely solely on the mathematics here. We need to develop more solid, definitive cell markers to distinguish these tumors reliably by immunohistochemical means.

D.J. Dabbs, M.D.

Molecular Analysis of Oral Lichen Planus: A Premalignant Lesion?

Zhang L, Michelsen C, Cheng X, et al (Univ of British Columbia, Vancouver; Simon Fraser Univ, Burnaby, BC; British Columbia Cancer Research Centre, Vancouver)

Am J Pathol 151:323–327, 1997 8–7

Introduction.—Oral lichens planus (OLP) is a common oral musosal disease that has been labeled as premalignant by the World Health Organization. Others contend that only lichenoid lesions with dysplasia are precancerous. Tumor suppressor genes are important in carcinogenesis. Their function must be lost if tumorigenesis is to occur. Allelic loss occurs in premalignant oral lesions, particularly on chromosome arms 3p, 9p, and 17p. Loss of heterozygosity (LOH) at 3p and 9p is associated with cancer risk. Microsatellite analysis was used to evaluate LOH at 3p, 9p, and 17p in OLP to determine whether OLP without dysplasia is premalignant.

Methods.—Specimens from archival paraffin blocks from 33 patients with OLP were assessed for allelic loss at 9 loci located on chromosomes 3p, 9p, and 17p. A set of specimens of oral dysplasias (10 mild, 11 moderate, 16 severe/carcinoma in situ), 22 oral squamous cell carcinomas, and 29 oral reactive lesions were also analyzed.

Results.—Loss of heterozygosity was observed in specimens as follows: 6% of OLP, 14% of reactive lesions, 40% of mild dysplasia, 46% of moderate dysplasia, 81% of severe dysplasia/carcinoma in situ, and 91%

of squamous cell carcinomas. LOH was seen on only a single arm in OLP and reactive lesions. It occurred on more than 1 chromosome in dysplasia and cancer. The frequency of this multiple LOH was significantly correlated with increasing degrees of dysplasia and progression into squamous cell carcinoma.

Conclusion.—These genetic findings indicate that OLP is not a lesion at risk for malignant transformation. The question remains whether OLP has an intrinsic tendency to become malignant vs. being a fertile ground for malignancy.

▶ The question asked in this study is, Is OLP a premalignant lesion, superceding squamous cell carcinoma of the oral cavity? The answer is important because OLP has a prevalence of approximately 1% in the general population. This question has been answered by genetic studies of LOH in OLP, compared with that of other reactive oral lesions and the entire spectrum of dysplasia from mild to severe. The results indicate that LOH is even less frequent in OLP than in reactive lesions, which does not support the idea of OLP as a premalignant lesion. The most important aspect of this study is the fact that the control samples were from reactive, dysplastic, and neoplastic lesions, supporting the premise that there are no more molecular abnormalities in OLP (in fact, there are less) than in reactive lesions.

D.J. Dabbs, M.D.

Suggested Reading

Holmstrup P: The controversy of a premalignant potential of oral lichen planus is over. *Oral Surg* 73:704–706, 1992.

Loval JGL, Harsanyi BBV, ElGeneidy AK: Oral lichenoid dysplasia: A clinicopathologic analysis. *Oral Surg* 68:57–63, 1989.

Epstein-Barr Virus Infection Is Associated With p53 Accumulation in Nasopharyngeal Carcinoma

Gulley ML, Burton MP, Allred DG, et al (Univ of Texas, San Antonio; Audie L Murphy Mem Veteran's Hosp, San Antonio, Tex; Univ of Hong Kong; et al)
Hum Pathol 29:252–259, 1998 8–8

Introduction.—In most patients with nasopharyngeal carcinoma, Epstein-Barr virus is found within the malignant cells, evidence that viral infection precedes malignant transformation. Nasopharyngeal carcinoma may also be associated with defects in the p53 oncoprotein. The association between Epstein-Barr virus infection and p53 accumulation in nasopharyngeal carcinoma was investigated.

Methods.—Using in situ hybridization to EBER1 transcripts, 83 patients with nasopharyngeal carcinoma were evaluated for the presence of Epstein-Barr virus. Immunostains using the D07 antibody, which detects native and mutant forms of the p53 protein, were used to detect p53 expression. There was histopathological diagnosis, detection of viral BZLF1 protein by immunohistochemistry, and statistical analysis. Eighteen potential premalignant lesions of the surface epithelium of the nasopharynx were also examined.

Results.—There were 77% of patients coexpressing both markers, demonstrating a highly significant association between Epstein-Barr virus infection and p53 overexpression. With respect to p53 accumulation, Epstein-Barr virus is not an innocent bystander. BZLF1 is not the factor responsible for p53 accumulation, judging by BZLF1's absence of colonization with p53 in these tumors. In the transition from metaplasia to carcinoma in situ, p53 accumulation might precede Epstein-Barr virus infection.

Conclusion.—There was a strong correlation between the presence of Epstein-Barr virus and the accumulation of p53 in nasopharyngeal carcinoma. To dissect stepwise progression of nasopharyngeal carcinogenesis, further studies are needed. Nasopharyngeal carcinomas from nonendemic and endemic regions of the world showed biological differences in tumor histology. These biological differences may underlie epidemiological variations in tumor prevalence.

The Clinical Importance of Cystic Squamous Cell Carcinomas in the Neck: A Study of 136 Cases

Thompson LDR, Heffner DK (Armed Forces Inst of Pathology, Washington, DC)

Cancer 82:944–956, 1998 8–9

Introduction.—The preoperative and operative diagnostic impression of squamous cell carcinomas discovered in the upper neck is often that of a branchial cleft cyst. A previous study concluded that bronchiogenic carcinomas may be cystic metastases in the neck from a tonsillary primary. A large series of patients were examined to determine whether the anatomic site of the primary carcinoma that produced the neck metastasis had a tonsillary primary, and whether the site can be predicted on the basis of the histologic features.

Methods.—There were 136 patients with cervical cystic squamous cell carcinoma in a 20-year period, with most having masses in the upper neck, involving the jugular digastric lymph nodes. Identification of a primary site and type of treatment received were recorded. A review was conducted of hematoxylin and eosin-stained slides for all patients. Histologic features were also reviewed.

Results.—The primary sites were found to be in the lingual or faucial tonsil in 64% of those patients where the primary site was discovered subsequently. The nasopharyngeal tonsillar tissue was the primary site for an additional 8% of patients. There generally was a difference in histologic appearance between those cases that did not originate in Waldeyer's tonsillar ring and those with tonsillar origins. Within an average of 12.4

months, the tonsillar primaries were discovered, but many were not found for up to 11 years. Most primaries were small, which indicated that there was a slower growth rate than is usually seen in squamous cell carcinomas. Patients with metastatic squamous cell carcinomas of other upper airway mucosal sites had a worse prognosis than those with carcinomas in the tonsillar region.

Conclusion.—The origin of the primary site in most patients with prominently cystic squamous cell carcinomas in the upper neck will be in faucial or lingual tonsillar crypt epithelium. More tailored therapy is possible with knowledge of the probable site of origin, allowing patients to be treated conservatively with surgical excision and subsequent field-limited radiation therapy. The 5-year survival with such treatment is 77%. Branchiogenic carcinoma was not found in any of the patients.

▶ With a thorough review of the literature and a consideration of the cases described by these authors, it seems that squamous cell carcinoma arriving in a branchiogenic cyst does not exist. Cystic squamous lesions in the upper neck may be very well differentiated, yet show accompanying evidence of squamous cell carcinoma as well. These lesions have previously been interpreted as demonstrating the development of squamous cell carcinoma in a branchiogenic cyst. However, as this article has convincingly demonstrates, almost all of these patients have a primary squamous cell carcinoma of low grade present in the faucial tonsil or lingual tonsil. In a significant proportion of such cases, the primary may be so small as to be occult, and may not even manifest itself for years. Thus, the indolent nature of many of these tumors is clear. All of the illustrations show convincing squamous carcinoma, particularly on a cytomorphologic basis. All of this means, of course, that needle aspiration of cystic lesions in the upper neck which show squamous epithelium would need to be completely excised for definitive diagnosis, except in the occasional case that shows poorly differentiated squamous carcinoma.

D.J. Dabbs, M.D.

9 Soft Tissue and Bone

Immunohistochemical and Molecular Genetic Approaches to Soft Tissue Tumor Diagnosis: A Primer

Hibshoosh H, Lattes R (Columbia Univ, New York)

Semin Oncol 24:515–525, 1997 9–1

Introduction.—In the past 2 decades, there have been incredible advances in the ability to detect patterns of differentiation and molecular events associated with neoplasia through an expanding list of immunohistochemical and molecular markers linked to histopathologically defined subtypes of tumors. These markers provide new insights and approaches to the classification of tumors, with important prognostic and/or therapeutic implications. The potentially diagnostic immunohistochemical and molecular markers of soft-tissue tumors were reviewed.

Markers of Soft-Tissue Tumors.—The immunohistochemical markers examined included vimentin, cytokeratin, desmin, HHF35, S100, myoD1, alpha 1–antitrypsin, vascular markers (factor VIII, CD31, CD34), MIC2, and others. Potentially diagnostic chromosomal translocations and associated genes detected in soft-tissue tumors include Ewing's/PNET, t(11;22) (q24;q12) (FLI-1;EWS), t(21;22) (q22;q12) (ERG;EWS); t(7;22) (p22;q12) (EVT1;EWS); desmoplastic small round cell tumor t(11;22) (p13;q12) (WT1;EWS); extraskeletal myxoid chondrosarcoma t(9;22) (q22;q12), TEC(CHN);EWS); malignant ectomesenchymoma t(11;22) (q24;12) (FLI1;EWS); alveolar rhabdomyosarcoma t(2;13) (q35;q14) (PAX-3;FKHR); t(1;13) (p36;q14) (PAX-7;FKHR); myxoid and round cell liposarcoma t(12;16) (q13;p11) (CHOP;TLS(FUS)); synovial sarcoma t(X;18) (p11;q11) (SSX1 and 2;SYT), and others.

Use of Markers.—The markers listed have been used to help confirm and substantiate relationships between certain types of tumors. Specific molecular markers are linked to histopathologically defined subtypes of tumors.

Conclusion.—Molecular markers expand the body of knowledge regarding soft-tissue tumors. These markers have potential diagnostic, prognostic, and/or therapeutic implications. The specificity and utility of molecular markers need further definition.

► This is an excellent summary/primer update of the latest in immunohistochemical knowledge and genetic abnormalities present in the entire World

Health Organization classification of soft-tissue tumors. I will keep a copy of it in the folder next to my microscope for quick reference.

D.J. Dabbs, M.D.

Core Needle Biopsy for Diagnosis of Extremity Soft Tissue Sarcoma
Heslin MJ, Lewis JJ, Woodruff JM, et al (Mem Sloan-Kettering Cancer Ctr, New York)
Ann Surg Oncol 4:425–431, 1997 9–2

Background.—Open biopsy is traditionally used for diagnosis of extremity masses suspicious for soft-tissue sarcoma. The disadvantages of this technique are cost, time, and morbidity. The advantages of core needle biopsy are minimal morbidity, cost, and time. However, the diagnostic accuracy of core needle biopsy has not been reliably established under these circumstances. The diagnostic accuracy of core needle biopsy was compared to that of open biopsy for the diagnosis of primary extremity masses suspicious for soft tissue sarcoma.

Study Design.—From 1990 through 1995, 164 patients with extremity masses suspicious for soft-tissue sarcoma were biopsied at a single institution. Two patients in this group underwent both types of biopsies. Of these 164 patients, 111 were derived from a prospective soft-tissue sarcoma database and 55 with a benign diagnosis were derived from a clinical information center. Pathology reports were reviewed. Statistical analyses were performed only for adequate biopsy specimens.

Findings.—For this group of 164 patients, the initial diagnostic approach was 60 core needle, 44 incisional, 36 frozen section, and 26 excisional biopsies. Two patients underwent 2 biopsy procedures. Of the core needle biopsy specimens, 93% were adequate for diagnosis. Of these adequate specimens, 95% correlated with the final resection diagnosis for malignancy, 88% for grade, and 75% for histologic subtype (Table 2). Of the frozen section biopsy specimens, 94% were adequate for diagnosis. Of these adequate specimens, 88% correlated with the final resection diagnosis for malignancy, 62% for grade, and 47% for histologic subtype. The false-negative rate for core needle biopsy was 5% and the false-positive

TABLE 2.—Overall Results of Biopsies

	Core	Incisional	Frozen section
n	60	45	36
Adequate (%)	93	100	94
Correct malignancy (%)	95	100	88
Correct grade (%)	88	96	62[a]
Correct histology (%)	75	84	47[a]

(Courtesy of Heslin MJ, Lewis JJ, Woodruff JM, et al: Core needle biopsy for diagnosis of extremity soft tissue sarcoma. *Ann Surg Oncol* 4:425–431, 1997.

TABLE 4.—Comparison of Biopsy Type for Grade of Adequate, Sarcoma Biopsy Specimens

Biopsy	Resection	Core (n = 40)	Incisional (n = 36)	Frozen section (n = 7)
High grade	High grade	17	23	3
High grade	Low grade	1	0	0
Low grade	High grade	2	1	1
Low grade	Low grade	20	13	3
Sensitivity (%)		89	96	
Specificity (%)		95	100	
Accuracy (%)		93	97	
Positive predictive value (%)		94	100	
Negative predictive value (%)		91	93	

Note: One core needle biopsy specimen and 1 incisional biopsy specimen (both from the same patient) could not be graded because of extensive necrosis. Grade could not be determined on 10 frozen section biopsy samples, and these were therefore excluded from analysis. Because of small numbers in the frozen section biopsy group, no analysis was performed.

(Courtesy of Heslin MJ, Lewis JJ, Woodruff JM, et al: Core needle biopsy for diagnosis of extremity soft tissue sarcoma. *Ann Surg Oncol* 4:425–431, 1997. Copyright © the Society of Surgical Oncology, Inc.)

rate was 0%. Two core needle biopsy specimens that were graded low were actually high and 1 graded high was actually low (Table 4).

Conclusions.—When read by an experienced pathologist, core needle biopsy is accurate for the preoperative diagnosis and grading of extremity

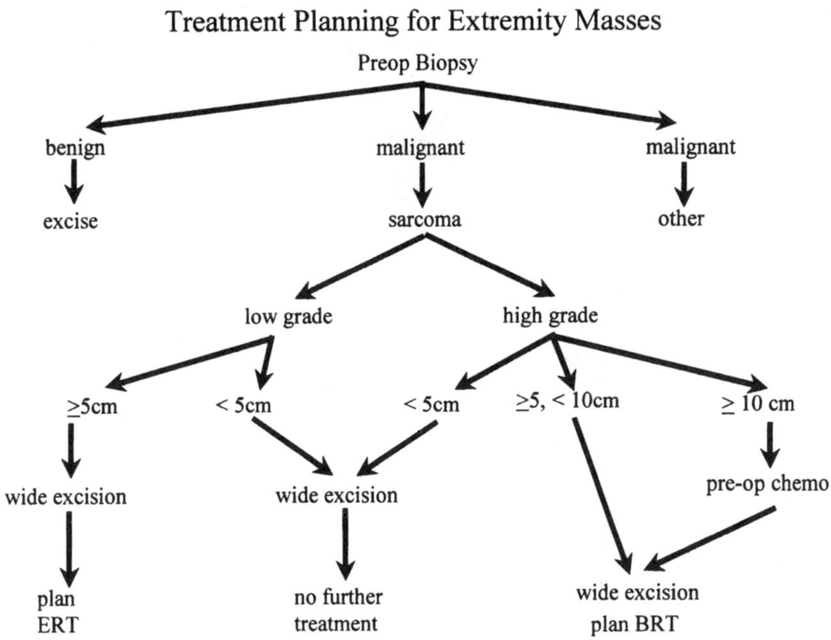

FIGURE 1.—Treatment planning for extremity masses suspicious for soft-tissue sarcoma at Memorial Sloan-Kettering Cancer Center. *Abbreviations: pre-op*, preoperative; *ERT*, external beam radiation therapy; *BRT*, brachytherapy. (Courtesy of Heslin MJ, Lewis JJ, Woodruff JM, et al: Core needle biopsy for diagnosis of extremity soft tissue sarcoma. *Ann Surg Oncol* 4:425–431, 1997. Copyright © the Society of Surgical Oncology, Inc.)

masses suspicious for soft-tissue sarcoma. If adequate tissue sampling cannot be achieved, open biopsy is required.

▶ With experience, a very high sensitivity, specificity, and positive predictive and negative predictive values can be obtained with the core biopsy for the primary diagnosis and treatment strategies of soft-tissue sarcomas. The results are excellent and comparable to those of open biopsy. This article does not address the use of fine needle aspiration biopsy, another technique, in the treatment strategy of patients with soft-tissue sarcomas. With respect to the treatment planning for patients (Fig 1), the results of this procedure are accurate and very efficient. To see how fine needle aspiration biopsies may complement this procedure, consult the suggested readings.

D.J. Dabbs, M.D.

Suggested Readings

Ackerman WH, Carlin B: Fine needle aspiration in the diagnosis of soft tissue tumors: A review of 22 years experience. *Cytopathology* 6:236–247, 1995.

Ayala AG, Ro JY, Fanning CV, et al: Core needle biopsy and fine needle aspiration in the diagnosis of bone and soft tissue lesions. *Hematol Oncol Clin North Am* 9:633–651, 1995.

Evaluation of Newer Prognostic Markers for Adult Soft Tissue Sarcomas

Levine EA, Holzmayer T, Bacus S, et al (Univ of Illinois, Chicago; Cell Analysis Systems, Elmhurst, Ill; Louisiana State Univ, New Orleans)

J Clin Oncol 15:3249–3257, 1997 9–3

Objective.—New molecular markers for soft tissue sarcomas (STS), including MDR-1 mRNA, *p*-glycoprotein (P-gp), Ki-67 expression, and DNA content expression, may improve prognosis. The ability of MDR-1/P-gp expression in adult STS, either singly or in combination with other known prognostic markers, to improve prognosis was evaluated.

Methods.—Specimens of STS from 65 patients (31 women), aged 13–80, were subjected to UIC-2 staining. DNA and MDR-1 mRNA were analyzed, and Ki-67 expression was determined. Patients were followed up on average for 83 months. Kaplan-Meier survival curves and 5-year survival rates were calculated and compared using the log rank test.

Results.—There were 9 stage I, 12 stage II, 23 stage III, and 11 stage IV tumors. Respective 5-year survival rates were 87%, 22%, 44%, and 16%. The rate differences were significant between all stages. The median survival times were 48 months for stage II, 39 months for stage III, and 23 months for stage IV tumors; the median survival for stage I tumors has not been reached. Overall survival and disease-free survival for patients with stage II and III disease are significantly better for P-gp–negative tumors. Patients with low MDR-1 mRNA expression had significantly better overall disease-free and 5-year survival rates than did patients with no expression. The survival rates of this latter group were significantly better than for patients with high expression. Patients with diploid tumors had significantly higher overall and 5-year survival rates than did patients with aneuploid tumors (51% and 52% vs. 31% and 27%). Patients with low Ki-67 expression had significantly longer overall and 5-year disease-free survival than did patients with high expression.

Conclusion.—P-gp expression and MDR-1 expression were found in 48% and 51% of adults with STS. Higher AJCC, aneuploidy, high Ki-67 expression, and P-gp expression were prognostic for a poor outcome.

► The identification of prognostic markers (i.e., those that predict outcome independent of treatment) is one of the major foci in tumor biology. Soft tissue tumors, despite their relative rarity, are no exception. This study highlights some of the difficulties in carrying out such studies. In this study the authors examined DNA ploidy, immunohistochemical markers (P-gp and Ki-67), and mRNA expression of MDR-1, in addition to staging. It is worth pointing out that staging of soft tissue tumors incorporates grading. The series of tumors examined was small (65 patients), and not all of the markers were performed on all of the patients. Further, but not unexpectedly, there were various histologic types, but only 7 were malignant fibrous histiocytomas, and several tumors that are not necessarily malignant (e.g., desmoid) were also examined. Examination of some of the markers was on frozen tissue, which limits applicability to other laboratories. Also of some concern, no pathologists were included in the study. Although statistically significant differences were identified, there was presumably overlap in the results, but the data are not provided; most of the data consists of Kaplan-Meier curves. Most important in this regard is the use of markers to the individual patient. Prognostic marker analysis is still a treacherous area. Hayes et al. provide one of the best articles in this regard.[1]

M.B. Cohen, M.D.

Reference

1. Hayes DF, Bast RC, Desch CE, et al: Tumor marker utility grading system: A framework to evaluate clinical utility of tumor markers. *J Natl Cancer Inst* 88:1456–1466, 1996.

Loss of RB and MTS1/CDKN2 (p16) Expression in Human Sarcomas

Cohen JA, Geradts J (Univ of North Carolina, Chapel Hill)

Hum Pathol 28:893–898, 1997 9–4

Introduction.—In the development of neoplasia, the loss of cell cycle control is a critical step. The loss of proliferation control has been linked to mutations in tumor-suppressor genes in a variety of tumors. In many types of carcinomas and other malignancies, loss of functional p16 or retinoblastoma protein (pRB) is frequent, and in some tumor types, the expression of both proteins may be inversely related. In human sarcomas, pRB and p16 may play an important role. The rate of disturbance in the p16/pRB pathway in aggressive mesenchyma neoplasms was determined.

Methods.—An immunohistochemical approach was used to analyze 59 primary, recurrent, or metastatic sarcomas and 23 lesions, with features of fibromatoses and other spindle cell neoplasms of low malignant potential, to determine whether p16 or pRB was abnormally expressed. Excisional biopsy and resection specimens were used. The histology of each specimen was reviewed.

Results.—In 16 of 59 sarcomas, p16 was abnormally expressed and in 14 of 59 sarcomas, pRB was abnormally expressed. The overall abnormality rate was 51%. There was a histologic variance of specific rates of abnormalities. Leiomyosarcomas were most commonly affected by loss of either tumor-suppressor gene product. There was no significant correlation between overall grade, mitotic grade, or tumor progressor for sarcomas and p16 or pRB. Abnormal p16 expression was not displayed in fibromatoses or other spindle cell neoplasms of low malignant potential. Loss of pRB was seen in 4 of 23 sarcomas that had fibromatoses or other spindle cell neoplasms of low malignant potential.

Conclusion.—One of the most common abnormalities in human sarcomas is loss of expression of these 2 tumor-suppressor genes.

▶ The all-important late G1 cell cycle check point is controlled by a complex of proteins, which includes p16, the product of the MTS1/CDKN2 gene, cyclin D1, CDK4/6, and pRB, the product of the retinoblastoma gene. The loss of functional p16 or pRB is common in many types of carcinomas and other malignancies, including malignant mesothelioma, pancreatic adenocarcinoma, and glioblastoma. The authors discover that more than 50% of sarcomas of high-grade type over-express either p16 or pRB by immunohistochemistry. The findings should open an avenue of investigation that includes the investigation of sarcoma mimics for p16 and pRB. This may turn out to be a fruitful approach to distinguishing sarcoma mimics (which, theoretically, should not contain over-expressed p16 or pRB) from sarcomas. Such studies are currently in progress—for example, examining the RB locus in osteosarcomas, to differentiate certain osteosarcomas from myositis ossificans.

D.J. Dabbs, M.D.

Suggested Reading

Belchis DA, Meece CA, Benko FA, et al: Loss of heterozygosity and microsatellite instability at the retinoblastoma locus in osteosarcomas. *Diagn Mol Pathol* 5:214–219, 1996.

Solitary Fibrous Tumor of Soft Tissue: A Report of 15 Cases, Including 5 Malignant Examples With Light Microscopic, Immunohistochemical, and Ultrastructural Data

Nielsen GP, O'Connell JX, Dickersin GR, et al (Harvard Med School, Boston; Vancouver Hosp, British Columbia)

Mod Pathol 10:1028–1037, 1997 9–5

Introduction.—Solitary fibrous tumors (SFTs), first described in 1931, are now thought to develop from submesothelial connective tissue cells. Recent studies have reported benign SFTs arising in soft tissues. In a review

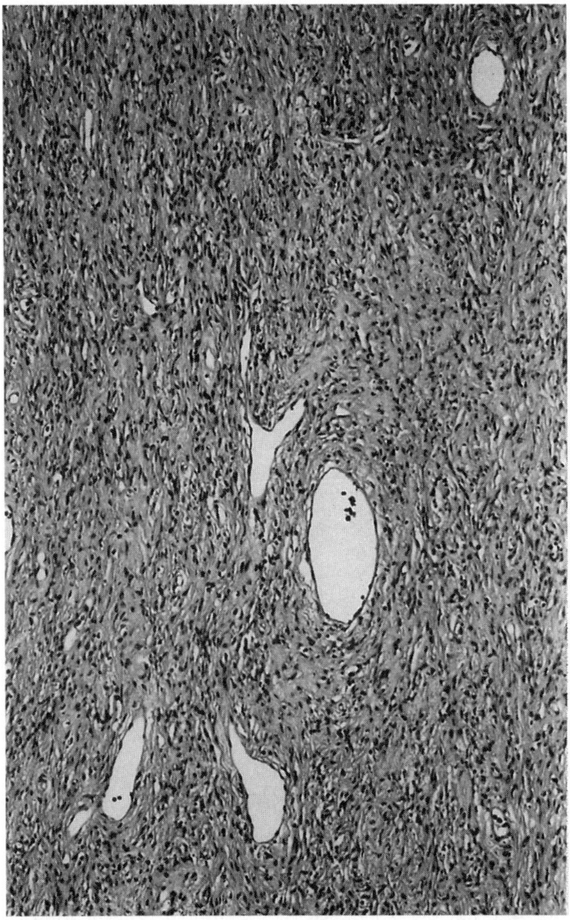

FIGURE 2.—Benign SFT. Bland spindle-shaped cells separated by extracellular collagen. There is prominent vascularity with a branching vessel in the center. *Abbreviation: SFT*, solitary fibrous tumor. (Courtesy of Nielsen GP, O'Connell JX, Dickersin GR, et al: Solitary fibrous tumor of soft tissue: A report of 15 cases, including 5 malignant examples with light microscopic, immunohistochemical, and ultrastructural data. *Mod Pathol* 10[10]:1028–1037, 1997.)

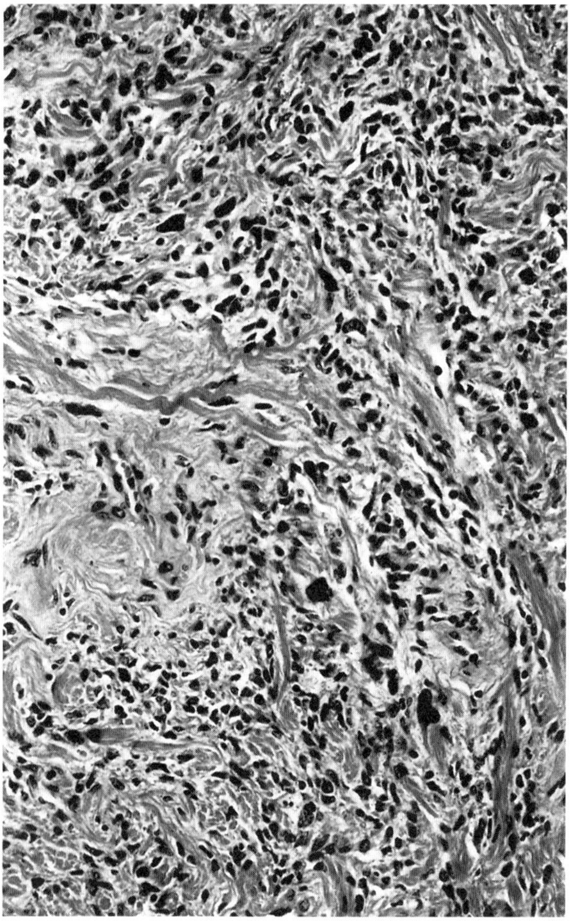

FIGURE 8.—Malignant SFT, showing a growth pattern similar to that of the benign tumors but with increased nuclear atypicality and pleomorphism. *Abbreviation: SFT*, solitary fibrous tumor. (Courtesy of Nielsen GP, O'Connell JX, Dickersin GR, et al: Solitary fibrous tumor of soft tissue: A report of 15 cases, including 5 malignant examples with light microscopic, immunohistochemical, and ultrastructural data. *Mod Pathol* 10[10]:1028–1037, 1997.)

of 15 soft-tissue SFTs, investigators describe the light microscopic, ultrastructural, and immunological findings in these tumors.

Methods.—The tumors were obtained from the pathology laboratory files of Massachusetts General Hospital and from consultation files. An average of 6 hematoxylin- and eosin-stained slides were examined per case. Tissue from 6 patients was processed for electron microscopy.

Results.—Patients were 9 men and 6 women, with a mean age of 50.6. Five malignant tumors were found in patients who were older (mean age, 58.6 years) than those with benign tumors (mean age, 46.7 years). Sites of benign tumors were the head and neck, thigh, vulva, upper arm, lower leg, and retroperitoneum. Malignant tumors arose in the thigh, abdominal wall, buttocks, and retroperitoneum. Benign tumors were treated by simple excision, and all but 1 of the malignant tumors were treated with wide local excision. Radiation therapy was administered to 2 patients with malignancy. Neither benign nor malignant tumors have recurred, and the malignant tumors have not metastasized.

Tumors had an average size of 4.6 cm (4.8 cm for benign and 4.3 cm for malignant cases). Microscopic examination of benign tumors (Fig 2) revealed areas of hyper-cellularity, with variable amounts of collagenous and myxoid stroma; amianthoid fibers were present in 1 case. Malignant tumors exhibited cytologically atypical cells (Fig 8) enmeshed in a collagenous or myxoid extra-cellular matrix. Ultrastructural findings in 3 benign and 3 malignant tumors included fibroblastic differentiation; 1 benign tumor showed myofibroblastic differentiation. All tumors examined immunohistochemically were immunoreactive for vimentin. Seven of 9 tumors were positive for CD34, including all malignant tumors examined.

Conclusion.—Although most SFTs arise within the pleural cavity, those described in this study offer additional evidence for the existence of soft-tissue tumors with morphological features of pleural-based SFTs. Two tumors arose in the vulva, a previously unrecognized site of SFTs.

▶ This article describes a series of 10 benign and 5 malignant solitary fibrous tumors, all but one of which were seen in consultation by 2 of the authors. These unusual tumors are currently thought to arise from submesothelial connective tissue, although they have been described in virtually all anatomic sites. The morphology is at once distinctive and not unique. Immunohistochemical findings indicate vimentin positivity (10/10) and variable CD34 positivity (7/9), but general negativity for actin, Leu-7, cytokeratin, desmin, S-100, epithelial membrane antigen, and smooth muscle-specific actin. The distinction between benign and malignant was based on cytologic atypia, chiefly because of nuclear enlargement, prominent nucleoli, and a higher mitotic rate. Follow-up of 4 benign tumors (12–21 months) did not reveal evidence of local recurrence, and follow-up of 4 malignant tumors (6–19 months) also revealed no evidence of recurrence or metastases.

M.B. Cohen, M.D.

Suggested Reading

Fukunga M, Naganuma H, Nikaido T, et al: Extrapleural solitary fibrous tumor: A report of seven cases. *Mod Pathol* 10:443–450, 1997.

Hyalinizing Spindle Cell Tumor With Giant Rosettes: A Distinctive Tumor Closely Resembling Low-grade Fibromyxoid Sarcoma

Lane KL, Shannon RJ, Weiss SW (Univ of Michigan, Ann Arbor)

Am J Surg Pathol 21:1481–1488, 1997 9–6

Introduction.—A number of distinct subtypes of fibrosarcoma have been identified in recent years. The previously undescribed tumor pre-

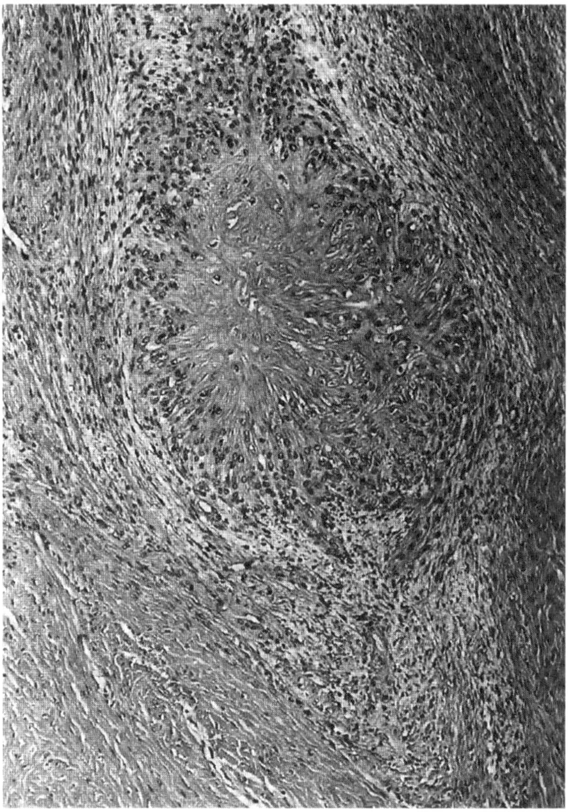

FIGURE 8.—Large collagen rosette arising abruptly from spindled stroma. (Courtesy of Lane KL, Shannon RJ, Weiss SW: Hyalinizing spindle cell tumor with giant rosettes: A distinctive tumor closely resembling low-grade fibromyxoid sarcoma. *Am J Surg Pathol* 21:1481–1488, 1997.)

sented here resembles a low-grade fibromyxoid sarcoma, but is distinguished by rosette-like structures.

Methods.—The 19 cases were referred for consultation between 1989 and 1996. At least a dozen possible diagnoses had been proposed. Hematoxylin and eosin-stained sections were available for review in all cases. Clinical data and follow-up information were sought from referring pathologists and surgeons.

Results.—Patients were 13 men and 6 women, with a mean age of 38. Most were seen initially with a painless, deep-seated, slowly growing mass that had been present for months or even years. All patients but 1 had solitary masses. In 1 case it was uncertain whether a single mass or 3 separate masses were present. Fourteen (74%) tumors occurred within or were attached to skeletal muscle. The mean size of the tumors was 6.3 cm (range 2.3–20.3 cm).

Although all lesions appeared grossly circumscribed, nearly all infiltrated adjacent soft tissue. The lesions consisted of a spindled stroma punctuated by large collagen rosettes which usually made up 10% to 15% of the tumor surface area (Fig 8). Rosette cells, in contrast to the stroma, expressed a number of antigens, including S-100 protein, neuron-specific enolase, and leu 22. Follow-up information was available for 12 patients, 7 of whom were treated by simple local excision and 5 by wide excision. With a mean follow-up of 39 months, there was 1 case of local recurrence. There were no other cases of recurrent or metastatic disease.

Conclusion.—The hyalinizing spindle cell tumor with giant rosettes appears to be a distinctive type of low-grade fibroblastic tumor. Given the behavior of neoplasms with similar appearance, wide surgical excision is recommended for local control.

▶ This article describes 19 cases of a soft-tissue tumor that resembles low-grade fibromyxoid sarcoma, all identified from the consultation files of the senior author. The stroma in these tumors varied in cellularity, both within and among the tumors, and was myxoid to hyalinized. The spindle cells lacked atypia. The characteristic feature was the rosettes (Fig 8). Immunohistochemical findings were not distinctive. Follow-up (1–78 months; 5 cases with no follow-up) suggests a low-grade neoplasm, with potential for local recurrence but no evidence of metastasis.

M.B. Cohen, M.D.

Leiomyosarcoma in Soft Tissue: Examination of *p53* Status and Cell Proliferating Factors in Different Locations

Konomoto T, Fukuda T, Hayashi K, et al (Kyushu Univ, Fukuoka, Japan)
Hum Pathol 29:74–81, 1998 9–7

Introduction.—Leiomyosarcoma (LMS), a relatively rare soft-tissue tumor, can arise from either deep soft tissue or superficial soft tissue. Although the histological features of these 2 subtypes are similar, the former carries a worse prognosis. Thirty-seven cases of LMS were analyzed (22 of the deep type and 15 of the superficial type) for factors, other than location, that might influence outcome.

Methods.—Patients were 20 men and 17 women, with an average age of 56.8 years. All had been treated by excision only. Tissue samples from the tumors were analyzed for cell proliferating factors (mitotic and Ki-67 indices) and *p53* status (as determined by both immunohistochemical staining and the presence or absence of mutation). Findings were correlated with patient outcome.

Results.—Tumors of the superficial type of LMS exhibited higher expression of both cell proliferating factors than did tumors of the deep type, but the differences were not significant. Similarly, there was a higher incidence of abnormal *p53* in the superficial type, but this difference between subtypes was not significant. Cases with abnormal *p53* showed a significantly poor prognosis (Fig 6) only in the deep type, but all 5 patients in the superficial subgroup who died of the disease were carrying abnormal *p53*.

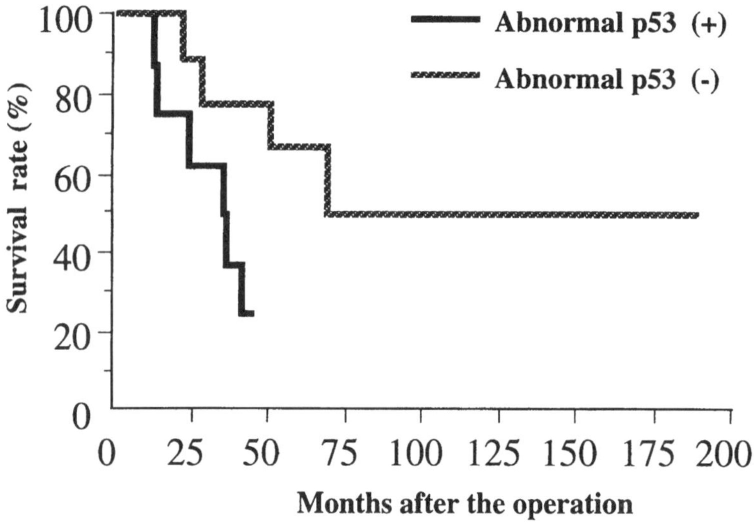

FIGURE 6.—Kaplan-Meier survival curves for patients with deep-type LMS. Overall survival is classified according to p53 abnormality. Patients with p53 abnormality showed a significantly poor prognosis (P = .0424, log rank test). *Abbreviation: LMS,* leiomyosarcoma. (Courtesy of Konomoto T, Fukuda T, Hayashi K, et al: Leiomyosarcoma in soft tissue: Examination of *p53* status and cell proliferating factors in different locations. *Hum Pathol* 29:74–81, 1998.)

Conclusion.—The location of LMS remains a good prognostic factor, for *p53* status and cell proliferating factors were essentially the same in deep and superficial subtypes. Potential prognostic factors are abnormal *p53* and a high Ki-67 index in the deep type, and a tumor larger than 6 cm in the superficial type.

► As noted by the authors, LMSs, like other sarcomas, may be superficially located or located deep within the body, and the second portends a worse prognosis. This study of 15 superficial and 22 deep leiomyosarcomas included histopathologic features and mitotic index (1,000 cells counted), MIB-1 staining, *p53* expression (Pab 1801), and *p53* mutations in exons 5–7. The histopathologic features were similar. Although differences in proliferation (MIB-1 staining) and *p53* expression were noted, these were not statistically significant. *p53* mutational analysis was only performed in a subset of the tumors (8 superficial and 8 deep); loss of heterozygosity was seen in 5 (3 superficial and 2 deep). However, *p53* mutation was associated with a markedly worse prognosis, regardless of location (Fig 6). There was relatively poor correlation between *p53* mutation and assessment of protein expression. Thus, it would appear that location remains a useful predictor of biologic behavior.

M.B. Cohen, M.D.

Peripheral Primitive Neuroectodermal Tumors in Adults: Documentation by Molecular Analysis

Lawlor ER, Mathers JA, Bainbridge T, et al (British Columbia's Children's Hosp, Vancouver; British Columbia Cancer Control Agency, Vancouver; Mem Sloan-Kettering Cancer Research Ctr, New York; et al)

J Clin Oncol 16:1150–1157, 1998 9–8

Introduction.—The peripheral primitive neuroectodermal tumors (pPNETs), the second most common group of malignant bone tumors in children and young adults, are rarely diagnosed in patients older than 40. Because pPNETs are often neglected in the differential diagnosis of primitive bone and soft tissue tumors in older patients, their incidence in this age group is unknown. Recent studies have shown that fusions between the EWS gene and different members of the ETS transcription factor family occur in virtually all pPNETs. Adults with suspected pPNETs were studied for the presence of EWS/ETS fusion gene expression as evidence of pPNETs.

Methods.—Tumor samples were obtained from 3 diagnostic molecular pathology laboratories. Clinical records and pathological materials were reviewed for all patients older than 40 who received a diagnosis of pPNETs. Nine patients with tumors positive for EWS/ETS gene fusion were identified: 7 men and 2 women, ranging in age from 40 to 65. Tumor tissue samples underwent histopathologic, cytogenetic, and molecular analysis.

Results.—Review of the pathologic material from all 9 patients revealed histologic features typical for pPNETs. The tumors exhibited diffuse sheets of primitive small round cells, with little or no evidence of differentiation. Six tumors showed histologic features of the Ewing tumor. No histologic features in the 9 adult pPNET cases would be considered atypical for childhood pPNETs. Eight samples from adult pPNETs showed EWS/FLII fusion transcripts typical of pPNETs; 1 showed the less common EWS/ERG fusion (Table 2).

Conclusion.—Adults found to have small round-cell tumors of bone or soft tissues are rarely examined for the possibility of pPNETs. Misdiagnosis can lead to inappropriate treatment and a poor prognosis. Identification of an EWS/ETS gene fusion by molecular analysis can provide evidence of pPNET in older patients.

▶ Primitive neuroectodermal tumors are believed to be part of the broader family of primitive tumors which includes Ewing's sarcoma, although age differences clearly exist among these tumors. The classification of these tumors was initially based on morphologic similarities, and, more recently, on immunohistochemical findings (e.g., O13 staining). In this multi-institutional report of 9 cases, the authors use molecular genetic analysis to document the commonality of these tumors. Specifically, a gene fusion product, presumably the result of translocation, allows one to identify the EWS/ETS gene product (a protein); this is similar to the BCR/ABL gene product in certain hematopoietic neoplasms. It provides an important mo-

TABLE 2.—Pathologic, Cytogenetic, and Molecular Characteristics

Case No.	Tissue Analyzed	DD_x	IHC O13	IHC NSE	Tumor Cytogenetics	Fusion
1	P	pPNET	+	+	NA	7–6
2	P	Metastatic carcinoma, lymphoma	+	+	NA	7–6
3	P, R	Lymphoma	+	+	46,XY,add(1)(p13),add(13)(p12),add(15)(q24),−16,add(18)(q23), +der(22)t(11;22)(q24;q12) [6]/47,XY,del(1)(q32),del(3)(p21), add(6)(q27),+mar1[cp4]	7–6
4	P	pPNET	+	NA	49,XY,+5,+7,+8,add(9)(p24),t(11;22;13)(q24;q12;q22), del(16)(q22) [2]/46,XY[36]	7–5
5	P	pPNET	+	+	47,XY,t(11;22)(q24;q12),+8,+(14)(q32)/46,idem,add(22)(q12)	7–6
6	P	Metastatic SRCT, NOS	+	−	NA	7–6
7	R	pPNET	+	−	NA	*EWS/ERG*
8	R	Neuroendocrine carcinoma	+	NA	NA	7–6
9	P	pPNET	+	NA	NA	7–9

Abbreviations: P, primary tumor; *R*, recurrence; *DDx*, differential diagnosis; *NOS*, not otherwise specified; *IHC*, immunohistochemistry; *NSE*, neuron-specific enolase; *NA*, not available; *fusion*, exons of EWS and FLII, respectively, fused in chimeric gene.

(Courtesy of Lawlor ER, Mathers JA, Bainbridge T, et al: Peripheral primitive neuroectodermal tumors in adults: Documentation by molecular analysis. *J Clin Oncol* 16:1150–1157, 1998.)

lecular marker of this group of tumors, which can be assayed by polymerase chain reaction. This finding also opens up the door into the pathogenesis of the disease, and to how the EWS/ETS gene product contributes to the biology of these tumors.

M.B. Cohen, M.D.

Risk of Malignancy and Death in Neurofibromatosis

Poyhonen M, Niemela S, Herva R (Oulu Univ, Finland)

Arch Pathol Lab Med 121:139–143, 1997 9–9

Objective.—Neurofibromatoses (NF) are precancerous hamartomatoses than can affect a variety of tissues. The most common type, NF1, a hereditary tumor syndrome, are neurofibromas. Because the course of NF varies widely, the risk for malignant progression and early death from NF was assessed in a large group of patients in northern Finland.

Methods.—Neurofibroma specimens from 69 NF1 patients were evaluated, including 34 females (3 months to 73 years). This is a subset of 197 identified patients (95 females) of which 106 were sporadic and 91 familial.

Results.—There were 15 (8%) malignant tumors (Table 1). Nine patients with NF1 died, 8 from their disease. The risk for death from malignancy in the general population was 1%.

TABLE 1.—Representative Malignancies Observed Among the 69 Biopsied Neurofibromatosis Type 1 Patients

Patient No.	Sex	Tumor Observed: Age at Detection, y	Tumor Observed: Location	Tumor Observed: Histology	Age at Most Recent Follow-up, y	Other
1	F	14	Peroneal nerve/ ischial nerve	MPNST	Died at 23	...
2	M	20	Ischial nerve	MPNST	Died at 23	Son of patient 5
3	F	23	Leg	MPNST	27	...
4	M	26	Pelvis	MPNST	Died at 26	...
5	F	48	Leg	MPNST	Died at 51	Mother of patient 2
		48	Eye	Melanoma		
6	M	49	Shoulder	MPNST	Died at 56	...
7	F	1	Kidney	Wilms' tumor	15	...
		15	Skin	Basal cell carcinoma		
8	F	37	Thalamus	GM	Died at 37	...
9	F	45	Breast	Ductal carcinoma	63	...
		54	Skin	Basal cell carcinoma		
		63	Adrenal medulla	Pheochromocytoma		
10	M	52	Rectum	Adenocarcinoma	54	...
		54	Adrenal medulla	Pheochromocytoma		
11	M	53	Cerebellum	Anaplastic astrocytoma	54	...

**Abbreviations: MPNST*, malignant peripheral nerve sheath tumor; *GM*, glioblastoma multiforme.

(Courtesy of Poyhonen M, Niemela S, Herva R: Risk of malignancy and death in neurofibromatosis. *Arch Pathol Lab Med* 121:139–143, 1997.)

Conclusion.—Patients with NF are at increased risk for malignancy, compared with the general population (8% vs. 1%). Patients with NF should be referred for genetic counseling and monitored carefully for sudden increase in size of an existing tumor.

▶ This study, which appears to be population-based in northern Finland, examined a series of patients with von Recklinghausen's disease NF, also known as NF1, as well as NF2 (the one with acoustic schwannomas), and NF5 (segmental NF). All but 6 patients had NF1. The risk of the development of malignancy was about 8%, as compared to 1% in the general population. As expected, most of the malignancies were malignant schwannomas (malignant peripheral nerve sheath tumors; see Table).

M.B. Cohen, M.D.

Neurofibroma and Cellular Neurofibroma With Atypia: A Report of 14 Tumors

Lin BT-Y, Weiss LM, Medeiros LJ (City of Hope Natl Med Ctr, Duarte, Calif)
Am J Surg Pathol 21:1443–1449, 1997 9–10

Introduction.—A patient with neurofibromatosis type 1 was found to have a neurofibroma with cytologic atypia, areas of increased cellularity, occasional mitotic figures, and no evidence of necrosis. Because the significance of neurofibromas with these findings has not been systematically assessed, researchers reviewed 14 such tumors from 6 patients.

Methods.—Patients were treated and studied at the institution from January 1989 to March 1997. Three patients had neurofibromatosis type 1. Three high-grade malignant peripheral nerve sheath tumors, all from patients with neurofibromatosis type 1, were also examined for comparison. Hematoxylin and eosin-stained slides were reviewed and immunohistochemical studies performed using standard methods. Paraffin-embedded tissue was analyzed to determine DNA content and S-phase fraction.

Results.—Patients were 4 women and 2 men, with a mean age of 40. Five tumors were from the head and neck area, 5 from the trunk, and 4 on the extremities. Tumors ranged in size from 0.5 to 5.0 cm, and all were excised conservatively. None of the patients received adjuvant chemotherapy or radiation therapy. Three patients had additional primary tumors. During follow-up ranging from 8 months to 6 years, none of the neurofibromas recurred or metastasized. All of these tumors had similar histopathological findings (Fig 1). Three tumors exhibited *p53* expression, but the remaining tumors were negative. Tumor cell proliferation rate, assessed by Ki-67 immunostaining, showed less than 5% cells in 13 tumors. All tumors had diploid DNA content; the mean S-phase fraction was 9.4%. In comparison, all 3 malignant peripheral nerve sheath tumors had high p53 and Ki-67 staining.

Discussion.—Clinically benign fibromas, both usual and cellular types, can have significant cytologic atypia, together with low mitotic activity.

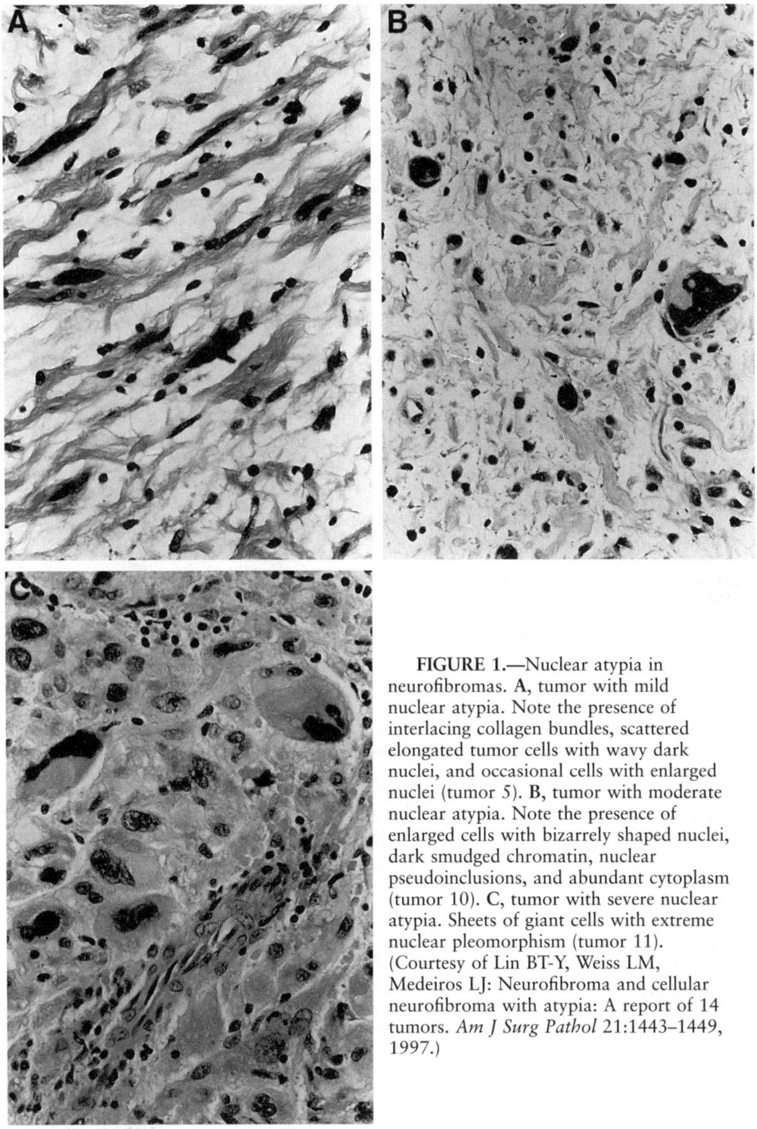

FIGURE 1.—Nuclear atypia in neurofibromas. **A**, tumor with mild nuclear atypia. Note the presence of interlacing collagen bundles, scattered elongated tumor cells with wavy dark nuclei, and occasional cells with enlarged nuclei (tumor 5). **B**, tumor with moderate nuclear atypia. Note the presence of enlarged cells with bizarrely shaped nuclei, dark smudged chromatin, nuclear pseudoinclusions, and abundant cytoplasm (tumor 10). **C**, tumor with severe nuclear atypia. Sheets of giant cells with extreme nuclear pleomorphism (tumor 11). (Courtesy of Lin BT-Y, Weiss LM, Medeiros LJ: Neurofibroma and cellular neurofibroma with atypia: A report of 14 tumors. *Am J Surg Pathol* 21:1443–1449, 1997.)

Prognosis is benign, and patients are adequately treated by conservative surgical excision.

► There has been little focus on the significance of cellularity or atypia in neurofibromas. These have been better studied in schwannomas and the malignant counterpart, malignant peripheral nerve sheath tumor. In this article about 14 cases from 6 patients, cellularity and atypia, as well *p53* staining (DO-7) and proliferation (S-phase fraction and MIB-1 staining), were assessed. Importantly 3 of 6 patients had neurofibromatosis type 1. The results of this study indicate that cellular and atypical neurofibromas may be treated conservatively. However, the definition of cellular and atypia are not well described, and so reproducibility may be a problem. In addition, this is a relatively small series, and the results will have to be confirmed by others. Lastly, follow-up ranged from 1 year to 6 years; follow-up for 10 of 14 cases was 2 years or less, which may be too short.

M.B. Cohen, M.D.

Kaposi's Sarcoma–associated Herpesvirus (KSHV)/Human Herpesvirus 8 (HHV8): A New Human Tumour Virus

Brooks LA, Wilson AJ, Crook T (London School of Hygiene and Tropical Medicine; Haddow Labs, Sutton, England)

J Pathol 182:262–265, 1997 9–11

Introduction.—At least 20% of human cancers are caused by viruses. Human herpesvirus 8 (HHV8) has been associated with the usually benign Kaposi's sarcoma (KS) that has become an aggressive tumor in those infected with HIV.

HHV8.—DNA sequences identified in KS skin lesions have been provisionally designated as HHV8. Human herpesvirus 8 is related to the oncogenic herpesvirus saimiri (HVS) and appears to have a lymphoid site of latency. Whereas HHV8 is more prevalent in AIDS patients with KS, the development of malignancy appears to require 1 or more cofactors.

Oncogenesis.—An additional HHV8 sequence resembles D-type cyclins and G-protein coupled receptors. Overexpression of D-type cyclins plays a role in carcinogenesis. Human herpesvirus 8 possibly functions by encoding RB-inactivating proteins, as do almost all other DNA tumor viruses, it appears to deregulate cell cycle arrest, and it may stimulate autocrine and paracrine growth factor (Fig 1).

Conclusion.—Human herpesvirus 8 appears to cause Kaposi's sarcoma by encoding proteins that deregulate growth and apoptosis. It may also be the causative agent for other diseases, particularly in immunocompromised individuals.

► This is a brief, relatively recent review article about a new virus believed to be etiologically important in KS. Although first described in the last century in elderly men of Mediterranean descent, KS is mostly associated with AIDS. The isolation of viral sequences, first reported in 1994 by Chang et al.,[1] from cutaneous cases of KS indicates homology to other human herpesviruses. More important, it provides strong supporting evidence of a viral origin of certain cancers, first reported by the Nobel laureate Peyton Rous at the beginning of this century. Finally, as illustrated in the accompanying figure, KSVH/HHV8 appears to exert its action via cell cycle control; more specifically, via the cyclin/cyclin-dependent kinase pathway(s). The future shows much promise. If, in fact, this virus is the cause of KS and a molecular understanding of its pathogenesis can be elucidated, then thera-

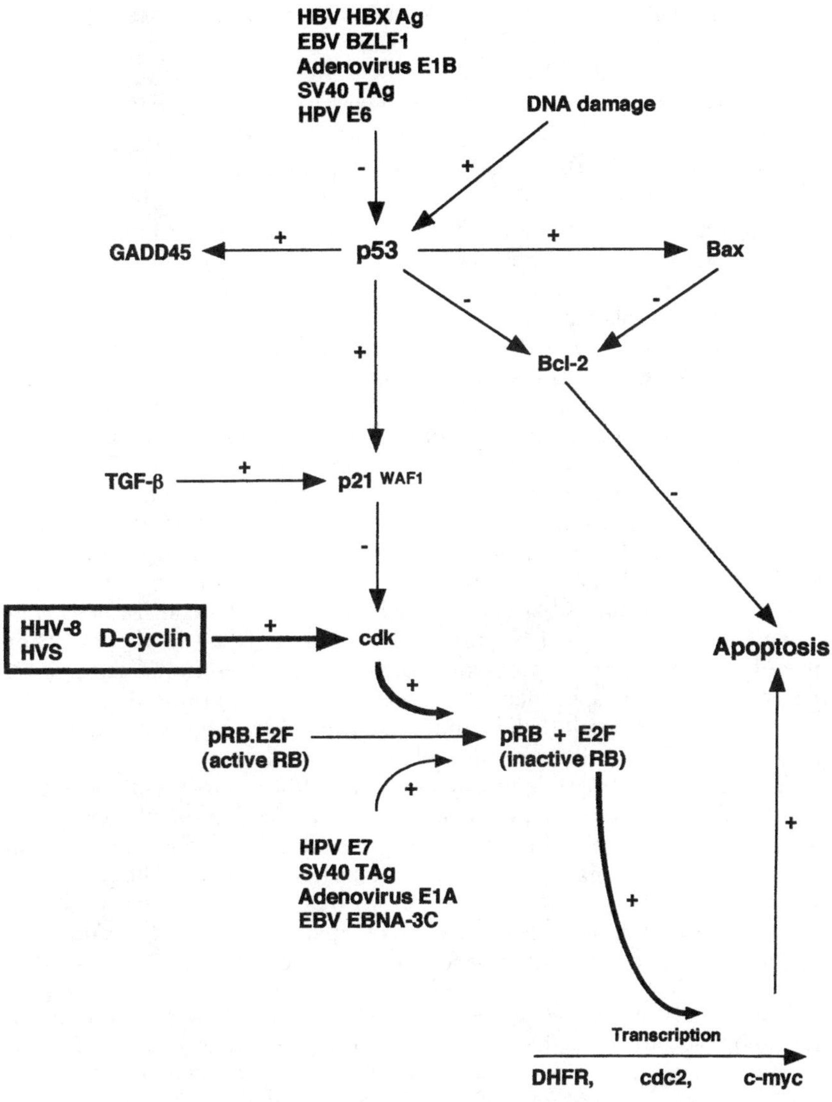

FIGURE 1.—A model of viral oncogenesis indicating one potential locus of HHV8 transforming function. (Reprinted by permission of John Wiley & Sons, Ltd., from Brooks LA, Wilson AJ, Crook T: Kaposi's sarcoma–associated herpesvirus (KSHV)/human herpesvirus 8 (HHV8): A new human tumour virus. *J Pathol* 182:262–265. Copyright 1997, John Wiley & Sons, Ltd.)

peutic strategies could be developed. In addition, KSVH/HHV8 could serve as a model for other tumor systems.

M.B. Cohen, M.D.

Reference

1. Chang Y, Cesarman E, Pessin MS, et al: Identification of herpesvirus-like DNA sequences in AIDS-associated Kaposi's sarcoma. *Science* 266:1865–1869, 1994.

An Immunohistochemical Analysis of Radiation Fibroblasts

Meehan SA, LeBoit PE (Univ of California, San Francisco)

J Cutan Pathol 24:309–313, 1997 9–12

Introduction.—There are acute, subacute, and chronic stages of radiation dermatitis. Transient erythema and epilation are seen in the early clinical manifestations. Little is known about radiation fibroblasts' immunophenotypical characteristics or their relationship to other populations of dermal dendritic cells. Biopsy specimens with radiation fibroblasts were examined to review the lineage of chronic radiation dermatitis and its potential for neoplastic transformation.

Methods.—There were 16 biopsy specimens that had radiation fibroblasts. Three antisera expressed by dermal mesenchymal cells, 1 antiserum to a nuclear protein found in actively cyclic cells, and 1 to the product of a tumor-suppressor gene that is commonly overexpressed in malignant neoplasms were used. The 3 antisera were FXIIIa, CD34, HHF-35; the proliferation marker was Ki-56, and the tumor-suppressor protein was p53.

Results.—For the markers of lineage used, radiation fibroblasts were largely negative. There was strong expression of FXIIIa in only 2 of 16 specimens, with 1 specimen showing weak expression. In 1 specimen, scattered radiation fibroblasts expressed CD34. Small, dendritic cells were stained in the superficial dermis by HHF-35, but not in the radiation fibroblasts. The tumor-suppressor protein was not seen in radiation fibroblasts in any of the specimens, but 2 specimens overexpressed it in endothelial cells. Rare endothelial and interstitial cells were stained by the proliferation marker but not the radiation fibroblasts.

Conclusion.—Dermal dendrocytes and myofibroblasts are immunophenotypically distinct from radiation fibroblasts. Radiation fibroblasts do not express high levels of the tumor-suppressor protein p53, despite their marked nuclear atypia, and appear to be noncycling cells. The possibility of their role as progenitors of atypical fibroxanthoma and dermatofibrosarcoma protuberans, which are associated with ionizing radiation-induced skin damage, is diminished by their phenotype.

▶ The framework for this article is elegant yet simple: what is the immunophenotypic profile of the atypical cells observed in tissues exposed to radiation, specifically targeting their cytoplasmic differentiation and proliferative abilities? The authors carried out the study with antibodies to FXIIIa, CD34, Ki-67, and p53. There was no appreciable immunostaining for any of these antibodies in the atypical radiation fibroblasts, and, more intriguingly, no nuclear staining for Ki-67. The microscopic findings of atypical cells in radiation fields sometimes raise the differential diagnosis of recurrent tumor or de novo sarcoma. The absence of proliferation in such cases may be useful in making a distinction. The authors conclude that the phenotype of radiation fibroblasts argues against their possible role as progenitors of atypical fibroxanthoma and dermatofibrosarcoma protuberans. These tumors are associated with ionizing radiation-induced skin damage, but based on these phenotypes, which are a photograph in time, it may be premature to completely exclude this radiation hit from being an initiating factor in the development of these 2 tumors.

D.J. Dabbs, M.D.

Atypical Decubital Fibroplasia: A Series of Three Cases
Baldassano MF, Rosenberg AE, Flotte TJ (Harvard Med School, Boston)
J Cutan Pathol 25:149–152, 1998 9–13

Background.—Atypical decubital fibroplasia (ADF) is a benign, reactive process that occurs as a result of prolonged tissue ischemia as the result of pressure. It is not the same as a decubital ulcer, although both have the same cause. Clinically and histologically, ADF may be confused with a sarcoma. These case reports describe the clinical and histologic findings in ADF and offer features to differentiate the benign ADF from other, malignant processes.

Clinical Features of Atypical Decubital Fibroplasia.—The authors describe ADF in 3 patients (2 men and 1 woman, aged 49, 66, and 89 years, respectively). Two were immobilized from other causes and 1 reported frequently lying on the affected area. The patients were seen with subcutaneous masses of 2.5, 3.0, and 7.0 cm, respectively, that developed over pressure points (greater trochanter, back, and right lateral chest wall over a rib). Only 1 mass was fixed, only 1 mass was painful, and only 1 patient had focal superficial ulceration. No patient had a history of trauma or of similar subcutaneous masses or decubitus ulcers, and no patient had a recurrence after respective follow-ups of 4, 5, and 91 months.

Pathologic Features of Atypical Decubital Fibroplasia.—Histologically, ADF lesions are ill-defined, tannish-yellow masses with focal hemorrhage and (typically) without ulceration. Dermal and cutaneous tissues are involved, with fibrinoid necrosis, reactive fibrosis, and myxoid degeneration centrally and prominent reactive neovascularization, atypical fibroblasts, and fat necrosis peripherally. The surrounding cellular zones contained both granulation tissue and ectatic vessels in the papillary dermis and deep in the subcutaneous tissue. Blood vessels contained fibrin thrombi and vessel walls were hyalinized. Red blood cell extravasation and hemosiderin deposition were substantial. The epidermis was not always ulcerated, but it was thinned and had elongated rete edges. Some inflammation was evident throughout the dermis and subcutaneous tissue. If the mass extended into muscle, the muscle tissue was degenerated.

Differentiating Atypical Decubital Fibroplasia From Other Conditions.—The condition must be differentiated from other pseudosarcomatous fibroblastic proliferations and from the sarcomas. It can be differentiated from myxoid malignant fibrous histiocytoma because tissues of histiocytoma are hypercellular, have atypical mitoses, and have a more atypical cytology. ADF can be differentiated from myxoid chondrosarcoma because there is no chondroid formation in ADF. As for differentiating liposarcomas from ADF, the vascular pattern and lipoblasts characteristic of liposarcoma are absent in ADF. Decubitus ulcer is marked by extensive ulcers that do not have the distinctive lobular pattern with central fibrinoid necrosis or the large, reactive-appearing fibroblasts typical of ADF.

▶ ADF is a recently described pseudosarcomatous process that occurs in association with decubital ulcers. The mass lesions are tan-yellow, ill-defined, and present in the dermis and subcutaneous tissues.

The microscopic findings described include central hypocellular fibrinoid necrosis, peripheral neovascularization, fat necrosis, and atypical reactive fibroblasts. Recognition of this entity is important, and this paper is a timely presentation. The major differential diagnosis to recognize is that of squamous cell carcinoma arising in a decubitus ulcer, and sarcoma. The microscopic features—including the fibroblasts with "ganglion-like nuclei," central fibrinoid necrosis, neovascularization, and fibrin thrombi within deep vessels—clearly distinguish this lesion from sarcomas, which will invariably demonstrate cytologic anaplasia and atypical mitoses.

D.J. Dabbs, M.D.

Suggested Reading

Montgomery EA, Meis JM, Mitchell MS, et al: Atypical decubital fibroplasia: A distinctive fibroblastic pseudotumor occurring in debilitated patients. *Am J Surg Pathol* 16:708, 1992.

Tumors Around Implants

Langkamer VG, Case CP, Collins C, et al (Bristol Royal Infirmary, England)
J Arthroplasty 12:812–818, 1997 9–14

Objective.—There have been 19 reports of tumors around implants, most containing cobalt-chrome alloy. Seven tumors were malignant. Metals such as nickel and chromium are known to cause malignant tumors in animals and in humans after chronic industrial exposure. Four case reports of tumors that developed around orthopedic implants are presented.

Case 1.—Woman, 77, who received a right total hip arthroplasty (THA) 2 years previously, had a 7.5 cm myxoid fibrosarcoma removed. Despite radiotherapy she had local recurrence and a pelvic mass 3 years later. She underwent chemotherapy and a right hindquarter amputation. She died of endocarditis 1 year later. A review immunochemical study confirmed leiomyosarcoma.

Case 2.—Man, 75, was found to have a fixed soft tissue mass in the left thigh and hip 20 months after a left THA. A malignant fibrous histiocytoma (MFH) was removed. Despite chemotherapy the patient died 2 months later.

Case 3.—Woman, 77, with a 16-year-old right THA, underwent revision surgery because of a loose prosthesis. After 42 months, she was readmitted with a mass in the lower hip that proved to be a high-grade leiomyosarcoma, which was excised.

Case 4.—Woman, 69, with a failed knee arthroplasty and *Staphylococcus aureus* infection, underwent arthrodesis. After 7 years she was readmitted with hip pain of 2 years' duration. A THA was performed, but 18 months later she was readmitted with a painful mass in the upper right thigh that proved to be a destructive lesion. She received palliative radiotherapy.

Discussion.—Studies have shown that the incidence of soft tissue sarcoma was not significantly increased in patients with THA. The most frequently diagnosed soft tissue sarcoma is MFH, which affects the lower limb ≤50% of the time. All 8 reports of MFH have occurred in conjunction with cobalt-chrome alloy or stainless steel implants. In vitro studies have established that particulate chromium and nickel induce local muscle necrosis, regeneration, and sarcoma formation.

▶ Although one is generally reluctant to include case reports, in this case 4, they can nonetheless be instructive. These cases were identified through the Bristol Bone Tumour Registry during a 12-year period. All four patients had had THAs. Two patients had leiomyosarcomas develop, and 2 developed MFHs. Although the incidence and mechanism of sarcoma development after prosthetic replacement is not known, there is clearly an association, as noted by the authors and the literature they have cited.

M.B. Cohen, M.D.

Osteocalcin and Osteonectin Immunoreactivity in the Diagnosis of Osteosarcoma

Fanburg JC, Rosenberg AE, Weaver DL, et al (Armed Forces Inst of Pathology, Washington, DC; Massachusetts Gen Hosp, Boston; Univ of Vermont, Burlington)

Am J Clin Pathol 108:464–473, 1997 9–15

Background.—Osteosarcomas are common primary malignant bone tumors. Most of these tumors are easily diagnosed by light microscopy, but, histologically, they can be difficult to distinguish from tumors with very different biological potentials and treatment protocols. Accurate diagnosis is important because osteosarcomas are treated by specific protocols that have been associated with improved survival. Diagnosis of these tumors involves the identification of malignant osteoblasts that produce neoplastic bone. Immunohistochemistry may be useful in the diagnosis because osteoblasts express specific marker proteins.

TABLE 1.—Observed Frequencies for Cytoplasmic Immunoreactivity Using Antiosteocalcin and Antiosteonectin

Tumor Type	Total No.	No. (%) Positive Antiosteocalcin	No. (%) Positive Antiosteonectin
Osteosarcoma	42	27 (64)	37 (88)
Fibroblastic	8	6 (75)	8 (100)
Osteoblastic	7	7 (100)	7 (100)
Chondroblastic	7	4 (57)	6 (86)
Giant cell–rich	5	3 (60)	5 (100)
Telangiectatic	3	1 (33)	3 (100)
Small cell	6	1 (16)	2 (33)
Low-grade	4	4 (100)	4 (100)
Extraskeletal	2	1 (50)	2 (100)
Benign primary bone-forming tumors	8	8 (100)	8 (100)
Fibrous dysplasia	4	4 (100)	4 (100)
Osteoma/osteoblastoma	4	4 (100)	4 (100)
Benign primary non–bone-forming tumors	7	0 (0)	7 (100)
Aneurysmal bone cyst	3	0 (0)	3 (100)
Giant cell of bone	4	0 (0)	4 (100)
Non–bone-forming sarcomas	25	0 (0)	16 (64)
Ewing's sarcoma	4	0 (0)	1 (25)
Rhabdomyosarcoma	3	0 (0)	3 (100)
Synovial sarcoma	5	0 (0)	2 (40)
Malignant fibrous histiocytoma or fibrosarcoma	5	0 (0)	5 (100)
Pleomorphic liposarcoma	1	0 (0)	0 (0)
Chondrosarcoma	7	0 (0)	5 (71)
Other tumors	24	0 (0)	4 (17)
Carcinomas	17	0 (0)	3 (18)
Spindle cell melanoma	3	0 (0)	1 (33)
Lymphoma	4	0 (0)	0 (0)

(Courtesy of Fanburg JC, Rosenberg AE, Weaver DL, et al: Osteocalcin and osteonectin immunoreactivity in the diagnosis of osteosarcoma. *Am J Clin Pathol* 108:464–473. Copyright 1997 by the American Society of Clinical Pathologists. Reprinted with permission.)

Methods.—The value of immunohistochemistry in the diagnosis of osteosarcomas was determined by examining 106 formalin-fixed, paraffin-embedded tumor specimens. Tumors were immunostained with monoclonal antiosteocalcin and antiosteonectin antibodies. The specimens consisted of 42 osteosarcomas; 25 non–bone-forming sarcomas; 24 other malignant tumors, including lymphomas, carcinomas, and melanomas; and 15 benign bone tumors.

Results.—Cytoplasmic staining with antiosteocalcin had 70% sensitivity and 100% specificity for bone-forming tumors. Staining with antiosteonectin had 90% sensitivity and 54% specificity for bone-forming tumors and consistently stained cell types other than osteoblasts (Table 1). Of the 42 osteosarcomas, 83% showed matrix staining with either antiosteocalcin or antiosteonectin, or both. In all osteosarcomas, dense collagen was negative for both antiosteocalcin and antiosteonectin (Table 2).

Discussion.—These findings indicate that although tumor cell cytoplasmic staining with monoclonal antiosteocalcin antibody cannot distinguish between benign and malignant bone tumors, it may be useful in distinguishing osteosarcomas from other malignancies. Monoclonal antiosteonectin antibody is not useful as a cytoplasmic marker in the diagnosis

TABLE 2.—Observed Frequencies of Matrix Immunoreactivity Using Antiosteocalcin and Antiosteonectin

Tumor/Type of Matrix	Total No.	No. (%) Positive Antiosteocalcin	Antiosteonectin	Either Antibody
Osteosarcoma				
Dense collagen	21	0 (0)	0 (0)	0 (0)
Neoplastic bone	35	20 (57)	20 (57)	29 (83)
Nonneoplastic bone	26	24 (92)	19 (73)	26 (100)
Benign primary bone-forming and non–bone-forming tumors				
Dense collagen	5	0 (0)	0 (0)	0 (0)
Neoplastic bone	10	10 (100)	6 (60)	7 (70)
Nonneoplastic bone	10	10 (100)	7 (70)	10 (100)
Non–bone-forming sarcoma				
Dense collagen	13	0 (0)	0 (0)	0 (0)
Neoplastic bone	0	0 (0)	0 (0)	0 (0)
Nonneoplastic bone	8	7 (88)	8 (100)	8 (100)
Other tumors				
Dense collagen	23	0 (0)	0 (0)	0 (0)
Neoplastic bone	0	0 (0)	0 (0)	0 (0)
Nonneoplastic bone	3	3 (100)	2 (67)	3 (100)

(Courtesy of Fanburg JC, Rosenberg AE, Weaver DL, et al: Osteocalcin and osteonectin immunoreactivity in the diagnosis of osteosarcoma. *Am J Clin Pathol* 108:464–473. Copyright 1997 by the American Society of Clinical Pathologists. Reprinted with permission.)

of osteosarcoma. Concurrent staining of matrix with antiosteocalcin and antiosteonectin may help distinguish neoplastic bone matrix from dense collagen, which is critical to the diagnosis of osteosarcoma.

▶ To date, there have been no antibodies available to reliably distinguish bone-forming cells from other cells. This study examines the usefulness of using antibodies to osteocalcin, a bone-specific protein produced by osteoblasts, and osteonectin, a connective tissue protein with high affinity for hydroxyapatite and type 1 collagen, found predominantly in bone tissue. As seen from the tables, the antibody to osteocalcin has 100% specificity in cytoplasmic reactivity of bone-forming tumors but is only good for distinguishing the osteoblastic phenotype, as it does not distinguish benign from malignant bone tumors. The osteonectin antibody is relatively nonspecific for cells of osteoblastic derivation and is not a useful cytoplasmic marker in the diagnosis of osteosarcoma, although the use of both antibodies concurrently may help distinguish neoplastic matrix from dense collagen, which we know can often mimic new bone matrix. Unfortunately, that nasty entity of small-cell osteosarcomas is not well studied but with the use of these antibodies, because of the very low sensitivity of both antibodies. This study showed a poor positive predictive value for osteonectin, but a good negative predictive value for cytoplasmic staining of bone-forming tumors.

D.J. Dabbs, M.D.

Suggested Reading

Serra M, Morini M, Scotlandi K, et al: Evaluation of osteonectin as a diagnostic marker of osteogenic bone tumors. *Hum Pathol* 23:1326–1331, 1992.

Schultz A, Jundt G, Berghauser K, et al: Immunohistochemical study of osteonectin in various types of osteosarcoma. *Am J Pathol* 132:233–238, 1988.

Takada J, Ishii S, Ohta T, et al: Usefulness of a novel monoclonal antibody against human osteocalcin in immunohistochemical diagnosis. *Virchows Arch* 420:507–511, 1992.

Vermeulen A, Vermeer C, Bosman F: Histochemical detection of osteocalcin in normal and pathologic human bone. *J Histochem Cytochem* 37:1503–1508, 1989.

Mesenchymal Chondrosarcoma of the Jaw Bones: Clinicopathologic Study of 19 Cases

Vencio EF, Reeve CM, Unni KK, et al (Mayo Clinic and Found, Rochester, Minn)

Cancer 82:2350–2355, 1998 9–16

Introduction.—Mesenchymal chondrosarcomas, neoplasms involving bone and soft tissue, are rarely encountered. In a series of 34 cases recorded at the Mayo Clinic, the most common site (9 cases) was the jaw bones. Most patients die of disease, but some experience long disease-free intervals. Nineteen cases of mesenchymal chondrosarcoma of the jaw bones were reviewed for clinical behavior.

Methods.—Six of the 19 cases were from Mayo Clinic files and 13 were from the authors' consultation files. Hematoxylin- and eosin-stained slides and radiographs were available in all cases. Clinical charts or correspondence from referring pathologists was the source of follow-up information. Patients had a mean age of 19 when initially seen; 10 were male and 8 were female. Only 3 patients were aged 30 or older. Eight tumors involved the maxilla and 11 were located in the mandible. Swelling was the most frequent reason for seeking treatment.

Results.—Treatment varied considerably and included surgical resection and adjuvant therapy. Local recurrences were seen in 7 patients from 1 to 10 years after the initial treatment. At the last follow-up, metastatic disease was known to have developed in 5 patients 3–22 years after initial treatment. Six patients died of disease, with a median survival of 6 years. Seven patients were alive without evidence of disease at 1–31 years after treatment. Histologically, all 19 tumors exhibited a bimorphic pattern composed of islands of well-differentiated hyaline cartilage juxtaposed with a small, round-cell undifferentiated malignancy (Fig 1). Mitotic activity of the neoplasms was low, however, and necrosis was absent in primary untreated tumors.

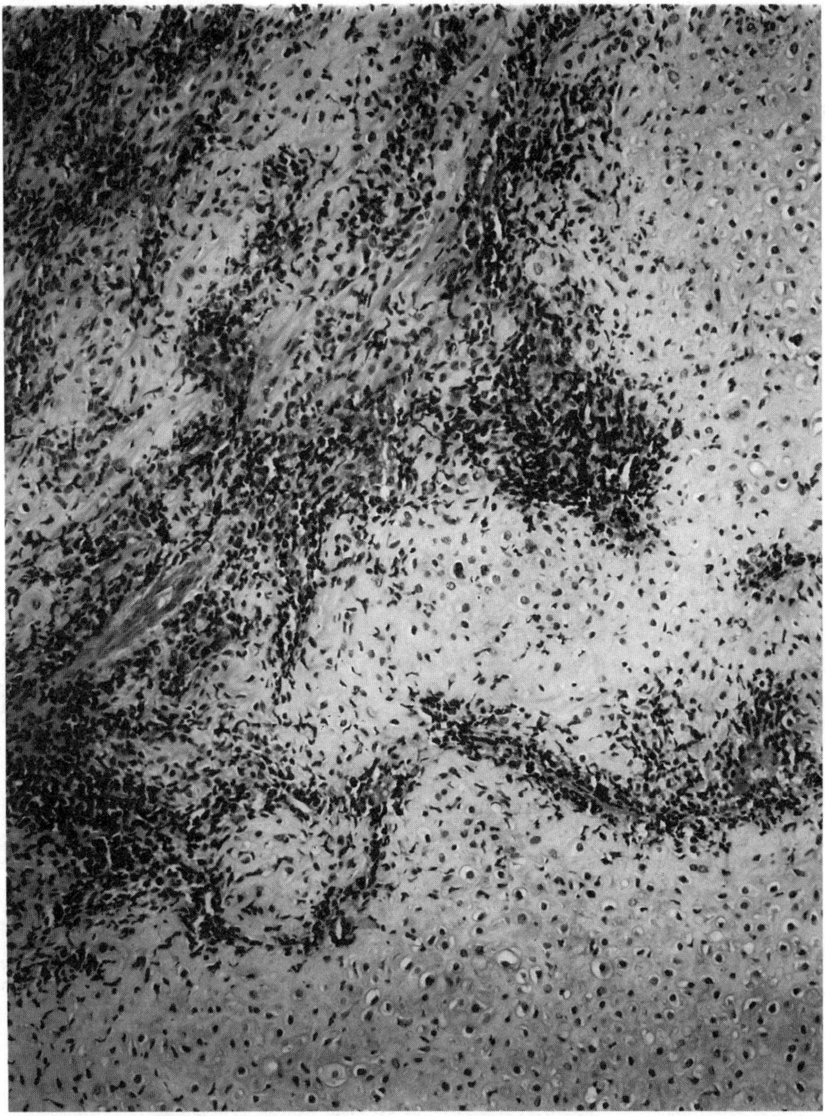

FIGURE 1.—Typical bimorphic pattern of mesenchymal chondrosarcoma, with well-differentiated hyaline cartilage sharply juxtaposed with a small, round-cell undifferentiated component (Hematoxylin-eosin; original magnification ×50). (Courtesy of Vencio EF, Reeve CM, Unni KK, et al: Mesenchymal chondrosarcoma of the jaw bones: Clinicopathologic study of 19 cases. *Cancer* 82[12]:2350–2355. Copyright 1998, American Cancer Society. Reprinted by permission of Wiley-Liss, Inc., a subsidiary of John Wiley & Sons, Inc.)

Conclusion.—Only 19 examples of mesenchymal chondrosarcoma were found among the more than 40,000 cases of bone tumors on file at the Mayo Clinic. The jaw bones are the most common location of this entity, and the course of disease appears to be more indolent than that of mesenchymal chondrosarcoma in other locations. Most patients are children and young adults. Radical local surgery is the recommended treatment.

▶ Mesenchymal chondrosarcomas are very rare, and typically arise within bone, but may also occur in soft tissue. The Mayo Clinic's experience suggests that the jaw bones (mandible and maxilla) are the most common site. This article includes 6 cases from the Mayo Clinic and 13 consultative cases of 1 of the authors. The morphologic findings were typical, and showed a biphasic pattern (Fig 1). The biology of these tumors in this location is different; they have a less aggressive course than similar tumors in other anatomic sites. Nonetheless, it is recommended that all of these tumors be treated with radical local surgery.

M.B. Cohen, M.D.

Association of Tumor Angiogenesis With Bone Marrow Micrometastases in Breast Cancer Patients

Fox SB, Leek RD, Bliss J, et al (Univ of Oxford, England; Inst of Cancer Research, Surrey, England; St George's Hosp, London)

J Natl Cancer Inst 89:1044–1049, 1997 9–17

Background.—Many patients with node-negative breast cancer will die of metastatic disease that is undetected by conventional techniques, even after apparently curative surgery. In patients with breast cancer, the presence of micrometastases in bone marrow and the degree of angiogenesis in primary tumors are both independent prognostic markers. Micrometastases occur as a result of interactions between the tumor cells and the surrounding neovasculature. The relationship between the extent of angiogenesis and the presence of micrometastases in breast cancer was analyzed.

Methods.—Before undergoing mastectomies or lumpectomies, 214 patients with breast cancer underwent bone-marrow aspiration from several sites to determine the presence or absence of micrometastases. Epithelial-membrane antigen expression and cell morphological analysis were performed to identify tumor cells. Tumor vascularity was graded semiquantitatively or quantitatively using the Chalkley point count after the cluster of differentiation 31 antigen expressed by the endothelial cells was stained by immunohistochemical methods. The vascular grading was validated as reproducible and accurate. Chi-square and logistic regression analyses were performed to determine associations between micrometastases and angiogenesis, along with other tumor characteristics.

Results.—Micrometastases were detected in the bone marrow of 20% of the patients, and 35% had high-vascular-grade tumors. The vascular grade of 35 tumors was assessed twice, and there was 86% agreement. Twenty-two of these tumors showed absolute concordance between the vascular grade and Chalkley point count. Tumor angiogenesis was significantly and positively associated with micrometastasis (P = 0.01), tumor grade (P =

0.003), and estrogen-receptor expression ($P = 0.007$). However, angiogenesis was unrelated to tumor size, lymph-node status, vascular invasion, menopausal status, or patient age. On multivariate analysis, the only factors significantly associated with the presence of micrometastases were tumor angiogenesis ($P = 0.016$) and vascular invasion ($P = 0.012$), each with an odds ratio of 2.7.

Conclusions.—In patients with breast cancer, assessing tumor vascularity and vascular invasion will provide reliable indicators of the risk of bone-marrow micrometastases. Both of these processes are likely to contribute to metastases. The extent of angiogenesis may be a useful indicator of the tumor's metastatic capability.

▶ Conclusions of this article are important and straightforward, but the way they are put in the context of overall tumor progression is thrilling. The conclusions are that tumor angiogenesis in the primary breast tumor is predictive of the presence of circulating tumor cells and tumor cells in the bone marrow. Is it the angiogenesis per se that is responsible for tumor-cell access to the circulation? No; in fact the processes are independent, although the neovessels made by the tumor may provide a framework for gaining access to the circulation. So, angiogenesis content causes metastatic behavior, right? No; the process of metastasis is independent of the phenotype/genotype for angiogenesis. In other words, both genotypes are required to generate metastasis, 1 providing the framework and the other providing a mechanism to penetrate the stroma. This may explain why there is a mixture of prognostic outcomes in patients with micrometastasis discovered in lymph nodes by immunocytochemistry, polymerase chain reaction, etc. These patient groups are probably a mixed bag: some patients may also have the metastatic genotype while others may not. The ones without a metastatic genotype exhibit the dormant behavior that we are all familiar with; for example, the breast cancer patients or melanoma patients who show up with lethal metastases 20–30 years following extirpation of their tumors. The premise of the article, then, becomes targeting the treatment of the patients with micrometastases with vascular proliferation inhibitors and watching for clinical progression with a measure of angiogenesis.

D.J. Dabbs, M.D.

Suggested Reading

Cote RJ, Rosen PP, Lesser ML, et al: Prediction of early relapse in patients with operable breast cancer by detection of occult bone marrow micrometastases. *J Clin Oncol* 9:1749–1756, 1991.

Diel IJ, Kaufmann M, Goerner R, et al: Detection of tumor cells in bone marrow of patients with primary breast cancer: A prognostic factor for distant metastasis. *J Clin Oncol* 10:1534–1539, 1992.

Osborne MP, Rosen PP: Detection and management of bone marrow micrometastases in breast cancer. *Oncology (Huntingt)* 8:25–31, 1994.

Pantel K, Izbicki JR, Angstwurm M, et al: Immunocytological detection of bone marrow micrometastasis in operable non-small cell lung cancer. *Cancer Res* 53:1027–1031, 1993.

Clinical and Pathologic Findings in Hemochromatosis Hip Arthroplasty

Montgomery KD, Williams JR, Sculco TP, et al (Lenox Hill Hosp, New York; Univ of Pittsburgh, Pa; Hosp for Special Surgery, New York)
Clin Orthop 347:179–187, 1998 9–18

Objective.—Hemochromatosis, abnormal deposition of iron in the body, can result in a variety of pathologic conditions, including arthropathy. Hip involvement affects approximately 25% of these patients. The clinical presentation, radiographic and histologic findings, and functional outcome of 15 patients with hemochromatosis after total hip arthroplasty are discussed.

Methods.—Between 1982 and 1992, 19 total hip arthroplasties were performed in 15 patients (6 women) with hemochromatosis, ages 48 to 68. Patients were followed up radiographically on average for 5.7 years to assess hip pain and function. Osteonecrosis was categorized as stage I, II, III, or IV.

Results.—The average preoperative Hospital for Special Surgery hip score was 15, and the average postoperative score was 30. Twelve (63%)

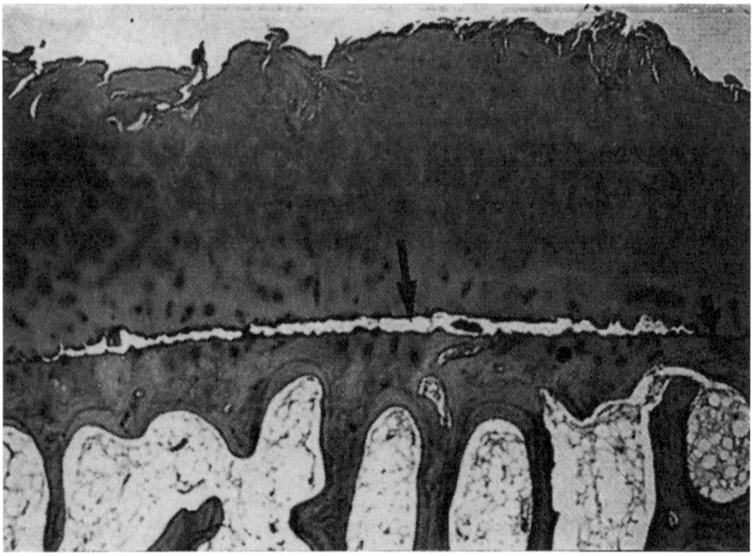

FIGURE 1.—This low power photomicrograph shows a split in the articular cartilage (*long arrow*) at the level of the tidemark (*short arrow*), the boundary between the noncalcified and calcified cartilage, with slight sclerosis of the end plate; hematoxylin-eosin; original magnification, ×5.) (Courtesy of Montgomery KD, Williams JR, Sculco TP, et al: Clinical and pathologic findings in hemochromatosis hip arthroplasty. *Clin Orthop* 347:179–187, 1998.)

femoral heads showed osteoarthritis, 8 (42%) had split cartilage at the tidemark level, and 7 (37%) had bone necrosis (Fig 1). Radiographs revealed subchondral sclerosis, joint space narrowing, or osteophyte formation. Iron deposition was found in the synovium of 5 patients. Only 3 of 7 patients with osteonecrosis showed such changes on radiographs. Radiographs revealed stage II disease in 1 femoral head, stage IV disease in 1 femoral head, and Stage I disease in 4 femoral heads. One patient had loosening and migration of a cemented acetabular component after 10 years, and 4 patients showed osteolysis. Five (26%) femoral heads showed calcium pyrophosphate deposits.

Conclusion.—Hemochromatosis should be suspected in patients with the appearance of degenerative joint disease and avulsion of the articular cartilage at the level of the tidemark. Only 5 patients had iron deposition in the synovium.

► Although this is a clinically focused study, it contains useful information for pathologists. The clinical recognition of joint, especially hip, disease in patients with hemochromatosis is not new, but there are relatively few pathologic descriptions. The authors' present experience with hip arthroplasty specimens from patients with hemochromatosis. Interestingly, 40% of the patients were women. The pathology revealed chiefly degenerative joint disease, most notably avulsion of the articular cartilage at the level of the tidemark, although 7 patients had evidence of avascular necrosis and 5 patients had deposition of calcium pyrophosphate. Importantly, iron deposition was seen in the synovium of only 5 patients. The authors propose a model for the pathophysiology of this process, but this remains a working hypothesis.

M.B. Cohen, M.D.

10 Neuropathology

Pituitary Carcinoma: A Clinicopathologic Study of 15 Cases

Pernicone PJ, Scheithauer BW, Sebo TJ, et al (Mayo Clinic and Found, Rochester, Minn; St Michael's Hosp, Toronto; Univ of Alabama, Birmingham; et al)

Cancer 79:804–812, 1997 10–1

Introduction.—Pituitary carcinomas are rare neoplasms, with only 64 cases (including 15 in this study) reported in the literature published in English. In a clinicopathologic study, investigators focused on the interrelationships of endocrine activity, hormone immunotype, tumoral proliferative activity, image morphometric assessment of DNA content, p53 gene expression, and tumor behavior.

Methods.—Six cases were from the files of the Mayo Clinic Tissue Registry and 9 were from consultation files. The presence of craniospinal and/or systemic metastases was used to distinguish pituitary carcinomas from invasive adenomas. Immunostaining was performed on 5 micron sections in all but 1 case.

Results.—Patients were 8 men and 7 women, with a mean age of 56. Seven patients, including 2 with Cushing's disease and 4 with Nelson's syndrome, had adrenocorticotropic hormone (ACTH) cell tumors. Another patient had mild ACTH elevation, but no clinical signs of Cushing's disease. A nonfunctioning tumor was present in 1 case. Seven patients with prolactin cell tumors were seen initially with headache and visual field deficits. Tumor extent was known in 10 patients, all of whom had invasive tumors. The mean interval from initial diagnosis of adenoma to that of carcinoma was 6.6 years. Among patients with Nelson's syndrome, however, the mean interval was 15.3 years. The rate of systemic metastasis was 71% for prolactin cell tumors and 57% for ACTH-producing tumors. Both systemic and craniospinal metastases were present in 13% of tumors. Nuclear pleomorphism and hyperchromasia were common findings, identified in half of the primary tumors and in the majority of metastases. Staining for p53 protein was seen in 57% of primary tumors and 88% of metastatic tumors. Initial treatment in all but 1 case was pituitary surgery; the remaining patient underwent radiation therapy after bilateral adrenalectomy. Metastatic disease was commonly treated with surgical decompression and/or radiation therapy. Of the 80% of patients who died of metastatic disease, two thirds died within a year of diagnosis.

Conclusion.—By definition, all pituitary carcinomas metastasize, and systemic metastasis is more common than craniospinal metastasis. Treatment with radiation and dopamine agonist therapy provides palliation, but prognosis is generally poor. When metastasis is not demonstrated, high mitotic and MIB-1 labeling indices and p53 immunoreactivity suggest the diagnosis of pituitary carcinoma.

▶ This is a good example of the continued desperate attempt to find meaning, in immunostaining for proliferation markers, where none exists. Pituitary carcinomas are rare tumors, which are diagnosed based on the presence of evident metastases, either craniospinal or distant. These tumors are so rare that a comprehensive, stastistically sound study of independent prognostic factors for metastasis in primary pituitary adenomas has not been performed. This article is 9 pages long, and, to my mind, the most accurate sentences appear near the end of the discussion, where the authors write about prognostic factors for these tumors: "Currently available parameters, such as mitotic and proliferation indices, cannot provide the precision required. The same is true of immunohistochemistry markers, such as p53 expression." Still, these authors advocate the identification of "adenomas of uncertain malignant potential" based on mitotic and MIB-1 indices and p53 immunoreactivity! Their data, based on such a small number of tumors, does not support this suggestion. Based on that data, one could predict tumor behavior just as well doing a mitotic index, which does not require special immunostaining. I agree with the author's last sentence: "Further studies will be needed to elucidate the pathogenesis of these unusual tumors further, to identify pathologic parameters that are reliable for prognosis and to develop more effective therapeutic modalities," I think it is premature to suggest an intermediate histologic category of adenomas based on the parameters they describe here.

D.M. Grzybicki, M.D., Ph.D.

Vascular Endothelial Growth Factor Expression and Vascular Density as Prognostic Markers of Survival in Patients With Low-grade Astrocytoma

Abdulrauf SI, Edvardsen K, Ho KL, et al (Henry Ford Hosp, Detroit)
J Neurosurg 88:513–520, 1998 10–2

Background.—The natural history of low-grade astrocytoma is unclear. Some patients survive for many years, while others survive for only a short period. Patients with short survival do not usually die of low-grade disease, but rather die after tumor transformation into a higher grade. To date, no biological markers indicating risk of malignant transformation of low-grade astrocytoma have been identified. Angiogenesis is important in the growth and spread of some malignant brain and systemic tumors, although there is no evidence that it can predict malignant transformation of low-grade astrocytoma.

Methods.—Seventy-four consecutive patients with diffuse supratentorial hemispheric fibrillary low-grade astrocytoma underwent surgery. Tumor tissue was studied using monoclonal antibodies to the antigens of proliferation-associated Ki-67, factor VIII, vascular endothelial growth factor, basic fibroblast growth factor, and epidermal growth factor. Mean follow-up was 6.1 years.

Results.—Overall survival at 5 years was 65%, and median survival was 7.5 years. At initial operation, all tumors had low proliferative potential, shown by a Ki-67 labeling index of less than 1.5%. Shorter survival was seen in patients with more than 7 microvessels in tumor tissue than in patients with 7 or fewer microvessels. Univariate and stepwise multivariate analyses showed that this difference in survival was significant. The incidence of malignant transformation was higher in tumors with a greater number of microvessels. Univariate and multivariate analyses showed that significant staining for vascular endothelial growth factor was associated with shorter survival and with a greater chance of malignant transformation. Median survival was 5.3 years for patients with tumors that were positive for vascular endothelial growth factor, and 11.2 years for patients with tumors negative for vascular endothelial growth factor. There was no association among basic fibroblast growth factor, epidermal growth factor, survival, or malignant transformation. Stepwise multivariate analyses included histological and clinical factors.

Conclusion.—These findings indicate that microvessel density and levels of vascular endothelial growth factor are independent predictors of survival in patients with fibrillary low-grade astrocytoma. It is proposed that fibrillary diffuse low-grade astrocytoma may not be a single pathological entity, but may consist of various tumors, each with a different potential for malignant transformation. This potential may be partly related to the inherent angiogenic potential of each tumor.

▶ This article caught my interest initially because I was relieved to find a report of potential brain tumor prognostic markers that were not cell proliferation antigens. In the ongoing quest for an independent histologic prognostic indicator for low-grade astrocytoma, the authors chose to concentrate on angiogenesis-related parameters. Angiogenesis is a hot (although not new) topic in tumor development/progression research, and the authors' rationale for investigating vascular growth factors and microvascular density is sound. Despite the majority of their data being a subjective assessment of immunostaining intensity for multiple specific growth factors, the authors appear to have attempted to objectify the analysis as much as possible. They provide nice details regarding their immunohistochemical grading scale and microvessel counting scheme. One weakness in their methods is that it appears only 1 observer counted the vessels and did the immunohistochemical grading. Their results would be even more convincing if they could show reproducibility among multiple observers in the grading and counting. Unlike many similar studies looking at proliferation markers, a strength of this study is that the authors not only perform univariate analyses with the individual angiogenic variables, but also perform multivariate analysis, using recognized clinical prognostic factors and the angiogenic variables together, to demonstrate that microvessel count and vascular endothelial growth factor are each independent prognostic factors for survival in these patients. These results lead the authors to suggest that there are 2 biological subgroups of low-grade astrocytoma, the "angiogenic" types associated with a significantly worse patient prognosis. This information is potentially important for future therapeutic strategies which may target tumor angiogenesis. Currently, the clinical management of adult patients with low-grade astrocytoma is controversial, and it is unclear how such prognosis-related information may practically be used in the clinical decision-making process.

D.M. Grzybicki, M.D., Ph.D.

Ganglioglioma: An Ultrastructural and Immunohistochemical Study

Hirose T, Scheithauer BW, Lopes MBS, et al (Mayo Clinic, Rochester, Minn; Univ of Virginia Health Sciences Ctr, Charlotteville; Univ of Bern, Switzerland)

Cancer 79:989–1003, 1997 10–3

Background.—Gangliogliomas are rare, usually benign tumors of the central nervous system that primarily affect children and young adults. Diagnosis depends on verifying the neoplastic nature of the neurons and excludes the possibility that they may represent entrapped preexisting elements. The ability of proliferation markers to predict more aggressive behavior or recurrence has not been systematically evaluated.

Methods.—The morphologic and immunophenotypic features of gangliogliomas, as well as features predictive of recurrence, were studied in 27 patients. Fourteen patients were male, and the age range was 3–52 years. Routine histochemistry was used in 27 specimens, immunochemistry in 21 specimens, and analysis at the ultrastructural level in 14 specimens.

Results.—Most gangliogliomas occurred in the temporal lobe. Local recurrence was seen in 3 patients. Microscopic examination showed well-differentiated, somewhat abnormal neurons and glial cells. The glial cells included fibrillary and pilocytic astrocytes. Two tumors had limited scant mitotic activity. In all tumors, glial cells were immunoreactive for glial fibrillary acidic protein, S-100 protein, and vimentin. The Ki-67 labeling indices were 0.6% to 10.5%. The p53 labeling indices were 1.1% to 42.4%. In recurrent tumors, the Ki-67 and p53 labeling indices were significantly higher than in nonrecurrent tumors. There was no anaplastic transformation. Immunohistochemical examination showed many neuronal cells positive for synaptophysin, Class 3 betatubulin, neurofilament protein, chromogranin A, S-100 protein, and, in some cases, vimentin. Ultrastructurally, the neuronal cells had numerous, 100- to 230-nanometer dense core granules in perikarya and cell processes, well-developed rough endoplasmic reticulum, microtubules within cell processes, and synapses associated with clear vesicles. Most astrocytic cells had abundant intermediate filaments; cell membranes were covered by basal lamina when abutting the stroma.

Conclusion.—These findings indicate that glial cells of gangliogliomas may be fibrillary or pilocytic. Neurons are characterized by immunoreactivity for chromogranin A, synaptophysin, and various neurotransmitters. The dense core granules in the neuronal peirkarya are distinct from the secretory structures of normal, mature neurons of the central nervous system. Higher Ki-67 and p53 labeling indices may be related to more aggressive behavior.

▶ This article provides an excellent review of the morphologic and immunophenotypic features of this subgroup of ganglion cell tumors. The authors don't provide any new information, but their description and discussion of the 27 cases they examined are highly detailed and comprehensive, including clinical correlation data as well as information regarding what is known about the molecular genetic abnormalities and histogenesis of this tumor. My one criticism of this article relates to the authors' conclusions regarding the possible prognostic significance of Ki-67 and p53 labeling in these tumors. The authors performed these immunohistochemical stains to investigate possible histologic features predictive of tumor recurrence. They report a statistically significant higher labeling index for both Ki-67 (using MIB-1 antibody) and p53 in the 3 recurrent tumors in their series, but the primary tumors were not available for study. Their conclusion "that the proliferative activity as well as p53 protein immunoreactivity of the neoplastic glial cells may be related to tumor recurrence" is unsupported by their data. The only conclusion they can make is that the 3 recurrent tumors have higher labeling indices for these antigens. *No* conclusions can be made regarding the prognostic significance of these markers, since the authors provide no data from the original tumors. This is an example of pathologists performing immunohistochemical stains on tumors "to see what happens" and then making far-reaching and scientifically unsupported conclusions based on their results.

D.M. Grzybicki, M.D., Ph.D.

Cerebrospinal Fluid Cytology: An 11-Year Experience With 5951 Specimens

Prayson RA, Fischler DF (Cleveland Clinic Found, Ohio)

Arch Pathol Lab Med 122:47–51, 1998 10–4

Background.—Examination of CSF specimens is useful in the diagnosis of many types of conditions. The findings on CSF cytology specimens from 1 institution collected during an 11-year period were retrospectively reviewed.

Study Design.—The cytology computer files were searched to identify all CSF cytology specimens from 1985 through 1995. There were a total

TABLE 1.—Summary of Tumor Diagnoses in Adult Patients (n = 276)

Tumor Type	No. of Cases (%)
Adenocarcinoma	114 (41.3)
Lymphoma	78 (28.3)
Leukemia	33 (12.0)
Carcinoma, not otherwise specified	10 (3.6)
Malignant unclassified neoplasm	9 (3.3)
Malignant melanoma	8 (2.9)
Glioblastoma mulitforme	7 (2.5)
Other*	17

* Includes astrocytoma (n = 3); malignant lymphoma/leukemia, not otherwise specified (n = 3); large cell carcinoma (n = 3); small cell carcinoma (n = 2); squamous cell carcinoma (n = 2); lymphoproliferative disorder, not otherwise specified (n = 2); pineocytoma (n = 1); and primitive neuroectodermal tumor (n = 1).

(Courtesy of Prayson RA, Fischler DF: Cerebrospinal fluid cytology: An 11-year experience with 5951 specimens *Arch Pathol Lab Med* 122:47–51, 1998.)

of 5,951 specimens, of which 390 were pediatric specimens. The diagnoses were reviewed and tabulated.

Findings.—Of the adult cases, 93% were negative for malignant cells. Of the pediatric cases, 90% were negative for malignant cells. Specific infectious organisms were identified in 26 adult specimens. The most common infectious agent was *Cryptococcus*. There was only 1 pediatric infection identified, a *Toxoplasma* infection. Tumor diagnoses in adults included metastatic tumors, lymphoma/leukemia, malignant unclassified neoplasms, and primary CNS neoplasms (Table 1). The most common pediatric neoplasm was medulloblastoma (Table 2). Atypical cells were detected in 2% of adult and pediatric samples. In adults, atypical lymphoid cells were most common.

Conclusions.—In this review of CSF cytology samples obtained during an 11-year period, infectious agents were not commonly identified in pediatric CSF specimens. The most commonly identified agent in adult samples was *Cryptococcus*. Metastatic neoplasms were the most commonly identified malignancy in adults, whereas medulloblastoma was most common in pediatric patients. Primary CNS neoplasms were more common in pediatric than in adult samples.

TABLE 2.—Summary of Tumor Diagnoses in Pediatric Patients (n = 31)

Tumor Type	No. of Cases (%)
Medulloblastoma/primitive neuroectodermal tumor	24 (77.4)
Lymphoma	2 (6.5)
Leukemia	2 (6.5)
Malignant ependymoma	1 (3.2)
Choroid plexus carcinoma	1 (3.2)
Germ cell tumor	1 (3.2)

(Courtesy of Prayson RA, Fischler DF: Cerebrospinal fluid cytology: An 11-year experience with 5951 specimens *Arch Pathol Lab Med* 122:47–51, 1998.)

▶ This study is simply a review of diagnoses from CSF cytology specimens reported at the authors' institution during an 11-year period, from 1985 to 1995. Although no surprising findings issue from this report, it is valuable to review because it reconfirms that, practically speaking, only a few diagnoses are commonly made on most CSF specimens from both adults and children. In adult patients, metastatic adenocarcinoma is by far the most common diagnosis, followed by metastatic hematopoietic neoplasms (Table 1). Other metastatic tumors (such as malignant melanoma) are uncommon, as are primary CNS tumors. In the pediatric population, small blue cell tumors (including medulloblastoma) are by far the most common, followed by metastatic hematopoietic neoplasms (Table 2). This report also emphasizes the well-known fact that the paucity of cells in many of these specimens complicates these seemingly straightforward observations; CSF specimens with one or a few "atypical" cells are a not uncommon diagnostic challenge in CSF cytology. However, knowing the clinical history of the patient, the precise location of a mass if present, and the most commonly seen lesions as reviewed by these authors can help at least minimize the potential difficulties with CSF cytology specimens.

D.M. Grzybicki, M.D., Ph.D.

Herpes Simplex Encephalitis (HSE) and the Immunocompromised: A Clinical and Autopsy Study of HSE in the Settings of Cancer and Human Immunodeficiency Virus–Type 1 Infection

Schiff D, Rosenblum MK (Mem Sloan-Kettering Cancer Ctr, New York)

Hum Pathol 29:215–222, 1998 10–5

Introduction.—Herpes simplex viruses (HSVs) are found often in the general population, but the incidence of herpes simplex encephalitis (HSE) is remarkably low. The yearly attack rates of this acute, febrile disorder are estimated at 2–4 cases per million inhabitants. When HSE occurs in immunocompromised patients, the disorder appears to be characterized by unusual clinical and neuropathologic features. Three cases of autopsy-proven HSE in immunocompromised patients were reviewed for clinical and pathological findings.

Methods.—Two of the patients had cancer; 1 was known to be HIV-1–seropositive, and another was suspected of having underlying HIV-1 infection. All 3 patients had fever, and exhibited changes in mental status and new, focal neurological deficits or worsening of established deficits. Two patients were receiving dexamethasone at the time of HSE onset. The patients' medical records, neurological scans, and autopsy findings were reviewed.

Findings.—The patients were women aged 24, 31, and 35. One (who was married to an IV drug abuser) had undergone subtotal resection of a left frontal lobe malignant lymphoma of B-cell immunoblastic type. A month later, she was transferred in a coma, after becoming increasingly unresponsive. Treatment had consisted of dexamethasone, cranial irradiation, and IV acyclovir, but the patient's condition deteriorated and she died approximately 6 weeks after surgery. The patient known to be HIV-1–seropositive came to an emergency room with fever and gross dehydration. Broad-spectrum antibiotics failed to bring improvement, and the patient deteriorated neurologically. Death came on the 19th hospital day after development of bilateral pulmonary infiltrates, hypotension, hypothermia, and disseminated intravascular coagulation. The third patient had undergone subtotal resection of a mass subsequently proven to be a glioblastoma. Whole brain irradiation was administered and she was discharged on dexamethasone maintenance. About 6 months later she was admitted with fever, confusion, and aphasia. Her condition worsened despite treatment, and generalized tonic-clonic seizures occurred. She died on hospital day 17.

Discussion.—None of these patients was clinically suspected of having HSE, but the disease, confirmed at autopsy, played a major role in all 3 deaths. This form of HSE is characterized by a noninflammatory, pseudo-ischemic histological presentation, with abundant and unexpected persistence of viral antigens. Because the diagnosis of HSE may be missed in immunocompromised patients, increased clinical suspicion is needed.

▶ This is a very well-written and complete article, which is important for 2 major reasons. First, it provides significant and interesting information regarding HSV infections in immunocompromised patients. The authors describe 3 such patients, with autopsy-proven HSE, who did exhibit clinical neurologic signs of HSE, but whose diagnoses were confounded because of radiologic studies nonsuggestive of HSE and because of non-inflammatory CSF studies. The neuropathologic findings described here support the idea that HSE is much more common in immunocompromised patients because of the ischemic, nonhemorrhagic, noninflammatory nature of the lesions, than is presently appreciated. Therefore, clinical suspicion for HSE can probably justifiably remain high in immunocompromised patients exhibiting neurologic signs of an acute encephalitis, even if the patients don't exhibit the expected CSF and radiologic changes. The generally accepted view has been that immunocompromise, including that occuring with HIV infection, does not predispose patients to typical HSE; one could conclude from this article that we are missing more cases of HSE in immunocompromised patients than we suspect. I agree with the authors' suggestion that empiric acyclovir treatment should probably be considered in these patients, while other diagnostic procedures, including HSV CSF polymerase chain reaction, are performed. Despite the high sensitivity of HSV polymerase chain reaction, which may yield false positive results in some cases, it appears to be indicated in immunocompromised patients to make the diagnosis. The second reason this is an important article is that it clearly illustrates the critical role the autopsy continues to play in revealing information which can significantly increase our knowledge about disease processes, and therefore have a positive impact on clinical diagnosis and patient management.

D.M. Grzybicki, M.D., Ph.D.

Pathogen-free Granulomatous Diseases of the Central Nervous System
Thomas G, Murphy S, Staunton H, et al (Beaumont Hosp, Dublin; Royal College of Surgeons in Ireland, Dublin)
Hum Pathol 29:110–115, 1998 10–6

Background.—The clinical and pathologic findings of pathogen-free granulomatous diseases of the CNS are protean. When the causative organism cannot be identified, diagnosis is difficult. The natural history of this disorder, as well as the nature and extent of disease outside the CNS, were investigated in a retrospective study.

Methods and Findings.—Eleven patients fulfilling the pathologic criteria for this condition were included in the analysis. Age at diagnosis ranged from 17 to 78 years, with a mean of 38.7 years. In 9 patients, the initial symptoms were neurologic. Neuroimaging demonstrated hydrocephalus in 54.5% of the patients, meningeal enhancement in 45.5%, and mass lesions in 45.5%. Antemortem CNS biopsies, performed in 7 patients, produced specimens showing noncaseating granulomas. Eight patients (72.7%) died. On postmortem evaluation, granulomatous involvement of the leptomeninges and cerebral parenchyma was present in all patients. Half had systemic involvement, mainly as noncaseating granuloma of the hilar nodes. The clinical, radiologic, and pathologic findings in 6 patients met the criteria for neurosarcoidosis. In the remaining 5 patients, unclassified pathogen-free granulomatous CNS disease was recorded (Table 4).

Conclusion.—Pathogen-free granulomatous diseases of the CNS carry a poor prognosis. Although some cases may be neurosarcoidosis, many are unclassifiable, making diagnosis and management difficult.

▶ The authors of this retrospective study provide interesting and useful information regarding this rare group of diseases. It is useful information

TABLE 4.—Comparison Between Neurosarcoidosis Subgroup and Unclassifiable Pathogen-Free Granulomatous Diseases Subgroup

	Neurosarcoidosis (N = 6)	Unclassifiable PFGD (N = 5)
Clinical features		
Clinical symptoms	Focal neurological deficits	Seizures Headaches
Systemic disease	Present	Absent
Mean duration from diagnosis to mortality	6.2 yr	2.5 yr
Histological features		
Granulomatous agniitis	Rare	Common
Spinal cord involvement	Rare	Common

(Courtesy of Thomas G, Murphy S, Staunton H, et al: Pathogen-free granulomatous diseases of the central nervous system. *Hum Pathol* 29:110–115, 1998.)

primarily because these cases are so rare. I have only seen 2 cases that I remember but, as the authors point out in their first sentence as characteristic of these diseases, they were very problematic for both the clinicians and neuropathologists. After doing all the appropriate testing for infectious causes, there is really nothing definitive the neuropathologist can offer, which is frustrating for clinicians trying to decide how to treat the patient.

In this series of 11 cases (collected from a 10-year review) the authors show that the cases tend to fall into 2 categories, with approximately half the patients in each category: patients in whom a diagnosis of neurosarcoidosis can be made based on the presence of systemic disease, and those without systemic disease who remain unclassifiable. Despite corticosteroid therapy, all the patients in the unclassifiable group had a poor long-term prognosis. The authors' comparison between these 2 subgroups, based on specific clinical and histologic features (see Table 4), provides potentially useful information for both clinicians and neuropathologists working up these rare but difficult cases.

D.M. Grzybicki, M.D., Ph.D.

Diagnostic Yield of Brain Biopsy in Neurodegenerative Disorders

Javedan SP, Tamargo RJ (Johns Hopkins Univ, Baltimore, Md)

Neurosurgery 41:823–830, 1997 10–7

Background.—Though the role of brain biopsy is well established in the diagnosis of patients with suspected neoplastic lesions, few authors have analyzed its diagnostic yield for idiopathic neurodegenerative disorders (meningoencephalitis, CNS vasculitis, and dementia syndromes). The current study determined the diagnostic yield of brain biopsy in these disorders.

Methods.—Forty-eight patients undergoing 50 consecutive brain biopsies between 1990 and 1995 were included in the analysis. Extensive laboratory and radiologic assessments were performed before surgery. Because diagnoses could not be established, brain biopsies were performed.

Findings.—Only 10 of the 50 biopsies resulted in diagnosis, for a diagnostic yield of 20%. Another 6% of the biopsies were suggestive of diagnoses. Findings on 66% of the biopsies were abnormal but not specific. Eight percent of the biopsies yielded normal findings. Minor complications associated with biopsy occurred in 10% of the patients. Only 4 of the 10 patients with diagnostic biopsies had a meaningful intervention as a result of the procedure. Thus the overall therapeutic benefit was only 4 (8%) of the 50 biopsies. A subgroup analysis showed that patients with focal MRI findings had the greatest likelihood of a diagnostic biopsy. Electroencephalography and laboratory abnormalities did not predict a diagnostic biopsy.

Conclusions.—The current diagnostic yield of brain biopsy for progressive neurodegenerative disorders was only 20% in this study, which is

TABLE 2.—Diagnostic Yield

		Odds Ratio	95% C.I.
All biopsies (n = 50) (%)			
Diagnostic	10 of 50 (20)		
Suggestive	3 of 50 (6)		
Nonspecific	33 of 50 (66)		
Normal	4 of 50 (8)		
Patient subgroups (%)			
Focal MR findings	8/27 (30)	4.00	0.75–21.3
Seizures/myoclonus	4/10 (40)	3.77	0.81–17.5
Dementia	5/13 (38)	3.75	0.87–16.2
Suspected Creutzfeldt	2/5 (40)	2.91	0.41–20.4
Elevated protein	6/26 (23)	1.35	0.33–5.56
Headache	2/9 (22)	1.11	0.19–6.39
Ataxia	3/14 (21)	1.05	0.23–4.83
Abnormal EEG	4/19 (21)	1.02	0.25–4.24
Suspected herpes	2/10 (20)	0.94	0.17–5.31
Fever	3/17 (18)	0.73	0.16–3.31
Suspected vasculitis	1/7 (14)	0.59	0.06–5.58
Pleocytosis	3/20 (15)	0.48	0.12–2.36

Abbreviations: C.I., confidence interval; *MR*, magnetic resonance; *EEG*, electroencephalography.
(Courtesy of Javedan SP, Tamargo RJ: Diagnostic yield of brain biopsy in neurodegenerative disorders. *Neurosurgery* 41:823–830, 1997.)

lower than that reported previously. The therapeutic benefits of brain biopsy in this population are limited.

▶ This report provides extremely important information regarding the overall low diagnostic yield of brain biopsies performed for neurodegenerative disorders. These results (summarized in Table 2) most likely concur with the majority of neuropathologists' experience, and they are in agreement with a recent study by Brainard et al.[1] which showed that frozen section evaluation of stereotactic brain biopsies is not very useful for nonneoplastic lesions, including suspected vasculitis. I think the most valuable piece of information from this study is that of the 48 patients undergoing biopsy, the information derived from the biopsy actually impacted patient treatment in only 2 cases. Similar critical reassessment of other well-established clinical and pathologic diagnostic procedures (which nevertheless may have questionable use or cost-effectiveness) is needed, as shrinking resources force us to limit procedures to those of proven value.

D.M. Grzybicki, M.D., Ph.D.

Reference

1. Brainard JA, Prayson RA, Barnett GH: Frozen section evaluation of stereotactic brain biopsies: Diagnostic yield at the stereotactic target position in 188 cases. *Arch Pathol Lab Med* 121:481–484, 1997.

Utility of the Apolipoprotein E Genotype in the Diagnosis of Alzheimer's Disease

Mayeux R, for the Alzheimer's Disease Centers Consortium on Apolipoprotein E and Alzheimer's Disease (Columbia Univ, New York; et al)

N Engl J Med 338:506–511, 1998 10–8

Introduction.—The finding of 1 or more ϵ4 alleles of the gene for apolipoprotein E (apoE ϵ4) in a patient with dementia has consistently been associated with Alzheimer's disease (AD). In a few small postmortem studies of the apoE genotype in clinical diagnosis, the specificity of the apoE ϵ4 allele was nearly 100%. Data pooled from 26 AD centers were reviewed to determine the value of the genotype in diagnosis of the disease.

Methods.—The study group included 2,188 patients who underwent evaluation for dementia. Clinical diagnoses and diagnoses obtained at autopsy were analyzed, and the sensitivity and specificity of the clinical diagnosis or the presence of an apoE ϵ4 allele were calculated. The standard for diagnosis was pathological confirmation of AD. A standard protocol at each center determined the apoE genotypes of genomic DNA from blood or other tissues.

Results.—The 2,188 patients represented 69% of those reviewed for eligibility; excluded patients had incomplete information. Patients had a mean age of 72 at clinical diagnosis, and a mean age of 77 at death. Most (97%) were white, and men and women were equally represented (49% and 51%, respectively). Autopsy confirmed AD in 1,770 patients; 1,833 had received a clinical diagnosis. At least 1 apoE ϵ4 allele was detected in 62% of patients with clinically diagnosed AD, and in 65% of those with pathologically confirmed AD. The sensitivity of the clinical diagnosis was 93%, whereas specificity was 55%. Sensitivity of the apoE ϵ4 allele was

TABLE 3.—Sensitivity and Specificity of the Clinical Diagnosis of Alzheimer's Disease According to the APOE Genotype

APOE Genotype	Both Clinical and Pathological Criteria for AD	Only Clinical Criteria for AD	Only Pathological Criteria for AD	Neither Clinical nor Pathological Criteria for AD	Sensitivity	Specificity
	no. of patients				%	
ϵ4/ϵ4	227	17	14	9	93	39
ϵ4/ϵ3	795	47	49	54	94	52
ϵ4/ϵ2	54	2	3	4	96	57
ϵ2/ϵ2	4	0	1	4	100	80
ϵ2/ϵ3	55	5	17	20	92	54
ϵ3/ϵ3	508	56	106	137	90	56
Total	1643	127	190	228	93	55

Abbreviations: AD, Alzheimer's disease; *APOE*, apolipoprotein E.

(Reprinted by permission of *The New England Journal of Medicine*, from Mayeux R, for the Alzheimer's Disease Centers Consortium on Apolipoprotein E and Alzheimer's Disease: Utility of the apolipoprotein E genotype in the diagnosis of Alzheimer's disease. *N Engl J Med* 338:506–511.)

65% and specificity was 68%. In patients who met clinical criteria for AD, addition of information about the apoE genotype reduced the false positive rate. Sensitivity and specificity for the clinical diagnosis were essentially unchanged (Table 3) when recalculated with stratification according to individual apoE genotypes.

Conclusion.—Both sensitivity and specificity are inadequate when apoE genotyping is used alone as a diagnostic test for AD. Because sequential use of the apoE genotype with clinical criteria significantly improved the specificity of the clinical diagnosis, apoE genotyping might be reserved for patients who meet clinical criteria for AD.

► The gold standard diagnostic test for AD has been and continues to be the postmortem examination. However, as genetic and molecular information about AD becomes increasingly available, great effort is being directed toward discovering how this basic scientific information may be applied to the premortem clinical diagnosis of AD. Additionally, because many asymptomatic family members of patients with AD desire information relating to their future risk of developing AD, such predictive biological markers are intensely sought. This article is a good example of such clinical application research, and it gives important information for neuropathologists and clinicians, as the diagnosis and treatment of AD evolve. The genetic testing for apoE has been one particular area of intense investigation, since an ϵ4 allele appears to confer an increased risk for AD. This article shows how apoE genotyping is useful only as an *adjunct* to clinical and other laboratory tests for Alzheimer's diagnosis, increasing the specificity of the diagnosis only under these conditions. Although the use of apoE genotyping will continue to be controversial, and although it will be used differently by different clinicians, this article is important because it clearly reveals the limitations of this test.

D.M. Grzybicki, M.D., Ph.D.

Diagnosis of Cerebral Amyloid Angiopathy: Sensitivity and Specificity of Cortical Biopsy

Greenberg SM, Vonsattel J-PG (Harvard Med School, Boston)

Stroke 28:1418–1422, 1997 10–9

Background.—Evaluating cortical tissue is important for diagnosing cerebral amyloid angiopathy (CAA). However, examination of a single tissue sample may yield false positive or false negative results. The sensitivity and specificity of cortical biopsy for diagnosing CAA as the cause of intracerebral hemorrhage were determined.

Methods.—Biopsy-sized cortical samples were obtained from postmortem brains to simulate CAA biopsy. The brains were known to have either

CAA-related bleeding or mild-to-severe CAA without bleeding. The specimens were stained, using methods routinely available in surgical pathology laboratories, and assessed blindly for vascular amyloid and amyloid-related vasculopathic changes.

Findings.—The finding of vascular amyloid was a sensitive marker for CAA-related hemorrhage, a marker present in all 28 samples from hemorrhagic brains. The appearance of fibrinoid necrosis in amyloid-laden vessels was relatively specific for CAA-associated bleeding, occurring in 46% of specimens from brains with hemorrhage, but in none of the 27 sections from brains with mild CAA, and in only 4 of 42 specimens with moderate-to-severe CAA without bleeding.

Conclusions.—Though there is marked section-to-section variability within each class of CAA, cases of CAA-related hemorrhage generally had more severe and widespread CAA pathologic findings than brains without hemorrhage. The current data will be useful in defining criteria for the diagnosis of CAA-related hemorrhage from surgical specimens.

► When I began reading this article, I thought it was going to report a study measuring the sensitivity and specificity of the surgical neuropathologic diagnosis of CAA. Instead, the authors' goal was to estimate the sensitivity and specificity of cortical biopsy for diagnosis of CAA-related hemorrhage, and they use only postmortem tissue from patients already given a postmortem diagnosis of CAA, with or without associated hemorrhage. I question the clinical usefulness of this information because, in practice, CAA is specifically searched for in hematoma evacuation specimens from patients who have already bled, not in cortical biopsy specimens. The diagnosis may therefore provide only a possible explanation for a lobar intracerebral hemorrage occuring in an elderly patient. Cerebral amyloid angiopathy may of course be diagnosed in cortical biopsies taken for other reasons from patients who have not bled, but what real impact this information has on patient management, particularly if found in elderly patients with Alzheimer's changes, is obscure. Also, while these authors do present sensitivity information regarding postmortem cortical biopsy, they do *not* provide any true specificity data. Specificity is defined as the number of true negative tests divided by the sum of the number of true negatives and the number of false positives. These authors designed their experiment to include histologic examination only from true positive tissue. No true negative tissue was examined. I was disappointed with this article; it not only does not address the question in which *I* was most interested, but it also is fundamentally flawed in its analysis of sensitivity and specificity. Finally, I am left wondering what the true goal of this study is, in terms of possible clinical applicability.

D.M. Grzybicki, M.D., Ph.D.

Neuropathologic Applications of Immunohistochemical Fiber Typing in the Non-neoplastic Muscle Biopsy

Rojiani AM, Cho E-S (Univ of South Florida, Tampa; Univ of Medicine and Dentistry, Newark, NJ)

Mod Pathol 11:334–338, 1998 10–10

Background.—Enzymatic histochemistry to detect adenosine triphosphatase (ATPase) is routinely used for fiber type analysis in non-neoplastic skeletal muscle biopsy specimens, but requires freshly prepared cryostat sections. A non-enzymatic method that could be performed on less-than-ideal specimens would be useful. MY-32, a commercially available antibody against fast twitch, myosin heavy chain, may have neuropathologic applications. The immunoreaction patterns of this antibody and the effect of fixation and processing, as well as tissue degradation on the immunoreaction were examined.

Methods.—Skeletal muscle biopsy specimens that were formalin fixed and paraffin embedded, acetone fixed, or formalin fixed were immunoreacted with MY-32 and assessed with ATPase preparations at pH 9.4 and 4.3 in parallel. Samples were also reacted after 24–48 hours of autolysis. Muscle biopsy specimens with a range of neuropathologic diagnoses were also evaluated for immunoreactivity.

Results.—The MY-32 monoclonal antibody specifically reacted with Type II (fast twitch) fibers. Immunoreactivity was most intense in cryostat sections fixed in acetone, but was also detectable and specific in formalin-fixed, frozen, or paraffin-embedded sections. Specific immunoreactivity could also be detected 48 hours after death.

Conclusions.—MY-32, a commercially available monoclonal antibody that is specific for fast twitch muscle fibers, was assessed for its use in neuropathology. Immunohistochemistry with MY-32 would be useful for evaluation of autopsy specimens with a long postmortem interval, formalin-fixed specimens, and archival material. This method cannot be used to identify Type II subfiber types, nor to visualize structural changes within myofibers. It does not replace enzymatic histochemical analysis but is a useful adjunct that can be used when enzymatic histochemical analysis is no longer informative.

► Occasionally skeletal muscle biopsies for non-neoplastic evaluation are inadvertently placed in formalin or are left at room temperature before processing. Under these conditions, fiber type distribution by enzyme histochemistry is either impossible or suboptimal. These authors describe a potentially very useful immunohistochemical method for demonstrating the 2 major fiber types, which addresses such problems. Using a commercially available antibody, they convincingly show that it specifically reacts with Type II fibers, with only minor differences in some cases in staining intensity compared with conventional enzyme histochemistry. This staining is retained in autopsy samples and in samples held up to 48 hours (the longest time investigated) after removal before processing. They demonstrate specific staining in both normal and pathologic specimens. In light of the limitations of this method (no fiber subtyping can be performed and certain morphological changes, such as fiber inclusions, cannot be seen), the authors provide a realistic list of practical, significant applications for this method (see abstract above). Although it cannot replace enzyme histochemistry, it would appear that this method could be a very useful adjunct method for demonstrating basic fiber type distribution in specimens that, for one reason or another, enzyme histochemistry is not possible.

D.M. Grzybicki, M.D., Ph.D.

Axonal Transection in the Lesions of Multiple Sclerosis

Trapp BD, Peterson J, Ransohoff RM, et al (Cleveland Clinic Found, Ohio; Haukeland Hosp, Bergen, Norway)

N Engl J Med 338:278–285, 1998 10–11

Objective.—The cause of multiple sclerosis (MS) is unknown, although environmental and genetic factors play a role in susceptibility. At the onset of MS, MRI scans may show breakdown of the blood-brain barrier. Even with anti-inflammatory or immunosuppressive therapy, progressive neurologic deterioration—perhaps reflecting axonal loss—occurs in most patients with this condition. One report suggested axonal accumulation of the amyloid precursor protein in MS lesions, possibly related to irreversible axonal damage. The pathologic changes of the axons in MS were analyzed by 3-dimensional imaging of brain sections.

Methods.—Autopsy specimens of brain from 11 patients with MS and 4 individuals without brain disease were studied. A total of 14 active MS lesions and 33 chronic active lesions were examined for demyelination and other abnormalities, along with samples of normal-appearing white matter. The finding of terminal axonal ovoids was used as an indicator of axonal transection.

Results.—MS lesions were consistently associated with transected axons. The more severe the inflammation within the lesions, the greater the frequency of transected axons.

Conclusions.—Axonal transection consistently follows demyelination in multiple sclerosis lesions in the brain. The axons appear to be a major target of disease in MS. The findings strengthen the rationale for early anti-inflammatory treatment in MS, because axonal transection is most frequent in inflamed areas. The ramifications of reduced *N*-acetyl aspartate in MS lesions need to be clarified, and new approaches to monitoring and treating the axonal pathologic changes are needed.

▶ This report by Trapp et al. is both important and elegant. An intimate anatomical association exists between axons and their myelin sheaths, and myelin is trophic for axons. Therefore, the idea that eventual secondary axonal damage most likely contributes to the nerve dysfunction and clinical neurologic impairment seen in MS has been accepted for a long time.

However, this study provides, for the first time, quantitative data showing that axonal transection occurs very commonly in MS lesions, and that it occurs commonly both in active lesions and in chronic active lesions. The authors suggest that this transection may be the correlate of the irreversible impairments seen with progressive disease. These findings support an adjustment in our thinking about the pathophysiology of MS and, as the authors also suggest, support a shift in research efforts to include diagnostic and therapeutic strategies aimed not only at the inflammatory component of MS but also specifically at the axonal pathology. In addition to the important neuropathologic information it provides, I think this is a valuable paper to read because it demonstrates how the use of basic (not to be confused with *easy*!) scientific methods—immunohistochemistry combined with careful microscopy and observation—can still be used to answer important and clinically relevant questions about disease processes.

D.M. Grzybicki, M.D., Ph.D.

Use of Perfusion Fixation for Improved Neuropathologic Examination

Adickes ED, Folkerth RD, Sims KL (Creighton Univ, Omaha, Neb; Brigham and Women's Hosp, Boston)

Arch Pathol Lab Med 121:1199–1206, 1997 10–12

Background.—In previous research on how to improve the timeliness and clinical value of autopsy, the authors used brain perfusion with 10% phosphate-buffered formalin to expediate neuropathologic assessment. The efficacy of this technique was further investigated.

Methods and Findings.—Four brains were examined immediately after removal. In each brain, 1 hemisphere was perfused with 10% buffered formalin for 15–20 minutes. The other hemisphere was treated with standard immersion fixation for 2 weeks in 10% formalin. The perfusion-fixation hemisphere was immediately available for evaluation. Histologic sections were processed immediately with the other necropsy tissue sections. Results indicated that the technical preparation, quality, and intensity of staining with both hematoxylin-eosin and silver, as well as immunoreactivity localization with a variety of immunohistochemical reactions in histologic sections from the hemispheres treated with perfusion fixation were at least as good as sections from the hemisphere treated conventionally.

Conclusion.—Immediate brain perfusion after death is an easy-to-do fixation technique with fixation equal to or better than that of prolonged immersion fixation. The new technique allows immediate complete neuropathologic assessment, enabling results to be reported in 3–5 days.

► The authors of this detailed report provide excellent histologic evidence that perfusion fixation is at least as good as—and is probably superior to in many cases—immersion fixation in the preparation of brains examined at autopsy. The side-by-side color photomicrographs comparing standard histologic and immunohistologic stains after use of both fixation methods are convincing by themselves, although the authors also provide data from a semiquantitative evaluation of histologic quality performed by a neuropathologist and a general pathologist. Their figures illustrating the perfusion apparatus and the technique itself are extremely helpful and provide all the information necessary to guide anyone wishing to try this technique.

Although using perfusion fixation clearly requires an investment in terms of assembling the proper apparatus and possible changes in established brain-cutting routines, the advantages—including shortened turnaround time for final autopsy diagnoses reporting—seem to be worth these initial adjustments. Even for practices in which relatively few autopsy brains are examined per year, the potential superior quality of the histology warrants investigation into this fixation method.

D.M. Grzybicki, M.D., Ph.D.

11 Hematolymphoid System

BCL2 Overexpression Associated With Chromosomal Amplification in Diffuse Large B-Cell Lymphoma

Monni O, Joensuu H, Franssila K, et al (Univ of Helsinki; Helsinki Univ)

Blood 90:1168–1174, 1997 11–1

Introduction.—Increased expression of bcl-2 protein and inhibition of apoptosis is considered a major mechanism in the genesis of follicular lymphomas. Translocation (14;18) is seen in most follicular lymphomas and in 20% to 30% of diffuse large-cell lymphomas. The role of gene amplification in non-Hodgkin's lymphoma is not well known. Diffuse, large B-cell lymphomas (large noncleaved cell lymphomas) were assessed to determine the mechanism and the frequency of bcl-2 amplification.

Methods.—Twenty-six frozen tissue specimens collected from 1989 to 1996 were evaluated by comparative genomic hybridization (CGH), Southern blot hybridization, Western analysis, immunohistochemistry, metaphase fluorescence in situ hybridization, and chromosome analysis.

Results.—The gain or high-level amplification of 18q was detected in 8 tumors (31%) by CGH. Southern analysis showed bcl-2 amplification in these tumors but not in tumors with normal chromosome 18 or t(14;18) (q32;q21). Western immunoblot analysis and immunohistochemistry showed a high-level expression of bcl-2 protein in tumors with bcl-2 amplification and t(14;18) (q32;q21). Translocation (14;18) (q32;q21) was not observed in any tumors with bcl-2 amplification.

Conclusion.—Amplification of the *bcl-2* gene is a significant mechanism for bcl-2 protein overexpression in diffuse large B-cell lymphoma. It is likely that other mechanisms influence bcl-2 overexpression.

bcl-2 and p53 Protein Expression in Follicular Lymphoma

Cooper K, Haffajee Z (South African Inst for Med Research, Johannesburg, South Africa; Univ of the Witwatersrand, Johannesburg, South Africa)

J Pathol 182:307–310, 1997 11–2

Introduction.—Recent trials have indicated that *bcl-2* is regulated by *p53*. Others have indicted that there may be an inverse relationship between p53 and bcl-2 protein in breast and colonic cancers and in several histologic subtypes of non-Hodgkin's lymphoma. The relationship between bcl-2 and p53 protein expression was assessed. These findings were correlated with the grade and cell type in follicular lymphoma (Revised European-American Lymphoma classification).

Methods.—Paraffin-embedded slides of tissue sections from nodal follicular lymphomas from 37 patients underwent bcl-2 and p53 immunohistochemistry using a 3-step ABC system. A 3-tiered scale was used to score positive immunostaining for p53 and bcl-2: +, less than 10% cells; ++, 10 to 50% cells; and +++, greater than 50% cells. The cutoff for negative cells was less than 10%. The mean patient age was 61.5 years.

Results.—The bcl-2 protein was expressed in all 3 grades in 97% of follicular lymphomas. The p53 protein expression had a pattern of increasing immunostaining with progression toward the high-grade follicular lymphoma: grade 1, 6% (1 of 16); grade 2, 48% (10 of 21); and grade 3, 100% (6 of 6). Five patients had varying combinations of grades.

Conclusion.—The varying combinations of grades suggests a role for *p53* mutation in the progression/transformation of follicular lymphoma. Because an inverse relationship was not observed between bcl-2 and p53, the mechanism in patients with follicular lymphoma may differ from that of breast and colonic cancers.

Prognostic Significance of Bcl-2 Protein Expression and Bcl-2 Gene Rearrangement in Diffuse Aggressive Non-Hodgkin's Lymphoma

Gascoyne RD, Adomat SA, Krajewski S, et al (Univ of British Columbia, Vancouver; Cancer Research Ctr, La Jolla, Calif)

Blood 90:244–251, 1997 11–3

Introduction.—There is controversy regarding the prognostic significance of bcl-2 protein expression and *bcl-2* gene rearrangement in diffuse large-cell lymphomas (DLCLs). Bcl-2 protein expression prevents apoptosis and may be important in clinical drug resistance. The presence of a *bcl-2* gene rearrangement in de novo DLCLs indicates a likely follicle center cell origin and perhaps a distinct clinical behavior more similar to low-grade non-Hodgkin's lymphoma. The impact of bcl-2 protein expression and *bcl-2* gene rearrangement (both mbr and mcr) on survival was examined in patients with advanced stage DLCLs (Working Formulation categories F, G, or H) and no prior treatment who were uniformly evaluated and treated with effective chemotherapy.

Methods.—Of 139 patients, 121 were treated with methotrexate, doxorubicin, cyclophosphamide, oncovin, prednisone, and gleomycin (MACOP-B) and 18 were treated with VACOP-B. The age range was 16–70 years. Polymerase chain reaction was used to analyze paraffin sections from diagnostic biopsy specimens for *bcl*-2 gene rearrangement, including mbr and mcr breakpoints; bcl-2 protein expression was analyzed by immunohistochemistry. Overall survival (OS), disease-free survival (DFS), and relapse-free survival (RFS) were assessed at a median follow-up of 81 months.

Results.—Analyzable DNA was present in 118 of 139 patients (85%). Fourteen exhibited a *bcl*-2 rearrangement (11 mbr, 3 mcr). All patients with *bcl*-2 gene rearrangement were in the cohort of 102 patients with a B-cell immunophenotype; the presence of the rearrangement had no significant influence on survival. One hundred sixteen patients (83%) had interpretable bcl-2 protein expression; immunopositivity was detected in 54 of the 116 (47%). Using a cutoff of greater than 10% bcl-2 immunopositive tumor cells for analysis, positive bcl-2 protein expression was observed in 28 of 116 patients (24%). The presence of this expression was associated with decreased 8-year OS (34% vs. 60%), DFS (32% vs. 66%), and RFS (25% vs. 59%).

Conclusion.—The *bcl*-2 gene rearrangement status did not have an impact on outcome, but bcl-2 protein expression was a strong significant predictor of OS, DFS, and RFS in patients with DLCLs.

▶ Good news for bcl-2 fans! These 3 papers (Abstracts 11–1, 11–2, and 11–3) form 3 additional pieces of the puzzle that, fitted together, can explain some common themes regarding bcl-2 and p53 in follicular lymphomas. The reason for bcl-2 protein expression by immunohistochemistry was originally believed to be caused by the (14;18) *bcl*-2 rearrangement. Other mechanisms clearly seem to be important, however, in the bcl-2 protein expression; a gain or high level amplification of 18q, in particular, was found to be an important associate of amplification in up to 31% of diffuse, large B-cell lymphomas. Indeed, the paper by Cooper et al. demonstrates increased level of expression of bcl-2 protein with increasing grade of follicular center lymphoma.

The importance of all of this bcl-2 business? Bcl-2 protein expression is a strong significant predictor of overall survival, disease-free survival, and relapse resurvival in diffuse large-cell lymphomas according to Gascoyne et al., and consistently in the paper by Gascoyne, and associates, *bcl*-2 gene rearrangement status could not be shown to have an impact on outcome. This, again, suggests other mechanisms for bcl-2 protein overexpression, consistent with the 18q high-level amplification.

D.J. Dabbs, M.D.

Primary Mediastinal Large B-Cell Lymphoma: A Clinicopathologic Study of 141 Cases Compared With 916 Nonmediastinal Large B-Cell Lymphomas, a GELA ("Groupe d'Etude des Lymphomes de l'Adulte") Study

Cazals-Hatem D, Lepage E, Brice P, et al (Hôpital Saint Louis, Paris; Hôpital Henri Mondor, Creteil, France; Hôpital Laennec, Paris; et al)

Am J Surg Pathol 20:877–888, 1996 11–4

Background.—Mediastinal involvement occurs in 15% to 25% of peripheral nodal non-Hodgkin's lymphoma (NHL), but primary NHL of the mediastinum is rare. Primary mediastinal large-cell lymphoma (PMLCL) is a distinct clinical entity, but recent reports regarding its treatment have dealt with only small series of patients. The clinicopathologic features and prognosis of PMLCL were compared with those of nonmediastinal large B-cell lymphoma (NMLCL).

Methods.—A series of 141 patients with PMLCL was compared with a cohort of 916 patients with NMLCL diagnosed during the same period. All the patients were treated uniformly in accordance with the NHL 87 trials by the Multicenter Cooperative Group (France) and the "Group d'Etude des Lymphomes de l'Adulte" (Belgium).

Results.—PMLCL was characterized by a predilection for young women, bulky tumors, high serum lactic dehydrogenase levels, and frequent extension to adjacent intrathoracic organs. Hematologic or extrathoracic dissemination was uncommon. All lymphomas were diffuse, large B-cell, nonimmunoblastic, nonanaplastic tumors. Histologically, PMLCL commonly showed the presence of fibrosis and large cells with clear cytoplasm, but these features did not prove to be prognostic indicators. Thirty percent of PMLCL expressed high levels of bcl-2 protein; only 2 of 41 specimens tested showed Epstein-Barr virus RNA.

The polychemotherapy regimen resulted in complete remission in 79% of patients with PMLCL and 68% of patients with NMLCL. Disease-free survival rates did not differ significantly, but 3-year survival rate was 66% for patients with PMLCL and 61% for patients with NMLCL. Overall and disease-free survival between groups did not differ when assessed by stratified analysis on the International Prognostic Index.

Conclusions.—PMLCL showed clinical features that were largely homogenous and distinct from those of NMLCL. On morphologic grounds, however, PMLCL can be combined with other diffuse large B-cell lymphomas. PMLCL can be managed like other high-grade lymphomas of the same histologic character, with a favorable response.

▶ This article provides an accurate assessment of the prognosis of PMLCL compared to the NMLCL. This is a large number of patients who have been followed up and treated fairly uniformly with precise morphologic criteria used for diagnosis. Once and for all, this study clearly demonstrates no appreciable prognostic difference between these 2 groups of patients. Importantly, the degree of sclerosis which is often present in these mediastinal lymphomas was not shown to have a prognostic significance in this large series of patients.

D.J. Dabbs, M.D.

Suggested Reading

Davis RE, Dorfman RF, Warnke RA: Primary large cell lymphoma of the thymus: A diffuse B-cell neoplasm presenting as primary mediastinal lymphoma. *Hum Pathol* 21:1262–1268, 1990.

Lamarre L, Jacobson JO, Aisenberg AC, et al: Primary large cell lymphoma of the mediastinum: A histologic and immunophenotypic study of 29 cases. *Am J Surg Pathol* 13:730–739, 1989.

Does Histology Influence Outcome in Childhood Hodgkin's Disease? Results From the United Kingdom Children's Cancer Study Group

Shankar AG, Ashley S, Radford M, et al (Royal Marsden Hosp, Surrey, England; Southampton Univ Hosp, England; Western Infirmary, Glasgow, Scotland)

J Clin Oncol 15:2622–2630, 1997 11–5

Introduction.—Children account for about 10% of patients with Hodgkin's disease. Distribution of histologic types may differ in the pediatric population. It is still unknown how much influence histology has on outcome in adults. There is little information regarding the distribution of the various histologic subtypes in children or prognostic impact. A group of children who were treated for Hodgkin's disease was analyzed.

Methods.—To evaluate overall survival, progress-free survival, and deaths according to stage and histology, 331 children treated for Hodgkin's disease were studied over a 10-year period. All children were clinically staged at diagnosis, and treatment for stage IA involved field-radiation alone. For other stages, treatment involved chlorambucil, vinblastine, procarbazine, and prednisolone chemotherapy with or without mediastinal radiation.

Results.—The most common histologic type was nodular sclerosing Hodgkin's disease (47%) uniformly distributed through all stages. The least common histologic subtype was lymphocyte-depletion Hodgkin's disease (1%). The highest relapse rate was seen with mixed-cellularity Hodgkin's disease, which was significant in stage I patients who received local irradiation alone. Among the various histologic subtypes, there was no other statistically significant difference in overall survival or progress-free survival. Stage was the most important prognostic factor and no effect of histology was seen.

Conclusion.—Histologic subtype does not influence outcome with effective multiagent chemotherapy. Mixed cellularity Hodgkin's disease is biologically aggressive, according to the high relapse rates for stage I mixed cellularity, and there may be a need for systemic treatment with or without local irradiation. There appeared to be no association of histology with the high relapse rate in stage IV patients.

▶ The ramifications of this article are easy to digest: histologic subtype of Hodgkin's disease does not influence outcome. In other words, subtype is not a prognostic factor. What is of prognostic significance is the stage of disease. Similar results were obtained more than a decade ago from a study of more than 800 patients, all adults, at Stanford. These studies give me the ability to make a fine needle aspiration biopsy lymph node diagnosis of Hodgkin's disease without having to worry about coming up with a specific phase or type (mixed cellularity, lymphocyte depleted, etc.). We may reassure our colleagues that when we make a fine needle aspiration biopsy diagnosis of Hodgkin's disease, stage and not the specific histologic type is the only true indicator of prognostic importance.

D.J. Dabbs, M.D.

Classical Hodgkin's Disease: Clinical Impact of the Immunophenotype

von Wasielewski R, Mengel M, Fischer R, et al (Pathologisches Institut der Medizinischen Hochschule, Hannover, Germany; Universität Köln, Germany; Universität Frankfurt, Germany)

Am J Pathol 151:1123–1130, 1997 11–6

Introduction.—Although immunohistochemistry has been described as an ideal tool for evaluating Reed-Sternberg cells in Hodgkin's disease, a diversity of immunophenotyping results has been found for classical Hodgkin's disease. The new technique of heat-induced epitope retrieval, however, has overcome limitations. The rate of false negative cases may be decreased with the use of a specific IgM secondary antibody and this new technique. The prevalence of the marker triplet CD15, −30, and −20 in classical Hodgkin's disease was investigated retrospectively.

Methods.—There were 1,751 patients with Hodgkin's disease who were retrospectively analyzed for the 3 markers, using microwave epitope retrieval to optimize staining sensitivity. After cells were counted, positivity was defined as 20% or more stained diagnostic cells. Clinical follow-up was available for 1,286 patients. Multivariate Cox regression using the 3 markers, age, sex, histology, stage, B-symptoms (fever, sweats, loss of more than 10% of body weight), hemoglobin, and erythrocyte sedimentation rate as factors was performed.

Results.—A classical immunophenotype (CD15+, CD30+, CD20−) was seen in 83% of the patients. Twelve patients lacked CD15 positivity, and 5% showed other combinations. In the clinical follow-up, significant differences were found in freedom from treatment failure. The lack of CD15 expression in classical Hodgkin's disease is an independent negative prognostic factor for relapses and survival. Patients with CD15− biopsies were older, predominantly men, and had higher clinical stages of diagnosis.

Conclusion.—Classical Hodgkin's disease patients with unfavorable clinical outcome can be identified by immunohistochemistry.

▶ The authors examine the prognostic significance of immunophenotyping in classical Hodgkin's disease. The strengths of the study are its large number of patients and the optimized immunohistochemical sensitivity, using both microwave epitope retrieval on formalin fixed tissue and specific IgM secondary antibody.[1] Controversial cases, such as borderline non-Hodgkin's lymphoma and Hodgkin's disease cases, were eliminated from the study population. A limited panel of immunohistochemical stains (CD20, CD15, CD30) were evaluated. CD45 (LCA) and T-cell markers, other antibodies routinely used in diagnostic workup of Hodgkin's disease, were not evaluated in this study

Although previous studies[2, 3] have not demonstrated a prognostic significance for CD15 positivity, the larger number of patients at all stages and the optimized immunohistochemical staining techniques may have enabled these authors to demonstrate the higher relapse rate and overall worse survival in the CD15 negative cases. It is interesting that the stage IV cases had a higher rate of CD15 negativity than the cases in other stages; however, the reason for this difference is not clear. Further analysis of patients within this large group will prove interesting.

J.F. Turner, Jr., M.D.

References

1. LeBrun DP, Kamel OW, Dorfman RF, et al: Enhanced staining for Leu M1 (CD15) in Hodgkin's disease using a secondary antibody specific for immunoglobulin M. *Hematopathol* 97:135–138, 1992.
2. deMascarel I, Trojani M, Eghbali H, et al: Prognostic value of phenotyping by Ber-H2, Leu-M1, EMA in Hodgkin's disease. *Arch Pathol Lab Med* 114:953–955, 1990.
3. Enblad G, Sundstrom C, Glimelius B: Immunohistochemical characteristics of Hodgkin and Reed-Sternberg cells in relation to age and clinical outcome. *Histopathology* 22:535–541, 1993.

Lymph Node Histology in Typical and Atypical Chronic Lymphocytic Leukemia

Bonato M, Pittaluga S, Tierens A, et al (Univ of Leuven, Belgium)
Am J Surg Pathol 22:49–56, 1998 11–7

Background.—The French-American-British (FAB) system classifies chronic lymphocytic leukemia (CLL) into 2 types, typical and atypical, and these types have different prognostic significance. The histologic findings associated with typical and atypical CLL were characterized.

Methods.—Lymph node biopsy confirmed CLL in 42 patients (35 men and 7 women; median age, 58 years). Most patients (35 of 42, or 83%) initially had generalized lymphadenopathy. Immunophenotyping and cytogenetic analysis were performed. Atypical CLL was divided into 2 subtypes: the CLL/PL (prolymphocytic leukemia) subtype had between 10% and 55% of prolymphocytes in peripheral blood, and the mixed cell subtype had small to large lymphocytes but less than 10% prolymphocytes in peripheral blood.

Findings.—Lymph node morphology was used to classify the cases into 2 groups. Group 1 (n = 14) had small lymphocytes with scant cytoplasm, a round nucleus with clumped chromatin, and ill-defined small pseudofollicles with few prolymphocytes or paraimmunoblasts. Group 2 (n = 28) included cells with small lymphocytes, round or irregular nuclei with or without chromatin clumping, and large pseudofollicles with many prolymphocytes or paraimmunoblasts. Twelve of the 14 cases in group 1 had a median white blood cell count of 35.4×10^9/L and a total lymphocyte count of 27,727/mm^3. Eighteen of the 28 patients in group 2 had a median white blood cell count of 28.65×10^9/L and a total lymphocyte count of 20,380/mm^3. Based on peripheral blood and bone marrow smears, 19 cases were diagnosed as typical CLL and 21 cases were classified as atypical CLL (6 cases of CLL/PL and 11 cases of CLL mixed cell type); in 2 cases the diagnosis was based on lymph node biopsy. When histologic and cytologic findings were compared, all 14 cases in group 1 were typical CLL, and all cases of atypical CLL were in group 2. Prominent pseudofollicles were evident in the lymph node in 5 of 6 cases of CLL/PL. Prominent pseudofollicles were evident in 3 of the 11 cases of CLL mixed cell type, and 7 cases had irregular nuclear outlines. Cytogenetic analysis revealed that both groups 1 and 2 had abnormalities of chromosomes 11 and 13, but only group 2 (atypical CLL) had trisomy 12. Median survival of patients with typical CLL was 69 months and survival with atypical CLL was 73 months (nonsignificant difference).

Conclusions.—A histologic counterpart to the FAB classification system of typical and atypical CLL was found. Atypical CLL was characterized by very large pseudofollicles consisting of prolymphocytes and paraimmunoblasts or by nuclear irregularities. Furthermore, trisomy 12 was associated only with atypical CLL. These histologic results support the belief that typical and atypical CLL are closely related, yet different, diseases.

▶ The majority of cases evaluated in this study have an absolute lymphocytosis, enabling the authors to accomplish their goal of identifying the histologic counterpart of the variants of CLL.[1] However, 12 of the cases selected for study have less than 5×10^9 lymphocytes/L and may be classified as small lymphocytic lymphoma rather than CLL.[2] Prominent pseudofollicles correlated with CLL/PL or the mixed cell variant of CLL that has less than 10% prolymphocytes, cytologic size variability, and irregular nuclear contours.[1] Lymph nodes exhibiting cells with irregular nuclear contours also correlated with this mixed cell type of CLL.

The authors failed to show a prognostic difference between typical CLL and atypical CLL. In fact, both categories of CLL have a shortened survival in this study. The poor survival for the morphologically typical CLL patients may be related to other factors such as an advanced stage, elevated peripheral blood count, or the pattern of bone marrow involvement. The prognostic significance of these other factors was not analyzed in this study.

J.F. Turner, Jr., M.D.

References

1. Bennett J, Catovsky D, Daniel M, et al: Proposals for the classifications of chronic (mature) B and T lymphoid leukaemias. *J Clin Pathol* 42:567–584, 1989.
2. Cheson B, Bennett J, Grever M, et al: National Cancer Institute–sponsored Working Group guidelines for chronic lymphocytic leukemia: Revised guidelines for diagnosis and treatment. *Blood* 87:4990–4997, 1996.

Suggested Reading

Ben-Ezra J, Burke JS, Swartz WG, et al: Small lymphocytic lymphoma: A clinicopathologic analysis of 268 cases. *Blood* 73:579–587, 1989.

Dick F, Maca R: The lymph node in chronic lymphocytic leukemia. *Cancer* 41:283–292, 1978.

Atypical Lymphocyte Morphology: An Adverse Prognostic Factor for Disease Progression in Stage A CLL Independent of Trisomy 12

Oscier DG, Matutes E, Copplestone A, et al (Royal Bournemouth Hosp, England; Derriford Hosp, Plymouth, England; Southampton Gen Hosp, England; et al)

Br J Haematol 98:934–939, 1997 11–8

Background.—Some risk factors have been identified for progressive disease in early (Binet stage A) chronic lymphocytic leukemia (CLL): a lymphocyte count of greater than 30×10^9/L, lymphocyte doubling within 1 year, hemoglobin level of less than 13 g/dL, diffuse marrow histology, and karyotypic abnormalities (particularly trisomy 12). However, up to 15% of patients who lack these features still have disease progression. Additional prognostic factors were sought by examining whether atypical cells were an independent risk factor for the progression of CLL.

Methods.—A total of 270 patients (mean age, 70 years) with stage A CLL who had greater than 30% lymphoid cells in bone marrow were studied. All patients underwent cytogenetic analysis and cytometric examination. All patients had positive reactions to monoclonal antibodies directed against CD5 and CD19, but none had strong surface immunoglobulin expression or a t(11;14) translocation. Atypical cells included CLL/prolymphocyte leukemia (between 10% and 55% prolymphocytes in peripheral blood) and mixed cell CLL (greater than 15% cleaved cells and/or lymphoplasmacytoid cells) that were found in patients whose blood contained mainly small lymphocytes with coarsely clumped chromatin. Disease progression was defined as an increase from stage A to stage B or C, the development of symptoms related to CLL, lymphocyte doubling within 1 year with decreases in hemoglobin levels or platelet counts, a requirement for treatment because of increased lymphadenopathy, or death from a cause related to CLL. Median follow-up was 70.2 months.

Findings.—Almost half the patients (46%) had an abnormal karyotype, with chromosome 13q14 abnormalities (17%) and trisomy 12 (15%) being the most common. Multivariate analysis indicated the following independent risk factors for disease progression (Table 2): atypical lymphocyte morphology, a high white blood cell count (greater than 30 × 10^9), a short lymphocyte doubling time (less than 1 year), and enlargement of 1 or more lymph nodes. Although trisomy 12 was associated with a greater risk for disease progression, most of this risk could be accounted for by the concomitant presence of atypical morphology. In fact, when controlling for atypical morphology, trisomy 12 was not a risk factor; but when controlling for trisomy 12, atypical morphology was still a risk factor.

TABLE 2.—Relative Hazards of Progression or Related Death With Chronic Lymphocytic Leukemia (*CLL*) Stage A (n = 270)

Variable	Unadjusted Relative hazard (95% CI)	*P* value	Adjusted* Relative hazard (95% CI)	*P* value
Sex				
Male	1·00	0·7761	1·00	0·7679
Female	0·93 (0·57. 1·52)		1·09 (0·63. 1·87)	
Age				
<65	1·00	0·0471	1·00	0·0633
≥65	0·60 (0·37. 0·99)		0·59 (0·34. 1·03)	
Stage				
A^0	1·00	0·0050	1·00	0·0016
A^{LN1}	2·18 (1·24. 3·84)		2·44 (1·31. 4·54)	
A^{LN2}	3·19 (1·35. 7·54)		4·43 (1·77. 11·11)	
Morphology				
Typical	1·00	0·0000	1·00	0·0298
CLL/PLL	6·74 (3·65. 12·47)		2·88 (1·18. 7·03)	
Mixed cell CLL	2·93 (1·43. 6·17)		2·28 (1·02. 5·07)	
Karyotype				
Normal	1·00	0·0000	1·00	0·1038
+12	2·84 (1·13. 7·12)		1·77 (0·73. 4·29)	
t(del)13	1·74 (0·73. 4·14)		1·39 (0·44. 4·39)	
Other	2·71 (1·18. 6·18)		2·90 (1·17. 7·21)	
Two abnormalities	4·79 (2·16. 10·62)		2·47 (0·93. 6·59)	
More than two abnormalities	5·69 (2·90. 11·15)		2·66 (1·11. 6·40)	
White blood cell count				
<30 × 10^9/l	1·00		1·00	0·0000
>30 × 10^9l	3·85 (2·24. 6·62)	0·0000	4·16 (2·17. 7·98)	
Lymphocyte doubling time				
>1 year	1·00	0·0000	1·00	0·0000
>1 year	12·60 (7·28. 21·79)		6·64 (3·25. 13·58)	

*Adjusted for all other variables in the Table.

Abbreviations: CI, confidence interval; *PLL*, prolymphocytic leukemia.

(Courtesy of Oscier DG, Matutes E, Copplestone A, et al: Atypical lymphocyte morphology: An adverse prognostic factor for disease progression in stage A CLL independent of trisomy 12. *Br J Haematol* 98:934–939. Copyright 1997, Blackwell Science Ltd.)

Conclusions.—The risk factors for progressive CLL include factors related to tumor load (lymphocyte count, diffuse marrow histology) and to biological characteristics (lymphocyte doubling time, lymphocyte morphology). Lymphocyte morphology, count, and doubling time and lymphadenopathy should be investigated in patients with stage A CLL to determine their prognosis. Whereas trisomy 12 has been linked to rapid disease progression, patients with abnormalities of chromosome 13q14 do not have a worse prognosis.

► The authors demonstrate the prognostic significance of atypical lymphocyte morphology in CLL as defined by the French-American-British (FAB) classification of CLL.[1] The patients evaluated were "early stage CLL," Binet stage A.[2] These patients are not anemic nor thrombocytopenic and have less than 3 designated sites of involvement. Although these patients should have a good prognosis according to the Binet staging system, 65 of 270 patients had progressive disease. While atypical lymphocyte morphology predicted progressive disease, other factors such as white blood cell count and leukocyte doubling time were other important clinical parameters for these patients.

The relatively simple examination of the peripheral blood smear provides prognostic information for patients with CLL. However, the presence of atypical lymphocyte morphology in an undiagnosed patient should also prompt exclusion of other chronic lymphoproliferative disorders such as the circulating phase of mantle cell lymphoma.

J.F. Turner, Jr., M.D.

References

1. Bennett JM, Catovsky D, Daniel MT, et al: Proposals for the classification of chronic (mature) B and T lymphoid leukaemias. *J Clin Pathol* 42:567–584, 1989.
2. Binet JL, Auquier A, Dighiero G, et al: A new prognostic classification of chronic lymphocytic leukemia derived from a multivariate survival analysis. *Cancer* 48:198–206, 1981.

Suggested Reading

Melo JV, Catovsky D, Gregory WM, et al: The relationship between chronic lymphocytic leukaemia and prolymphocytic leukaemia. *Br J Haematol* 65:23–29. 1987.

Vallespi T, Montserrat E, Sanz MA: Chronic lymphocytic leukaemia: Prognostic value of lymphocyte morphological subtypes. A multivariate survival analysis in 146 patients. *Br J Haematol* 77:478–485, 1991.

Anaplastic Large Cell Lymphoma: A Distinct Molecular Pathologic Entity. A Reappraisal With Special Reference to p80$^{NPM/ALK}$ Expression

Nakamura S, Shiota M, Nakagawa A, et al (Aichi Cancer Ctr Research Inst, Nagoya, Japan; Univ of Tokyo; Nagoya Univ Hosp, Japan; et al)

Am J Surg Pathol 21:1420–1432, 1997 11–9

Background.—An important contributor to the pathogenesis of anaplastic large-cell lymphoma (ALCL) is p80$^{NPM/ALK}$ expression, activated by the t(2;5) (p23;q35) translocation. The clinicopathologic significance of identifying p80 in patients with ALCL is still uncertain, however. In addition, difficulty in differentiating ALCL and Hodgkin's disease (HD) histologically and immunophenotypically often complicates the clinicopathologic assessment and treatment of these entities.

Methods and Findings.—Sixty-seven ALCL and 63 HD specimens were immunostained using anti-p80 antibody and other relevant markers on paraffin sections. Sixty-four percent of the ALCL specimens had p80 expression, but none of the HD specimens did. The p80^{+} ALCL specimens made up a homogenous group of tumors, occurring in a much younger group of patients and associated with a somewhat more favorable clinical course than that of the p80^{-} ALCL specimens. This homogenous group demonstrated p80, CD30, and epithelial membrane antigen positivity, and CD15, *bcl*-2, and Epstein-Barr virus negativity, with T- and null-cell phe-

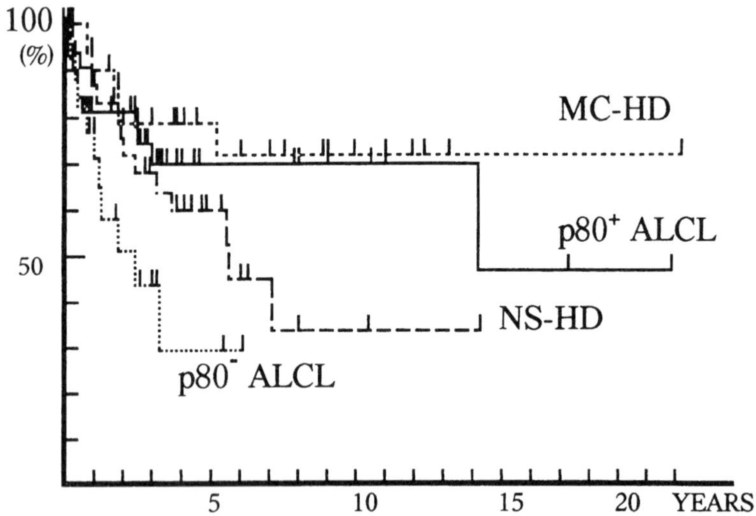

FIGURE 2.—Actuarial survival (after Kaplan and Meier) of patients with p80^{+} ALCL (p80^{+} ALCL) (n = 40), p80^{-} ALCL (p80^{-} ALCL) (n = 22), 29 HD of the nodular-sclerosing type (NS-HD) (n = 29), and HD of the mixed-cellularity type (MC-HD) (n = 28). Survival time was calculated from the time of diagnosis. The patients with p80^{+} ALCL had a protracted and relatively favorable prognosis compared with patients with p80^{-} ALCL (P less than .05 by the log-rank test), although there was no significant difference between NS-HD and MC-HD patients. (Courtesy of Nakamura S, Shiota M, Nakagawa A, et al: Anaplastic large cell lymphoma: A distinct molecular pathologic entity: A reappraisal with special reference to p80$^{NPM/ALK}$ expression. *Am J Surg Pathol* 12:1420–1432, 1997.)

notype. Distinct morphologic features were the indented nuclei, often termed *reniform*, embryolike and horseshoe-like; multiple, irregular, but indistinct nucleoli; and few reactive cells of eosinophils and epithelioid cells. By contrast, the 24 $p80^-$ ALCL specimens, with positive epithelial membrane antigen and *bcl*-2 in 33% and 55%, formed a heterogenous group. These included 11 cases of HD-like ALCL, 6 of $p80^-$ common ALCL, 3 of secondary ALCL, 2 of primary cutaneous ALCL, and 2 of primary classical ALCL lacking p80 expression (Fig 2).

Conclusions.—The immunohistochemical detection of p80 is very important in distinguishing the biologically distinct entity of primary classical ALCL from various diseases, including HD and HD-like ALCL, that show morphologic and immunohistologic overlap. These findings also verify that $p80^+$ ALCLs occur primarily in young patients and are associated with favorable outcomes.

ALK-positive Lymphoma: A Single Disease With a Broad Spectrum of Morphology

Benharroch D, Meguerian-Bedoyan Z, Lamant L, et al (CHU Purpan, Toulouse, France; Institut Gustave Roussy, Villejuif, France; John Radcliffe Hosp, Oxford, England; et al)

Blood 91:2076–2084, 1998 11–10

Background.—Anaplastic large-cell lymphoma (ALCL) has been associated with the t(2;5)(p23;q35) translocation, which results in the expression of a chimeric NPM-ALK protein detectable by the ALK1 monoclonal antibody. The morphologic and phenotypic spectrum of a large series of lymphomas expressing ALK protein was described.

Methods.—One hundred twenty-three cases of lymphoma expressing ALK protein were selected from 145 cases with morphologic features of ALCL expressing both CD30 and epithelial membrane antigen and no B-cell markers. Mean patient age was 21.3 years.

Findings.—A variety of morphologic patterns was detected in the current series. In some patients, different subtypes coexisted in 1 biopsy or in successive biopsies from 1 patient. All cases showed a very characteristic large cell, with an eccentric nucleus and an eosinophilic paranuclear region. Another feature of these tumors was a perivascular pattern of neoplastic cell infiltration, present in a significant number of patients. All tumors also expressed epithelial membrane antigen and lacked CD15. In 84% of the cases, malignant cells demonstrated both a cytoplasmic and nuclear staining for ALK1, and were thus presumably carrying the 2;5 translocation (Figs 1 and 4).

Conclusions.—These data provide strong evidence that the morphologic patterns of ALCL reported previously as possible subtypes of ALCL are morphologic variants of the same entity. Because the morphology of ALK-

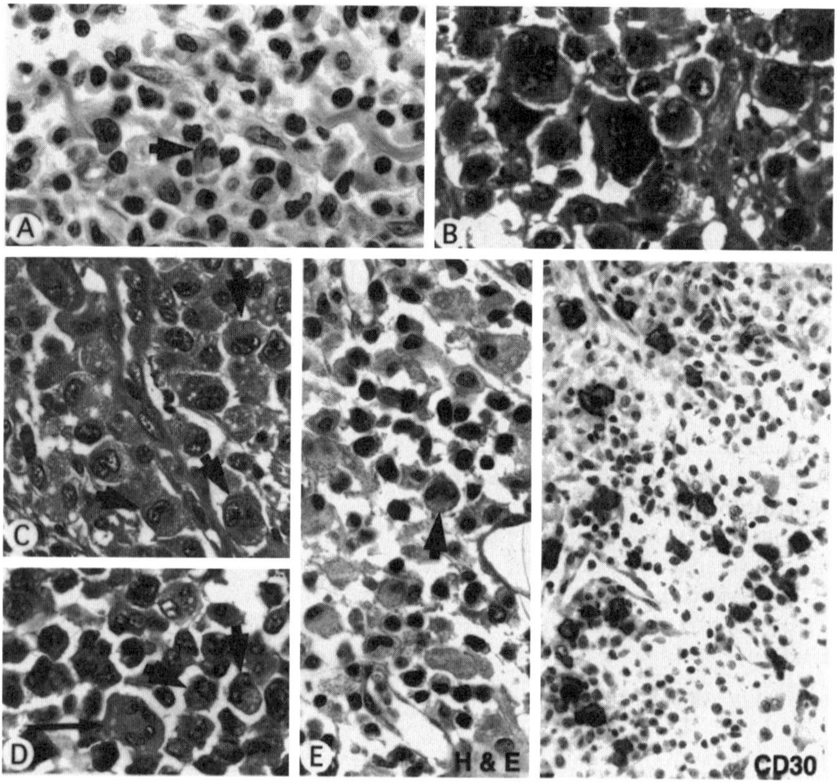

FIGURE 1.—ALK-positive anaplastic large-cell lymphomas (*ALCLs*) show a wide morphologic spectrum. **A**, small-cell pattern. A predominant population of small cells with irregular nuclei is associated with scattered large hallmark cells (*arrow*) showing eccentric lobated nuclei. **B**, giant-cell–rich pattern, showing striking cellular pleomorphism. **C**, common-type ALCL showing several hallmark cells (*arrows*). **D**, common-type ALCL showing several hallmark cells (*arrows*). **D**, common-type ALCL showing several hallmark cells (*arrow*) and also a cell with crown-like nuclei (*long arrow*). **E**, lymphohistiocytic variant showing, in the hematoxylin- and eosin-stained section, a single hallmark cell (*arrow*). Note the eosinophilic paranuclear area. Other cells are nonneoplastic, including histiocytes and plasma cells. Immunostaining of this case for CD30 highlights the scattered malignant cell population. (Courtesy of Benharroch D, Meguerian-Bedoyan Z, Lamant L, et al: ALK-positive lymphoma: A single disease with a broad spectrum of morphology. *Blood* 91:2076–2084, 1998.)

positive neoplasms is often neither anaplastic nor large cell, these neoplasms should be termed ALK lymphomas.

► Since its initial description in 1985,[1] the common form of ALCL has become recognized by its sinusoidal growth pattern of pleomorphic cohesive cells and by its reaction with the CD30 immunohistochemical stain. Its morphologic appearance may simulate a nonhematopoietic neoplasm or the syncytial variant of Hodgkin's disease, nodular sclerosis type. Fortunately, a battery of immunohistochemical stains will usually resolve the differential diagnosis.

More recently, several less common morphologic variants of ALCL have been described. These variants include the monomorphic, lymphohistio-

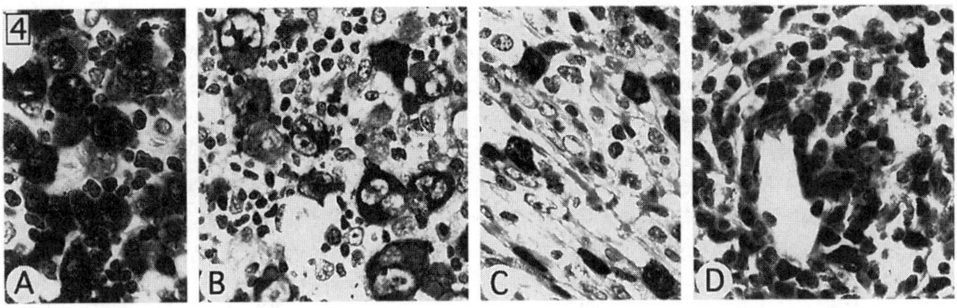

FIGURE 4.—Patterns of expression of ALK protein. **A,** both cytoplasmic and nuclear expression of the protein was seen in most tumors. **B,** ALK staining was confined to the cytoplasm of neoplastic cells in a few cases. This case was of common type, but showed Hodgkin's-like areas. **C,** lymphohistiocytic variant showing scattered positive cells, some of them with a fibroblast-like appearance. **D,** small-cell variant, showing strong staining of large anaplastic cells, associated with only moderate or weak nuclear staining in the small cells. (Courtesy of Benharroch D, Meguerian-Bedoyan Z, Lamant L, et al: ALK-positive lymphoma: A single disease with a broad spectrum of morphology. *Blood* 91:2076–2084, 1998.)

cytic, small-cell, sarcomatoid, giant-cell–rich, neutrophil-rich, and Hodgkin's-like types. Since other lymphomas with nonanaplastic morphology can be CD30-positive, and anaplastic cells are not frequent in some of these variants, the criteria for diagnosis of anaplastic large cell lymphoma become less clear. In addition, the relationship of Hodgkin's disease–like ALCL to Hodgkin's disease is controversial. Distinguishing these latter entities is of particular importance because of the differing therapeutic implications of a diagnosis of Hodgkin's disease vs. a diagnosis of a non-Hodgkin's lymphoma.

These 2 articles (Abstracts 11–9 and 11–10) more clearly define ALCL by analyzing a large number of patients with the novel immunohistochemical stains, $p80^{npm\text{-}alk}$ [2] and ALK1.[2] These stains detect expression of the ALK protein that correlates with the (2;5) translocation observed in ALCL. This protein has not been demonstrated in normal lymphoid cells and its expression is relatively specific for the (2;5). Only a rare case expressing the ALK protein by immunohistochemistry had a variant (1;2) translocation.[2]

Both studies reveal a distinct clinicopathologic entity. Frequent expression of the p80 and ALK1 protein occurs in the ALCL of children or young adults. The lymphoma presents mainly at nodal sites, although occurrence at extranodal sites, including the skin, is also possible. The prognosis is more favorable in these $p80^+$ and $ALK1^+$ positive cases than in the $p80^-$ lymphomas that occur mainly in older adults.

The morphologic features of ALCL are better defined by these studies. The $p80^+$ and $ALK1^+$ cases have a characteristic $CD30^+$ atypical large mononuclear cell. This cell has an indented, eccentric nucleus, multiple irregular indistinct nucleoli, and an eosinophilic paranuclear region. In addition to the common sinusoidal location of the large neoplastic cells, Benharroch et al observed a perivascular distribution of these cells. This pattern was evident in approximately half of all their cases, with a higher frequency in the small-cell and lymphohistiocytic variants.

The relationship of the different variants of ALCL to the "common type of ALCL" is clarified. Features of the small-cell, lymphohistiocytic, giant-cell, and Hodgkin's-like variants were noted in the same biopsies with the "common type of ALCL." The predominant histologic features changed over time, with different patterns occurring in some patients who relapsed.

CD30 positivity occurring in a membranous and Golgi pattern, as well as epithelial membrane antigen (EMA) positivity are characteristics of ALK1$^+$/p80$^+$ ALCL. EMA positivity was a selection criterion for the cases of Benharroch et al. and Nakamura et al. found EMA positivity in 95% of their p80$^+$ cases. Nakamura et al. extended the immunophenotypic profile of the p80$^+$ cases. Virtually all cases were CD15$^-$, bcl-2$^-$ and EBV$^-$. In addition, the lymphomas were either T- or null-cell phenotype. No p80$^+$ B-cell ALCLs were detected.

Although the study of Benharroch et al. was restricted to ALK$^+$ ALCL, the study of Nakamura et al. demonstrated immunophenotypic and clinical heterogeneity of p80$^-$ ALCL. Only 33% of these cases were EMA$^+$ and 55% were bcl-2$^+$. The clinical manifestations varied from primary cutaneous presentations to lymphomas consisted with a prior lymphoproliferative disorder. Although the presentations were heterogenous, the lymphomas generally occurred in an older age group, and carried a poorer prognosis.

Nakamura et al. demonstrate lack of p80 expression in all 63 specimens of Hodgkin's disease. This finding is congruent with most other reports that demonstrate the lack of the (2;5) translocation in Hodgkin's disease. The absence of p80 expression in the 11 cases of Hodgkin's-like ALCL examined by Nakamura et al. as well as the variable expression of CD15 and EBV, suggests that Hodgkin's-like ALCL is more closely related to Hodgkin's disease than to ALCL. Other studies have also shown absence of ALK1 in the majority of these Hodgkin's disease-like cases.[3] However, Benharroch et al. identified rare cases with typical features of ALK1$^+$ ALCL that had areas of a Hodgkin's-like pattern. In these areas, the large cells were CD15$^-$, EBV$^-$ and ALK1$^+$. Further studies of the cases that have overlapping features of Hodgkin's disease and ALCL are necessary to determine whether Hodgkin's-like ALCL is a distinct entity.

J.F. Turner, Jr, M.D.

References

1. Stein H, Mason DY, Gerdes J, et al: The expression of the Hodgkin's disease associated antigen Ki-1 in reactive and neoplastic lymphoid tissue: Evidence that Reed-Sternberg cells and histiocytic malignancies are derived from activated lymphoid cells. *Blood* 66:848, 1985.
2. Pulford K, Lamant L, Morris SW, et al: Detection of anaplastic lymphoma kinase (ALK) and nucleolar protein nucleophosmin (NPM)–ALK proteins in normal and neoplastic cells with the monoclonal antibody ALK1. *Blood* 89:1394–1404, 1997.
3. Shiota M, Fujimoto J, Takenaga M, et al: Diagnosis of t(2;5)(p23;q35)-associated Ki-1 lymphoma with immunohistochemistry. *Blood* 84:3648–3652, 1994.

Suggested Reading

Arber DA, Sun L-H, Weiss LM: Detection of the t(2;5)(p23;q35) chromosomal translocation in large B-cell lymphomas other than anaplastic large cell lymphoma. *Hum Pathol* 27:590–594, 1996.

De Bruin PC, Beljaards RC, Van Heerde P, et al: Differences in clinical behaviour and immunophenotype between primary cutaneous and primary nodal anaplastic large cell lymphoma of T-cell or null cell phenotype. *Histopathology* 23:127–135, 1993.

DeCoteau JF, Butmarc JR, Kinney MC, et al: The t(2;5) chromosomal translocation is not a common feature of primary cutaneous CD30+ lymphoproliferative disorders: Comparison with anaplastic large-cell lymphoma of nodal origin. *Blood* 87:3437–3441, 1996.

Bone Marrow Involvement in T-cell–rich B-cell Lymphoma

Skinnider BF, Connors JM, Gascoyne RD (Univ of British Columbia, Vancouver)

Am J Clin Pathol 108:570–578, 1997 11–11

Introduction.—Proper diagnosis of T-cell–rich B-cell lymphoma depends on the immunohistochemical identification of the scattered large malignant cells as B-cells amid small reactive T-lymphocytes. It is still unknown whether T-cell–rich B-cell lymphoma represents a distinct clinicopathologic entity or an unusual morphologic subtype of conventional large B-cell lymphoma. Advanced-stage disease is often seen in the initial examination of patients with T-cell–rich B-cell lymphoma, with bone marrow involvement as high as 67%. The histopathologic features of the bone marrow in patients with T-cell–rich B-cell lymphoma were investigated to differentiate it from morphologically similar entities and to explore its possible relationship to diffuse lymphocyte-predominant Hodgkin's disease and histiocyte-rich B-cell lymphoma.

Methods.—There were 13 patients with a previous tissue-based diagnosis of T-cell–rich B-cell lymphoma who had specimens from their bone marrow biopsies examined histologically and immunohistochemically.

Results.—In 62% (8 of 13 patients), bone marrow involvement was found and was often paratrabecular (Fig 1). The differential diagnosis included Hodgkin's disease and peripheral T-cell lymphoma, and the histologic appearance was not pathognomonic of T-cell–rich B-cell lymphoma. A pale low-power appearance was typically seen in the infiltrates, resulting from histiocytic infiltration or relative hypocellularity. The infiltrates were suggestive of Hodgkin's disease because there was a presence of a polymorphous infiltrate of scattered large atypical cells amid a mixed infiltrate of small lymphocytes and histiocytes (Fig 2). The large atypical cells and CD20 reactivity, with an absence of CD15 and CD30 reactivity, supported the diagnosis of T-cell–rich B-cell lymphoma. In all positive

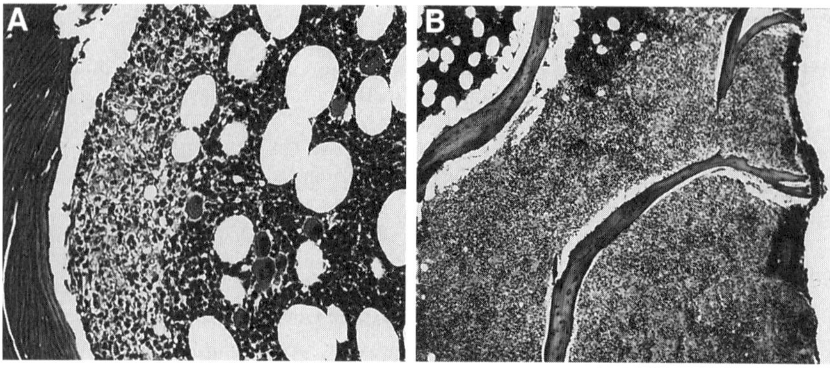

FIGURE 1.—Bone marrow trephine biopsy specimens. **A**, case 3, tumor infiltrates occur most commonly as paratrabecular lesions (hematoxylin-eosin, ×180). **B**, case 6, tumor infiltrates also occur as large deposits occupying the intertrabecular spaces, a pattern that resembles bone marrow involvement with Hodgkin's disease on low power (hematoxylin-eosin, ×45). (Courtesy of Skinnider BF, Connors JM, Gascoyne RD: Bone marrow involvement in T-cell-rich B-cell lymphoma. *Am J Clin Pathol* 108:570–578. Copyright 1997 by the American Society of Clinical Pathologists. Reprinted with permission.)

bone marrow biopsy specimens, a prominent small T-cell infiltrate accompanying the large atypical cells was observed. De novo B-cell diffuse large-cell lymphoma has a decreased incidence of bone marrow involvement, compared to that found in T-cell–rich B-cell lymphoma, a contrast which suggests a possible biologic difference between the 2 entities.

Conclusion.—There are some similar clinicopathologic features shared by T-cell–rich B-cell lymphoma and diffuse lymphocyte-predominant Hodgkin's disease, paragranuloma type.

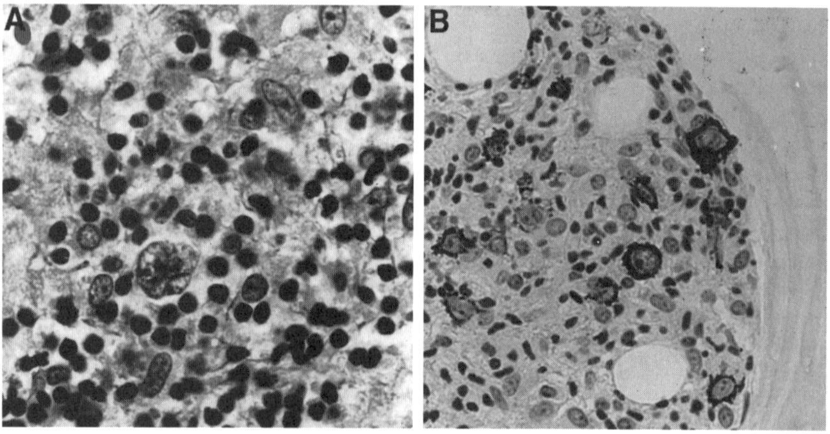

FIGURE 2.—Detail of neoplastic infiltrate. **A**, case 6, scattered large malignant cells are accompanied by an infiltrate of small lymphocyte and histocytes. The malignant cells include cells resembling lymphocytic and histiocytic (L&H) cells (hematoxylin-eosin, ×720). **B**, case 3, the malignant cells are accentuated by L26 staining (immunoperoxidase, hematoxylin counterstain, ×450). (Courtesy of Skinnider BF, Connors JM, Gascoyne RD: Bone marrow involvement in T-cell-rich B-cell lymphoma. *Am J Clin Pathol* 108:570–578. Copyright 1997 by the American Society of Clinical Pathologists. Reprinted with permission.)

▶ The authors nicely describe the morphologic and immunophenotypic appearance of bone marrow involvement in T-cell–rich B-cell lymphoma. For primary nodal or extranodal diagnosis, the authors chose strict criteria for defining the relative percentage of the neoplastic large cell population and the reactive small lymphoid cells (less than 10% large neoplastic B cells, greater than 90% small reactive T cells). In addition, the majority of their cases (10 of 13) were also histiocyte rich, a common but not often emphasized feature of this variant of diffuse large B-cell lymphoma.

The authors found morphologic concordance between the bone marrow and the primary diagnostic site in individual cases. The appearance of the neoplastic cells and the background reactive infiltrate were similar. The neoplastic cells may be either multilobated (lymphocytic and histiocytic-like) or immunoblast-like. The multilobated cells make lymphocyte-predominant Hodgkin's disease a consideration. When the immunoblast-like cells occur in the polymorphic background of lymphocytes and histiocytes, classical Hodgkin's disease, as well as peripheral T-cell lymphoma, enter the differential diagnosis. This broad morphologic differential diagnosis makes an initial diagnosis from the bone marrow difficult. Immunohistochemical studies for diagnosis and demonstration of B-cell monoclonality may be necessary in cases with only focal bone marrow involvement. In difficult cases, confirmation of lymphoma in an extramedullary site may be necessary.

A higher rate of bone marrow involvement (62%) was noted in this series than in other series reported in the literature (23% average per literature review in this study). The more stringent criteria for diagnosis of T-cell–rich B-cell lymphoma may have given the authors a more uniform group of patients than the groups in more heterogenously defined studies.

J.F. Turner, Jr., M.D.

Ruptured Spleens With Expanded Marginal Zones Do Not Reveal Occult B-Cell Clones

Kroft SH, Singleton TP, Dahiya M, et al (Univ of Michigan, Ann Arbor; Loyola Univ Med Ctr, Maywood, Ill)
Mod Pathol 10:1214–1220, 1997 11–12

Introduction.—Splenic marginal zone lymphoma recapitulates the architectural, cytologic, and immunophenotypic features of the normal splenic marginal zone, and typically afflicts older individuals seen with prominent splenomegaly. It was determined whether chronic immune stimulation manifesting as splenic marginal zone lymphoma could produce occult B-cell clones and predispose the patient to splenic marginal zone lymphoma.

Methods.—The study included 58 men and 33 women, ranging in age from 17 to 87, with a mean age of 40. Seventy patients had splenectomies for blunt trauma, 7 for penetrating trauma, 13 for surgical misadventures, and 1 for spontaneous rupture, resulting in 91 traumatically ruptured spleens that were examined for the presence of marginal zone hyperplasia and for Ig heavy chain gene rearrangements with polymerase chain reaction. These spleens were stained for CD20, CD43, and κ and λ light chains with polymerase chain reaction. The spleens were classified by whether they had expanded marginal zones or were more than 12 cell layers thick. The average spleen weighed 183 g.

Results.—Expanded marginal zones were seen in 27 (30%) of 91 patients. There were no significant differences in age, sex, spleen weight, or reason for excision in the patients with and without marginal zone expansion. There was a variance in germinal centers, from absent to inactive to floridly reactive. Twenty-four patients had paraffin blocks available, and 20 patients with amplifiable DNA were polyclonal by polymerase chain reaction. Lymphoma did not develop in any of the 25 patients with expanded marginal zones, although 1 patient's spleen was morphologically suspicious for lymphoma. This spleen had involvement of the red pulp by marginal zone-type B-cells. No evidence of lymphoma was seen in this patient's 3-year follow-up. Only 2 patients showed the presence of B-cells in a subendothelial location, despite the common finding of subendothelial infiltration of trabecular veins by T cells.

Conclusion.—Occult B-cell clones do not seem to be harbored in traumatically ruptured spleens with expanded marginal zones. It is rare to find spleens containing low-stage splenic marginal zone lymphoma.

▶ Does splenic marginal zone lymphoma enter the differential diagnosis of splenectomy specimens without enlargement? Yes, but infrequently. This article did not identify any cases of lymphoma among 91 traumatically ruptured spleens. However, 1 case was morphologically suspicious for splenic marginal zone lymphoma, but ancillary studies and the relatively short clinical follow-up did not give supportive evidence for lymphoma.

Marginal zone hyperplasia (defined arbitrarily by Farhi[1] as a marginal zone expansion beyond 12 cell layers) does occur without resultant splenic enlargement. Another interesting finding is that marginal zone hyperplasia may occur focally without concomitant hyperplasia of the germinal centers.

When should we consider splenic marginal zone lymphoma as a possibility in a spleen of normal weight? The lymphoma is evidently a rare occurrence, given that only 2 reports are cited in the current literature. However, morphologic clues are expanded, monotonous-appearing marginal zones without the accompanying normal tripartite architecture of the white pulp. Additional atypical findings are marginal zone cells replacing the periarteriolar lymphoid sheaths, and increased aggregates of monocytoid cells within the red pulp.[2, 3]

J.F. Turner, Jr., M.D.

References

1. Farhi DC, Ashfaq R: Splenic pathology after traumatic injury. *Am J Clin Pathol* 105:474–478, 1996.
2. Rosso R, Neiman RS, Paulli M, et al: Splenic marginal zone cell lymphoma: Report of an indolent variant without massive splenomegaly presumably representing an early phase of the disease. *Hum Pathol* 26:39–46, 1995.

3. Dunphy CH, Bee C, McDonald JW, et al: Incidental early detection of a splenic marginal zone lymphoma by polymerase chain reaction analysis of paraffin-embedded tissue. *Arch Pathol Lab Med* 122:84–86, 1998.

Clinical Utility of Heteroduplex Analysis of TCR Gamma Gene Rearrangements in the Diagnosis of T-Cell Lymphoproliferative Disorders
Chhanabhai M, Adomat SA, Gascoyne RD, et al (Univ of British Columbia, Vancouver)
Am J Clin Pathol 108:295–301, 1997 11–13

Introduction.—The detection of monoclonality in lymphoproliferative disorders is useful to distinguish benign from malignant disease. Molecular genetic analysis of immunoglobulin and T-cell receptor gene rearrangement is widely used for this purpose in the clinical investigation of lymphoproliferative disorders. The T-cell receptor has 4 components: alpha, beta, delta, and gamma chains, which are glycoprotein heterodimers linked by disulfide bonds. Juxtaposing the individual gene segments with looping out and excision of the intervening DNA is part of the rearrangement process. Southern analysis and polymerase chain reaction can establish the presence of immunoglobulin or T-cell receptor rearrangement. However, Southern analysis is labor intensive and expensive. Polymerase chain reaction methods are less expensive and less labor intensive. The clinical usefulness of heteroduplex analysis of polymerase chain reaction products for Tγ gene rearrangements in the diagnosis of T-cell lymphoproliferative disorders, using a single set of consensus primers, was examined.

Methods.—Fresh or frozen tissue was analysed from 103 patients, including 62 patients with T-cell lymphoproliferative disorders, 25 with B-cell lymphoproliferative disorders, 3 with anaplastic large cell lymphomas of undefined lineage, and 13 with reactive disorders who served as the negative control group. A comparison was made of all patients with T-cell lymphoproliferative disorders, using Tβ Southern analysis and heteroduplex Tγ polymerase chain reaction analysis. Ten patients with postthymic T-cell lymphoma were also studied, using paraffin-embedded tissue.

Results.—In 51 of 57 patients who were rearranged by Tβ Southern analysis, heteroduplex Tγ polymerase chain reaction was positive. Of the 10 patients with T-cell lymphoma which was analyzed using paraffin-embedded tissue, 8 were positive. No false positive results were seen.

Conclusion.—In the clinical laboratory, this method is an effective screening test. The need to perform Southern analysis is obviated by a positive result. In 89% of patients who also had a rearrangement by Tβ Southern analysis, Tγ HDX polymerase chain reaction detected clonal T cells. A single set of consensus primers will detect the vast majority of clonal rearrangements using this method.

▶ The 89% diagnostic sensitivity and the 100% specificity for detection of T-cell monoclonality make heteroduplex analysis of T-cell receptor gamma gene rearrangement a potentially useful initial test for those cases that have been traditionally evaluated by Southern blot hybridization analysis. The utility of this test was evaluated over a wide range of T-cell lymphoproliferative disorders, as well as reactive disorders and B-cell lymphoproliferative disorders. Although only a small number of paraffin-embedded tissue samples were analyzed, positivity in 8 in 10 cases evaluated demonstrates the test's potential utility.

J.F. Turner, Jr., M.D.

The Spectrum of Multiple Myeloma: Diagnostic and Biological Implications

Larson RS, Sukpanichnant S, Greer JP, et al (Vanderbilt Univ, Nashville, Tenn; Mahidol Univ, Bangkok, Thailand; Univ of New Mexico, Albuquerque)

Hum Pathol 28:1336–1347, 1997 11–14

Introduction.—A common hematopoietic neoplasm, multiple myeloma is diagnosed in fulminant form. Because of the focality of marrow involvement early in the disease and overlap in manifestations with other diseases, myeloma may be difficult to diagnose. At presentation, myeloma has an array of clinical and laboratory findings, including widespread skeletal lesions, paraprotein production, infiltrative marrow process, anemia, and susceptibility to infection. The clinical and pathological findings of patients with myeloma were documented and analyzed to enhance the understanding of the diversity of myeloma, including its earliest forms.

Methods.—There were 145 patients with myeloma in a 14-year period. All patients had histological sections, paraffin immunoperoxidase studies, clinical information, and laboratory findings available at presentation. Age, sex, bone lesions, M-type peak on serum electrophoresis, anemia, infections, plasmacytoma of soft tissue, renal insufficiency, presence of amyloid, peripheral neuropathy, and unusual clinical features were recorded. A marrow examination was also conducted.

Conclusions.—There are at least 2 distinct subtypes of myeloma: 1 with an infiltrative growth pattern and the other with bone lesions. Both types appear to arise in the marrow, but the relationship of these 2 forms to plasma cell biology is not clear. Eighty-five percent of the patients with myeloma were identified according to the criteria used in this study. To establish the diagnosis in patients with early marrow involvement, immunoperoxidase studies are required. Younger and older patients have similar clinical and pathological characteristics of myeloma. Factors such as dysplasia, immunoglobulin type, and leukemic phase were evenly distributed among clinical presentations, and did not identify clinicopathological subtypes of myeloma.

► This article nicely describes the clinical and histologic spectrum of multiple myeloma, and presents data from a large series of patients. The histologic findings in bone marrow biopsies are emphasized. The authors correlate the morphologic patterns of infiltration with the common clinical findings of patients with myeloma, noting that the nodular growth pattern correlates with bone lesions and that an infiltrative pattern frequently occurs in patients seen with anemia alone. These patterns may represent different myeloma biologic subtypes. However, the number of patients seen with anemia alone is small in this study and there is some overlap between the histologic patterns, and the clinical presentations. An attempt to correlate prognosis with these individual patterns was not made in the current article, but was addressed by these authors previously. The patients with "packed" marrow had a shorter median survival (15.2 months) than patients with the other nodular, infiltrative, or mixed patterns (40.4–29.7).[1]

The authors proposed diagnostic criteria for myeloma were tested in a previous study.[1] The finding of interstitial clusters of plasma cells, which expand at least 1 interfatty space, is a helpful morphologic feature in cases without sheets of plasma cells. If immunohistochemistry proves these nodules to be monoclonal, they would be considered diagnostic of myeloma. However, immunohistochemistry is probably not necessary in those cases with monoclonality proven by serum immunofixation.

The authors confirm the heterogenous cytologic appearance of multiple myeloma. They grade the cytologic atypia in terms of mild, moderate, or severe dysplasia. Their previous study indicated that this cytologic scheme is useful for prognosis. Similar studies emphasizing the cytologic features on aspirate sections have also shown that attention to cytologic detail can aid in predicting outcome.[2, 3, 4]

J.F. Turner, Jr., M.D.

References

1. Sukpanichnant S, Cousar JB, Leelasiri A, et al: Diagnostic criteria and histologic grading in multiple myeloma: Histologic and immunohistologic analysis of 176 cases with clinical correlation. *Hum Pathol* 25:308–318, 1994.
2. Fritz E, Ludwig H, Kundi M: Prognostic relevance of cellular morphology in multiple myeloma. *Blood* 63:1072–1079, 1984.
3. Greipp PR, Raymond NM, Kyle RA, et al: Multiple myeloma: Significance of plasmablastic subtype in morphological classification. *Blood* 65:305–310, 1985.
4. Bartl R, Frish B, Fateh-Moghadam A, et al: Histologic classification and staging of multiple myeloma: A retrospective and prospective study of 674 cases. *Am J Clin Pathol* 87:342–355, 1987.

T-Cell Subset Analysis of Peripheral T-Cell Lymphomas by Paraffin Section Immunohistology and Correlation of CD4/CD8 Results With Flow Cytometry

Macon WR, Salhany KE (Vanderbilt Univ Med Ctr, Nashville, Tenn; Univ of Pennsylvania Med Ctr, Philadelphia)
Am J Clin Pathol 109:610–617, 1998 11–15

Introduction.—Peripheral T-cell lymphomas are a clinically, morphologically, and immunologically heterogeneous group of mature T-cell malignant neoplasms, which are often diagnosed after T-cell lineage–related antigen expression has been demonstrated on neoplastic lymphocytes by flow cytometry, frozen section immunoperoxidase, or paraffin immunoperoxidase. Paraffin immunoperoxidase, however, has not been previously used for complete T-cell subset analysis for helper, suppressor/cytotoxic, αβ, and γδ phenotypes. T-cell subset–related antigen expression on 31 peripheral T-cell lymphomas was examined with paraffin immunoperoxidase.

Methods.—In 31 peripheral T-cell lymphomas, previously studied for CD4 and CD8 by flow cytometry, paraffin immunoperoxidase was performed for CD4, CD8, T-cell intracellular antigen, and βF1 expression. A comparison was made of the CD4 and CD8 results from both methods. Paraffin immunoperoxidase was used to study all βF1-peripheral T-cell lymphomas for T-cell receptor.

Results.—There was a 71% correlation with the 21 peripheral T-cell lymphomas that had distinct CD4+CD8− or CD4−CD8+ phenotypes by flow cytometry with paraffin immunoperoxidase. The sensitivity for CD4 expression was 64% and for CD8 expression was 90%. Flow cytometry found tumor cells in 4 of 6 peripheral T-cell lymphomas, with no clear CD4 or CD8 predominance or coexpression of these antigens, yet paraffin immunoperoxidase showed them to be CD4+CD8− or CD4−CD8+. Paraffin immunoperoxidase demonstrated 12 (39%) peripheral T-cell lymphomas to be cytotoxic phenotypes, including 8 CD4−CD8+, 1 CD4+CD8− and 3 CD4−CD8− instances. Paraffin immunoperoxidase found that of 30 immunoreactive peripheral T-cell lymphomas, 26 (87%) were αβ (β F1+). Paraffin immunoperoxidase found that both large cell cases among 4 βF1− peripheral T-cell lymphomas were T-cell receptor γδ+, including 1 γδ+ case confirmed by flow cytometry.

Conclusion.—Paraffin immunoperoxidase can assign CD4 and CD8 T-cell subsets for most peripheral T-cell lymphomas, with CD4 showing moderate and CD8 showing strong correlation with flow cytometric results. In the peripheral T-cell lymphomas in which flow cytometry produces inconclusive results, paraffin immunoperoxidase can also define CD4 or CD8 expression on tumor cells. T-cell intracellular antigen-1 can easily identify cytotoxic peripheral T-cell lymphomas, and it can also distinguish cytotoxic from "suppressor" CD8+ peripheral T-cell lymphomas. Some large cell γδ peripheral T-cell lymphomas may be identified by paraffin immunoperoxidase, but most peripheral T-cell lymphomas are derived from αβ T-cells.

▶ An increasing number of antibodies are becoming available for immunophenotypic analysis of paraffin embedded tissue. This article provides a timely evaluation and discussion of these markers for T-cell subset analysis of T-cell lymphoproliferative disorders. Whereas the CD8 antibody showed a 90% sensitivity and 100% specificity on paraffin tissue, as compared to the flow cytometrically analyzed standard, the CD4 antibody was less favorable. The CD4 sensitivity was only 64%. The major cause for the low sensitivity was the CD4 antibody's failure to react with either the neoplastic cells or residual normal cells in 8 of 31 cases. Only 1 case, an intestinal T-cell lymphoma, was potentially CD4 false positive. This case was $CD8^+/CD4^-$ by flow cytometric analysis, and dual $CD4^+/CD8^+$ by immunohistochemistry. As the authors suggest, this discrepancy may result from differences in the particular epitope of CD4 detected by each antibody. Some CD4 positive T cells may not react with all antibodies.

The use of TIA-1, a cytotoxic granule associated protein, allows separation of the $CD8^+$ T cells into cytotoxic and suppressor subsets. As the authors comment, this distinction may prove clinically relevant, because T-cell lymphomas with a cytotoxic phenotype have been considered aggressive. Ones with a T-suppressor phenotype have been considered low grade.

The major advantage for immunophenotyping specimens from paraffin tissue is the better morphologic assessment of the neoplastic population. In this study, the neoplastic T-cell subset was unclear by flow cytometric analysis in 6 cases, and in 5 of these cases, the neoplastic subset was determined by the immunohistochemical technique.

J.F. Turner, Jr., M.D.

Extranodal Lymphomas Associated With Hepatitis C Virus Infection

Ascoli V, Lo Coco F, Artini M, et al (Università La Sapienza, Rome, Italy; Univ Hosp, Geneva)

Am J Clin Pathol 109:600–609, 1998 11–16

Introduction.—During the course of chronic hepatitis C virus infection, clonal B-cell expansions and non-Hodgkin's lymphomas may develop. A group of heterogenous disorders ranging from nonlymphomatous infiltrates to high-grade lymphomas to hepatitis C virus-related lymphocyte proliferations usually involve peripheral blood, bone marrow, lymph nodes, and extranodal sites. However, there is still a lack of consensus on lymphoma classification and criteria used to define true hepatitis C virus-associated non-Hodgkin's lymphoma. Eight cases of B-cell non-Hodgkin's lymphoma originating in extranodal sites that occurred during noncryoglobulinemic hepatitis C virus infection were described.

Methods.—There were 8 cases of B-cell extranodal non-Hodgkin's lymphoma occurring in hepatitis C virus-positive persons: low-grade of mucosa-associated lymphoid tissue-type, diffuse large cell, Burkitt, and diffuse small cell. Nested reverse transcriptase-polymerase chain reaction was used to assess the presence of hepatitis C virus RNA in serum and ascitic fluid, with primers derived from the highly conserved 5' noncoding region of the prototype hepatitis C virus RNA sequence. A semi-quantitative, strand-specific reverse transcriptase-polymerase chain reaction was used to assess the presence and relative amount of either strand of the hepatitis C virus RNA in total tissue RNA for the tumor specimens.

Results.—The extranodal sites were the liver, liver and spleen, spleen, peritoneal cavity, parotid gland, nasopharynx, and eyelid. Clonal immunoglobulin gene rearrangements were exhibited in 4 lymphomatous specimens available for molecular analysis, and they lacked *bcl*-2, *bcl*-6, *c-myc* genes, and *p53* alterations. They also lacked replicative intermediate hepatitis C virus RNA, as documented by a strand-specific reverse transcriptase-polymerase chain reaction. In a single hepatic lymphoma, low levels of positive-strand hepatitis C virus RNA, suggesting the presence of the virus in residual hepatocytes, were detected.

Conclusion.—The antigen-driven properties of hepatitis C virus-associated B-cell malignant neoplasms may be considered for hepatic mucosa-associated lymphoid tissue-type lymphoma, which may have originated from lymphoid tissue acquired during long-standing hepatitis C virus infection.

► Circumstantial evidence is accumulating that hepatitis C virus (HCV) may be involved in the pathogenesis of non-Hodgkin's lymphomas. As pointed out by Lai and Weiss[1] in their editorial accompanying this article, the prevalence of HCV serologic positivity is increased in patients with lymphomas. In addition, HCV is reported to be lymphotrophic and to have the capability to stimulate B-cells.

Although this circumstantial evidence exists, there is little direct evidence that HCV contributes to the pathogenesis of non-Hodgkin's lymphoma. This study examined 8 cases of non-Hodgkin's lymphoma that occurred in patients with HCV-related hepatic disease (chronic hepatitis and cirrhosis). Only 1 of these patients had HCV-RNA detected from the lymphomatous tissue. In this case of hepatic lymphoma, the titer of positive strand HCV-RNA was low, and the positivity may reflect infected hepatocytes rather than lymphoma. However, another study had contradictory results, finding HCV-RNA in predominantly low-grade non-Hodgkin's lymphomas.[2] In addition, a single study has demonstrated HCV associated proteins within lymphoma cells by immunohistochemical techniques.[3] Clearly, further studies of these lymphomas, with in-situ techniques for HCV, are needed.

J.F. Turner, Jr., M.D.

References

1. Lai R, Weiss LM: Hepatitis C virus and non-Hodgkin's lymphoma. *Am J Clin Pathol* 109:508–509, 1998.
2. Luppi M, Grazia FM, Bonaccorsi G, et al: Hepatitis C virus infection in subsets of neoplastic lymphoproliferations not associated with cryoglobulinemia. *Leukemia* 10:351–355, 1996.
3. Sansonno D, De Vitra S, Cornacchiulo V, et al: Detection and distribution of hepatitis C virus related protein in lymph nodes of patients with type II mixed cryoglobulinemia and neoplastic and non-neoplastic lymphoproliferation. *Blood* 88:4638–4645, 1996.

Cytotoxic Protein Expression in Natural Killer Cell Lymphomas and in αβ and γδ Peripheral T-Cell Lymphomas

Boulland M-L, Kanavaros P, Wechsler J, et al (Hôpital Henri Mondor, Créteil, France; Univ Hosp of Heraklion, Greece; Institut Gustave Roussy, Villejuif, France)

J Pathol 183:432–439, 1997 11–17

Introduction.—Peripheral T-cell lymphomas usually express the αβ T-cell receptor, and rare peripheral T-cell lymphomas express the γδ T-cell receptor. Up to 30% of peripheral T-cell lymphomas express neither T-cell receptor, and are referred to as T-cell receptor silent peripheral T-cell lymphomas, which include sinonasal tumors that are considered as natural killer cell lymphomas. The possibility that at least some peripheral T-cell lymphomas are derived from lymphocytes with cytotoxic potential was investigated.

Methods.—Immunohistochemistry was used to study 60 patients with peripheral T-cell lymphomas, including 27 expressing the αβ T-cell receptor, 15 expressing the T-cell receptor γδ, and 18 expressing neither T-cell receptor, as well as 14 natural killer-cell lymphomas, studied for the expression of T-cell intracellular antigen-1, perforin, and granzyme B proteins. Expression of T-cell intracellular antigen-1 is characteristic of cytotoxic cells regardless of their activation status and expression of perforin and granzymes is highly increased in activated cytotoxic cells, correlating with the induction of cytolytic activity.

Results.—T-cell intracellular antigen-1, perforin, and granzyme B in most tumors were expressed by all natural killer-cell lymphomas, comprising 11 sinonasal and 3 systemic patients. T-cell intracellular antigen-1 protein in most tumors was expressed for all γδ peripheral T-cell lymphomas. There was a different cytotoxic antigen profile in hepatosplenic γδ peripheral T-cell lymphomas (T-cell intracellular antigen-1+, perforin−, granzyme B−) and in non-hepatosplenic γδ peripheral T-cell lymphomas (3 nasal, 1 skin, 1 lung), which expressed the 3 cytotoxic proteins. Cytotoxic lymphocytes, with the expression of at least 1 cytotoxic protein in tumor cells, seem to be the cause for 15 (33%) of the 45 patients with αβ and T-cell receptor silent peripheral T-cell lymphomas. The site of localization appeared to be related to this cytotoxic protein expression, because 54% extranodal and only 25% nodal αβ and T-cell receptor silent peripheral T-cell lymphomas expressed T-cell intracellular antigen-1. There is also a relation to histology: this pattern was seen in a proportion of anaplastic (75%) and pleomorphic (47%) lymphomas, but not in the angioimmunoblastic-type non-Hodgkin's lymphomas.

Conclusion.—Natural killer cell lymphomas represent tumors of activated cytotoxic natural killer cells, and non-hepatosplenic γδ peripheral T-cell lymphomas represent tumors of γδ T cells. Hepatosplenic γδ peripheral T-cell lymphomas represent tumors of non-activated cytotoxic γδ T cells. Tumors of cytotoxic T cells represent a small proportion of αβ and

T-cell receptor silent peripheral T-cell lymphomas, mostly extranodal cases, or nodal anaplastic lymphomas.

▶ TIA-1, granzyme B, and perforin are granule-associated cytotoxic proteins normally present in cytotoxic T cells and in natural killer cells. The recent development of monoclonal antibodies against these proteins enabled the authors to study a moderately large number of peripheral T-cell lymphomas and natural killer cell lymphomas. While B-cell lymphomas are better studied and have been segregated according to their normal counterpart within the lymphoid system, segregation of the T-cell neoplasms is less clear. Studies such as this one may reveal distinct lymphoma subtypes. For example, the authors did note that nonhepatic γδ T-cell lymphomas differ from the hepatic γδ T-cell lymphomas by having an activated phenotype indicated by expression of granzyme B and perforin. This phenotype was present in the 3 nonhepatic γδ T-cell lymphomas studied in this article and was confirmed in a subsequent study of 11 patients.[1]

J.F. Turner, Jr., M.D.

Reference

1. Anaulf B, Copie-Berman C, Delfau-Larue M-H, et al: Nonhepatosplenic γδ T-cell lymphoma: A subset of cytotoxic lymphomas with mucosal or skin localization. *Blood* 91:1723–1731, 1988.

Suggested Reading

Barekman CL, Fair KP, Cotelingam JD: Comparative utility of diagnostic bone-marrow components: A 10-year study. *Am J Hematol* 56:37–41, 1997.

▶ This study confirms the utility of 4 components that are necessary for an optimum bone marrow examination. The aspirate clot section and touch preps of the core biopsy provide morphologic information that is complimentary to the aspirate smears and core biopsy sections. Occasionally, the aspirate clot section or the touch preps of the core biopsy will contain the only diagnostic material. Therefore, their inclusion as part of the bone marrow examination is warranted. This study also provides data supporting the performance of bilateral core biopsies for staging of lymphoma or carcinoma.

J.F. Turner, Jr., M.D.

Wilson CS, Traweek ST, Slovak ML, et al: Myelodysplastic syndrome occurring after autologous bone marrow transplantation for lymphoma: Morphologic features. *Am J Clin Pathol* 108:369–377, 1997.

▶ Although only a small number of patients with myelodysplastic syndrome (MDS) were evaluated, this study illustrates the dyspoietic findings that occur in patients receiving several different chemotherapeutic combinations and autologous bone marrow transplantation for lymphoma. Many of the dyspoietic findings are subtle and may overlap with nonclonal dyspoietic findings associated with the transplantation process. It may be difficult to initially detect these patients with "indolent" MDS without performing cytogenetic analysis. It is easier to recognize patients with "aggressive" MDS because of the greater qualitative and quantitative trilineage dyspoieis seen in those patients.

NO POSTAGE
NECESSARY
IF MAILED
IN THE
UNITED STATES

BUSINESS REPLY MAIL
FIRST-CLASS MAIL PERMIT NO 135 ST LOUIS MO

POSTAGE WILL BE PAID BY ADDRESSEE

SUBSCRIPTION SERVICES
MOSBY, INC.
11830 WESTLINE INDUSTRIAL DRIVE
ST. LOUIS MO 63146-9988

NO POSTAGE
NECESSARY
IF MAILED
IN THE
UNITED STATES

BUSINESS REPLY MAIL
FIRST-CLASS MAIL PERMIT NO 135 ST LOUIS MO

POSTAGE WILL BE PAID BY ADDRESSEE

SUBSCRIPTION SERVICES
MOSBY, INC.
11830 WESTLINE INDUSTRIAL DRIVE
ST. LOUIS MO 63146-9988

Want to speed up the process?

To order a *Year Book* or *Advances*, you also may call 1-800-426-4545

To subscribe to a journal today, call toll-free in the U.S.:
1-800-453-4351
or fax 314-432-1158
Outside the U.S., call: 314-453-4351

Visit us at: *www.mosby.com/periodicals*

Mosby, Inc.
Subscription Services
11830 Westline Industrial Drive
St. Louis, MO 63146 U.S.A.

Mosby

Because both MDS and acute leukemia can occur following treatment for other malignancies, it is not surprising that MDS occurred in some of these previously treated patients with lymphoma. It is interesting to note the varied clinical course in these patients with clonal cytogenetic abnormalities. The greater dyspoiesis seems to correlate with a more aggressive course, similar to the FAB classification of MDS.

J.F. Turner, Jr., M.D.

12 Kidney

A Locus for Inherited Focal Segmental Glomerulosclerosis Maps to Chromosome 19q13: Rapid Communication

Mathis BJ, Kim SH, Calabrese K, et al (Oklahoma State Univ, Tulsa; Univ of Chicago; Harvard Med School, Boston)

Kidney Int 53:282–286, 1998 12–1

Introduction.—Focal segmental glomerulosclerosis (FSGS) is a pathologic finding in various renal disorders that are characterized by proteinuria and progressive degeneration in renal function. Linkage analysis was performed to map the disease gene in a previously identified large family with FSGS.

Methods.—All family members were clinically re-evaluated and peripheral blood samples were collected to determine lymphoblastoid cell lines, DNA extraction, and serum creatinine measurements.

Results.—This family demonstrated variable expression of the gene defect. Some family members developed end-stage renal disease by the fourth decade or had severe proteinuria, and others developed only mild microalbuminuria. One family member with mild microalbuminuria had 2 daughters who were severely affected. The disease gene was mapped to a region of chromosome 19q13.

Conclusion.—With a high degree of certainty, it can be stated that the gene responsible for FSGS is located on chromosome 19q13.

▶ The occurrence of familial FSGS is well documented in the literature, although it is distinctly unusual to see this condition in clinical practice. The morphology of this familial FSGS is identical to the other sporadic forms, as well as to secondary forms of FSGS. In this study of a very large family, the inherited condition was documented to be autosomal dominant, and with detailed molecular mapping, the chromosome was finally located. Whether this locus is a pure genetic influence with variable penetrance remains to be seen, but it clearly at least represents a very serious risk factor or marker for the occurrence of FSGS. Further studies on the sporadic form of the disease, and in patient populations with the secondary form of FSGS, would be of interest, possibly clarifying whether the gene is present in those cases as well.

D.J. Dabbs, M.D.

Suggested Reading

Faubert PF, Porush JG: Familial focal segmental glomerulosclerosis: Nine cases in four families and review of the literature. *Am J Kidney Dis* 30:265–270, 1997.

Glicklich D, Haskell L, Senitzer D, et al: Possible genetic predisposition to idiopathic focal segmental glomerulosclerosis. *Am J Kidney Dis* 12:26–30, 1988.

An 11-Month-Old With Anti-Glomerular Basement Membrane Disease

Bigler SA, Parry WM, Fitzwater DS, et al (Univ of Mississippi, Jackson)

Am J Kidney Dis 30:710–712, 1997 12–2

Introduction.—Anti-glomerular basement membrane (GBM) disease is rare in children. Hallmarks of this disease are increased circulating anti-GBM antibodies and linear immunofluorescence for IgG in glomeruli. The authors report the youngest known patient with anti-GBM disease.

Case Report.—Infant, 11 months, was treated with amoxicillin for otitis media. She returned 2 weeks later with persistent fever. Family history was free of renal disease, and parental history free of occupational exposure to hydrocarbons, solvents, or other potential toxic agents. On physical examination, the patient was pale, and had a temperature of 99°F and blood pressure of 95/53 mm Hg. Her hemoglobin was 7.0 g/dL, serum creatinine 159 μmol/L, urea nitrogen 10.4 mmol/L urea, erythrocyte sedimentation rate 70 mm/hr, and protein 3+ with numerous erythrocytes. A spot urine protein to creatinine ratio was 2 and anti-GBM antibody titer was 1:7,640. Her renal function deteriorated quickly. She was treated with 20 mg/kg methylprednisolone. Renal biopsy revealed 7 glomeruli with florid cellular crescents and segmental necrosis of glomerular tufts on light microscopy. An interstitial infiltrate of lymphocytes and scattered neutrophils was observed. No obsolescent glomeruli or significant interstitial fibrosis was seen. Immunofluorescence showed intense linear staining with antibodies to IgG and C3. Crescents were positive for fibrinogen, and tubular basement membranes were negative for all immunoglobulins and complement components. Cellular crescents and absence of immune complex deposits were seen on electron microscopy. Plasmapheresis was begun on day 9 and cyclophosphamide was added on day 20. The patient's clinical condition worsened and she was started on chronic peritoneal dialysis. Her titers of antibodies to glomerular basement membranes gradually diminished. At 12 months after initial evaluation, she underwent kidney transplantation. At 16 months after transplantation, she had good preservation of renal function, serum creatinine of 53.01 μmol/L, and urea nitrogen of 7.14 mmol/L urea.

Conclusion.—Anti-glomerular basement membrane disease has a poor prognosis, especially in children. The very high titers of anti-GBM antibodies in this patient indicate precocious development of mature basement membranes or development of autoimmunity to a different antigen.

► There are only 9 documented cases of anti-GBM disease in children younger than 15 years. The youngest previously reported patient was 2.5 years, and this patient was 11 months. The Goodpasture antigen is now recognized to be the NC1 domain of the alpha 3 chain of Type IV collagen. Precisely what triggers the disease is unknown, but interestingly the development of anti-GBM disease tends to be age dependent. This suggests that the Goodpasture antigen "matures" and appears with age, since it has been found that immune serum from patients with Goodpasture's disease does not react with kidneys from patients younger than 3 months. A key point then for the nephropathologist in the audience is the possibility of anti-GBM disease in the infant.

D.J. Dabbs, M.D.

Allergic Nephropathy Associated With Norfloxacin and Ciprofloxacin Therapy: Report of Two Cases and Review of the Literature

Hadimeri H, Almroth G, Cederbrant K, et al (Eksjö County Hosp, Sweden; Univ Hosp, Linköping, Sweden; AB Astra Safety Assessment, Södertälje, Sweden)

Scand J Urol Nephrol 31:481–485, 1997 12–3

Introduction.—Acute interstitial nephritis (AIN) is a potential complication of drug therapy. This article describes a case of AIN associated with norfloxacin treatment and another case of AIN associated with ciprofloxacin treatment.

Case 1.—Woman, 68, presented with loin pain, fever, and glucosuria. Norfloxacin treatment was initiated. Symptoms gradually disappeared but recurred on the seventh day. Serum creatinine increased. Renal biopsy revealed edema, acute interstitial inflammation with eosinophils, and a histopathological appearance that was consistent with drug-induced AIN. Norfloxacin was discontinued and the patient gradually improved. No corticosteroid treatment was employed.

Case 2.—Woman, 70, had 1 course of chemotherapy. The second course was delayed because of fever and angiitis, treated with ciprofloxacin. Serum creatinine level, white cell count, erythrocyte sedimentation rate and C-reactive protein level became elevated. Renal biopsy revealed histopathologic appearance compatible with drug-induced AIN. Ciprofloxacin was discontinued. Corticosteroid treatment was not employed. The patient gradually improved.

Conclusions.—Clinicians should be aware of the possibility of quinolone-associated AIN, a rare but potentially serious renal complication.

▶ Here we go again: a new class of antibiotics and yet a new class of antibiotics associated with AIN as a toxic reaction. These quinolone antibiotics are widely used nowadays in the treatment of urinary tract, respiratory tract, and soft tissue infections, as well as osteomyelitis. As with any drug, the potential for a renal untoward reaction is possible. Clinical features for the diagnosis of AIN may not be readily apparent, and a diagnosis must be established by a renal biopsy. Biopsies in these cases demonstrate an interstitial infiltrate composed mostly of lymphocytes, with varying degrees of eosinophils and plasma cells. The eosinophils predominated in these cases, along with lymphocytes associated with destruction of tubular epithelium. The precise immunologic mechanism for these changes is not readily apparent, although it is considered to be in the plane of hypersensitivity allergic reaction. Of course, peripheral eosinophilia and/or eosinophiluria can also be helpful in establishing a diagnosis.

D.J. Dabbs, M.D.

Suggested Reading

Anderson I, Sjöström P: Ciprofloxacin can cause allergic interstitial nephritis with acute renal failure. *Läkartidningen* 88:1298–1299, 1991.

Bailey JR, Trott SA, Philbrick JT: Ciprofloxacin-induced acute interstitial nephritis. *Am J Nephrol* 12:271–273, 1992.

Hootkins R, Fenves AZ, Stephens MK: Acute renal failure secondary to oral ciprofloxacin therapy: A presentation of three cases and a review of the literature. *Clin Nephrol* 32:75–78, 1989.

Oritz A, Plaza JJ, Egido J: Ciprofloxacin-associated tubulointerstitial nephritis with linear tubular basement membrane deposits. *Nephron* 60:248, 1992.

Analysis of Fine-Needle Aspiration Biopsies by Flow Cytometry in Kidney Transplant Patients

Oliveira JGG, Ramos JP, Xavier P, et al (Hosp S João, Porto, Portugal; Tissue Typing Ctr, Porto, Portugal)
Transplantation 64:97–102, 1997 12–4

Introduction.—Short- and long-term outcome has improved for kidney transplant recipients. Core renal biopsy is the most commonly accepted method for diagnosing acute rejection. It has a small, yet significant, rate of false results. Fine-needle aspiration biopsy (FNAB) has a similar diagnostic yield to core renal biopsy. Fine-needle aspiration biopsy allows comparison of the number and activation status of mononuclear cells present in the aspirated sample with those observed in the circulation.

Aspiration biopsy samples were analyzed in conjunction with peripheral blood lymphocytes (PBL) by flow cytometry to determine the diagnostic reliability of FNAB in patients with acute rejection crisis.

Methods.—Lymphocytes from PBL and aspiration biopsies from 83 consecutive renal transplant recipients were analyzed. Fifty-one patients who were stable and rejection free for the first 6 months were compared with 32 patients with 40 acute rejection episodes. Comparisons were made of FNAB findings on day 7 and day 30 after transplantation.

Results.—The aspiration biopsy samples revealed significant differences for several lymphocyte subpopulations in stable patients and patients with rejection. The PBL analysis was not useful in differentiating the 2 patient groups. The expression of several activation markers inside the graft were combined with CD3DR and CD3CD25 aspiration biopsy to peripheral blood ratios, producing a sensitivity of 83.9% and a specificity of 90.5%. The positive predictive value for dysfunctional graft rejection was 85.8%.

Conclusion.—Flow cytometry study of aspiration biopsy samples of kidney transplant patients may be considered a reliable, rapid, and useful method for diagnosing acute rejection episodes. Cytofluorometric analysis provides the FNAB to PBL ratios for some subpopulations and significantly improves FNAB's performance as a diagnostic tool.

▶ The principles of this study are simple: Obtain peripheral blood from patients not more than 2–3 months after renal transplantation and obtain FNAB samples from the kidneys. Compare the ratios of the T-cell subsets in the kidney to peripheral blood to examine for selective homing of cells that would be involved in rejection. The sensitivity was found to be about 84% and the specificity 91%, with a positive predictive value of rejection of about 86%. Only this select group of patients could benefit by bypassing the core renal biopsy. From my frame of reference, it is important to realize that a negative result by this method in this group of patients should immediately prompt a core tissue biopsy. Other relevant lesions to look for in this setting obviously include tubular necrosis, vascular (humoral) rejection, and the morphologic stigmata of viral infection.

D.J. Dabbs, M.D.

Suggested Reading

Bogman MJTT: Fine-needle aspiration biopsy of the renal transplant: Is it worthwhile or a waste of time? *Nephrol Dial Transplant* 10:2182, 1995.

Gray DWR, Richardson A, Hughes D, et al: A prospective, randomized, blind comparison of three biopsy techniques in the management of patients after renal transplantation. *Transplantation* 53:1226, 1992.

Utility of Standardized Histological Classification in the Management of Acute Rejection

Gaber LW, Moore LW, Gaber AO, et al (Univ of Tennessee–Memphis; Univ of Cincinnati, Ohio; McGill Centre for Clinical Immunobiology and Transplantation, Montreal; et al)

Transplantation 64:376–380, 1998 12–5

Background.—An important criterion for diagnosing rejection in immunosuppression clinical trials is standardized histologic grading of transplant kidney biopsies. The value of such classification in the management of acute rejection was investigated.

Methods.—Twelve transplant centers in North America, Europe, and Australia participated in an assessment of kidney transplant rejection. Data from the 1995 Efficacy Endpoints Conference were analyzed to determine the frequency of Banff schema adoption.

Findings.—Seventy-three percent of 953 patients had histologically confirmed rejection episodes. The adoption of Banff criteria increased between 1992 and 1995. Banff grades were significantly associated with clinical rejection severity, though nadir creatinine levels were similar. The response rates of patients with Banff grades I and II rejection to steroid treatment did not differ. However, only 42% of those with grade III rejection responded to such therapy. Banff grade III was correlated with decreased graft survival at 1 year. These rates were 86% in patients with grade I rejection, 88% in those with grade II, and 70% in those with grade III (Table 4).

Conclusions.—Standardized histologic classifications such as the Banff schema can be used reliably to determine patients' risk of treatment failure. The current findings support the use of Banff criteria in clinical trials.

► Renal transplant pathology used to be a specialty unto itself. However, many practicing pathologists now see such biopsies, and still with some anxiety. This article describes the results of a 19-center international trial at grading acute rejection using the Banff schema and is based on a 1995 endpoint.[1] Ultimately, the utility of any histologic grading scheme is its

TABLE 4.—Correlation of Clinical Signs with Biopsy Grades

Symptoms	Borderline n (%)	Grade I n (%)	Grade II n (%)	Grade III n (%)	Total n*
No UV decrease†	7 (4)	68 36	88 (47)	25 (13)	188
UV decrease†	2 (3)	20 (26)	27 (35)	28 (36)	77
No fever	6 (3)	88 (45)	73 (38)	27 (14)	194
Fever‡	3 (3)	24 (25)	42 (44)	27 (28)	96

Note: P = 0.0007, χ^2 difference without borderline cases. P = 0.0022 χ^2 difference without borderline cases.
*Total number of cases responding to this query.
†UV = urine volume.
‡Temperature equal to or greater than 38.5°.
(Courtesy of Gaber LW, Moore LW, Gaber AO, et al: Utility of standardized histological classification in the management of acute rejection. *Transplantation* 64[3]:376–380, 1998.)

correlation with key clinical parameters. This study did find a significant correlation between the Banff criteria and serum creatinine and graft survival (probably the most important parameter); correlation with steroid response was not impressive. One key aspect that is not fully addressed is the interinstitutional and interpathologists variability in applying these criteria. Whereas it can be argued that utility within an institution is most important, it is also critical that these criteria should be more widely applicable and be useful to other, non-renal, pathologists. Perhaps this is the focus of a future publication.

M.B. Cohen, M.D.

Reference

1. Solez K, Axelsen RA, Benediktsson H, et al: International standardization of criteria for the histologic diagnosis of renal allograft rejection: The Banff working classifications of kidney transplant pathology. *Kidney Int* 44:411, 1993.

Mechanisms of Drug-induced Lupus: III. Sex-specific Differences in T Cell Homing May Explain Increased Disease Severity in Female Mice

Yung R, Williams R, Johnson K, et al (Univ of Michigan, Ann Arbor)

Arthritis Rheum 40:1334–1343, 1997 12–6

Introduction.—The mechanisms responsible for the increased immune responsiveness and sex-specific disease manifestations of systemic lupus erythematosus are unknown. A lupus-like disease was induced in a D10 murine model to correlate sex-specific disease manifestations with differences in T-cell homing between male and female recipients.

Methods.—Six- to 8-week-old female and male AKR mice underwent splenectomy and oophorectomy or orchiectomy. Mice were injected with procainamide-treated T-cell clones. Trafficking was analyzed by labeling the injected cells with ^{51}Cr or 5-chloromethylfluorescein diacetate.

Results.—Autoimmune liver disease developed in more females than males. Females had greater titers of anti-DNA antibodies and 2–7 times more cells accumulated in the spleen than males. The development of autoantibodies and renal and liver disease were prevented by splenectomy. In females, oophorectomy reduced the splenic homing, autoantibody titer, and liver disease severity to levels observed in males.

Conclusion.—Sex-specific differences in the number of T cells homing to the spleen were detected in this murine model of drug-induced systemic lupus erythematosus. This explains the increased disease severity in female mice. Splenectomy has increased survival and improved disease severity in human lupus.

► I like this paper because it speculates considerably into the future regarding the possible mechanisms explaining why females predominate in connective tissue disease, specifically lupus. In this experimental model, lupus was induced in mice with procainamide, and it was discovered that the spleen was necessary to disease induction. However, most interesting was the observation that T-cell homing in the spleen is different between male and female mice. The speculation is that this may be a sex-specific disease because of these differences in lymphoid homing, presumably because of sex steroids.

This article particularly caught my eye because estrogen-receptor protein may be observed by the immunoperoxidase technique in subsets of lymphoid cells in normal lymph nodes. A few of the lymphocytes observed are on the interfollicular zone, but there are substantial numbers as well in the germinal center areas of lymphoid follicles. As mentioned in the article, it is of interest to speculate regarding triggering mechanisms that may be involved with estrogen receptor at the transcriptional level in lymphoid cells that are encountering specific types of antigen. The finding of estrogen receptor proteins in human lymphoid cells is not a well-known phenomenon, although they have been observed in certain leukemia cell lines that have, in fact, been responsive to estrogen receptor blockade. I am sure we will hear more about this tantalizing subject in the future.

D.J. Dabbs, M.D.

Renal Vasculitis With HIV Seropositivity: Potential Manifestation of Cytomegalovirus Infection

Chertow GM, Rennke HG, Curhan GC, et al (Brigham and Women's Hosp, Boston; Harvard Med School, Boston)

Am J Kidney Dis 30:428–432, 1997 12–7

Introduction.—Relationships among HIV infection, focal segmental glomerulosclerosis, and the latter's variant, "collapsing glomerulopathy," are well-known precursors of chronic renal failure. In patients who are HIV-seropositive, such immune complex–mediated glomerular diseases as postinfectious glomerulonephritis, IgA nephropathy, and membranoproliferative glomerulonephritis can also develop. A patient with pauci-immune necrotizing renal vasculitis and HIV seropositivity was described.

Case Report.—Male, 54, was hospitalized with nausea, vomiting, watery diarrhea, and diffuse abdominal pain of 2 days duration. This followed a week of pharyngitis, myalgia, and a purpuric rash of the lower extremities. He had a known history of cocaine and ethanol abuse, infectious hepatitis, chronic prostatitis, arthritis, hypertension, hypercholesterolemia, and HIV seropositivity. On admission, the patient was volume depleted and hypotensive. He responded to treatment with broad-spectrum antibiotics. A skin biopsy specimen revealed leukocytoclastic vasculitis, and corticosteroid therapy was started. The abdominal pain recurred during the next several days and the purpuric rash advanced to bullae and ulcers.

An abdominal paracentesis was performed; findings suggested peritonitis, but Gram's stain and cultures were negative. Serum creatinine concentration increased gradually. Gastrointestinal bleeding intensified. Upper and lower endoscopies revealed superficial ulcerations of the esophagus, stomach, and colon. Biopsy specimens had nonspecific findings. Renal function deteriorated over the next 2 weeks, with serum creatinine concentrations increasing gradually to 2.8 mg/dL. Percutaneous renal biopsy sampling revealed a proliferative and focal necrotizing glomerulonephritis, with infiltrating cells that consisted mainly of mononuclear leukocytes.

The patient continued to have low-grade fevers, refractory gastrointestinal bleeding, and ventricular ectopy. He required ultrafiltration and hemodialysis for pulmonary edema and worsening azotemia. On hospital day 38, the patient had an asystolic cardiac arrest and died. Postmortem examination showed multiorgan involvement with cytomegalovirus, extensive pulmonary hemorrhage with invasive and cavitary aspergillosis, and findings consistent with *Pneumocystis carinii*. A diagnosis of pauci-immune necrotizing renal vasculitis was made.

Conclusion.—Pauci-immune necrotizing glomerulitis and vasculitis with associated cytomegalovirus infection should be considered in the differential diagnosis of acute renal failure in patients who are seropositive. This diagnosis may be more prevalent in the white race and in persons who are HIV seropositive without frank AIDS.

▶ The panoply of glomerulopathies in HIV-positive patients includes the classic HIV nephropathy, focal segmental glomerulosclerosis and its variant, "collapsing glomerulopathy," as well as immune complex–related glomerulopathies including postinfectious glomerulonephritis, IgA nephropathy, and membranoproliferative glomerulonephritis. The last can be associated with hepatitis, especially hepatitis C.

This paper goes 1 step further in describing another probable infection-related glomerulopathy, that of a pauci-immune necrotizing glomerulonephritis and vasculitis associated strongly with cytomegalovirus infection. Vasculitis associated with cytomegalovirus infection is not an uncommon finding in other tissues, and finding it in the kidney is not surprising. Unique in this paper, of course, is the concurrent necrotizing glomerulonephritis reflecting capillary vasculitis. This is another glomerulopathy to keep in mind when examining renal biopsy specimens from patients with HIV infection.

D.J. Dabbs, M.D.

Localization of Hepatocyte Growth Factor and Tubulointerstitial Lesions in IgA Nephropathy

Taniguchi Y, Yorioka N, Yamashita K, et al (Hiroshima Univ, Japan)

Am J Nephrol 17:413–416, 1997 12–8

Introduction.—Hepatocyte growth factor (HGF) may be associated with tubular damage in primary glomerulonephritis, including IgA nephropathy. Tubulointerstitial lesions (TILs) affect the serum creatinine (s-Cr) level and the glomerular filtration rate. The TILs occur frequently in various types of glomerulonephritis and may have prognostic importance. The relationship between localization of HGF and TILs in the cortical area of renal biopsy specimens was evaluated in 35 patients with IgA nephropathy.

Methods.—Renal biopsy specimens underwent immunohistochemical examination. The correlation between HGF positivity and the extent of histologic damage and the TIL grade was determined. The relationship between HGF positivity and various clinical findings was analyzed. Total daily urinary protein excretion (TUP), s-Cr, serum β_2-microglobulin, urinary β_2-microglobulin, and creatinine clearance were analyzed at the time of renal biopsy.

Results.—Histologic damage was mild, moderate, and severe in 12, 15, and 8 patients, respectively. The TIL grade was negative, +1, +2, and +3 in 14, 11, 6, and 4 patients, respectively. Localization of HGF was detected primarily on epithelial cells in the renal tubules; no HGF was observed in the glomeruli. Fourteen of 35 patients tested positive for HGF. The correlation between HGF positivity and severity of histologic damage was significant. Histologic damage and TIL grade were significantly correlated with HGF staining. In patients positive for HGF, TUP, s-Cr, serum β-$_2$-microglobulin, and urinary β_2-microglobulin were significantly higher and creatinine clearance was significantly lower. Mean age did not differ in patients positive for HGF, but increased in parallel with TIL grade. Compared with patients with a TIL grade of 2+ or 3+, patients with negative TIL grade had significantly higher TUP, s-Cr, and serum β_2-microglobulin and significantly lower creatinine clearance.

Conclusion.—HGF positivity in patients with IgA nephropathy may be correlated with sites of histologic damage and tubular damage. The presence of HGF may influence exacerbation of IgA nephropathy.

▶ In a series of 35 patients with IgA nephropathy of various severities, the authors examined the relationship between the presence of tubular epithelial HGF and the severity of tubulointerstitial damage. It seems as though the authors were looking for a prognostic factor to determine the outcome in patients with IgA nephropathy. Although their results, presented in table form, clearly show significant differences between the patients who are HGF-negative and HGF-positive—specifically, total urine protein in grams per day, s-Cr, serum β_2-microglobulin, urinary β_2-microglobulin, and creatinine clearance—a causal relationship is readily apparent to me.

Clearly, patients who have HGF-positive tubular epithelial cells have worse functional parameters, but I see no appreciable difference between semiquantitative tubulointerstitial damage assessment by the authors and the presence of HGF. The HGF is probably a response to damage, and, therefore, seemingly correlates with tubulointerstitial damage. The same prognostic information can be obtained from merely assessing TILs in a semiquantitative fashion.

D.J. Dabbs, M.D.

Suggested Reading

Taniguchi Y, Yorioka N, Yamashita K, et al: Hepatocyte growth factor localization in primary glomerulonephritis and drug-induced interstital nephritis. *Nephron* 73:357–358, 1996.

Wang H, Tomino Y, Fukui M, et al: Correlation between tubulointerstitial changes and prognosis in patients with primary membranous nephropathy. *Nephron* 67:362, 1994.

Association of Vasculitic Glomerulonephritis With Membranous Nephropathy: A Report of 10 Cases

Tse WY, Howie AJ, Adu D, et al (Queen Elizabeth Hosp, Edgbaston, Birmingham, England)

Nephrol Dial Transplant 12:1017–1027, 1997 12–9

Introduction.—Except for patients with systemic lupus erythematosus, vasculitis or crescentic glomerulonephritis rarely occurs in association with membranous nephropathy. There are few data on the clinical course, treatment, and renal outcomes of patients with this unusual combination of nephritis. Ten patients with concomitant vasculitic glomerulonephritis and membranous nephropathy were described.

Patients.—The patients were 9 men and 1 woman, with a median age of 64 years, seen during a 14-year period. In each case, renal biopsy led to a diagnosis of membranous nephropathy and vasculitic glomerulonephritis in the absence of systemic lupus erythematosus. All specimens showed a vasculitic glomerulonephritis with an accumulation of cells in Bowman's space, and thus met conventional criteria for crescentic glomerulonephritis. The clinical presentation was acute renal failure in 3 patients, nephrotic syndrome in 4, and nonnephrotic range proteinuria and renal insufficiency in 2. The patients had a median serum creatinine level of 296 µmol/L at diagnosis. Except for 1 patient with vasculitic transformation from membranous nephropathy during a 5-year period, all patients had vasculitic glomerulonephritis and membranous nephropathy presenting together. Eight patients were treated with oral prednisolone and cyclophosphamide; 1 received plasma exchange as well. One patient received oral prednisolone and azathioprine, and 1 patient with histologic evidence of chronic renal damage received no specific immunosuppressive therapy. Four of 9 patients had positive serologic results for antineutrophil cytoplasmic antibodies (ANCA). The patients were followed up for a median of 3.5 years.

Outcomes.—Three patients had improvements in renal function, 2 had stable renal function, and 2 required renal replacement therapy. The remaining 3 patients died, 2 of sepsis and 1 ANCA-negative patient of a systemic vasculitis.

Conclusions.—The unusual combination of membranous nephropathy complicated by vasculitic glomerulonephritis appears to be clinically more aggressive than membranous nephropathy alone and may be associated with ANCA. For patients with membranous nephropathy who have an acute or accelerated decline in renal function, a repeat biopsy should be performed to assess the possibility of superimposed vasculitic transformation. Immunosuppressive therapy may be helpful in patients with this condition.

▶ Vasculitis associated with a primary membranous glomerulopathy is distinctly uncommon. This paper adds 10 additional cases to the prior 19 cases of membranous nephropathy that have been reported to be associated with crescentic glomerulonephritis. The patients described in this paper had either active vasculitis of the glomerulus exemplified by crescent transformation, or evidence of healed segmental glomerular vasculitis. Several of the patients had associated systemic vasculitis, but the majority did not have a systemic disease. Prior reported cases demonstrated anti–glomerular basement membrane (GBM) antibodies in almost half of the patients, whereas in this case series none of the patients had anti-GBM disease. Whereas some patients may have ANCA-positive serologic reaction, the majority of patients did not. Therefore, the association of crescents with membranous glomerulopathy may or may not be associated with a primary systemic vasculitis affecting other organs, and may be associated with ANCA. The fact that glomerular necrosis with crescent transformation is so uncommon in membranous glomerulonephritis suggests that when it occurs, the idiotypes of antigen-antibody reaction somehow set off a cascade of inflammatory cytokines that result in capillary rupture, spillage of fibrin into the urinary space, and subsequent crescent formation. Clinically, all of these patients had a rapidly progressive glomerulonephritis, which is what one would expect. As an aggressive, rapid progression of renal failure, the patients tend to respond to the antivasculitis regimens of steroids and cytotoxic agents. Of course, it is important to exclude an underlying lupus membranous nephritis giving rise to vasculitic lesions.

D.J. Dabbs, M.D.

Suggested Reading

Gaber LW, Wall BM, Cooke CR: Coexistence of anti-neutrophil cytoplasmic antibody-associated glomerulonephritis and membranous glomerulopathy. *Am J Clin Pathol* 99:211–215, 1993.

Kurki P, Helve T, Von Bonsdorff M, et al: Transformation of membranous glomerulonephritis into crescentic glomerulonephritis with glomerular basement membrane antibodies. Serial determinations of anti-GBM before the transformation. *Nephron* 38:134–137, 1984.

Moorthy AV, Zimmerman SW, Burkholder PM, et al: Association of crescentic glomerulonephritis with membranous glomerulonephropathy: A report of three cases. *Clin Nephrol* 6:319–325, 1976.

X-linked Alport Syndrome in Females

Meleg-Smith S, Magliato S, Cheles M, et al (Tulane Univ, New Orleans, La; Children's Mercy Hosp, Kansas City, Mo; Univ of Minnesota, Minneapolis)

Hum Pathol 29:404–408, 1998 12–10

Introduction.—The diagnosis of Alport syndrome (AS) is challenging, especially in females with mild symptoms and thin glomerular basement membrane (GBM). The clinical presentation is variable, and the ultrastructure changes are not identical in all patients. Immunostaining for GBM expression of α5 (IV) was assessed as an adjunctive diagnostic method using renal biopsy specimens from 8 female patients with clinical symptoms suggestive of AS.

Methods.—The patients' ages ranged from 7 to 36 years; 6 of 8 patients were aged 12–15 years. A semiquantitative Alport Index was developed by quantification of severity and extent of ultrastructural GBM changes to express variability of the ultrastructural GBM changes.

Results.—Findings of light microscopy were variable, ranging from no pathologic findings to severe chronic changes of glomerular sclerosis and interstitial fibrosis. A continuous linear pattern was observed along the GBM in normal kidneys and was absent in renal biopsy specimens from male X-linked AS. An interrupted, discontinuous linear pattern for α5 (IV) in glomeruli was seen in all 8 patients in this series, confirming the diagnosis of X-linked AS. The ultrastructural Alport Index varied between 6 and 47, demonstrating the heterogeneity in severity of GBM changes, even in patients aged 12–15 years. The predominant change was thin GBM and an Alport Index below 20 in 3 patients.

Conclusions.—Immunohistochemistry for α5 (IV) in renal biopsy specimens may be used to determine female patients heterozygous for X-linked AS. Using this technique made it possible to diagnose AS in female patients with predominant ultrastructural changes of thin basement membrane.

▶ The diagnosis of AS has always been a challenge and has always relied on semiquantitative evaluation of electromicrographs when taken into account with the clinical presentation in laboratory findings. The laminated and basket-weave abnormalities of the GBM, along with areas alternating with thinning and thickening by themselves are notoriously nonspecific, but when seen globally in all glomeruli in the proper clinical context, the diagnosis of AS can be made. Even more difficult with this X-linked disorder is making the diagnosis in females because of the heterozygous nature of expression. Because the basic defect in all AS is the result of one of several new mutations in the collagen IV genes, identification of the abnormal isoform would be ideal. This is what the authors have done in this study, showing that immunohistochemistry for α5 (IV) in renal biopsy specimens can identify the abnormal α5 (IV) collagen staining patterns.

It might be of interest to examine other tissues that might be more readily accessible than the kidney for documentation of this disorder.

D.J. Dabbs, M.D.

Suggested Reading

Lee CS, Southey MC, Slater H, et al: Primary cutaneous Ewing's sarcoma/peripheral primitive neuroectodermal tumors in childhood: A molecular, cytogenetic and immunohistochemical study. *Diagn Mol Pathol* 4:174–181, 1995.

Handling and Evaluation of Pediatric Renal Tumors

Zuppan CW (Loma Linda Univ, Calif)

Am J Clin Pathol 109:S31–S37, 1998 12–11

Introduction.—Pathologic evaluation of pediatric renal tumors is similar in some ways to evaluation of adult renal tumors, but it also has some unique features. Many of the special considerations in pediatric renal tumors involve the use of specialized classification, grading, or staging systems and participation in ongoing collaborative clinical and biologic studies. The author reviews some important considerations in the pathologic handling and evaluation of these tumors.

Pediatric Renal Tumors.—The differential diagnosis of pediatric renal tumors should be considered preoperatively. The diagnostic considerations vary for unilateral vs. bilateral tumors, for patients of different ages, and other clinical considerations. The author presents an overview of the handling of surgical specimens, including the intact specimen, bivalving, frozen section analysis, and fixation. Certain special studies may be indicated, including snap-frozen specimens, electron microscopy, and touch preparations. However, examination of specimens stained with hematoxylin and eosin remains the mainstay of diagnosis. Guidelines for submitting histologic sections address the need to establish the diagnosis, evaluate tumor spread, detect focal lesions, and define any developmental lesions that may be present. Special attention to the renal capsule is required, as this is a problem area in evaluation of tumor stage. Areas of suspected margin involvement should be documented with appropriate sections. Some type of specimen map should be used to document the location of the sections.

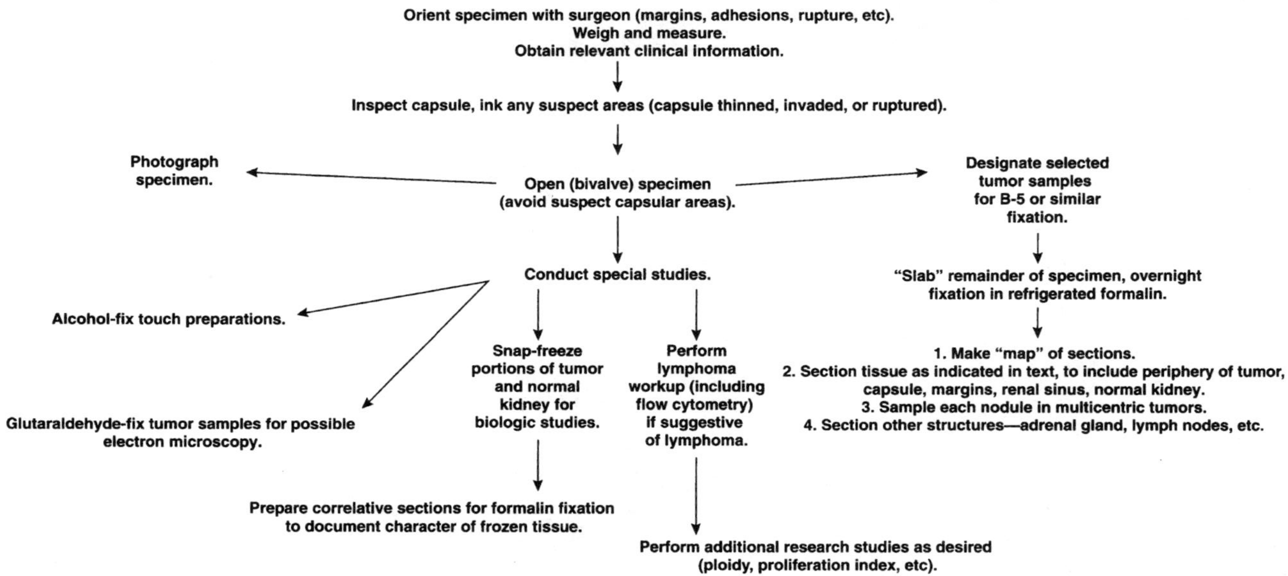

FIGURE 1.—Handling of pediatric renal tumors. (Courtesy of Zuppan CW: Handling and evaluation of pediatric renal tumors. *Am J Clin Pathol* 109:S31–S37. Copyright 1998 by the American Society of Clinical Pathologists. Reprinted with permission.)

For most pediatric renal tumors, the staging criteria for Wilms' tumor apply. Key staging features include the integrity of the renal capsule and the status of the tumor sinus. If the capsule is ruptured, staging depends on whether the tumor spillage was localized or extensive, involving peritoneal contamination. The pathologist should be alert for "toothpasting," or artifactual tumor spread outside the kidney after sectioning, which may be confused with true extrarenal tumor extension. Other important considerations in staging include the status of an intravenous tumor thrombus and careful lymph node examination. The pathology report must be delivered in a timely fashion and should include the diagnosis with relevant modifying factors, factors affecting tumor stage, and additional findings (e.g., nephrogenic rests or developmental dysplasia).

Discussion.—The pathologic handling and evaluation of pediatric renal tumors differ in some important ways from those of adult renal tumors. This article reviews some important issues in gross evaluation, tissue sampling for special studies, and selection of tissue blocks for examination with the light microscope. Illustrations of the most frequently encountered pediatric renal tumors are also included. Expert consultation should be sought in problematic cases.

▶ The College of American Pathologists (CAP) Cancer Committee and the Association of Directors of Anatomic and Surgical Pathology (ADASP) have tried to help practicing pathologists in standardizing the handling of tumor resection specimens. Pediatric renal tumors represent a somewhat specialized area that is likely not to be covered by these groups. This article therefore is a welcome addition and fills an important niche. Figure 1 provides a practical algorithm, and additional details may be found within the body of the text. In this regard, the checklist type of approach by the CAP and ADASP is more user friendly.

M.B. Cohen, M.D.

13 Male Genital Tract and Urinary Bladder

Testicular Germ-Cell Cancer
Bosl GJ, Motzer RJ (Mem Sloan-Kettering Cancer Ctr, New York; Cornell Univ, New York)
N Engl J Med 337:242–253, 1997 13–1

Purpose.—Germ-cell tumors account for 95% of malignant tumors arising in the testis. The cure rate for patients with newly diagnosed germ-cell tumors exceeds 90%, but delayed diagnosis leads to an advanced disease stage at presentation. With advances in cisplatin-based combination chemotherapy, the treatment of germ-cell tumors has changed greatly during the past 20 years. Recent advances in understanding and treatment of testicular germ-cell tumors were reviewed.

Epidemiology and Biology.—The incidence of germ-cell tumors appears to be increasing worldwide. These tumors occur mainly in whites; although predisposing factors have been identified, the cause is usually unknown. A precursor carcinoma in situ usually develops into an invasive germ cell tumor in a median of 5 years. About half of testicular germ-cell tumors are seminomas, usually occurring in the fourth decade of life. Nonseminomatous germ-cell tumors include embryonal carcinomas, teratomas, choriocarcinomas, and yolk-sac carcinomas.

Diagnosis.—Most patients with primary testicular tumor come to medical attention with diffuse testicular pain, swelling, and/or hardness. If symptoms do not resolve, ultrasound is performed. All patients with suspected testicular tumors undergo radical inguinal orchiectomy with ligation of the spermatic cord at the internal ring. Abdominal and pelvic CT and chest radiography are performed to seek metastases. Serum tumor markers, including α-fetoprotein and human chorionic gonadotropin, are evaluated before, during, and after treatment and during long-term follow-up. The tumor-node-metastasis system of classification of germ-cell tumors was recently revised by the American Joint Committee on Cancer and the Union Internationale contre le Cancer.

Treatment.—For patients with low-stage germ-cell tumors, radical inguinal orchiectomy is followed by retroperitoneal and ipsilateral pelvic lymph node irradiation. Ninety-nine percent of these patients are cured.

For patients with stage I nonseminomatous tumor, treatment may consist of either surveillance—based on the high cure rate of chemotherapy for relapse—or nerve-sparing retroperitoneal lymph node dissection. The latter option is preferred for patients with lymphatic, vascular, scrotal, or spermatic cord invasion. For stage II nonseminomatous tumors, treatment can consist of retroperitoneal lymph node dissection or chemotherapy. The decision depends on the extent of disease, the serum tumor marker concentration, and the presence of tumor-related symptoms.

About one third of patients with germ-cell tumors require initial chemotherapy. For "good-risk" patients, 4 cycles of standard etoposide and cisplatin or 3 cycles of bleomycin, standard etoposide, and cisplatin are effective and well tolerated. In combination with adjunctive surgery, the cure rate of approximately 90% is achieved for such patients. New approaches are being studied for the treatment of poor-risk patients, i.e., those with hepatic, osseous, or brain metastases; high serum concentrations of tumor markers; or mediastinal nonseminomatous primary tumors. In some situations, surgical resection of residual disease is necessary after chemotherapy. Second- or third-line chemotherapy is needed for patients who do not achieve a complete remission after first-line chemotherapy, or who have relapsed disease. In some cases, high-dose chemotherapy with stem cell rescue is needed.

Summary.—The biology, diagnosis and classification, and treatment of germ-cell tumors were reviewed. With the availability of cisplatin-containing combination chemotherapy to treat advanced disease, a very high cure rate is obtained for patients with these common cancers.

► The authors of this well-written and well-rounded review article are 2 oncologists. While the pathology is adequately covered, this article will be of interest to pathologists because of the clinical aspects that are covered. These include the evolution of the identification of molecular genetic alterations in the disease, the pattern of metastases, the role of serum tumor markers, staging, therapy, and its sequelae.

M.B. Cohen, M.D.

Carcinosarcoma and Sarcomatoid Carcinoma of the Bladder: Clinicopathological Study of 41 Cases

Lopez-Beltran A, Pacelli A, Rothenberg HJ, et al (Cordoba Univ, Spain; Mayo Clinic, Rochester, Minn)

J Urol 159:1497–1503, 1998 13–2

Introduction.—Carcinosarcoma of the bladder is a rare malignancy that sometimes arises in patients with a history of radiation therapy or chemotherapy. Because fewer than 50 cases have been reported, there is uncertainty regarding treatment and prognosis. The records of 15 patients with carcinosarcoma and 26 with sarcomatoid carcinoma of the bladder were reviewed to determine the clinical value of differentiating these 2 neoplasms.

Methods.—Cases were obtained from a review of surgical pathology files at the Mayo Clinic from 1936 to 1995. Carcinosarcoma consisted of an intimate admixture of carcinoma and sarcoma, whereas sarcomatoid carcinoma was characterized by spindle cell malignancy with or without coexistent overt urothelial carcinoma. Pathology slides were examined without knowledge of the patients' clinical course.

Results.—The carcinosarcoma group had a mean age of 66 and a male-to-female ratio of 2:1. Nine patients had urothelial carcinoma, small cell carcinoma, 3 had squamous cell carcinoma, and 2 had more than 1 type. Four had undergone cyclophosphamide treatment, and 1 had a history of radiation therapy. All had high-stage disease at diagnosis; the most common presenting sign was hematuria (77%). Eleven patients underwent cystectomy, and 4 were treated with transurethral resection. Five of 15 also had radiation therapy. Follow-up was available for 14 patients, 11 of whom had died of cancer at a mean of 17.2 months. The sarcomatoid carcinoma group had a male-to-female ratio of 4:1 and a mean age of 66.5. Eighteen of 26 patients had urothelial carcinoma, and 25 had high-stage disease at diagnosis. Seventeen were treated with transurethral resection and cystectomy was performed in 5; 9 had radiation therapy and 2 received chemotherapy. With a mean follow-up of 49 months (21 cases), 17 patients had died of cancer at a mean of 9.8 months. Pathological stage was the main predictor of patient survival. Treatment was predictive of survival only when the 2 patients with sarcomatoid carcinoma who were treated with chemotherapy were included. Otherwise, treatment did not affect survival, nor did gender or histological type.

Conclusion.—Both carcinosarcoma and sarcomatoid carcinoma of the bladder are highly aggressive malignancies. The histological findings that distinguish these tumors appear to have no clinical significance, and survival is limited regardless of treatment.

▶ This study describes the approximately 60-year experience of patients at the Mayo Clinic who had carcinosarcoma and sarcomatoid carcinoma of the urinary bladder. Sarcomatoid carcinomas were defined as carcinomas consisting of a spindle cell malignancy with or without coexistent overt urothelial carcinoma, and carcinosarcomas were defined as neoplasms with an intimate admixture of carcinoma and sarcoma. Some generalities emerge from this study, including a male predominance of these 2 histologic types, a variety of different morphologic entities, and a poor prognosis. The latter point could potentially be debatable since treatment has altered significantly over the 60 years encompassed in this study. As with more conventional types of tumors in this location. (i.e., urothelial carcinomas), stage remained the most useful predictor of outcome—in this case, patient survival. Immunohistochemistry was performed using a panel of antibodies (2 pan-cytokeratins, vimentin, muscle-specific actin, desmin, and S100 protein); however, their utility in distinguishing carcinosarcoma from sarcomatoid carcinoma was not impressive. The conclusions of this study might also call into question the importance of distinguishing between these 2 morphologic types since the prognosis, regardless of treatment, was poor.

M.B. Cohen, M.D.

Adenocarcinoma of the Urachus and Bladder Expresses a Unique Colonic Epithelial Epitope: An Immunohistochemical Study

Pantuck AJ, Bancila E, Das KM, et al (Robert Wood Johnson Med School, New Brunswick, NJ)

J Urol 158:1722–1727, 1997 13–3

Background.—Primary adenocarcinoma of the urachus and bladder is believed to result from glandular metaplasia of the bladder and urachal urothelium. Immunohistochemical analysis was used to test whether benign and malignant epithelial tissues would react with a monoclonal antibody developed against a unique colonic epithelial epitope.

Methods.—Retrospective review identified 16 specimens of carcinoma of the bladder or urachus (5 adenocarcinomas, 7 transitional cell carcinomas, and 4 squamous cell carcinomas) and 10 specimens with benign colonic metaplasia or epithelial proliferation. Malignant and benign tissues underwent immunoperoxidase assay to determine their reactivity with $7E_{12}H_{12}$ monoclonal antibody, an IgM isotype previously determined to be unique to colonic epithelium.

Findings.—All 5 of the adenocarcinomas had a strong reaction with the $7E_{12}H_{12}$ monoclonal antibody (Table). Reactivity occurred regardless of the histologic variant and regardless of whether the adenocarcinoma originated from the bladder or urachus. No reactivity occurred in transitional cell or squamous cell carcinomas. In the specimens with benign metaplasia, reactivity to the $7E_{12}H_{12}$ monoclonal antibody correlated with the type of epithelial proliferation in the tissue: Normal urothelium and Brunn's nests had no reactivity, whereas some tissues with cystitis cystica reacted and some did not. In cystitis glandularis and frank colonic intestinal metaplasia, reactivity was consistently positive.

TABLE.—Immunohistochemical Reactivity With $7E_{12}H_{12}$ Monoclonal Antibody

Tissue Specimen	No. Blocks	No. Pos.	No. Neg
Urachal adenoca	2	2	0
Bladder adenoca	3	3	0
Bladder squamous cell Ca	4	0	4
Bladder transitional cell Ca	7	0	7*
Colonic metaplasia	2	2	0
Cystitis cystica	4	1	3
Cystitis glandularis	7	7	0

Note: There was focal positive staining in an area of adjacent cystitis glandularis in 1 block and in a small area of glandular differentiation in 1.

(Courtesy of Pantuck AJ, Bancilla E, Das KM, et al: Adenocarcinoma of the urachus and bladder expresses a unique colonic epithelial epitope: An immunohistochemical study. *J Urol* 158[5]:1722–1727, 1997.)

Conclusions.—Adenocarcinoma of the bladder and urachus shares with benign epithelial metaplasia a unique colonic epitope for $7E_{12}H_{12}$ monoclonal antibody. Reactivity in benign tissues increased in a stepwise fashion as the proliferation progressed, suggesting that these progressive changes are a pathway for the development of adenocarcinoma of the bladder and urachus. Thus, reactivity to $7E_{12}H_{12}$ may be useful in studying the histogenesis of these cancers.

► Primary adenocarcinoma of the bladder is very rare, probably accounting for approximately 1.5% of all bladder malignancies. Adenocarcinomas of the urachus are even rarer. In this single institution study, spanning nearly 20 years, the authors identified 5 such cases, 2 arising from the urachus and 3 in the urinary bladder, confirming the rare nature of this tumor. The most intriguing aspect of this study is the identification of an antigen, recognized by a monoclonal antibody ($7E_{12}H_{12}$) that recognizes an epitope typically found on colonic epithelial cells. Immunoreactivity was identified in all 5 of the adenocarcinomas but also in both cases of colonic metaplasia and in selected cases of cystitis cystica/glandularis (Table). This raises the intriguing possibility that adenocarcinoma as in this anatomical site may share certain commonalities with colonic adenocarcinomas, and the molecular genetic alterations identified in the latter may be worth further study in these tumors.

M.B. Cohen, M.D.

Bladder Carcinoma With Lymphoepithelioma-like Differentiation: A Report of 9 Cases

Holmäng S, Borghede G, Johansson SL (Sahlgrenska Univ, Göteborg, Sweden; Univ of Nebraska, Omaha)

J Urol 159:779–782, 1998 13–4

Background.—Lymphoepithelioma (undifferentiated carcinoma with lymphoid stroma) of the bladder is quite rare, with only 14 cases reported to date. The optimal treatment of and long-term prognosis for patients with this disease are not known. These authors describe lymphoepithelioma-like differentiation of bladder cancer in a further 9 patients.

Methods.—A prospective, population-based study in western Sweden identified 3 cases of bladder carcinoma with lymphoepithelial features from a total of 713 patients with bladder tumors seen over a 2-year period. Furthermore, another 6 cases with these features were retrospectively identified from 816 patients with bladder cancer who were treated at the authors' institution over a 28-year period. There were 4 men and 5 women (mean age at diagnosis, 70 years) whose tumors matched the criterion for epithelioma-like differentiation (i.e., tumors were histopathologically identical to lymphoepithelioma of the nasopharynx). The extent of the lymphoepithelium-like features in these 9 cases was graded as pure (100%;

n = 3), predominant (more than 50%; n = 3), or focal (less than 50%; n = 3).

Findings.—Tumors were well demarcated (median, 3 cm) and with 1 exception, they were solitary. They appeared on the posterior wall (3 cases), right lateral wall (2 cases), left lateral wall (2 cases), anterior wall (1 case), and the dome (1 case). Tumors invaded to muscle in 7 cases and to the deep lamina propria in the other 2 cases. Each patient had undergone bladder resection or partial cystectomy with or without radiotherapy, but none had received systemic chemotherapy or intravesical therapy. Among the 6 cases with pure or predominant lymphoepithelioma-like carcinoma of the bladder, there was only 1 death due to intercurrent disease 18 years after diagnosis. Tumor staging in this case was T2. The other 5 cases (tumor stages T1–T3) remained free of disease during follow-up that lasted up to 104 months. But of the 3 patients with focal disease, each died of the disease within 9–68 months of diagnosis. Tumor staging in these cases was T1, T3, and T3.

Conclusions.—In its early stages, lymphoepithelioma-like carcinoma of the bladder has a more favorable long-term prognosis. According to these data and a review of the literature, lymphoepithelioma-like carcinoma of the bladder should be treated like other bladder carcinomas, i.e., stage by stage.

▶ According to the authors, only 14 cases of the unusual lymphoepithelioma-like carcinoma of the urinary bladder have previously been reported. This report, based on material in Sweden, is important because it is based on a population-based sampling and therefore the 9 cases (out of 713 patients) better indicate the relative incidence of this rare tumor. All but two of the tumors had invasion of the muscularis propria, and 4 of 9 died of their disease, including both patients who had only T1 disease. As defined by Amin et al.,[1] 3 patients had pure lymphoepithelioma-like carcinomas (100%), and the remaining patients had evidence of this morphologic feature (between 20% and 80%), representing predominantly and focal. The limited data from this study would suggest that these patients have a less aggressive course than those with the usual urothelial carcinoma, but their tumors should be treated like the usual urothelial carcinoma.

M.B. Cohen, M.D.

Reference

1. Amin MB, Ro JY, Lee KM, et al: Lymphoepithelioma-like carcinoma of the urinary bladder. *Am J Surg Pathol* 18:466–473, 1994.

Transitional Cell Carcinoma In Situ of the Seminal Vesicles: 8 Cases With Discussion of Pathogenesis, and Clinical and Biological Implications

Montie JE, Wojno K, Klein E, et al (Univ of Michigan, Ann Arbor; Cleveland Clinic Found, Ohio)

J Urol 158:1895–1898, 1997 13–5

Background.—The cause of transitional cell carcinoma in situ of the seminal vesicles is an enigma. The lining of the seminal vesicles (columnar epithelium of wolffian duct origin) makes it unlikely that the disease originates here. It is also unlikely that cancer cells sloughed in the urine could be implanted in the vesicle mucosa. These authors examined whether the mucosal spread of transitional cell carcinoma in situ from the bladder, prostate, or upper urinary tract could cause this disease in the seminal vesicles.

Methods.—Over a 2-year period, 8 cases of transitional cell carcinoma in situ of the seminal vesicles were identified from 84 cases of carcinoma of the bladder. The clinical courses and pathologic findings in these 8 cases were examined in detail.

Findings.—The time from diagnosis to cystectomy ranged from 1 month to 12 years, and 5 of the 8 patients had undergone intravesical therapy. In all 8 cases, carcinoma in situ was found in the prostate ducts; in half of these the stroma was also involved. In 4 of the 8 cases, the urethra was positive. In 3 cases at least 1 of the ureters was positive, and in 2 cases nodes were positive.

Conclusions.—On the basis of this circumstantial evidence, the intramucosal migration of carcinoma in situ from the bladder or the prostate into the prostatic ducts and then into the seminal vesicles seems likely. Carcinoma in situ was found in the nodes, ureter(s), prostate, and urethra even after intravesical therapy, which would indicate that the primary bladder or prostate cancer had not been completely destroyed. These findings warrant a reexamination of strategies to preserve the bladder in grade III disease, because perhaps only cystectomy can prevent disease progression to more distal sites.

▶ The staging of urothelial (transitional cell) carcinoma may be problematic, particularly when it extends into the prostate and, as reported in this study, into the seminal vesicle. Perhaps the most important distinction to be made is that between in situ disease, which is thought to represent migration of the pagetoid type, and invasive disease beyond the basement membrane into the supporting stromal tissue of the prostate (or seminal vesicle). This study reports 8 cases of urothelial carcinoma in situ of the seminal vesicle, which presumably arose from extension in the urinary bladder through the prostatic ductular system. The importance of this study includes the fact that this may be another hiding place for carcinoma in situ in the "urinary" system, particularly in light of a positive urinary cytologic specimen. In addition, treatment of this disease may be problematic. The only point with which issue is to be raised is that a monoclonal origin of bladder cancer is suggested, but such a conclusion awaits molecular analysis.

M.B. Cohen, M.D.

Has There Been a Recent Shift in the Pathological Features and Prognosis of Patients Treated With Radical Prostatectomy?

Soh S, Kattan MW, Berkman S, et al (Baylor College of Medicine, Houston; The Methodist Hosp, Houston)

J Urol 157:2212–2218, 1997 13–6

Introduction.—Now that more clinical stage T1c prostate tumors are being detected with prostate specific antigen (PSA) testing, there is concern that radical surgery will be performed for cancers of low biological potential. A series of patients with clinical stages T1 to T3NXM0 prostate cancer treated with radical prostatectomy during a 13-year period was reviewed to determine whether there was a significant change in pathologic features or prognosis with time.

Methods.—Two groups of patients were analyzed. The first included 2,326 patients who underwent staging pelvic lymphadenectomy for clinically localized prostate cancer at a teaching hospital between 1984 and 1995. The 759 consecutive patients in the second group were treated with radical retropubic prostatectomy by a single surgeon between 1983 and 1995; morphometric analysis was possible in 754 cases. Methods of diagnosis, pathologic features, and prognosis of these 754 patients were analyzed by year of diagnosis.

Results.—Analysis of the first patient group indicated a decrease in the proportion with lymph node metastases and an overall shift away from regional stage disease at diagnosis. There was a marked decrease in the proportion of cancers initially detected by transurethral detection after 1989 and an increase in nonpalpable cancers detected by PSA after 1990. Although there was a marked increase in the annual number of radical prostatectomies over time, preoperative serum PSA, tumor volume, and pathologic stage did not change significantly during the study period. The proportion of patients with Gleason sum 7 cancer increased significantly after 1991. Fewer patients had an advanced cancer at diagnosis during recent years, but there was no increase in the proportion of patients with indolent or clinically unimportant cancers. When the study years were grouped into 3 periods (1983 to 1987, 1988 to 1991, and 1992 to 1995) the actuarial probability of progression after surgery showed no change.

Conclusion.—There have been considerable changes in method of detection and number of patients treated each year for prostate cancer, but no changes in pathologic stage or rate of progression were observed in patients treated between 1983 and 1995. These findings suggest that few radical procedures are being performed for small, indolent cancers.

► With the introduction of PSA screening in the late 1980s, considerable attention has focused on the possibility that a stage migration has occurred, i.e., that PSA allows one to identify lower-stage disease. This is a single institution study—actually a single urologic surgeon's practice—encompassing 754 consecutive patients seen in a 13-year time span. Not unexpectedly, the number of radical prostatectomies performed increased during this period, particularly for cancers detected by PSA elevations only.

This study concludes that there was no change in pathologic stage during this period. Some changes in grade were noted. More important, prognosis, as defined by progression rate, was not altered between 1983 and 1995. Thus, this study would add to the growing literature stating that the increased detection of prostate cancer does not lead to increased numbers of patients being unnecessarily treated. Other studies, using additional methodologies, including "biomarkers," will be needed to confirm these findings.

M.B. Cohen, M.D.

Incidence and Clinical Significance of High-grade Prostatic Intraepithelial Neoplasia in TURP Specimens

Gaudin PB, Sesterhenn IA, Wojno KJ, et al (Johns Hopkins Med Insts, Baltimore, Md; Armed Forces Inst of Pathology, Washington, DC; Univ of Michigan, Ann Arbor)

Urology 49:558–563, 1997 13–7

Introduction.—There is considerable evidence for a relationship between high-grade prostatic intraepithelial neoplasia (PIN) and prostatic adenocarcinoma, particularly when PIN is present in needle biopsy specimens. The significance of high-grade PIN in specimens obtained from transurethral resection of the prostate (TURP) has received less attention.

Methods.—A review of TURP specimens was conducted to determine the frequency with which high-grade PIN is found in those specimens that do not contain adenocarcinoma of the prostate. Eighty-five cases of PIN 2 and PIN 3 were identified; slides stained with hematoxylin-eosin were reviewed in 82 cases. At low magnification, high-grade PIN is seen as prostatic ducts or acini with a micropapillary, papillary, cribriform, or flat architecture. Secretory cells show hyperchromasia, nuclear enlargement, and prominent nucleoli at high magnification.

Results.—Patients had a mean age of 70 years at the time of TURP; 74% were 65 years of age or older. Follow-up clinical information was available in 48% of cases. The median post-TURP follow-up was 52 months. Four patients had died of unrelated diseases and with no evidence of prostate cancer. Repeat TURP or follow-up needle biopsy was performed in 14 patients (34%), discovered adenocarcinoma of the prostate in 8; an additional case was diagnosed at the time of surgery for transitional cell carcinoma of the urinary bladder (Fig 3). The mean time between TURP and diagnosis of adenocarcinoma was 44 months. Patients with focal+ or diffuse high-grade PIN at TURP were more frequently found to have

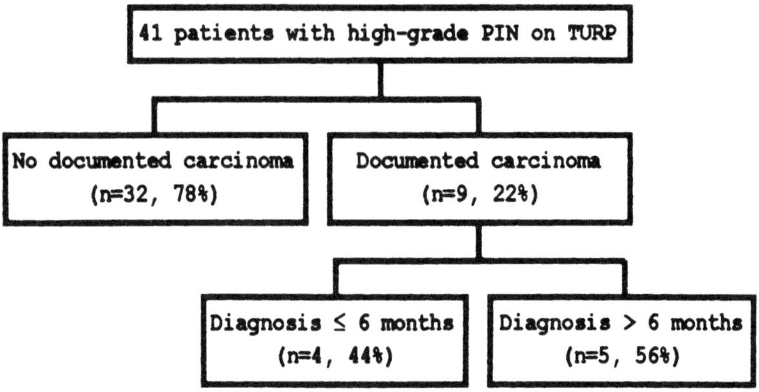

FIGURE 3.—Flow chart summarizing the outcome of patients with high-grade prostatic intraepithelial neoplasia or transurethral resection of the prostate. (Reprinted by permission of the publisher from Gaudin PB, Sesterhenn IA, Wojno KJ, et al: Incidence and clinical significance of high-grade prostatic intraepithelial neoplasia in TURP specimens. *Urology* 49:558–563. Copyright 1997, with permission from Elsevier Science, Inc.)

adenocarcinoma that those with focal high-grade PIN, but the difference was not statistically significant. The estimated incidence of high-grade PIN was 2.3% in all TURP specimens and 3.2% in those without invasive carcinoma.

Conclusion.—The finding of high-grade PIN in specimens obtained via TURP is relatively uncommon and occurs primarily in men 70 years or older. Approximately one fifth of the patients in this series for whom follow-up information was available were subsequently given a diagnosis of adenocarcinoma of the prostate. The risk of prostatic cancer is less than that associated with high-grade PIN in needle biopsy specimens.

► According to McNeal, there are distinct differences between the transition zone and the peripheral zone. In this study, TURP specimens (transition zone specimens), were examined for the incidence and significance of high-grade PIN. The study included specimens taken at Johns Hopkins Medical Institutions and diagnosed over approximately 4-year period in the early to mid-1980s which did not contain adenocarcinoma, but which did contain either grades PIN 2 or PIN 3. In addition, cases from several other institutions were included.

Sampling of the TURP specimens was not discussed in the Materials and Methods section, raising some question about the interpretation of the data. Another concern regarding this study is that follow-up was only available in approximately half (48%) of the patients and is summarized in the accompanying figure. High grade PIN is relatively uncommon in this location, but when present it does appear to be associated with adenocarcinomas. The finding of high-grade PIN in TURP specimens would warrant submission of additional tissue for histologic evaluation, but deeper sections of the already embedded material might also be pursued.

M.B. Cohen, M.D.

Application of the Principle of Marginal Analysis to Sampling Practice Using Prostatic Chippings as a Model

Langlois NEI, Donaldson C (Univ of Aberdeen, Scotland)
J Clin Pathol 51:104–107, 1998 13–8

Objective.—Because health care resources are limited, decision-making about the best practices needs to be based on economic principles. Marginal costs of sampling entire specimens for histopathologic analysis were calculated to minimize opportunity costs.

Methods.—The median sample size of transurethral resections of prostate specimens was calculated using a mathematical model. The median number of chips necessary for detecting each cancer, and the associated costs, were determined.

Results.—Each transurethral resection of prostate specimen (median weight, 12.0 g) yielded an average of 60 chips, with 9 chips in each tissue cassette. The cost for detecting each cancer ranged from £47 to £151, depending on whether the fraction of malignant cells in the sample was 2.5% or 10%. When an entire 24-g sample was processed and examined, the cost escalated to more than £10,000.

Conclusion.—Because marginal costs take into account more than just the £2.50 for producing an extra histologic section (including extra tissue cassettes), the mathematical model demonstrates a way to evaluate the optimal handling of pathologic specimens.

▶ The article by Langlois and Donaldson attempts to apply "outcomes analysis" to histopathology. This is very important, because it provides a mathematical model which may be more generally applicable to other areas of pathology, particularly anatomic pathology. As with all strategies, there are pros and cons to how resources are allocated for the determination of a specific outcome, in this case adenocarcinoma of the prostate. While argument may be raised about the outcome studied (detection of cancer) and the cost ascribed to these different evaluations, this study does serve as a useful model for more rigorous evaluation of the optimal handling of pathological specimens, including their microscopic evaluation. It is hoped that this may be more generally applied to other areas of anatomic pathology, much as critical analysis has been applied to clinical pathology (laboratory medicine).

M.B. Cohen, M.D.

Prognostic Implications of Extracapsular Extension of Lymph Node Metastases in Prostate Cancer

Griebling TL, Özkutlu D, See WA, et al (Univ of Iowa, Iowa City; Iowa City Veterans Affairs Med Ctr, Iowa)
Mod Pathol 10:804–809, 1997 13–9

Objective.—Neither the Whitmore-Jewett nor the primary tumor–regional node–metastasis staging system accurately takes account of the presence of perinodal tumor extension. The incidence and clinical significance of extracapsular perinodal tumor extension in patients with regionally metastatic prostate cancer was reviewed retrospectively.

Methods.—Records of 69 patients, aged 45–79, who received a diagnosis (between July 1985 and July 1994) of regional lymph node metastasis from prostate cancer, were reviewed. Clinical data were subjected to multiple regression analysis to identify independent predictors of survival.

Results.—An average of 9.3 lymph nodes per patient were excised. According to primary tumor, regional nodes, metastasis staging, 20 (33.3%) of 60 patients had stage N1 disease and 40 (66.6%) had stage N2 disease. Extracapsular disease was diagnosed in 42 of 60 patients. The 5-year adjusted cumulative survival rate was 54.6% for patients with perinodal tumor extension, significantly lower than the 71.4% rate for patients with histologically confined disease. Multivariate analysis revealed that Gleason score was the strongest predictor of patient survival, and margin status of the regional lymph nodes was the second strongest independent predictor (Table 3).

Conclusion.—Extracapsular extension of lymph node metastases is a strong predictor of survival in patients with node-positive prostate cancer.

► The importance of extracapsular extension of lymph node metastasis has been found to be an important prognostic indicator in a number of other

TABLE 3.—Forward Stepwise χ^2 Multivariate Correlation With Disease-specific Survival (Wilcoxon Analysis)

Variable	χ^2	*P* value
Primary tumor grade (Gleason sum score)	9.9019	.0017*
Presence of extracapsular perinodal tumor extension	14.5759	.0306*
Age	16.7564	.1398
Nodal stage (N1, N2, N3)	17.9165	.2814
Lymphadenectomy technique (open *vs.* laparoscopic)	18.1563	.6243
Adjuvant hormonal therapy	18.2015	.8316
Number of nodes with metastatic tumor	18.2335	.8581
Total number of nodes excised	18.2544	.8852

Note: Two pathologic strata: positive and equivocal perinodal extension *vs.* no perinodal extension.
*Statistically significant ($P < .05$).
(Courtesy of Griebling TL, Özkutlu D, See WA, et al: Prognostic implications of extracapsular extension of lymph node metastases in prostate cancer. *Mod Pathol* 10[8]:804–809, 1997.)

malignancies, particularly carcinomas. This article attempts to assess that feature in prostatic adenocarcinoma. I must admit up front, however, that I feel somewhat awkward in including a study in which I have participated. Nonetheless, the results of this study, which suggest that this histopathologic finding portends a poor prognosis in prostate cancer as well, are of importance. However, they will need to be confirmed by other investigators from other institutions. One potential caveat is that this study encompasses patients from a relatively long period, during which treatment modalities evolved, and thus does not represent a homogeneous patient population. However, these data do suggest that extracapsular extension of lymph node metastasis is an important prognostic factor, in both univariate and multivariate analysis, with respect to disease-specific survival. If these findings are confirmed, refinement of the staging system may be warranted.

M.B. Cohen, M.D.

Microvessel Density in Core Biopsies of Prostatic Adenocarcinoma: A Stage Predictor?

Rogatsch H, Hittmair A, Reissigl A, et al (Univ of Innsbruck, Austria)
J Pathol 182:205–210, 1997 13–10

Objective.—Although microvessel density (MVD) has been shown to be correlated with tumor stage in prostate cancer, its use as a predictor of metastatic disease is less clear. The use of neovascularization of prostatic adenocarcinomas in core biopsies and corresponding prostatectomies to predict tumor stage, and to discriminate between organ-confined and organ-extending neoplasms, was investigated.

Methods.—Of 322 core biopsies, performed before radical prostatectomy on 46 patients, aged 61–73, 116 biopsies contained malignant tissue. There were insufficient core biopsy samples in 10 patients. Microvessels were detected using a monoclonal antibody against the CD31 antigen, and MVD was determined from biopsy tissue and 36 prostatectomy specimen tissues, using light microscopy at × 400 magnification. Microvascular counts in organ-confined and organ-extending tumors were compared statistically.

Results.—When the 36 tumors were pathologically staged, there were 16 pT2 and 20 pT3 tumors. The median Gleason scores, 6 in core biopsies and 7 in prostatectomy specimens, were significantly correlated with tumor stage for both biopsy and prostatectomy samples. The median MVD in benign hyperplasia samples was 18.5, whereas the median MVD in tumor areas was 35.5. MVD in biopsies and prostatectomy specimens were highly correlated (Fig 2). MVD was also significantly correlated with tumor stage, and could be used to distinguish between organ-confined and organ-extending disease, with a sensitivity of 85%, a specificity of 93.7%, and positive predictive value of 94.4%.

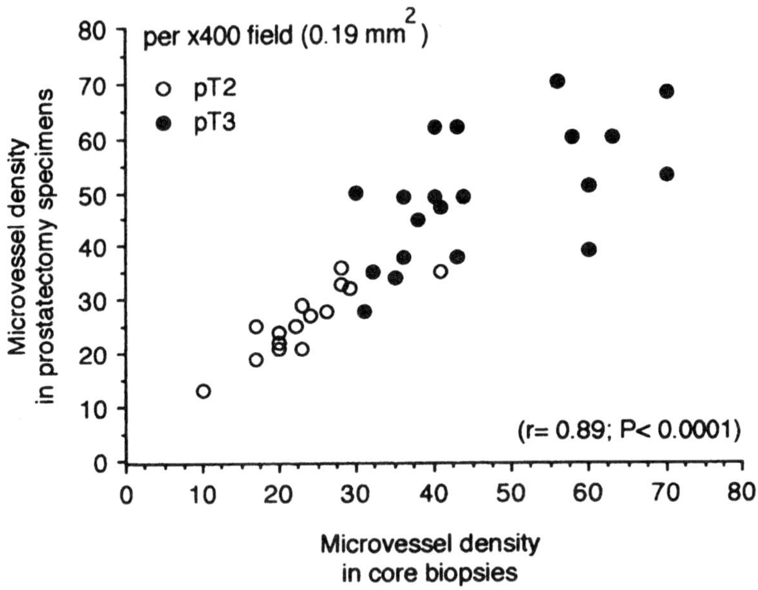

FIGURE 2.—Correlation between tumor MVD in core biopsies and corresponding prostatectomies of 36 patients. Individual MVD values represent the highest number of microvessels immunoreactive for the CD31 antigen, identified within a single × 400 field, per case (r−0.89; P less than 0.0001). (Reprinted by permission of John Wiley & Sons, Ltd., from Rogatsch H, Hittmair A, Reissigl A, et al: Microvessel density in core biopsies of prostatic adenocarcinoma: A stage predictor? *J Pathol* 182:205–210. Copyright 1997, John Wiley & Sons, Ltd.)

Conclusion.—Microvessel density in core biopsy specimens correlates highly with tumor stage, and can be used to predict which patients can be cured by surgery alone.

▶ Much attention (too much?) has focused on the importance of angiogenesis, pathologically related to MVD, in a number of human malignancies, including prostatic adenocarcinoma. This article focuses on the identification of MVD in biopsy specimens as a useful marker for predicting stage. These findings support other studies previously reported in the literature. Three hundred twenty-two total biopsies, 116 of which contained adenocarcinoma, from 46 patients formed the basis of this study. CD31 antigen staining was used to identify the blood vessels, and the methodology described previously by Weidner et al. was used.[1] A correlation between MVD and stage of disease (pT2 or pT3) was noted. However, as with all markers to date, there was overlap among individual cases. Consequently, the utility of this type of marker in individual patients will need refinement, likely with the combination of other markers.

M.B. Cohen, M.D.

Reference

1. Weidner N, Folkmann J, Pozza F, et al: Tumor angiogenesis: A new significant and independent prognostic factor in early-stage breast carcinoma. *J Natl Cancer Inst* 84:1875–1887, 1992.

The Prognostic Value of Neuroendocrine Differentiation in Adenocarcinoma of the Prostate in Relation to Progression of Disease After Endocrine Therapy

Krijnen JLM, Bogdanowicz JFAT, Seldenrijk CA, et al (Erasmus Univ, Rotterdam, The Netherlands; Reiner de Graaf Hosp, Delft, The Netherlands)

J Urol 158:171–174, 1997 13–11

Background.—The functional role of neuroendocrine cells in prostatic adenocarcinoma is unknown. There is little information on how neuroendocrine differentiation affects the prognosis of prostatic adenocarcinoma. However, several lines of evidence suggest that a high incidence of neuroendocrine tumor cells before endocrine therapy for metastatic prostate cancer could be associated with early treatment failure. The prognostic significance of neuroendocrine differentiation was examined retrospectively in terms of response to treatment.

Methods.—A total of 72 patients who had transurethral resection followed by endocrine therapy for prostate cancer were studied. The patients' progression-free interval was monitored for 44–95 months' follow-up. The surgical specimens were analyzed to determine the pattern of distribution and proportion of neuroendocrine cells, based on immunoreactivity for chromogranin A. Neuroendocrine differentiation was analyzed as a prognostic factor for disease progression during endocrine therapy.

Results.—Disease progression occurred in 32 patients, 27 of whom died of prostate cancer. Overall, 55% of the cancers showed chromogranin A–positive cells. Neuroendocrine differentiation was negatively correlated with progression-free survival on Cox proportional hazards analysis. The prognostic impact of neuroendocrine differentiation was independent from that of the Gleason score.

Conclusions.—The presence of neuroendocrine differentiation in prostatic carcinoma is a significant prognostic factor for disease progression during endocrine therapy. This and other studies suggest that neuroendocrine differentiation is not associated with a higher Gleason score. The increased incidence of neuroendocrine tumor cells in cancers that are prone to failure of endocrine therapy could be an epiphenomenon, rather than reflecting a paracrine stimulatory role.

► For some time there has been an increasing literature which would suggest that neuroendocrine differentiation in prostatic adenocarcinoma portends a poorer prognosis. This study, which is based on transurethral prostatectomy material, includes patients with established prostatic adenocarcinoma who subsequently underwent hormonal therapy. Neuroendocrine differentiation was determined by immunohistochemical identification of chromogranin A (LK2H10, an antibody obtained from Eurodiagnostica). Positive cells were counted as scattered or as cell clusters (2 or more positive cells) and counted in a defined tumor area. Fifty-five percent of the tumors had positive immunoreactivity and was typically noted as single cells and only clustered in 13 patients. The total number of positive cells ranged from 0 to approximately 21 per square millimeter of tumor, in reality a small number. Thus, one conclusion from this study is that neuroendocrine positivity may be identified in a significant number of patients but is a relatively uncommon finding with respect to the number of tumor cells present. Kaplan-Meier curves did find differences in survival in those without and with chromogranin A–positive cells. The finding in this report, as has been previously reported, supports the notion that the identification of neuroendocrine differentiation is an adverse prognostic indicator and may be important in androgen-independent disease.

M.B. Cohen, M.D.

Pseudomyxoma Ovariilike Posttherapeutic Alteration in Prostatic Adenocarcinoma: A Distinctive Pattern in Patients Receiving Neoadjuvant Androgen Ablation Therapy

Tran T-A, Jennings TA, Ross JS, et al (Albany Med College, NY)
Am J Surg Pathol 22:347–354, 1998 13–12

Purpose.—Neoadjuvant androgen ablation therapy with leuprolide and flutamide can cause histologic changes in prostatic tissues, nontumoral and cancerous. In some cases, this treatment may lead to a distinctive appearance resembling that of pseudomyxoma ovarii in prostatic adenocarcinoma (Fig 1, B). This change may be the only sign of tumor regression and could be mistaken for mucinous carcinoma. The prevalence, features, and significance of posttreatment pseudomyxoma ovarii–like change in prostatic adenocarcinoma were analyzed.

Methods.—Participants were 53 patients with clinically localized prostatic adenocarcinoma who received 3–5 months of treatment with leuprolide and flutamide. The patients' mean age was 65 years; mean follow-up after surgery was 31 months. Radical prostatectomy specimens obtained after neoadjuvant therapy were analyzed for changes from the pretreatment needle biopsy specimens. Immunohistochemical studies were performed as well.

Results.—Consistent with previous reports, all specimens showed therapy-associated changes in benign and malignant elements. Twenty percent showed distinctive pseudomyxoma ovarii–like changes that were not present on the initial biopsy. The change consisted of very small to large pools of extravasated secretions dissecting through the prostatic stroma. At low-power magnification, the secretions had an infiltrative appearance. Seventy-seven percent of cases with pseudomyxoma ovarii–like changes had associated, recognizable tumor. In routine sections, the secretions were

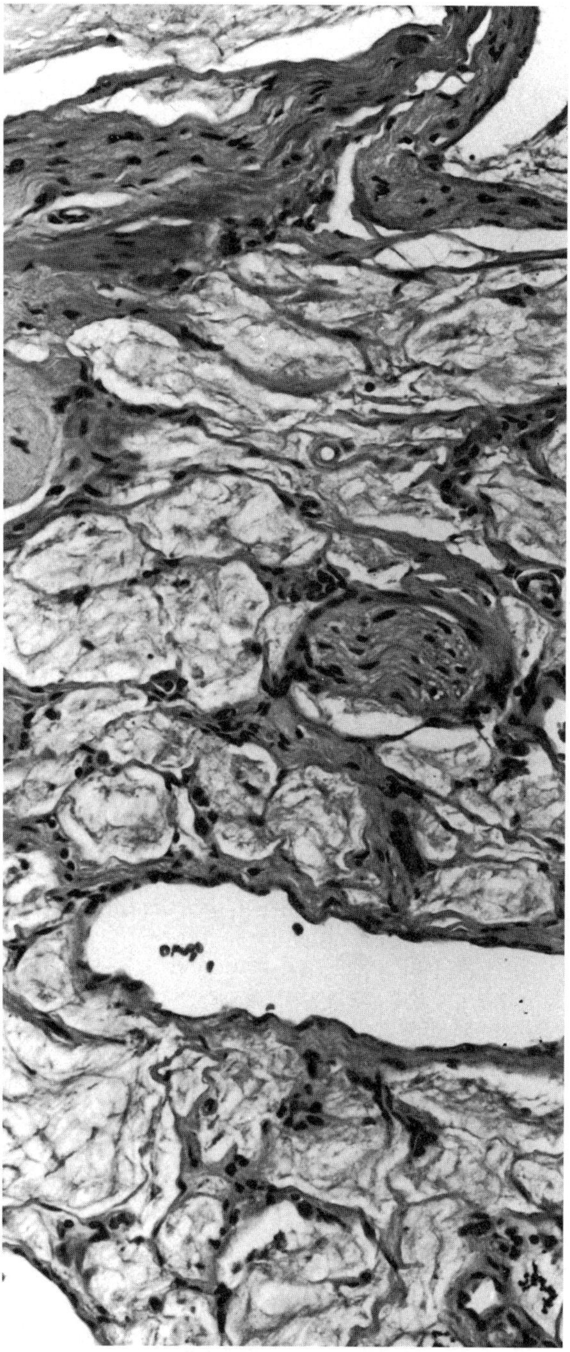

FIGURE 1, B.—Intermediate-power view of pseudomyxoma ovariilike posttherapeutic alteration in prostatectomy specimens. (Courtesy of Tran T-A, Jennings TA, Ross JS, et al: Pseudomyxoma ovariilike posttherapeutic alteration in prostatic adenocarcinoma: A distinctive pattern in patients receiving neoadjuvant androgen ablation therapy. *Am J Surg Pathol* 22:347–354, 1998.)

basophilic with occasional degenerated cells. Very few pancytokeratin-positive cells were apparent at the secretion/stroma interface. Staining for the high–molecular weight keratin 34 beta E-12 was consistently negative. Further analysis of the secretions showed that they were periodic acid–Schiff positive after diastase digestion and were mucicarminophilic and reactive with Alcian blue at a pH of 2.5.

In 5 of the 13 cases, the distinctive change made up less than 5% of the tumor; in another 5, it accounted for up to 40% of the tumor. In the remaining 3 cases, 1 or 2 foci of change measuring less than 1.0 mm constituted the only evidence of treated tumor. The finding of pseudomyxoma ovarii–like change was unrelated to the dose or duration of neoadjuvant therapy, clinical course after prostatectomy, original or final Gleason score or pattern, or disease stage.

Conclusions.—About 20% of prostatic adenocarcinomas show a pseudomyxoma ovarii–like change after neoadjuvant combination endocrine therapy. Features of this change, which is often intimately associated with residual carcinoma on the radical prostatectomy specimen, include extravasated acid mucin with a lack of prostatic basal cells. This distinctive change probably reflects tumor regression caused by androgen ablation and tumor cell attrition.

▶ The treatment of adenocarcinoma of the prostate, as with other malignancies, is an evolving concept, and efforts continue to obtain better end results. One such current approach is to use neoadjuvant combination hormonal therapy before definitive surgical therapy. This intervention may lead to morphological alterations in the subsequently resected prostate. One such change, as described in the study by Tran et al., is the identification of pseudomyxoma ovarii–like alterations (Fig 1, B). This finding was identified in approximately 20% of cases and included the identification of extravasated acid mucin lacking basal cells and typically intimately associated with prostatic adenocarcinoma. It is likely that this represents a direct effect of the hormonal intervention but makes the diagnosis of prostatic adenocarcinoma difficult. Although not specifically addressed in this study, such alterations also make the grading in radical prostatectomy specimens a considerable problem.

In a related study by Bazinet et al.,[1] the authors note that there may be considerable morphological alterations, including regression, which make the evaluation of prostatic adenocarcinoma difficult. This is most notable in attempts determining the stage of disease, particularly the identification of involvement of tumor at the surgical margin and/or capsular penetration. Both of these articles, therefore, document the significant alterations that can occur with hormonal therapy, and the difficulties that may arise in evaluation of subsequently resected specimens.

M.B. Cohen, M.D.

Reference

1. Bazinet M, Zheng W, Bégin LR, et al: Morphologic changes induced by neoadjuvant androgen ablation may result in underdetection of positive surgical margins and capsular involvement by prostatic adenocarcinoma. *Urology* 49:721–725, 1997.

Atypical Small Acinar Proliferation Suspicious for Malignancy in Prostate Needle Biopsies: Clinical Significance in 33 Cases

Iczkowski KA, MacLennan GT, Bostwick DG (Mayo Clinic, Rochester, Minn)

Am J Surg Pathol 21:1489–1495, 1997 13–13

Introduction.—As the number of prostate needle biopsies increases, so does the likelihood of encountering unusual lesions that could lead to misinterpretation. An example is the occasional finding of an atypical small acinar proliferation (ASAP), which is suspicious for adenocarcinoma but not diagnostic (Fig 1). There are inadequate histologic and clinical data on this lesion. A series of 33 such cases was reviewed.

Findings.—The patients, whose mean age was 62 years, all had at least 1 follow-up needle biopsy performed at a median of 9 months. These biopsy specimens revealed adenocarcinoma in 45% of patients, with a mean Gleason score of 6. In another 6% of patients, repeat biopsies led to repeat diagnoses of ASAP. The likelihood of cancer on follow-up biopsy could not be predicted by digital rectal examination, serum prostate-specific antigen, or histologic findings.

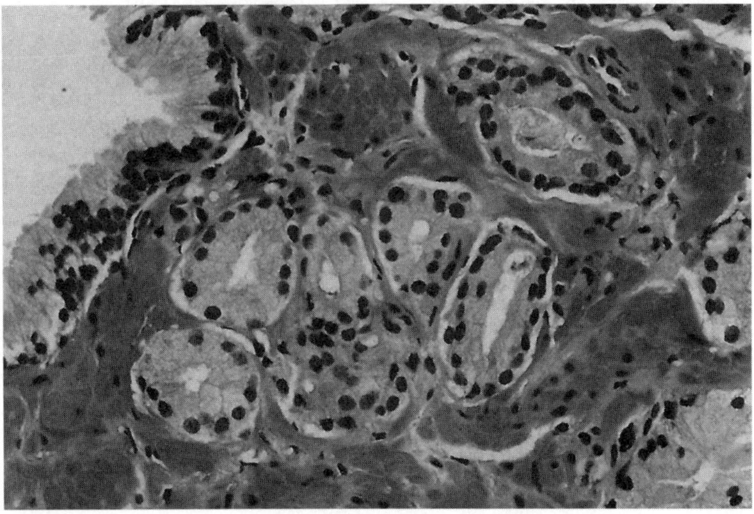

FIGURE 1.—Atypical small acinar proliferation in needle biopsy. Architectural features suggest infiltration and distortion of acini, and the basal cell layer is absent. (Courtesy of Iczkowski KA, MacLennan GT, Bostwick DG: Atypical small acinar proliferation suspicious for malignancy in prostate needle biopsies: Clinical significance in 33 cases. *Am J Surg Pathol* 21:1489–1495, 1997.)

The mean number of biopsy cores was 5.5, the mean number of acini per focus of ASAP was 8, and the mean number of foci was 1. The acini varied in size. Nuclear enlargement was absent in 12% of cases, mild in 45%, moderate in 33%, and severe in 10%; nucleolar enlargement was absent in 27% of specimens, mild in 46%, and moderate in 27%. Thirty-nine percent of cases showed luminal mucin, 6% showed crystalloids, and 64% showed focal chronic inflammation. All lesions were associated with adjacent atrophy, and 42% with high-grade prostatic intraepithelial neoplasia (PIN). Subsequent cancer was found in 20% of cases of ASAP without PIN stratified as "favor benign" and 256% of those stratified as "uncertain," compared with 60% of those interpreted as "favor carcinoma." However, this stratification was not significant.

Conclusions.—Patients with prostate needle biopsy specimen showing ASAP have a high rate of cancer diagnosed on subsequent biopsy specimen. The authors believe that the finding of ASAP often reflects underdiagnosis of cancer and should be an indication for repeat biopsy. The use of ASAP to designate cases that are neither "atypical but benign" or cancer will help to ensure adequate surveillance and follow-up.

▶ With the increasing use of prostate-specific antigen, an increasing number of patients are undergoing biopsy to determine whether this prostate-specific antigen elevation is the result of prostatic adenocarcinoma. As such, pathologists are increasingly faced with making diagnoses of adenocarcinoma on relatively smaller foci of glandular proliferations. This study documents that, like other areas of pathology, a gray zone exists, in this case, ASAPs suspicious for prostatic adenocarcinoma. An example of this is shown in Figure 1. In our own institution we have been using similar terminology for some time. While a number of features may help to define this entity, it is likely to be best viewed as a threshold phenomenon, i.e., the quantitative and or qualitative features required to definitively diagnose adenocarcinoma are not entirely met. Follow-up of the 33 study cases show that 45% had diagnosable adenocarcinoma and an additional 6% had an essentially similar diagnosis on repeat biopsy. Attempts at stratification, i.e., the determination of the level of suspicion, was only somewhat predictive.

In summary, this diagnostic category, by whatever term or terms are used, will continue to exist and warrant further evaluation. None of the criteria examined, either alone or in combination, helps to seperate out those foci that eventually were diagnosed as adenocarcinoma.

M.B. Cohen, M.D.

Correlation of Prostate Needle Biopsy and Radical Prostatectomy Gleason Grade in Academic and Community Settings

Steinberg DM, Sauvageot J, Piantadosi S, et al (The Johns Hopkins Hosp Med Insts, Baltimore, Md)

Am J Surg Pathol 21:566–576, 1997 13–14

Objective.—Several studies have examined the correlation between grading of prostate biopsy and radical prostatectomy (RP). However, these studies have all used material from academic settings and have not analyzed the reasons for discrepancies in grading. With the growing use of the Gleason grading system, such correlation studies are easier to perform. The correlation between prostate needle biopsy and RP grade was assessed in academic and community-practice settings.

Methods.—A total of 499 specimens from RPs performed at 1 academic hospital during 1994 were analyzed. All specimens were graded by the Gleason scoring system. The results were compared with the Gleason grade of the needle biopsy performed at the same institution. In 390 cases, comparison with the Gleason biopsy grade assigned at an outside institution was possible as well.

Results.—Within the academic center, agreement between biopsy and RP grades was exact in 58% of cases and within 1 digit in 93%. For outside institutions, agreement was 34% and 67%, respectively. For further analysis, the cases were placed into clinically meaningful groups, with Gleason scores of 2–4, 5–6, 7, and 8–10. With this grouping, the rate of exact agreement was 66% within the academic center and 45% outside. The percentage of biopsy specimens graded 2–4 was 1% within the academic center vs. 22% outside, suggesting that the outside centers undergraded more frequently. None of the cases graded 2–4 on biopsy, inside or outside the academic setting, received the same grade on RP. Of biopsy specimens graded 2–4 at outside centers, 55% proved to have capsular penetration, seminal vesicle involvement, or lymph node involvement. In contrast, all specimens graded 2–4 within the academic center proved to be organ confined. Correlation between the needle biopsy grade and the pathologic stage was better at the academic center than at outside centers.

Accuracy in predicting the grade or stage of RP was not significantly affected by the extent of cancer in the biopsy specimen. Examination by a genitourinary pathologist did not increase the accuracy of biopsy grading within the academic center. Eighty-eight percent of biopsy specimens with a score of 7 or greater scored in the same category at RP, compared with 64% of specimens scoring less than 7. Some of the noted discrepancies reflected biopsy findings that were on the borderline between 2 Gleason scores. The main source of discrepancy was sampling error; the high-grade component noted on RP was often missing from the biopsy specimen, or the component of cancer seen on biopsy made up only a small percentage of the RP specimen.

Conclusions.—Prostate needle biopsy specimens tend to be undergraded in community practice settings. Small amounts of tumor obtained by needle biopsy can be graded just as well as samples with substantially larger amounts of tumor. Discrepancies between biopsy grading and RP grade can result from pathology error, borderline cases, reverse sampling error, and sampling error. The data suggest that the Gleason grading system is relatively easy to teach and learn.

► The documentation of interobserver and intraobserver agreement in grading prostatic adenocarcinoma, most commonly using the Gleason system, has received variable attention in the literature, with a recent upswing. This study contains a large amount of data but is based on a single institutional study of a relatively large series of RP specimens. Four major causes of discrepancies were identified: pathology error, borderline cases, reverse sampling error, and sampling error. The usual cause for pathology error was undergrading. Borderline cases were defined as those in which biopsy samples bridged 2 of the grades and were subjectively categorized into 1 or another category. Reverse sampling error was defined as those cases in which a minor component of the tumor in the prostatectomy specimen was present in the biopsy and, as a result, this minor component was not incorporated in the final grade of the prostatectomy. Sampling error was defined as those cases in which a major component of the tumor in the prostatectomy specimen was not present in the biopsy samples. With this background, the conclusion clearly indicates that sampling error was the major source of discrepancy and was often due to a higher-grade component in prostatectomy specimen not being present in the biopsy samples. Thus, limitations of the Gleason grading system in biopsy specimens will continue to plague pathologists but should also be well recognized by physicians taking care of these patients.

M.B. Cohen, M.D.

Transitional Cell Carcinoma of the Prostate: Clinicopathologic Study of 50 Cases

Cheville JC, Dundore PA, Bostwick DG, et al (Mayo Clinic, Rochester, Minn)
Cancer 82:703–707, 1998 13–15

Introduction.—There is currently no accepted staging system for transitional cell carcinoma (TCC) of the prostate, implying that it is a high-stage cancer with a poor prognosis. There are few data on the prognostic factors and biological behavior of this tumor in the absence of invasive bladder carcinoma. Clinical and histologic factors related to outcome in patients with TCC of the prostate without invasive bladder cancer were evaluated.

Methods.—The histologic and clinical findings of 50 patients with prostatic TCC but without invasive bladder carcinoma were analyzed. The patients were treated with radical cystoprostatectomy during a 3-year period. Four patients had TCC in situ (CIS) of the prostatic urethra, 15 had CIS of the prostatic ducts and acini, 21 had TCC with invasion of the prostatic stroma, 3 had extraprostatic extension and/or seminal vesicle involvement, and 7 had lymph node metastases. Survival distributions for these categories of locoregional disease were calculated by the Kaplan-Meier method, and the survival curves were compared by the log rank test.

Results.—The patients had an overall 5-year disease-specific survival of 52%. Five-year disease-specific survival was 100% for patients in the combined category of CIS of the prostatic urethra and prostatic ducts and acini. This compared with 45% for patients with stromal invasion, 0% for those with extraprostatic extension, and 30% for those with lymph node metastases. The survival advantage of the CIS group, compared with the other groups, was significant.

Conclusions.—Locoregional involvement has an important impact on survival for patients with TCC of the prostate without invasive bladder carcinoma. Five-year disease-specific survival is significantly lower for patients with involvement of the prostatic stroma, extraprostatic tissues, seminal vesicles, and lymph nodes than for those with CIS. Prostatic TCC is commonly associated with CIS of the urinary bladder; urethral recurrences of the CIS are frequent.

► Adenocarcinomas of the prostate account for greater than 95% of all primary malignancies in this location. TCC of the prostate is therefore clearly a relatively rare occurrence in this anatomical site and most commonly arises as a result of in situ spread from the urinary bladder into the prostatic ductular system. Primary transitional cell carcinoma in the prostatic ducts may also occur, and from both of these invasion into the prostatic stroma may occur.

This study of 50 patients from the Mayo Clinic represents an approximately 30-year time span. Not unexpectedly, 42% of the patients had a previous history of CIS involving the urinary bladder, and 64% had concurrent CIS of the bladder. As has been previously reported and well recognized in various staging schemes, prostatic stromal invasion portends a much poorer prognosis. In this study, stromal invasion was identified in 42% of the patients. In addition, extension to extraprostatic tissues, including the seminal vesicles and metastatic disease to lymph nodes, worsened the 5-year disease-specific survival. In reality, however, the distinction between extensive in situ disease and invasive disease, particularly on limited pathologic material, may be problematic, and is clearly of importance both therapeutically and prognostically. Diagnostic features that address this difficult problem are not extensively discussed.

M.B. Cohen, M.D.

Human Glandular Kallikrein 2 (hK2) Expression in Prostatic Intraepithelial Neoplasia and Adenocarcinoma: A Novel Prostate Cancer Marker

Darson MF, Pacelli A, Roche P, et al (Mayo Clinic and Found, Rochester, Minn; Hybritech Inc, San Diego, Calif)

Urology 49:857–862, 1997 13–16

Background.—Prostate-specific antigen (PSA), or human glandular kallikrein 3, is the most useful marker for diagnosis and monitoring of prostate cancer. However, its sensitivity and specificity are limited. Human glandular kallikrein 2 (hK2) is very similar to PSA and is also under androgen control; however, it appears to be differentially regulated. Human glandular kallikrein 2 was evaluated as a potential marker for diagnosis and monitoring of prostate cancer.

Methods.—A total of 257 radical prostatectomy specimens from patients with pathologic stage T2 adenocarcinoma were studied. All patients had undergone serum PSA evaluation within 120 days before surgery. Immunohistochemical studies were performed to evaluate cytoplasmic expression of hK2, PSA, and prostatic acid phosphatase (PAP) in benign tissue, high-grade prostatic intraepithelial neoplasia (PIN), and adenocarcinoma. The analysis used 2 monoclonal antibodies specific for hK2, in addition to antibodies against PSA and PAP.

Results.—All cases showed intense epithelial cytoplasmic immunoreactivity for both hK2 monoclonal antibodies, as well as for PSA and PAP. The prostate cancers showed greater intensity and extent of hK2 expression than did specimens of high-grade PIN, whereas expression was greater in high-grade PIN than in benign epithelium. Nearly every cell of Gleason primary grade 4 and 5 cancers stained for hK2; lower grades showed more heterogeneous patterns of staining. The benign epithelium showed the most intense immunoreactivity for PSA and PAP, compared with PIN and carcinoma. Cancer recurrence was not predicted by the number of immunoreactive cells for hK2 and PSA.

Conclusions.—These findings suggest that all prostate cancers express hK2. Expression of this marker is higher in high-grade PIN than in benign epithelium, and higher in adenocarcinoma than in PIN. The reverse pattern is apparent for PSA and PAP immunoreactivity. Expression of hK2 appears to be localized to the prostate and associated with tumor, and regulated independently of PSA and PAP. The value of hK2 immunoreactivity in diagnosis and monitoring of prostate cancer remains to be defined.

► PSA is now known to be a member of a family of related proteins (kallikreins) and is referred to as hK3. More recently, hK2 has been identified, and intense study is underway to determine its utility as both a clinical and pathologic marker for prostate cancer. This immunohistochemical study evaluated a series of 257 radical prostatectomy specimens and examined the expression of a number of prostate-related antigens, including 2 against hK2—both of which are mouse monoclonal antibodies developed by Hybritech. Expression of hK2 appeared to increase from benign through PIN to cancer, although significant overlap occurred among individual cases; the converse appeared to be true for expression of PSA and PAP. Another point worth emphasizing is that the PSA antibody used in this study, also obtained from Hybritech, does not cross-react with hK2, which is not true for some other anti-PSA antibodies. The importance of hK2 expression either in serum or in tissue sections remains to be determined but is a rapidly evolving area.

M.B. Cohen, M.D.

Characteristics of Prostate Cancer in Families Potentially Linked to the Hereditary Prostate Cancer 1 (*HPC1*) Locus

Grönberg H, Isaacs SD, Smith JR, et al (Johns Hopkins Univ, Baltimore, Md; NIH, Bethesda, Md; Umeå Univ, Sweden)

JAMA 278:1251–1255, 1997 13–17

Purpose.—Mutations of relevant susceptibility genes are now thought to account for about 9% of cases of prostate cancer, and for up to half of early cases of prostate cancer. Other than age at diagnosis, no distinct clinical, phenotypic, or pathologic characteristics of inherited cases of prostate cancer have been identified. Differences between inherited prostate cancer and cases occurring in the general population were identified.

Methods.—A total of 74 North American families with hereditary prostate cancer were studied. Thirty-three families, including 133 cases, were regarded as potentially linked (PL), and thus likely to have an altered *HPC1* gene. The other 41 families, with 172 cases, were regarded as potentially unlinked (PUL), based on *HPC1* haplotype analysis. The findings of the 2 groups were compared, including age at diagnosis, serum prostate-specific antigen levels, digital rectal examination findings, stage, grade, primary treatment, and occurrence of other cases. For comparison with a nationwide reference population, prostate cancer patients from the National Cancer Data Base were identified.

Results.—Mean age at diagnosis was 64 years in the PL families and 66 years in the PUL families, compared with 72 years in the nationwide reference population. Cases from the PL families were more likely to have higher grade cancers. Forty-one percent of these patients had advanced-stage disease, compared with 31% of those in the PUL families and in the reference population. None of the other clinical variables analyzed was significantly different between groups. The PL families had a nonsignificantly increased risk of breast and colon cancers, compared with the PUL families.

Conclusions.—Cases of prostate cancer potentially linked to the *HPC1* locus are, in most regards, clinically indistinguishable from nonhereditary cases. However, cases from PL families tend to have a younger age at diagnosis, higher grade tumors, and more advanced-stage disease. Thus it is particularly important to identify prostate cancers as early as possible in men with prostate cancer susceptibility genes. The findings support the recommendation to begin screening at 40 years of age for men with a family history of prostate cancer.

▶ The identification of a prostate cancer gene, much like the hunt for a breast cancer gene, has received intense attention. It is estimated that approximately 5% to 10% of prostate cancers might be familial, and the search has been on to identify a *BRCA* analogue for prostate cancer, e.g., *HPC1*. In a previous study by the authors,[1] such a potential gene was identified on chromosome 1. In the current study, further investigation into the *HPC1* locus was performed. Families that have evidence for segregation of an altered *HPC1* gene are characterized by multiple cases of prostate cancer that by most criteria appear to be similar to nonhereditary prostate cancer cases, indicating that *HPC1* may not be the answer. Three important features of patients with *HPC1* were, however, demonstrated, including younger age at diagnosis, higher tumor grade, and more advanced stage of disease.

In a related study by McIndoe et al.[2] a series of 49 "high risk" families were studied for the *HPC1* locus. The results of this study do not confirm the linkage reported to the previous study, alluded to above, or a similar study by another group of investigators, led by Carter.[3] In summary, the identification of a familial prostate cancer locus is likely to exist but probably accounts for only a small fraction of all prostate cancers that are identified (less than 5%). The prostate cancer genes have not yet been found.

M.B. Cohen, M.D.

References

1. Smith JR, Freije D, Carpten JD, et al: A genome-wide search reveals a major susceptibility locus for prostate cancer on chromosome 1. *Science* 274:1371–1373, 1996.
2. McIndoe RA, Stanford JL, Gibbs M, et al: Linkage analysis of 49 high-risk families does not support a common familial prostate cancer–susceptibility gene at 1q24–25. *Am J Hum Genet* 61:347–353, 1997.
3. Carter BS, Bova GS, Beaty TH, et al: Hereditary prostate cancer: Epidemiologic and clinical features. *J Urol* 150:797–802, 1993.

Localized Amyloidosis of the Seminal Vesicle: Possible Association With Hormonally Treated Prostatic Adenocarcinoma

Unger PD, Wang Q, Gordon RE, et al (The Mount Sinai Hosp, New York)
Arch Pathol Lab Med 121:1265–1268, 1997 13–18

Introduction.—Although identified in almost every organ system, localized amyloidosis is an uncommon finding in the genitourinary tract. A review of more than 200 prostate needle biopsies, seminal vesicle biopsies, and prostatectomy specimens from surgical pathology files yielded 6 cases of localized seminal vesicle amyloidosis. An examination of these cases suggests that hormonal therapy may lead to the production of amyloid.

Methods.—Three of the cases were found in the seminal vesicle biopsy group. Before biopsy, all 3 patients had received androgen deprivation hormonal therapy for prostatic adenocarcinoma. One of 2 cases obtained from prostatectomy specimens was that of a patient treated with androgen deprivation. The sixth case of seminal vesicle amyloidosis was found in a biopsy for benign prostatic hyperplasia. This patient had also received hormone therapy. None of the patients had a chronic inflammatory disorder, serum or urine protein abnormalities, or other identifiable masses.

Results.—With the exception of the patient with benign prostatic hyperplasia, all patients with localized amyloidosis of the seminal vesicle had prostatic carcinoma. Hormonal treatment (leuprolide acetate with flutamide) had been employed in 4 of the 5 carcinoma cases, and 1 patient received radiotherapy. Amyloid deposits were limited to the seminal vesicle lamina propria; there was no involvement of vesicle walls. All cases had Congo red amyloid staining sensitive to potassium permanganate. None was positive for AA amyloid, β_2-microglobulin, or κ and λ light chains.

Conclusion.—Findings in these 6 cases raise the possibility that localized amyloidosis of the seminal vesicle is related to previous androgen deprivation hormonal therapy. The seminal vesicle epithelial cells may be stimulated to produce amyloid by alteration of the normal hormonal milieu.

▶ This relatively small study (6 cases) describes the identification of localized amyloidosis in the seminal vesicle, identified on biopsy material (4 cases) as well as radical prostatectomy specimens (2 cases). These 6 cases add to the relatively small literature previously reported, which includes 7 cases, according to the authors. The possibility that some of these cases of localized amyloidosis were the result of prior hormonal therapy is raised, but no compelling evidence supports this contention. Thus, this article appears to present a rare but interesting finding.

M.B. Cohen, M.D.

The Significance of Intraluminal Crystalloids in Benign Prostatic Glands on Needle Biopsy

Henneberry JM, Kahane H, Humphrey PA, et al (The Johns Hopkins Med Insts, Baltimore, Md; Dianon Systems, Stratford, Conn; Washington Univ, St Louis)

Am J Surg Pathol 21:725–728, 1997 13–19

Introduction.—Intraluminal prostatic crystalloids have been associated with adenocarcinoma of the prostate, and were recently identified in benign glands adjacent to tumor. A review of 56 prostate needle biopsy results was conducted to determine whether, when intraluminal crystalloids are found in benign glands, a repeat biopsy is needed to rule out malignancy (Fig 1).

Methods.—Excluded from the biopsy results were glands that were markedly atypical and suspicious for carcinoma, cases with high-grade

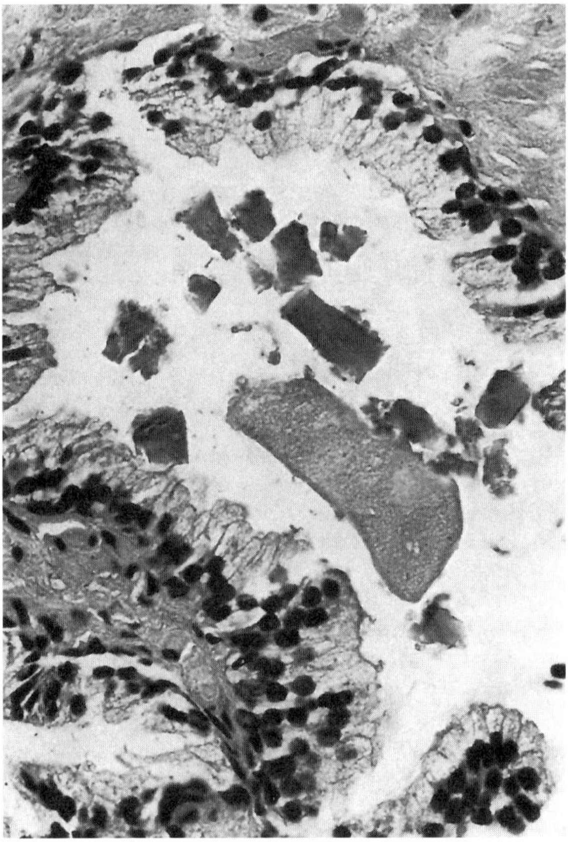

FIGURE 1.—Benign prostatic gland with numerous rectangular intraluminal crystalloids. (Courtesy of Henneberry JM, Kahane H, Humphrey PA, et al: The significance of intraluminal crystalloids in benign prostatic glands on needle biopsy. *Am J Surg Pathol* 21:725–728, 1997.)

prostatic intraepithelial neoplasia, and cases in which crystalloids were identified in the benign glands of adenosis. Follow-up data included subsequent biopsy reports and serum prostate-specific antigen levels.

Results.—At Johns Hopkins Hospital, the overall incidence of intraluminal crystalloids in benign glands was 1.5% in a consecutive series of 473 benign needle biopsy samples. Thirty-one (55%) of 55 men in this study underwent a repeat biopsy, 7 (23%) had adenocarcinoma, and 1 (3%) had high-grade prostatic intraepithelial neoplasia. The remaining men had benign diagnoses. Those with and without cancer on repeat biopsy did not differ in prostate-specific antigen values. In a control group of 360 men with a benign first biopsy and no crystalloids, a repeat biopsy yielded a cancer incidence of 16.2%. This incidence did not differ significantly from that of the study group.

Conclusion.—Because crystalloids are found frequently in adenocarcinoma and rarely in benign glands, some studies have suggested that crystalloids in benign glands (excluding adenosis) indicate the need for repeat biopsy. The findings of this study, however, suggest that crystalloids in benign glands are not associated with an increased risk for concurrent carcinoma.

▶ Intraluminal crystalloids are eosinophilic, refractile structures that were initially described in 1977 and thought to be a useful marker for the diagnosis of prostatic adenocarcinoma. In this article by Henneberry et al., and in the related article by Anton et al.,[1] intraluminal prostatic crystalloids were identified in benign prostatic glands on needle biopsies. Henneberry's article presents a series of 56 consecutive needle biopsies. Thirty-one men underwent repeat biopsies; nearly three quarters (23) had benign diagnoses, and approximately one quarter (7) had adenocarcinoma. In the study by Anton and colleagues, comprising 331 patients who underwent 1–3 subsequent biopsies, 5% of patients had crystalloids on the initial biopsy and 38% of these (6 patients) subsequently were diagnosed with carcinoma, whereas the remaining 10 patients had benign diagnoses. The conclusion from Henneberry indicates that the finding of intraluminal crystalloids in benign prostatic glands does not significantly increase the risk of having cancer on repeat biopsy. Similar data were found in the study by Anton. Taken together, therefore, the finding of intraluminal crystalloid in benign prostatic glands does not appear to be a marker of adenocarcinoma of the prostate.

M.B. Cohen, M.D.

Reference

1. Anton RC, Chakraborty S, Wheeler TM: The significance of intraluminal prostatic crystalloids in benign needle biopsies. *Am J Surg Pathol* 22:446–449, 1998.

Partial Atrophy in Prostate Needle Cores: Another Diagnostic Pitfall for the Surgical Pathologist

Oppenheimer JR, Wills ML, Epstein JI (The Johns Hopkins Med Insts, Baltimore, Md; Prost-Data, Inc [J.R.O.], Edmond, Okla)

Am J Surg Pathol 22:440–445, 1998 13–20

Objective.—Complete atrophy of benign lesions has been shown to mimic intermediate-grade prostate cancer. Partial atrophy, also sometimes misconstrued as well-differentiated prostate cancer, is discussed.

Methods.—When original slides of prostate needle biopsies performed between 1991 and 1995 were reviewed for partial atrophy, 51 cases were identified. The index slide and current slides were examined for the presence of adenocarcinoma and atypical cells.

Results.—Partial atrophy was characterized by a crowded collection of pale staining cells (Fig 1). Irregular nuclei were present in 23.5% of specimens, nucleoli in 25.4%, and unidentifiable or difficult-to-find basal cells in 62.7% (Table 2). Intraluminal pink amorphous debris was present in about one third of samples. Adenocarcinoma or suspect adenocarci-

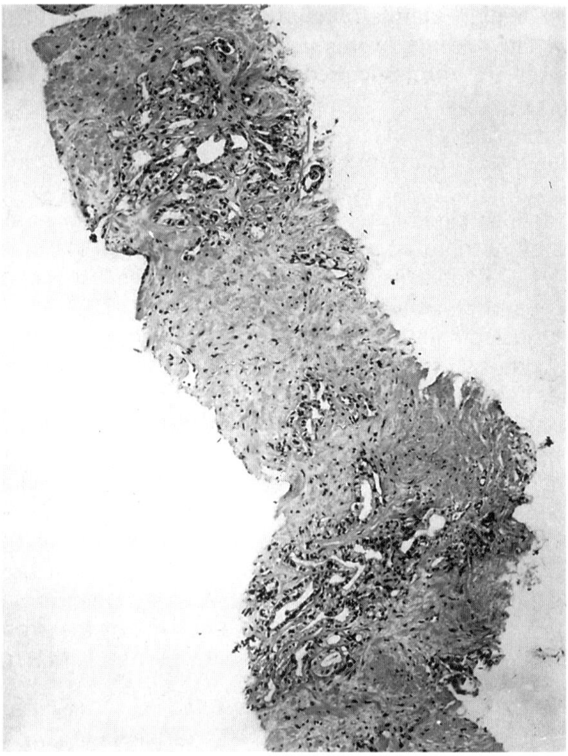

FIGURE 1.—Two lobular foci of partial atrophy consisting of crowded pale staining glands. (Courtesy of Oppenheimer JR, Wills ML, Epstein JI: Partial atrophy in prostate needle cores: Another diagnostic pitfall for the surgical pathologist. *Am J Surg Pathol* 22:440–445, 1998.)

noma was found in 8 (15.6%) biopsies. Coexisting significant atrophy was present in 35.3% of samples, in 22.2% of samples in one 10× field, in 11.1% of samples in more than one 10× field, and with a partial transition to atrophy in 66.7% of cases.

Conclusion.—The characteristics of partial atrophy include little cytoplasm, irregular nuclei, and pale cytoplasm. Recognizing them can prevent a misdiagnosis of adenocarcinoma.

▶ The Hopkins group continues to identify (potential) pitfalls for the diagnosis of prostatic adenocarcinoma. In this article, "partial" atrophy is the basis of study. A number of morphologic parameters were assessed (see Table 2), and an example from the paper is illustrated in the Fig 1. It is important to note that the vast majority of cases (47 of 51) were seen in consultation by the senior author. Although some clues for recognizing partial atrophy are discussed, this entity may often end up under the rubric of atypical small acinar proliferation, as discussed in another abstract in this section.

M.B. Cohen, M.D.

TABLE 2.—Histologic Features of Partial Atrophy.

Histoligic feature	Number (1%)
Nuclear irregularity	
None	8 (15.7)
Rare	14 (27.5)
Occasional	17 (33.3)
Frequent	12 (23.5)
Visible nucleoli	
None	24 (47)
Rare	14 (27.5)
Frequent	13 (25.4)
Nuclear: cytoplasmic ratio >0.5	
<50% of cells	16 (31.3)
50–90% of cells	21 (41.2)
>90% of cells	14 (27.5)
Visibility of basal cells	
Not identifiable	14 (27.4)
Hard to identify	18 (35.3)
Easy to identify	19 (37.3)
Adjunctive findings	
Intraluminal pink amorphous debris	33.3
Blue-tinged mucinous secretions	0
Crystalloids	0

(Courtesy of Oppenheimer JR, Wills ML, Epstein JI: Partial atrophy in prostate needle cores: Another diagnostic pitfall for the surgical pathologist. *Am J Surg Pathol* 22:440–445, 1998.)

Diagnostic Effect of Complete Histologic Sampling of Prostate Needle Biopsy Specimens

Reyes AO, Humphrey PA (Washington Univ, St Louis)
Am J Clin Pathol 109:416–422, 1998 13–21

Objective.—What constitutes an adequate core needle sample of prostatic tissue, and the appropriate number of sections and slides to be prepared, have not been standardized. Most pathologists obtain at least 3 slides with several sections. The effect of examination of additional slides on the detection of high-grade prostatic intraepithelial neoplasia (PIN) and adenocarcinoma of the prostate in needle biopsy specimens was evaluated prospectively.

Methods.—All needle biopsy samples of 100 patients with atypia (60 with high-grade PIN, 36 with focal glandular atypia [FGA], and 4 with both) and 100 with benign prostatic tissue results were evaluated histologically and compared. Three slides of each were reviewed initially. Each paraffin block was completely sectioned and stained with hematoxylin and eosin, yielding an average of 30 slides, with an average of 4 sections per slide.

Results.—There were 5,574 slides and 20,872 sections reviewed. There were 2,913 slides and 10,680 sections in the atypical group, and 2,661 slides and 10,192 sections in the benign control group. In the atypical group, 17 patients showed new morphologic abnormalities, including 4 new cases of adenocarcinoma. Four patients received diagnosis of invasive carcinoma on the fourth slide, after a diagnosis of FGA was made after the first 3 slides. Four patients in the benign control group had additional changes in additional slides, including 2 cases of high-grade PIN and 2 of FGA. None of the control patients received diagnosis of cancer with additional slides after benign prostatic tissue was diagnosed on the basis of findings in the first 3 slides.

Conclusion.—When FGA is diagnosed on the basis of the first 3 slides, it is recommended that an additional 3-μm section slide be prepared. When PIN is diagnosed on the basis of information obtained in the first 3 slides, it is not necessary to prepare a fourth slide.

▶ This article presents a carefully designed prospective study attempting to aid the pathologist in the optimal handling of prostate needle biopsy specimens to diagnose adenocarcinoma. Given the importance of making the correct diagnosis, the authors have come up with the following recommendation: "We recommend 3 initial slides with several sections per slide per prostate needle biopsy specimens, with preparation of a single additional slide with several 3-micron sections when a diagnosis of 'focal glandular atypia' is given on the initial 3 slides. Generation of an additional slide does not seem necessary after initial diagnosis of pure high grade PIN." As in other articles reviewed in this section, these small glandular proliferations are problematic and are worthy of further, but not exhaustive, evaluation. It is worth noting, though, that PIN typically involves large, pre-existing glandular/ductular structures.

M.B. Cohen, M.D.

14 Cardiovascular System

Prevalence of Myocarditis at Autopsy in Turin, Italy

Passarino G, Burlo P, Ciccone G, et al (Univ of Torino, Italy; San Giovanni Hosp, Italy; Ospedale Civile Santa Croce, Mondovì, Cuneo, Italy)

Arch Pathol Lab Med 121:619–622, 1997 14–1

Objective.—The frequency of myocarditis in the general population is not known. The prevalence of postmortem diagnosis of myocarditis in the San Giovanni Battista General Hospital in Turin, Italy, was investigated retrospectively.

Methods.—Records of 17,162 autopsies performed between 1965 and 1994 were reviewed, and retrospective and prospective investigations were compared.

Results.—There were 157 diagnoses of myocarditis, but only 91 were confirmed by means of the Dallas criteria. Polymorphonuclear infiltrate was present in 36 cases and lymphocytic infiltrate in 34. In addition 12 hearts were rheumatic, 6 showed fungal infections, and 3 were granulomatous. All hearts showed some degree of hypertrophy. The prevalence of myocarditis was significantly higher between 1985 and 1994 and was found significantly more frequently in patients aged 20–39. The incidence for the two sexes was similar. Previously reported prospective data showed a significantly higher frequency than did the present retrospective data (5.1 vs. 0.5%, respectively). The prevalence in the present study is 5 times higher than that found retrospectively.

Conclusion.—Myocardial sampling must be standardized to avoid underestimating the proportion of the population with myocarditis.

▶ Relatively few (retrospective) studies have attempted to assess the prevalence of myocarditis without selection for cause of death. This study is one of them. Myocarditis was defined according to the "Dallas criteria"[1] and was identified in 0.53% (95% CI 0.4–0.7). Briefly, this was a microscopic focus of inflammation with associated myocardial injury (necrosis or degeneration), which was atypical for ischemic injury. This figure is well within the previous reported ranges (0.11% to 5.5%). This higher prevalence is similar to that found in a prospective analysis by the same authors in a series of 605 autopsies, where the prevalence of myocarditis was 5.1%. Sampling and definition of criteria appear to be the key aspects in this approximately fivefold "discrepancy." Taken together, myocarditis may be underdiagnosed.

However, these data demonstrating histologic evidence of myocarditis do not translate to clinical disease or cause of death from myocarditis.

M.B. Cohen, M.D.

Reference

1. Aretz HT, Billingham ME, Edwards WD, et al: Myocarditis: A histopathologic definition and classification. *Am J Cardiovasc Pathol* 1:3–14, 1986.

Coronary Risk Factors and Plaque Morphology in Men With Coronary Disease Who Died Suddenly

Burke AP, Farb A, Malcom GT, et al (Armed Inst of Pathology, Washington, DC; Louisiana State Univ, New Orleans; Univ of Maryland, Baltimore)

N Engl J Med 336:1276–1282, 1997 14–2

Objective.—Although cigarette smoking and high serum cholesterol level increase the risk of atherosclerotic heart disease, their role in triggering acute coronary thrombosis in not known. The part, if any, that cigarette smoking and abnormal cholesterol values play in causing acute coronary thrombosis and sudden death from either rupture of vulnerable coronary plaques or erosion of plaques was investigated.

Methods.—The coronary arteries of 113 men (27 black), average age 50, who died suddenly were prospectively examined if they were more than 50% occluded. Hearts were divided into 2 groups: hearts with acute thrombi (n = 59) and hearts without acute thrombi (n = 54). Hearts with acute thrombi were subdivided into hearts with ruptured plaques (n = 41) and hearts with eroded plaques (n = 18). Serum samples were analyzed for total cholesterol, HDL cholesterol, and thiocyanate. Blood cells were analyzed for glycosylated hemoglobin. The number of vulnerable plaques was compared with smoking status, race, presence or absence of hypertension, and serum cholesterol level (Fig 2).

Results.—The average age of men dying with acute thrombi was significantly lower than for men dying with stable plaque (47 vs. 53). Smokers were significantly younger than nonsmokers (47 vs. 54), men with hypertension were significantly older than men without hypertension (55 vs. 48), and men with elevated cholesterol levels were significantly younger than men without elevated cholesterol levels (48 vs. 53). Men dying of acute thrombosis were significantly more likely to be smokers (75% vs. 41%) than men dying with stable plaques. Men with acute thrombosis had significantly higher ratio of total cholesterol to HDL cholesterol than men without acute thrombosis (8.5 vs. 5.5). According to multivariate analysis, the ratio of total cholesterol to HDL cholesterol was significantly related to the presence of plaques vulnerable to rupture.

Conclusion.—Men with coronary disease who died suddenly as a result of plaque rupture were more likely to have elevated ratios of total choles-

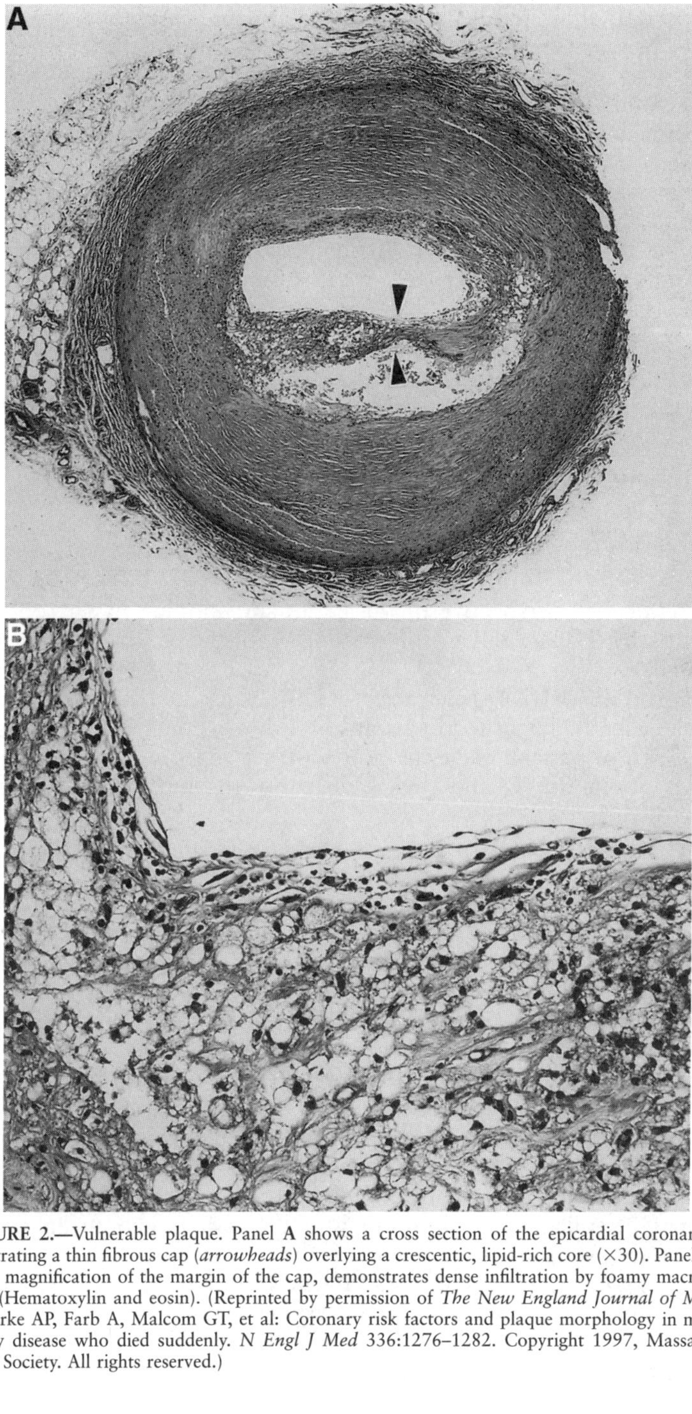

FIGURE 2.—Vulnerable plaque. Panel **A** shows a cross section of the epicardial coronary artery demonstrating a thin fibrous cap (*arrowheads*) overlying a crescentic, lipid-rich core (×30). Panel **B**, with a higher magnification of the margin of the cap, demonstrates dense infiltration by foamy macrophages (×300) (Hematoxylin and eosin). (Reprinted by permission of *The New England Journal of Medicine*, from Burke AP, Farb A, Malcom GT, et al: Coronary risk factors and plaque morphology in men with coronary disease who died suddenly. *N Engl J Med* 336:1276–1282. Copyright 1997, Massachusetts Medical Society. All rights reserved.)

terol to HDL cholesterol. Patients dying of acute thromboses were more likely to be cigarette smokers.

► This pathologic study, centered at the Armed Forces Institute of Pathology, examined 113 hearts from men who had sudden cardiac deaths. An acute coronary thrombus was identified in 52% of the men; 71% of these were the result of rupture of a vulnerable plaque (fibrous cap less than 65 μm thick with a macrophage infiltrate; see Fig 2) and 29% were the result of erosion of a fibrous plaque. In addition, a stable plaque (cross-sectional luminal narrowing of at least 75% in the absence of a thrombus) was seen in 48%. The epidemiologic studies indicated a correlation between cholesterol and vulnerable plaques, and between cigarette smoking and acute thrombosis.

M.B. Cohen, M.D.

Hypertrophic Cardiomyopathy
Maron BJ (Minneapolis Heart Inst Found)
Lancet 350:127–133, 1997 14–3

Objective.—A perspective of the issues surrounding hypertrophic cardiomyopathy (HCM) and a profile of HCM for the practicing clinician are presented.

Background.—HCM is characterized by a thickened and nondilated left ventricle, usually diagnosed by means of 2-dimensional echocardiography. About 75% of patients have the non-obstructive form. The prevalence of HCM is about 0.2%, and this is probably the most common familial cardiac disorder.

Genetic Defects.—HCM is a mendelian autosomal dominant inherited disorder resulting from mutation in any 1 of 4 genes that encode proteins of the sarcomere. Although DNA diagnosis is expensive because of the heterogeneity involved in the disorder, pedigree studies have established the presence of disease-causing mutations in symptom-free children. Affected adults without phenotypic expression are rare. The variety of hypertrophic patterns observed suggests that phenotypic expression of HCM is strongly influenced by modifier genes or environment.

Morphological Characteristics.—Hypertrophy is asymmetrical most of the time but almost always involves the anterior ventricular septum. Significant left ventricular remodeling typically occurs during growth periods, and decrease in left ventricular wall thickness is associated with aging. Cellular structure is disorganized, the mitral valve may be malformed, and there may be collagen distribution within the wall and abnormal intramural coronary arteries with thickened walls.

Pathophysiology.—Symptoms include exertional dyspnea, fatigue, orthopnea, and paroxysmal nocturnal dyspnea.

Natural History and Treatment.—The natural history is variable and treatment is determined by the clinical course of the disease. Sudden and unexpected death commonly occurs between the ages of 12 and 35. Congestive symptoms typically begin in midlife and are treated with β-blockers, verapamil, or disopyramide and possibly a diuretic. Atrial fibrillation is the most common arrhythmia indicative of disability or increased risk of adverse clinical incident. Patients who do not respond to drug therapy have been treated with ventricular septal myotomy-myectomy.

► This review article briefly covers various aspects of this cardiac disorder, including: nomenclature and prevalence, genetic defects, morphology (gross and microscopic), pathophysiology, and clinical aspects. In addition, it includes approximately 75 references.

M.B. Cohen, M.D.

Human Neutrophil Elastase in Temporal (Giant Cell) Arteritis: Plasma and Immunohistochemical Studies

Génèreau T, Peyri N, Berard M, et al (Hôpital St-Louis, France; Groupe Hospitalier Pitie-Salpêtrière, France; Hôpital St-Antoine, Paris; et al)

J Rheumatol 25:710–713, 1998 14–4

Objective.—Temporal arteritis (TA) is a mononuclear cell infiltration that destroys the internal elastic lamina. Because human neutrophil elastase (HNE) can hydrolyze elastin, its role in the pathogenesis of TA was investigated by measuring HNE-α_1 levels and prospectively studying its localization within temporal artery walls in patients undergoing temporal artery biopsy because of suspected TA.

Methods.—Between July and December 1994, temporal artery biopsy was performed in 33 patients (11 men), aged 47–91 years, with suspected TA, and in 19 healthy age-matched controls. TA was diagnosed in 15 patients (TA group). The remaining 18 patients were placed in the non-TA group. Blood cell counts, erythrocyte sedimentation rate, and plasma HNE (pHNE)–α_1 complex concentration were determined using venous blood samples. Immunohistochemical analysis was performed on biopsy specimens.

Results.—The average pHNE-α_1 level was significantly higher in the TA group than in the control group (84 vs. 51 μg/L). Levels for the non-TA and control groups were similar. The sensitivities of pHNE-α_1 levels >50 μg/L and of temporal artery biopsy were 100% and 60%, respectively, whereas the specificities were 60% and 100%, respectively. The negative predictive value of pHNE-α_1 levels <50 μg/L was 100%. The temporal arteries of patients with TA contained mononuclear inflammatory infiltrates with fragmented internal lamina in 6 of 7 patients. No HNE was detected in the temporal artery of any patient by immunohistochemistry.

Conclusion.—High levels of pHNE-α_1 complexes were found in the temporal arteries of patients with TA. The sensitivity and specificity of pHNE-α_1 levels >50 μg/L were 100% and 60%. Because HNE was not found in the temporal artery walls of any patient, its role in the pathogenesis of TA is unknown.

► This study of 15 patients with histologically proven TA focuses on additional means of diagnosing this rare and intriguing disease. Like other vasculitides, (e.g., ANCA), there is keen interest in novel markers. In this study, the authors examined a link between TA and HNE in serum and in lesional tissue. Higher levels of HNE were found in serum of patients with TA than those without TA, including a subset that had temporal artery biopsies, although there was overlap among individual patients. In addition, immunohistochemical staining of sections did not identify HNE in any of the sections. Thus it would appear that HNE may be a useful serum marker. It remains to be determined if HNE is involved in the pathophysiology of TA.

M.B. Cohen, M.D.

15 Dermatopathology

Proliferation Marker Ki-S5 as a Diagnostic Tool in Melanocytic Lesions

Rudolph P, Schubert C, Schubert B, et al (Univ of Kiel, Germany; Inst of Dermatopathology; Buchholz, Germany)

J Am Acad Dermatol 37:169–178, 1997 15–1

Introduction.—It is difficult to differentiate the various melanocytic lesions because a substantial percentage cannot be diagnosed by conventional histology. There is a need to improve diagnostic accuracy. Using proliferation-specific monoclonal antibody Ki-S5, which is directed against a formalin-resistant epitope of the Ki-67 antigen, the proliferative behavior of a broad spectrum of benign and malignant melanocytic lesions was examined by immunohistochemistry. The mean growth fractions of junctional nevi were compared with those of melanomas in situ, and compound nevi and invasive melanomas were also compared. The proliferative activity in various types of melanocytic neoplasms was determined and its value as a diagnostic adjunct appraised.

Methods.—Using the monoclonal antibody Ki-S5 directed to the Ki-67 antigen, the growth fraction was assessed immunohistochemically in 398 melanocytic lesions. The lesions were classified as dermal congenital nevi, common nevi, Spitz nevi of the junctional type, melanomas in situ, common compound, Spitz nevi of the compound type, and invasive melanomas. There were 112 lesions of equivocal histology that were used to define and apply a cut-off level. The clinical courses were correlated to the revised diagnoses.

Results.—Significantly different proliferation indices and distinctive distribution patterns of cycling cells were exhibited by common nevi, Spitz nevi, and melanomas (Fig 4). In 68% of patients with uncertain diagnosis, malignancy diagnosed on the basis of a growth fraction greater than 5% was confirmed by disease progression.

Conclusion.—Conventional histology may be usefully complemented by determination of the proliferative activity in melanocytic lesions, and diagnostic accuracy improved. A discrimination between benign and malignant lesions can be made on the basis of a cut-off level of 5% proliferating cells, according to statistically significant differences between nevi and melanomas.

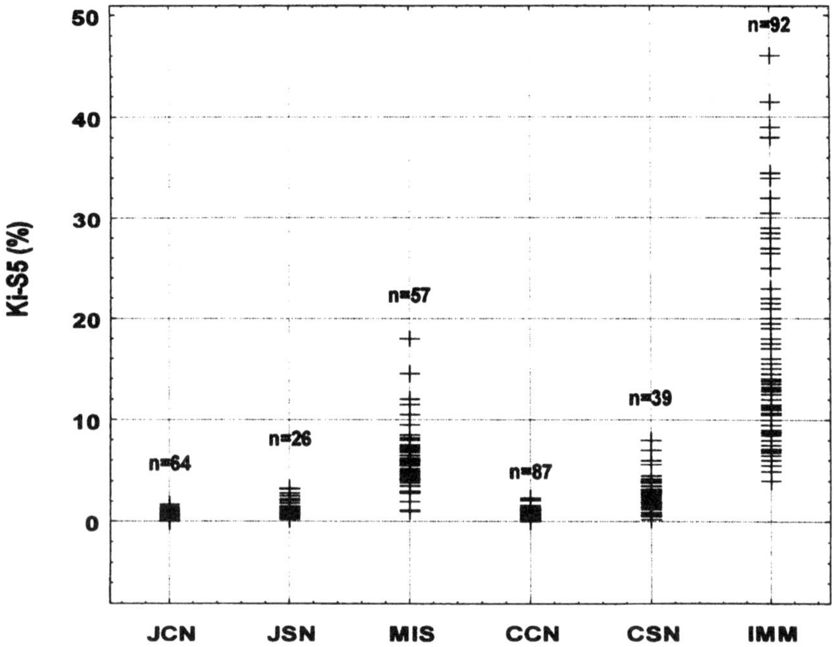

FIGURE 4.—Ki-S5 labeling indices in various types of melanocytic lesions. *Abbreviations: JCN*, junctional common nevi; *JSN*, junctional Spitz nevi; *MIS*, melanoma in situ; *CCN*, compound common nevi; *CSN*, compound Spitz nevi; *IMM*, invasive malignant melanomas. The wide scatter of values in the latter group is partly because of differences in tumor thickness (0.3–4.4 mm, Clark level II–IV). (Courtesy of Rudolph P, Schubert C, Schubert B, et al: Proliferation marker Ki-S5 as a diagnostic tool in melanocytic lesions. *J Am Acad Dermatol* 37: 169–178, 1997.)

▶ Common problems in pigmented lesions of the skin almost always include the distinction between the Spitz nevus and malignant melanoma. In this study, the authors used the antibody to a Ki-67 antigen on formalin-fixed paraffin-embedded tissues of 112 lesions of equivocable histology. The distribution of proliferative nuclear labeling that was found could be characterized into 2 broad zones. For Spitz nevi, the nuclear proliferative immunostaining was "top heavy," with preponderance of staining of the tumor cells within the intraepidermal or junctional areas. In contrast, malignant melanomas in the radial growth phase and vertical growth phase showed a more random distribution of nuclear immunostaining, with a tendency towards nuclear immunostaining around the invasive aspects of the tumor cells ("bottom heavy"). As with most immunostaining studies, there is a zone of overlap, and the authors caution that it is critical to pay attention to morphology. Nevertheless, this article and some other recent studies of proliferative activity in pigmented lesions show the future holds promise for distinguishing some of these difficult lesions.

D.J. Dabbs, M.D.

Suggested Reading

Kanter-Lewensohn L, Hedblad MA, Wejde J, et al: Immunohistochemical markers for distinguishing Spitz nevi from malignant melanomas. *Mod Pathol* 10:917–920, 1997.

Niemann TH, Argenyi ZB: Immunohistochemical study of Spitz nevi and malignant melanoma with use of antibody to proliferating cell nuclear antigen. *Am J Dermatopathol* 15:441–445, 1993.

Vascular Density in Melanoma Xenografts Correlates With Vascular Permeability Factor Expression But Not With Metastatic Potential

Westphal JR, van't Hullenaar RGM, van der Laak JAWM, et al (Univ Hosp Nijmegen, The Netherlands)

Br J Cancer 76:561–570, 1997 15–2

Introduction.—Recently, it has been found that the vascular density of a number of tumor types can be predictive for the metastatic capacity of the primary tumor. An important factor in tumor biology is tumor angiogenesis. The production of angiogenic factors by tumor cells is the most prominent feature that facilitates angiogenesis. In a human xenograft model, the relation between tumor vascular density and tumor growth rate, metastatic incidence, and vascular permeability factor mRNA levels was examined.

Methods.—The human xenograft model consisted of a panel of cultured melanoma cell lines which formed a local tumor after subcutaneous injection into nude mice. There was variance in growth rates and in capacity to form spontaneous lung metastases among the resulting xenograft. The cell lines used were 530, 1F6, M14, Mel57, MV1, MV3, and BLM, which were derived from surgically removed human melanoma metastases. Automated image analysis was used to determine vascular density.

Results.—The highest mean vascular density, the highest in vivo growth rate, high vascular permeability factor mRNA levels, and rapid development of lung metastases were seen in xenograft derived from cell lines BLM and MV3. A significantly lower degree of vascularization was observed in xenograft of cell lines M14, Mel57, and MV1, but these cell lines formed lung metastases with an incidence similar to those of BLM and MV3. Lung metastases were not formed in xenograft from cell line 1F6. However, tumors derived from a spontaneous mutant of 1F6, which was designated as 1F6m, developed lung metastases to the same extent as Mel57, M14, and MV1 tumors. There were similar mean vascular density values in 1F6 and 1F6m xenograft, vascular permeability factor mRNA levels, and in vivo growth rates of 1F6 and 1F6m xenograft.

Conclusion.—Vascular density correlated with in vivo growth rate and in vitro vascular permeability factor mRNA levels, but it did not correlate with the ability to metastasize, in this melanoma xenograft model.

▶ For many tumors, a correlation between high vascular density and occurrence of metastases with poor clinical prognosis has been reported. These tumors include breast carcinoma, prostate carcinoma, non-small-cell lung carcinoma, malignant melanoma, and others. This study is informative because it is, at least in part, intuitive. We know that most tumors produce angiogenesis factors, the most powerful of which are vascular endothelial growth factor and basic fibroblast growth factor. In addition to providing abundant nourishment for tumor cells, these vessels may also act as routes of access to the vasculature. However, the presence of the vasculature is not an obligatory step for entry of tumor cells into the vascular space, and this study supports this concept. Metastases require a whole set of different capabilities, including the ability to digest basement and matrix components. From a teleologic viewpoint, however, one may suspect that if a tumor can elaborate vascular endothelial growth factor and stimulate its own blood vessel supply, it is supporting viability of the immortal cells which, through neoplastic progression, can acquire a genetic abnormality necessary to punch through basement membrane and digest extracellular matrix.

D.J. Dabbs, M.D.

Suggested Reading

Liotta LA, Steeg PS, Stetler-Stevenson WG: Cancer metastasis and angiogenesis: An imbalance of positive and negative regulation. *Cell* 64:327–336, 1991.

Cytokeratins, CEA, and Mucin Histochemistry in the Diagnosis and Characterization of Extramammary Paget's Disease

Battles OE, Page DL, Johnson JE (Vanderbilt Univ, Nashville, Tenn)
Am J Clin Pathol 108:6–12, 1997 15–3

Introduction.—Extramammary Paget's disease, superficial spreading malignant melanoma, and squamous cell carcinoma in situ are the differential diagnoses of a cutaneous neoplasm. Immunohistochemical stains have been useful in differentiating extramammary Paget's disease from superficial spreading melanoma and squamous lesions. The differential diagnosis is complicated by any nearby solid tumors. Specimens of extramammary Paget's disease were examined to identify a sensitive marker and the histochemical and immunohistochemical features that suggest occult pelvic cancer in the patients.

Methods.—The specimens were from 16 patients with extramammary Paget's disease who had 30 surgical procedures. Two patients had pelvic malignancies, 1 with a rectal adenocarcinoma and another with transitional carcinoma. Their specimens were stained for alcian blue/periodic acid-Schiff, AE1/AE3, mucicarmine, cytokeratin 7, cytokeratin 20, cytokeratin CAM 5.2, carcinoembryonic antigen, S-100, and prostate-specific antigen.

Results.—All specimens were marked with cytokeratin 7. The specimens were marked by mucins that were sensitive but focal, which is a potential problem in small biopsy specimens. A unique staining profile, carcinoembryonic antigen- and mucin-negative, was seen in the transitional tumor. Paget cells associated with rectal cancer were strongly marked by cytokeratin 20. A large bowel lesion is suggested by its presence, but it is not specific. Prostate-specific antigen was not expressed by any of the specimens. In a man, its presence suggests prostatic carcinoma.

Conclusion.—In the specimens of extramammary Paget's disease, cytokeratin 7 was 100% sensitive, including a specimen associated with large bowel malignancy, which usually expresses cytokeratin 20 and is cytokeratin-7-negative. In the differentiation of extramammary Paget's disease from melanoma and squamous carcinoma in situ, keratin antibodies, mucins, and carcinoembryonic antigens are useful.

► The old problem of identifying Paget's disease in the skin is approached with a new battery of antibodies that can help to discern the origin of the tumor. As shown previously, low molecular weight or simple cytokeratins identify the adenocarcinoma cells within the squamous epithelium, and in this study it was cytokeratin 7. Other cytokeratins work as well, especially CAM 5.2. Depending on the location of the tumor, the immunostaining can be very helpful in suggesting a primary. In the perineal region, cytokeratin 20-positive Paget's cells that are carcinoembryonic antigen-positive, S100-negative, and GCDFP15-negative most likely represent metastatic colorectal carcinoma. Cytokerin 7-positive cells, cytokeratin 20-negative results, and a positive GCDFP15 may represent a primary skin adenocarcinoma in the form of an adnexal tumor or, of course, in the vicinity of breast, a primary breast adenocarcinoma. Perineal carcinomas in males may be prostate-specific antigen-positive with origin in the prostate. An appropriate battery of immunostains to use then would include cytokeratins 7, 20, carcinoembryonic antigen, S100 protein, GCDFP 15, and possibly prostate-specific antigen.

D.J. Dabbs, M.D.

The Diagnostic Yield of Histologic Examination of Seborrheic Keratoses

Eads TJ, Hood AF, Chuang T-Y, et al (Indiana Univ, Indianapolis)

Arch Dermatol 133:1417–1420, 1997 15–4

Introduction.—Seborrheic keratoses are common, benign tumors that may be cosmetically disfiguring, but not life threatening. Electrodesiccation, curettage, shave biopsy, excision, and cryotherapy with liquid nitrogen are some of the treatments. Because these treatments are destructive and do not allow for histologic examination, it was not known whether histologic confirmation of seborrheic keratoses would be necessary or cost-effective. Lesions clinically diagnosed as seborrheic keratoses were histologically evaluated and their frequency of malignancy was compared with that of biopsy specimens clinically diagnosed as melanocytic nevi.

Methods.—There were 577 cutaneous pathology specimens that had a preoperative clinical diagnosis of seborrheic keratosis with or without a modifier. They were compared to a group of specimens with the clinical diagnosis of melanocytic nevus. A retrospective review, conducted on preoperative and postoperative diagnoses, was based on information given to the laboratory by the clinician on the subsequent histopathologic diagnosis. The microscopic diagnosis was compared to the preoperative clinical diagnosis.

Results.—A histological diagnosis of malignant tumors was ascribed to 37 of 577 specimens clinically diagnosed and submitted as seborrheic keratosis (6.4%). When clinical information suggested findings beyond the classic clinical presentation, such as irritation, or when a malignant tumor was considered in the differential diagnosis, the rate of malignant tumors increased. This group had 2 lesions that proved to be melanomas histologically. Seborrheic keratoses were more likely to be malignant tumors than were melanocytic nevi. Clinically diagnosed melanocytic nevi were less likely to be melanomas than clinically diagnosed seborrheic keratoses submitted by dermatologists.

Conclusion.—The rate of malignant tumors differed between nondermatologists and dermatologists. Clinically diagnosed, surgically removed melanocytic nevi are less likely to be malignant tumors than clinically diagnosed, surgically removed seborrheic keratoses.

▶ If you ever wondered why we look at seborrheic keratoses microscopically, here is the answer. The central question of this study is what is the importance of submitting clinically diagnosed seborrheic keratoses for histologic examination? The authors found an overall rate of 6.4% for malignant tumors in this group. The rate increased to nearly 20% when there was a clinical suspicion of malignancy of a seborrheic keratosis. Is it a cost-effective procedure? Yes. The outcome measurement and cost were felt to be justifiable.

D.J. Dabbs, M.D.

Immunohistochemical Markers for Distinguishing Spitz Nevi From Malignant Melanomas

Kanter-Lewensohn L, Hedblad M-A, Wejde J, et al (Karolinska Hosp, Stockholm)

Mod Pathol 10:917–920, 1997 15–5

Introduction.—Spitz nevi are difficult to distinguish from malignant melanoma because the clinical characteristics of Spitz nevi are usually not distinctive enough. Some patients with Spitz nevi may develop malignant melanoma. The exact nature of these lesions and a method to classify them still has not been explored. It was determined whether immunohistochemi-

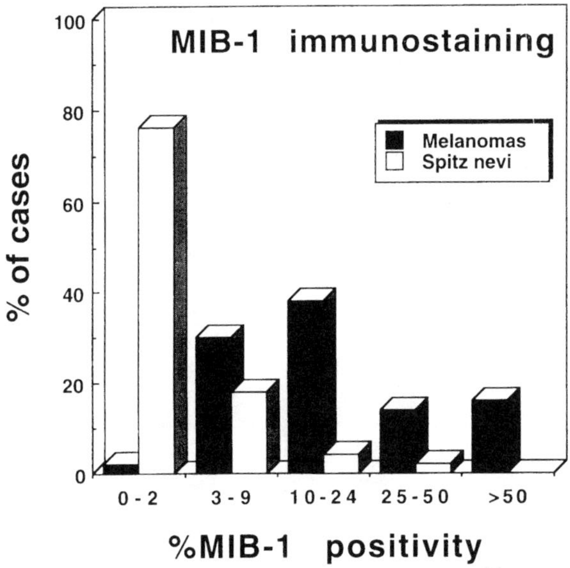

FIGURE 2.—MIB-1 immunoreactivity in the dermal component of malignant melanoma and Spitz nevi. The distribution of percentages of MIB-1 immunoreactivity is shown. (Courtesy of Kanter-Lewensohn L, Hedblad M-A, Wejde J, et al: Immunohistochemical markers for distinguishing Spitz nevi from malignant melanomas. *Mod Pathol* 10[9]:917–920, 1997.)

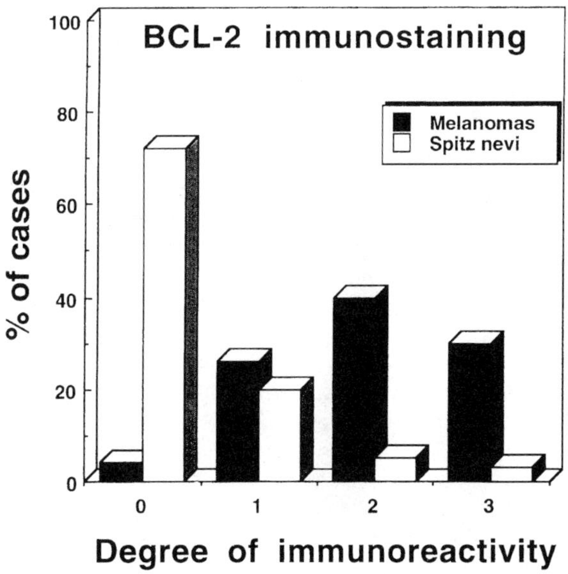

FIGURE 3.—bcl-2 immunoreactivity in 50 malignant melanomas and 46 Spitz nevi. The intensity of immunostaining in the dermal component was evaluated. The distribution of bcl-2 immunoreactive intensity is shown. The mean value for melanomas was +2.0 (± 0.9) and for Spitz nevi +0.4 ± 0.9). (Courtesy of Kanter-Lewensohn L, Hedblad M-A, Wejde J, et al: Immunohistochemical markers for distinguishing Spitz nevi from malignant melanomas. *Mod Pathol* 10[9]:917–920, 1997.)

cal analysis, on the basis of assessing the proliferation and expression of oncogene and tumor suppressor gene, can be used to differentiate Spitz nevi from malignant melanomas.

Methods.—Immunoreactivity of MIB-1 was compared to that of bcl-2 in the intradermal component of lesions in 46 patients with Spitz nevi and 50 with vertical growth-phase melanomas (Clark III-V). There was an independent review by 2 pathologists.

Results.—A low percentage of MIB-1 immunoreactivity (0.2%) was seen in as many as 76% of the Spitz nevus patients (Fig 2). Only 2% of the patients with malignant melanomas showed such a low MIB-1 index. In malignant melanomas, the average MIB-1 index was 29.7%, and in Spitz nevi, it was 4%. The average bcl-2 index was 4% in the malignant melanomas and 72% in the Spitz nevi. The differences were highly significant according to statistical analyses. As many as 96% of the melanomas expressed a bcl-2 positivity and exhibited a MIB-1 index exceeding 2% in the dermal component, considering the immunoreactivity for MIB-1 and bcl-2 in the individual patients (Fig 3). In the Spitz nevi patients, the corresponding value was as low as 6%.

Conclusion.—To distinguish compound Spitz nevi from malignant melanomas, immunostaining with MIB-1 and anti–bcl-2 is a useful tool. It was confirmed that benign nevocellular nevi express a high bcl-2 immunoreactivity in the dermal component.

▶ This article represents a progressive step in determining the distinction between Spitz nevi and malignant melanoma. As a useful guide, MIB-1 and bcl-2 are both expressed to a great degree in malignant melanoma, but to a much lesser degree in Spitz nevus. By looking at the "immunocytograms," one can see that for MIB-1 positivity, values above 24% are clearly a superior determinant, and for bcl-2, values above 2%. While these values are useful together, there is a substantial group of patients at the low end of the spectrum of both MIB-1 and bcl-2 in which absolute distinction may not be possible on the basis of these immunocytochemistry tests. That is why we will continue to have a category of atypical Spitz nevus of an uncertain malignant potential.

D.J. Dabbs, M.D.

Superficial Angiomyxoma (Cutaneous Myxoma): A Clinicopathologic Study of 17 Cases Arising in the Genital Region

Fetsch JF, Laskin WB, Tavassoli FA (Armed Forces Inst of Pathology, Washington, DC; Northwestern Univ, Chicago)

Int J Gynecol Pathol 16:325–334, 1997 15–6

Introduction.—Superficial angiomyxoma (cutaneous myxoma) is a rare, incompletely characterized lesion that can arise in various anatomic sites as an isolated event or as a component of Carney's complex. The clinical and histopathologic features of 17 patients with superficial angiomyxoma arising in the genital region are described.

Methods.—Archival material from tumors of the soft tissues of the pelvis, perineum, vulva, inguinal region, scrotum, and retroperitoneum were examined. Follow-up data were obtained by questionnaires mailed to the contributing pathologist, the patient's surgeon, gynecologist, or the family practitioner. Some patients were contacted by telephone.

Results.—Of 17 patients, 13 were women and 4 were men. Sites of involvement for women were: 6 labium majus or labium, 4 vulva, 2 groin, and 1 mons pubis. All lesions in men involved the scrotum. Most patients sought medical attention for a slow-growing painless mass. Tumors were present for 2 months to 4 years before undergoing local excision. Nine patients were able to be studied for a mean of 135 months (median, 95 months). Three patients developed recurrence at 8 months, 7 years 11

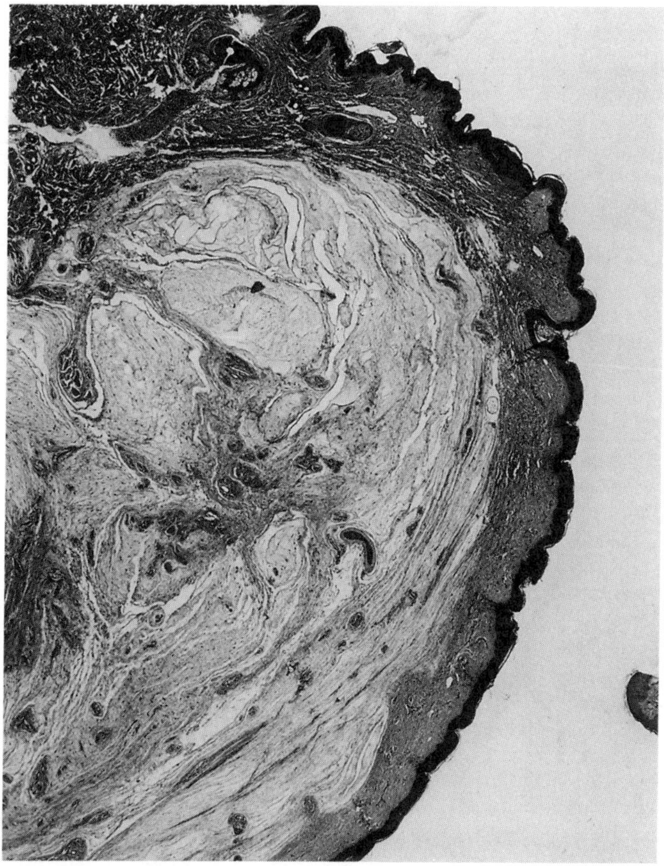

FIGURE 2.—A low-power view of a superficial angiomyxoma (cutaneous myxoma) involving the dermis. Note the lobular contour, relative hypocellularity, and abundant myxoid matrix forming acellular clefts. (Courtesy of Fetsch JF, Laskin WB, Tavassoli FA: Superficial angiomyxoma [cutaneous myxoma]: A clinicopathologic study of 17 cases arising in the genital region. *Int J Gynecol Pathol* 16:325–334, 1997.)

months, and 20 years, respectively. No patients had Carney's complex. Histologic examination showed variably demarcated, moderately to sparsely cellular, angiomyxoid nodules within the dermis or subcutis, or both sites (Fig 2). The tumors contained bipolar and stellate stromal cells with bland to mildly pleomorphic nuclei, and several had a "smudgy," somewhat hyperchromatic cromatin pattern (Fig 5). Tumors were immunoreactive for vimentin (11/11), CD34 (11/11), muscle-specific actin (8/12), smooth muscle actin (9/11), S100 protein (5/13), and Factor XIIIa (5/9). No immunoreactivity was detected for desmin, glial fibrillary acidic protein, estrogen receptor, or progesterone receptor.

Conclusion.—Superficial angiomyxomas can be optimally managed with a conservative but complete excision to minimize the possibility of local recurrence.

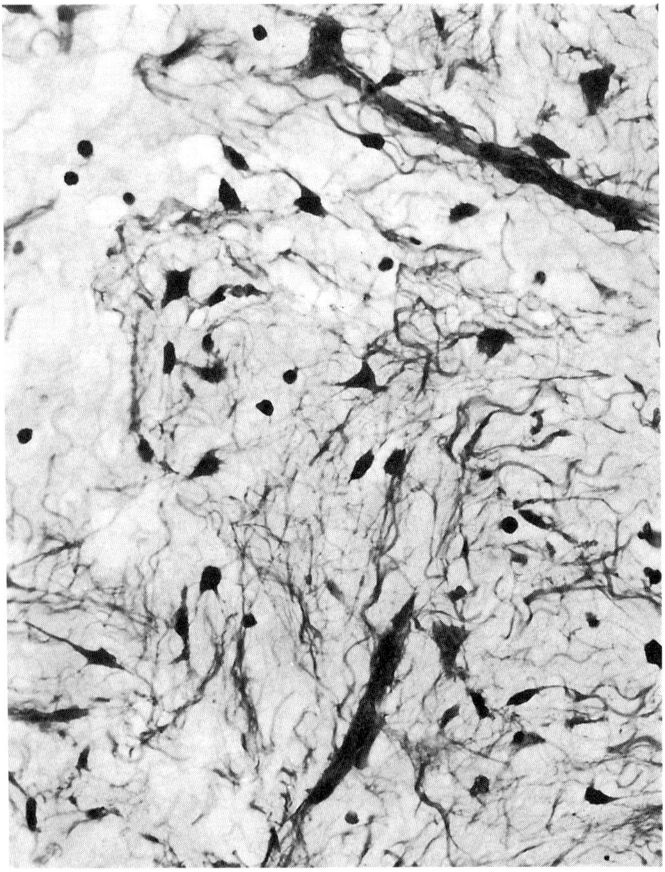

FIGURE 5.—A high-power view of superficial angiomyxoma demonstrating stellate and spindled tumor cells with "smudgy" chromatin, embedded in abundant myxoid matrix with capillary-sized vessels. (Courtesy of Fetsch JF, Laskin WB, Tavassoli FA: Superficial angiomyxoma [cutaneous myxoma]: A clinicopathologic study of 17 cases arising in the genital region. *Int J Gynecol Pathol* 16:325–334, 1997.)

► The cutaneous myxoma is a poorly characterized lesion that can arise in a variety of sites, and can occur in the setting of Carney's complex. In a superficial dermal/subcutaneous location, the lesion can be confused with focal mucinosis, angiomyofibroblastoma, neurothekeoma, myxoid neurofibroma, myxoid smooth muscle tumors, aggressive angiomyxoma, or myxoid malignant fibrous histiocytoma. This lesion is fairly common in women, and must be differentiated histologically from the lesions above. The key differential points are the very superficial location, paucity of vascularity, abundant acid mucin within the dermis forming pools and microcysts, and overall lobular contour. The other lesions in the differential diagnosis lack these features. Local recurrence has been described in 3 of the 17 patients in this study, but no recurrence has been associated with local destructive behavior.

D.J. Dabbs, M.D.

Differential Expression of the Intermediate Filament Peripherin in Cutaneous Neural Lesions and Neurotized Melanocytic Nevi

Prieto VG, McNutt NS, Lugo J, et al (Duke Univ, Durham, NC; New York Hosp)

Am J Surg Pathol 21:1450–1454, 1997 15–7

Introduction.—Peripherin is an intermediate filament involved in the growth and development of the peripheral nervous system. It is generated by neurons and the β cells of the islets of Langerhans. Some malignant melanomas and melanocytic nevi have recently demonstrated expression of peripherin. It is not known if Schwann cells, which are derived from the neural crest, express peripherin. A variety of cutaneous lesions that contain a proliferation of Schwann cells were analyzed for peripherin expression.

Methods.—Data were retrieved from archives and tissue blocks were recut so that all diagnoses could be confirmed on review. The diagnoses included 26 neurofibromas (NF), 10 schwannomas (SCH), 7 granular cell tumors, and 5 palisaded encapsulated neuromas (PEN). Thirteen neurotized melanocytic nevi (NMN) were also assessed because they contain Wagner-Meissner like structures and type C nevus cells that exhibit a "schwannian" phenotype.

Results.—Peripherin was observed only within elongated cell processes corresponding to axons in both normal cutaneous nerves and in nerves associated with the lesions. Numerous axons were seen throughout the lesions in NF and PEN. In NF, axons were concentrated near the periphery of lesions, compared to an even distribution of PEN axons. Only rare axons were immunolabeled in SCH, and predominantly at the periphery of lesions. Only nerves were observed within the lesions in granular cell tumors. Peripherin was expressed only by axons in NF, PEN, SCH, and granular cell tumors. Expression of peripherin was absent or restricted to rare scattered epithelioid melanoma, located in the superficial portion of the lesion, in most NMN. Most nevus cells, including the deep areas with the Wagner-Meissnerlike processes or type C cells, were not labeled. Numerous axons were seen in the Wagner-Meissnerlike areas. Elongated cell processes in cutaneous nerves were immunolabeled in skin next to lesions. Immunoreactive cells were not detected in the epidermis or adnexae, so keratinocytes, normal resting adult melanocytes, Merkel cells, and Langerhans cells did not express peripherin.

Conclusion.—Analysis of peripherin expression may be helpful in the differential diagnosis of NR, PEN, SCH, and NMN.

▶ Add peripherin to the family of intermediate filaments. The family consists of cytokeratins, vimentin, glial fibrillary acidic protein, the neural filaments, and now peripherin. With a molecular weight of 56 kd, peripherin is recognized as derived from the neural tube and neural crest, and as present in neurons as well as the β cells of the islets of Langerhans. While the function of these intermediate filaments is unknown, it is speculated that they may be useful, at least in part, in the regeneration of axonal processes. There appears to be a peripherin dynamic, with peripherin variably staining melanocytes within nevi, and disappearing in the neurotized deeper portions of nevi. Like glial fibrillary acidic protein, peripherin does not decorate Schwann cells, although it does a wonderful job of decorating neurons and axonal processes.

D.J. Dabbs, M.D.

Primary Metaplastic Carcinoma (Carcinosarcoma) of the Skin: A Clinicopathologic Study of Four Cases and Review of the Literature

Patel NK, McKee PH, Smith NP, et al (St John's Inst of Dermatology, London; Harvard Med School, Boston)

Am J Dermatopathol 19:363–372, 1997 15–8

Introduction.—Metaplastic carcinoma is a relatively uncommon tumor, composed of malignant epithelial and mesenchymal elements, which has been found in a variety of organs, including the uterus, ovary, lung, bladder, breast, and larynx. It is rarely found on the skin, but all cutaneous metaplastic carcinomas have malignant sweat gland or adnexal tumors as the epithelial component. Four patients with these exceedingly rare skin tumors are described.

Methods.—Four patients had cutaneous metaplastic carcinoma, and 3 cases developed in association with squamous cell carcinoma. One patient had an eccrine porocarcinoma. The clinical features, histology, and role of immunocytochemistry were recorded. A 71-year-old man had an ulcerate lesion, which was excised, on the upper right eyelid. A 74-year-old man had a solitary ulcerated lesion, which was excised on the scalp, and the patient had postoperative radiotherapy, with no recurrence 19 months later. An 83-year-old man had a scalp tumor which was excised. There was no adjuvant therapy, and he died of unrelated causes 20 months later. A 67-year-old man had a smooth reddish nodule, which was excised, on the right side of his nose. He had adjuvant radiotherapy, and 2 months later a 5-mm nodule, which was a benign epithelial inclusion cyst, developed. After 16 months of follow-up, there was no evidence of recurrence.

Results.—Malignant osteosarcoma, chondrosarcoma, leiomyosarcoma, and rhabdomyosarcomas were the heterologous malignant mesenchymal elements. Metaplastic carcinomas arising in the skin do not appear to have a very aggressive manner, in contrast to metaplastic carcinomas arising in visceral sites. In the skin the recurrence rate is 22%, the metastasis rate is 22%, and the overall mortality is 11%. However, the number of patients studied was very small and the follow-up period was short.

Conclusion.—In view of the possible histogenesis of these tumors, "metaplastic carcinoma," rather than "carcinosarcoma," should be used as the appropriate term to describe these very rare cutaneous neoplasms.

▶ You are familiar with the terms "carcinosarcoma," "malignant mixed tumor," and "metaplastic carcinoma," but "metaplastic carcinoma" is the preferred term for the group of neoplasms that we recognize as having both epithelial and mesenchymal differentiation. Yes, they occur primarily in the skin, as described in this article, which adds 4 cases to the English literature. These cases, primary in the skin, are obviously very rare, but have a morphologic fellowship with other tumors, occurring in the uterus, ovary, lung, bladder, breast, and larynx. In each of these cutaneous cases, the malignant mesenchymal components were in continuity with adnexal carcinomas of different types, and the mesenchymal components included undifferentiated spindle cell sarcomas, chondroid and osteoid differentiation, osteoclast-like giant cells, and skeletal muscle as well as smooth muscle. Only neural differentiation was not observed. This panoply of morphologic findings, of course, is characteristic for these tumors when they occur primarily in the uterus. Unlike the mortality with tumors at other sites, the mortality has been low, although follow-up is somewhat less than optimal in this small series of cases. Nevertheless, it would always be prudent to exclude a metastasis to the skin from 1 of the other more common sites. A key point of recognition would be the underlying adnexal carcinoma.

D.J. Dabbs, M.D.

Suggested Reading

Wick MR, Fitzgibbon J, Swanson PE: Cutaneous sarcomas and sarcomatoid neoplasms of the skin. *Semin Diagn Pathol* 10:148–158, 1993.

The Differential Diagnosis of Pagetoid Cells in the Epidermis

Kohler S, Rouse RV, Smoller BR (Stanford Univ, Calif)

Mod Pathol 11:79–92, 1998 15–9

Introduction.—Paget's cells show glandular differentiation on the basis of histochemical, immunophenotypic, and ultrastructural studies. There is a wide and varied differential diagnosis for intraepidermal pagetoid cells,

TABLE 1.—The Differential Diagnosis of Intraepidermal Pagetoid Cells

Mammary Paget's disease
Extramammary Paget's disease
Pagetoid squamous cell carcinoma *in situ*
Superficial spreading malignant melanoma
Pagetoid Spitz nevus
Clear cells of Toker
Pagetoid dyskeratosis
Clear cell papulosis
Sebaceous carcinoma
Merkel cell carcinoma with pagetoid intraepidermal spread
Eccrine porocarcinoma
Cutaneous T-cell lymphoma
Histiocytosis X
Langerhans' cell microabscess
Epidermotropic metastasis

(Courtesy of Kohler S, Rouse RV, Smoller BR: The differential diagnosis of pagetoid cells in the epidermis. *Mod Pathol* 11[1]:79–92, 1998.)

because cells of epithelial, melanocytic, neuroendocrine, lymphoid, and histiocytic differentiation can all show pagetoid spread (Table 1). Clinical correlation and immunophenotypic studies are required for accurate diagnosis. The clinical, histopathologic, and immunophenotypic features of Paget's disease and lesions that can give to rise to intraepidermal pagetoid cells are summarized.

Mammary Paget's Disease.—An eczematous eruption of the nipple and/or areola is the clinical presentation of mammary Paget's disease, which is often accompanied by pain or pruritus. Paget's disease will develop in up to 4% of female patients with breast carcinoma. Neoplastic cells with large nuclei, prominent nucleoli, and abundant pale-to-amphophilic cytoplasm scattered throughout the entire epidermal thickness are the histologic characteristics of mammary Paget's disease. Pagetoid squamous cell carcinoma in situ, superficial spreading malignant melanoma in situ, and clear cells of Toker are the histologic differential diagnosis of mammary Paget's disease. The distinction among these 3 entities is usually readily achieved with mucin stain and immunophenotyping (Table 2).

Other Diseases.—Other diseases include extramammary Paget's disease, which is initially seen as a nonhealing, well-circumscribed, erythematous-to-gray-white plaque; pagetoid squamous cell carcinoma in situ, seen as well-demarcated erythematous plaque that is characteristically located on sun-exposed skin; superficial malignant melanoma, which has pagetoid upward scatter and is the most common form of melanoma, accounting for about 80% of cases; pagetoid Spitz nevus noted as a pigmented macule measuring less than 0.5 cm; clear cells of Toker, which are smaller than Paget's cells but larger than adjacent keratinocytes; pagetoid dyskeratosis, with cells that are most frequently located suprabasally and extend as high as the stratum corneum; clear cell papulosis; sebaceous carcinoma; Merkel cell carcinoma with pagetoid intraepidermal spread;

TABLE 2.—Pagetoid Neoplasms of the Skin: Immunophenotypic Features

Diagnosis	EMA	CEA	S100	AE1/AE3	CAM5.2	GCDFP-15	LCA	CD3
Mammary Paget's disease	++	+	+/−	++	++	+	−	−
Extramammary Paget's disease	++	++	−	+	+	+	−	−
Squamous cell carcinoma	++	−	−	++	−	−	−	−
Melanoma/Spitz nevus	−*	+/−	++	−	−*	−	−	−
Clear cells of Toker	+/−	ND	−	ND	+	ND	ND	ND
Pagetoid dyskertosis	ND	−	−	+	ND	ND	ND	ND
Clear cell papulosis	++	++	−	++	ND	++	ND	ND
Sebaceous carcinoma	++†	−	−	++	ND	−	−	−
Merkel cell carcinoma	++	−	−	++‡	++‡	ND	−	−
Eccrine porocarcinoma	++	−§	−	++	++	−	−	−
Cutaneous T-cell lymphoma	+/−	−	−	−	−	−	++	++
Histiocytosis X	−	−	++	−	−	−	+	−

*Some series report as much as 10% reactivity.
†Microvacuolar cytoplasmic staining.
‡Paranuclear dotlike stain.
§Highlights ductal lumina.
Abbreviations: CEA, carcinoembryonic antigen; *EMA*, epithelial membrane antigen; *LCA*, leukocyte common antigen; *ND*, not determined; ++, 80% to 100% positive staining; +, 50% to 80% positive staining; +/−, 10% to 50% positive staining; =, no staining or just focal and weak.
(Courtesy of Kohler S, Rouse RV, Smoller BR: The differential diagnosis of pagetoid cells in the epidermis. *Mod Pathol* 11[1]:79–92, 1998.)

eccrine porocarcinoma; cutaneous T-cell lymphoma; histiocytosis X; Langerhans' cell microabscess; and epidermotropic metastasis.

Conclusion.—The presence of discrete non-Malpighian or abnormal Malpighian cells, occurring singly or in nests within the epidermis, is the common denominator of these diseases. Pagetoid cells can represent the only histologic change, as in pagetoid squamous cell carcinoma in situ or superficial spreading malignant melanoma in situ. Pagetoid cells can also be an expression of an associated dermal or internal malignancy.

▶ This is a superb review article on the morphologic and immunohistochemical differential diagnostic features of pagetoid cells in the epidermis. Table 1 shows the differential diagnosis of intraepidermal pagetoid cells, while Table 2 shows the immunocytochemical reagents that are helpful in making the appropriate distinctions. These 2 tables alone are very handy to keep at your side.

D.J. Dabbs, M.D.

Primary Cutaneous Ewing's Sarcoma: Immunophenotypic and Molecular Cytogenetic Evaluation of Five Cases

Hasegawa SL, Davison JM, Rutten A, et al (Brigham & Women's Hosp, Boston; Harvard Med School, Boston; Dermatohistopathologisches Gemeinschaftslabor, Friedrichshafen, Germany)

Am J Surg Pathol 22:310–318, 1998 15–10

Introduction.—Small blue cell tumors of the skin are rare in children and young adults and typically encompass either primary neuroendocrine, adnexal, melanocytic, or lymphoproliferative tumors, and include metastatic spread from neuroblastoma or small cell carcinoma. Most extraosseous Ewing's sarcoma (ES)/malignant primitive neuroectodermal tumor (MPNET) are found in the deep soft tissues of the paraspinal region, chest wall, or lower extremities. Primary cutaneous ES/MPNET is rare and has been reported primarily in the dermatologic literature. A series of 5 patients with extraskeletal ES/MPNET occurring as primary neoplasms in the superficial dermis was described.

Methods.—Four-micrometer thick sections were prepared from formalin-fixed, paraffin-embedded archival tissue from 5 patients with ES/MPNET who had a solitary dermal node in the lower extremities. Immunohistochemical stains and fluorescence in situ hybridization (FISH) were performed.

Results.—The age range of 4 females and 1 male patient was 8–50 years (median, 18 years). All tumors appeared as raised, usually painless superficial nodules. Disease was polypoid in 3 patients. All tumors were made up of nodular proliferations of monomorphous, small blue cells with round, vesicular nuclei and scant-to-moderate cytoplasm immunoreactive for the CD99 cell surface glycoprotein in a characteristic membranous pattern. One tumor was not able to be evaluated by FISH. Three of 4 tumors were positive for a chromosomal translocation involving the *EWS* locus at 22q12 observed in greater than 90% of ES/MPNET cases. All patients underwent local excision, and 2 received postoperative chemotherapy and radiotherapy. At a median follow-up of 33 months, no patients had evidence of local recurrence or metastases.

Conclusions.—Extraskeletal ES/MPNET may occur infrequently in cutaneous locations and seem to be associated with a favorable outcome. Even though unlikely, diagnosis of extraskeletal ES/MPNET should be considered when a primary cutaneous small blue cell tumor is found.

▶ Pathologists beware of the small blue cell tumor of skin. In this paper, the authors describe in detail 5 cases of ES/MPNET occurring as primary cutaneous malignant neoplasms. The cases are documented immunohistochemically and by FISH. Superficial locations originally described by Angervall and Enzinger, included the forearm, hip, and plantar surface of the foot as primary ES/MPNET. Obviously this occurrence is distinctly uncommon but should add to the pathologists differential diagnosis of small blue cell tumors of the dermis/subcutaneous tissue. The age range may be broad, including children or adults, and a differential diagnosis to consider includes Merkel cell carcinoma, metastatic small cell carcinoma, adnexal tumors such as eccrine spiradenoma, malignant melanoma, and metastatic neuroblastoma. These tumors can be differentiated from each other by a panel of immunohistochemical antibodies; however, the CD-99 antibody should not be relied on completely because CD-99 can be seen in a wide variety of tumors and is not specific for ES/MPNET. It is important to correlate carefully the entire clinical picture for small cell tumors of the skin. The diagnosis of small cell tumors of skin may need to be substantiated by molecular methods.

D.J. Dabbs, M.D.

16 Pathology Outcomes Analysis

Interinstitutional Comparison of Frozen Section Turnaround Time: A College of American Pathologists Q-Probes Study of 32 868 Frozen Sections in 700 Hospitals

Novis DA, Zarbo RJ (Wentworth-Douglas Hosp, Dover, NH; Henry Ford Hosp, Detroit)

Arch Pathol Lab Med 121:559–567, 1997 16–1

Objective.—The Q-Probes Study was initiated to establish a frozen section (FS) turnaround time (TAT) and to determine what variables affect TAT.

Methods.—From June to October 1995, information on 32,868 FS from elective surgery patients was provided by 700 hospitals in North America, Australia, New Zealand, the United Kingdom, Hong Kong, Mexico, and Norway. Pathologists completed a questionnaire about their practice characteristics. Aggregate 90% and institutional FS block completion times (the number of minutes for the fastest 90% of all FS blocks to be completed and results communicated) and outlier FS block TAT were determined, benchmarks were established, and TAT performance was evaluated.

Results.—Fifty percent of all FS blocks were completed within 10 minutes, 75% within 15 minutes, and 90% within 20 minutes. The 8.3% (2,728) FS outliers occurred mainly in large hospitals or in small hospitals. FS TAT was more likely to exceed the 20-minute outlier threshold when more than 1 pathologist was involved, when medical students and residents were involved, when the pathologist received other samples for FS, when the pathologist could not make a diagnosis, or when technical problems interfered with processing. The institutional 90% completion times were shorter for hospitals with 300 or fewer occupied beds than for hospitals with more than 300 occupied beds.

Conclusions.—The data show that 90% of FS can be prepared and results reported within 20 minutes.

► Although it is important to know the ideal FS TAT, I think more important questions to ask are: Why do we do so many FSs in the first place, and when does FS TAT matter? The concept of a low TAT should matter only in specific situations, such as one in which a low TAT improves a specific patient outcome (and I include a low cost as a good patient outcome). I do not intend to bash the study by Novis and Zarbo because it is another good Q-probes assessment of how multiple institutions behave. I think it is a good starting point to measure other important issues in the area of FS. For example, in the Novis and Zarbo study, why were 16.7% of all FSs (the second-highest number next to skin) performed on breast material? How were these breast FSs affecting patient care? I think that breast FSs should rarely be performed. In addition, could touch preparations lower intraoperative consultation TAT and replace the FS? Do surgeons really need to have a FS completed in 20 minutes? Are low FS TATs associated with more error? Even though we know how many institutions behave, it does not mean that we should behave similarly, particularly if the behavior is dysfunctional.

S.S. Raab, M.D.

Amended Reports in Surgical Pathology and Implications for Diagnostic Error Detection and Avoidance: A College of American Pathologists Q-Probes Study of 1 667 547 Accessioned Cases in 359 Laboratories

Nakhleh RE, Zarbo RJ (Henry Ford Hosp, Detroit)

Arch Pathol Lab Med 122:303–309, 1998 16–2

Background.—The College of American Pathologists sponsored this Q-Probes study to examine the rates and types of amendments to surgical pathology reports. The influence of error detection methods on error rate was also examined.

Study Design.—The study participants consisted of 359 laboratories, 96% in the United States, who participated in the Q-Probes quality improvement program from February to June 1966. Laboratories documented amended reports involving patient misidentification, final diagnosis errors, preliminary diagnosis errors, and other diagnostic errors that would have a significant effect on patient management or prognosis. Laboratories also documented the method of error detection. Each laboratory participated for 5 months or 50 amended reports. Each laboratory also completed a questionnaire on practice and policy related to amended reports.

Findings.—During the study period there were 1,667,547 surgical pathology specimens accessioned at the 359 participating laboratories. Of these, there were 3,147 amended reports, for an aggregate mean amended report rate of 1.9 per 1,000 cases. Among these errors, 19.2% were patient identification errors, 38.7% were final diagnosis changes, 15.6% were preliminary diagnosis changes, and 26.5% were changes in other clinically significant information. The most common method of error detection followed a request from a clinician to review a case (Table 4). A higher amended report rate was associated with a routine diagnostic slide review performed after completion of the pathology report. The lowest rate was

TABLE 4.—How Errors Were Actually Detected

Means of Error Detection	Frequency of All Amended Reports, n (%)	Patient ID Errors (%)	Original DX Changes (%)	Preliminary DX Changes (%)	Other DX Changes (%)
Following additional clinical information	277 (8.7)	8.85	10.28	5.07	8.58
Clinician requested review of case	649 (20.5)	18.85	20.07	2.64	32.66
During slide review of all malignancies	16 (0.5)	0.16	0.49	0.20	0.95
During slide review of set percentage of cases	118 (3.7)	0.66	5.87	0.61	4.65
During slide review of all cases	22 (0.7)	0.16	1.31	0.41	0.36
During slide review of cases for conference	111 (3.5)	0.49	3.43	0.41	7.39
Following intradepartmental consultation	182 (5.7)	0.98	8.65	3.45	6.32
Following extradepartmental review, requested by you	512 (16.1)	0.82	16.39	50.51	6.67
Following review at another institution for follow-up care	58 (1.8)	0.82	1.71	2.64	2.26
Following review at another institution for tumor registry	2 (0.1)	0.00	0.08	0.20	0.00
Following review of text (not slides) in report	309 (9.7)	22.13	6.44	4.46	8.70
Following review of special stains, decals, or other studies	403 (12.7)	0.00	14.03	25.56	12.51
Error detected by chance	82 (2.6)	10.49	0.82	0.61	0.60
Don't know	103 (3.2)	3.28	4.40	1.22	2.74
Other	293 (9.2)	31.48	4.49	1.01	4.89
Multiple methods of detection	35 (1.1)	0.82	1.55	1.01	0.72

Abbreviations: ID, identification; *DX*, diagnostic.

(Courtesy of Nakhleh RE, Zarbo RJ: Amended reports in surgical pathology and implications for diagnostic error detection and avoidance: A College of American Pathologists Q-Probes study of 1 667 547 Accessioned Cases in 359 Laboratories. *Arch Pathol Lab Med* 122:303–309, 1998.)

associated with institutions that had routine diagnostic slide review performed before completion of the pathology report.

Conclusions.—A large study of more than 1.6 million accessioned surgical pathology reports was conducted to determine the amended report rate. The median laboratory produces 1.46 amended reports per 1,000 cases. There was an association between a lower amended report rate and routine diagnostic slide review before the completion of the pathology report.

► In this Q-Probe study, Nakhleh and Zarbo measure surgical pathology laboratory amended report rates and attempt to correlate these rates with laboratory "errors." In my opinion, not all amended reports represent errors, and for those that do represent errors, the significance of those errors is uncertain. In addition, by measuring amended report rates, the level at which an error occurred is uncertain (e.g., if the error resulted from patient identification, this error could have occurred before the tissue even reached the pathology laboratory; by a physician assistant or pathologist in the gross room; or by a computer glitch). Knowing where the error occurred is important in fixing the problem (or at least in assigning blame!). Of the amended report types included in the analysis, one type was an amended report to a change in diagnosis, secondary to a special stain (e.g., a Gomori methenamine silver stain showing fungi). I hardly think this counts as a diagnostic error, because in my practice I often issue a preliminary report with a statement that the diagnosis may change after other stains or material are examined. This is an issue of turnaround time, not error.

Nonetheless, despite some drawbacks, this manuscript makes for an interesting read and presents lots of data. The authors systematically present amended error report rates, how "errors" were detected (more than 20% of amended reports resulted from a clinician requesting review; see Table 4), and how changes in reports were communicated to the clinicians. It would be great to see a follow-up study on how patient management was affected by an amended report.

S.S. Raab, M.D.

A Questionnaire-based Survey of Errors in Diagnostic Histopathology Throughout the United Kingdom

Furness PN, Lauder I (Univ of Leicester, England)

J Clin Pathol 50:457–460, 1997 16–3

Objective.—Results of error studies in diagnostic histopathology have varied widely, and none have addressed the circumstances under which the errors have occurred. A questionnaire was sent to all consultant histopathologists in the United Kingdom identified in the *Handbook of the Royal College of Pathologists* to provide information for use in designing a definitive study.

Methods.—Responses were anonymous. The responder was to provide a description of the mistake and the circumstances surrounding it.

Results.—There were 202 (19.8%) of 1,021 questionnaires returned. There were 169 (17.1%) completed responses. A total of 244 errors were reported by 119 pathologists, 183 errors (75%) involved small diagnostic biopsies, and 61 (25%) involved therapeutic resections. Fifty-one errors (21%) were made in teaching hospitals, 234 (96%) had the potential to change management, 102 (42%) did change management, and 173 (71%) represented a benign/malignant error. Most pathologists blamed human error or excessive workload for the errors. Most errors were made with gastrointestinal tract, skin, breast, gynecologic, and lymph node specimens. Most errors were made by locum consultant pathologists.

Conclusions.—This potentially biased study indicated that a pathologist is aware of making approximately 1 serious error a year. A larger, significantly more expensive study would appear to be desirable in light of these results.

▶ In the aviation industry, how many airplane crashes per year are permissible? How much passenger baggage may be lost or mangled before we stop flying that airline because of baggage handling "error"? Mistakes occur in every industry and ours is no exception. Despite instituting a number of quality control measures (particularly in cytology), errors still occur and there really has been no effort to establish national practice guidelines or serious investigation to monitor surgical pathology errors and their effects. Is it that to do so puts us too far "out there" and it is better to leave errors concealed? We need to move beyond the interobserver variability and investigate the meaning of differences in opinion and failures.

In the surgical pathology "error" literature, there have been studies about peer review and consensus conference error rates,[1, 2] but this United Kingdom study attempted to measure surgical pathology error by a survey method. Albeit highly anecdotal, and exhibiting a horrible participant response rate, their data indicated pathologists commit a serious error approximately every year or 1 every 5,000 specimens. We need to further investigate the validity of these data, perform a much more rigorous statistical error analysis (as the authors advocate), and ask ourselves the tough question of how to monitor ourselves and what are acceptable error rates.

S.S. Raab, M.D.

References

1. Safrin RE, Bark CJ: Surgical pathology signout: Routine review of every case by a 2nd pathologist. *Am J Surg Pathol* 17:1190–1192, 1993.
2. Lind AC, Bewtra C, Healy JC, et al: Prospective peer review in surgical pathology. *Am J Clin Pathol* 104:560–566, 1995.

Pathology Slide Review in Gynecologic Oncology
Santoso JT, Coleman RL, Voet RL, et al (Univ of Texas, Dallas)
Obstet Gynecol 91:730–734, 1998 16–4

Background.—The importance of interinstitution pathology consultation was analyzed for gynecologic oncology patients.

Study Design.—All 720 interinstitutional gynecologic pathology consultations from 1987 through 1995 at a tertiary care hospital were reviewed. Discrepancies between original and consultant diagnoses were categorized as none, minor, and major. Major discrepancies were defined as diagnostic differences that altered clinical intervention. The cost of pathology review was calculated using a standard billing fee of $150 per case.

Findings.—Among these 720 specimens, there were no diagnostic discrepancies in 601, minor discrepancies in 104, and major discrepancies in 15 consultations (Table 2). After reviewing these 15 discrepancies, 6 surgeries were cancelled, 2 surgeries were modified, 1 adjuvant radiation treatment was added, 1 chemotherapy treatment was modified, and 5 adjuvant chemotherapy treatments were cancelled. There was no systematic error associated with either tissue type or method of obtaining the specimen. The total cost of consultation for all 720 specimens was $108,000. The cost/discrepancy was $720/discrepancy.

Conclusions.—This review of 720 inter-institution gynecologic pathology consultations demonstrated a 2% rate of diagnostic discrepancy significant to alter care. The cost per/discrepancy was $7200.

► It sits well with me that a group of gynecologists publishes (in the gynecologic literature) a report recommending that before treatment is initiated, patients who had their pathologic diagnoses elsewhere should have their slides reviewed "in house." This is not a cost-effectiveness study, but the authors conclude that costs of the pathologic review are outweighed by the value of the information gained. It's interesting that the gynecologists wrote that pathologic services are "globally expensive." I'm sure they view themselves as a bargain in comparison. At least Santoso and colleagues thought that our services are necessary, echoing reports detailing interinstitutional variation already in the literature.[1, 2] The 15 major discrepancies are reproduced here (see Table 2). I presume that the majority of cases with major discrepancies were from patients originally seen at smaller hospitals that were referred to the University of Texas Southwestern Medical Center. I wondered whether if some of the discrepancies could be explained by interobserver variability, rather than error. This would mean that other large university practices may agree with the original diagnoses! Also, the issue of who pays the costs of the review was not examined. Should the patients, gynecologic department, or pathology departments foot the bill?

S.S. Raab, M.D.

TABLE 2.—Patients With Major Diagnostic Differences That Altered Treatment

Patient #	Age (y)	Cancer site	Specimen type	Original diagnosis	Consultant diagnosis	Treatment alteration
1	31	Cervix	Cervical biopsy	Adenocarcinoma	Adenocarcinoma in situ	Surgery modified
2	22	Cervix	Cervical biopsy	CIN III	CIN I	Surgery cancelled
3	28	Ovary	TAH-BSO	Cystadeno-carcinoma grade 2	Low malignant potential	Adjuvant chemotherapy cancelled
4	70	Ovary	TAH-BSO	Adenocarcinoma	Granulosa cell tumor	Different chemotherapy
5	29	Ovary	TAH-BSO	Adenocarcinoma grade 2	Low malignant potential	Adjuvant chemotherapy cancelled
6	54	Ovary	TAH-BSO	Cystadeno-carcinoma	Low malignant potential	Adjuvant chemotherapy cancelled
7	34	Ovary	TAH-BSO	Adenocarcinoma	Low malignant potential	Adjuvant chemotherapy cancelled
8	67	Uterus	TAH-BSO	Stage IA, grade 1 adenocarcinoma	Stage IIB, grade 1 adenocarcinoma	Adjuvant radiation added
9	29	Uterus	Endometrial biopsy	Adenocarcinoma grade 1	Hyperplasia	Surgery cancelled
10	26	Uterus	Dilation and curettage	Choriocarcinoma	Hydatidiform mole	Adjuvant chemotherapy cancelled
11	67	Vagina	Vaginal biopsy	Focal squamous carcinoma	Squamous carcinoma in situ	Surgery cancelled
12	41	Vulva	Vulvar biopsy	VIN III	VIN I	Surgery cancelled
13	75	Vulva	Vulvar biopsy	VIN III	Hyperplastic dystrophy	Surgery cancelled
14	44	Vulva	Vulvar biopsy	VIN III	Hyperplastic dystrophy	Surgery cancelled
15	39	Vulva	Vulvar biopsy	Squamous carcinoma	VIN III	Surgery modified

Abbreviations: CIN, cervical intraepithelial neoplasia; *TAH-BSO*, total abdominal hysterectomy and bilateral salpingo-oopherectomy; *PSST*, placental site trophoblastic tumor; *VIN*, vulvar intraepithelial neoplasia.

(Courtesy of Santoso JT, Coleman RL, Voet RL, et al: Pathology slide review in gynecologic oncology. *Obstet Gynecol* 91:730–734, 1998. Reprinted with permission from the American College of Obstetricians and Gynecologists.)

References

1. Abt AB, Abt L, Olt GJ: The effect of interinstitution anatomic pathology consultation on patient care. *Arch Pathol Lab Med* 119:514–517, 1995.
2. Epstein JI, Walsh PC, Sanfilippo F: Clinical and cost impact of second-opinion pathology. *Am J Surg Pathol* 20:851–857, 1996.

A Survey of General Practitioners' Views on Autopsy Reports

Karunaratne S, Benbow EW (Univ of Manchester, England)
J Clin Pathol 50:548–552, 1997 16–5

Objective.—Attitudes of the public and of general practitioners underlie the decline in autopsy rates over the last decades. The opinions of general practitioners regarding the quality and utility of routine autopsy reports and of autopsies in general were evaluated at the Manchester Royal Infirmary.

Methods.—Between May 1 and October 30, 1995, autopsy reports sent routinely to general practitioners were accompanied by a questionnaire that solicited opinions on the content and quality of the reports.

Results.—Of the 395 autopsy reports, 256 were on patients who died in the community, 129 were on patients who had died in the hospital, and 10 were clinical interest autopsies. There were 135 (34.2%) usable questionnaires returned. More than 93% of general practitioners found the reports useful, and 73.4% felt that the patient's family would also find the report useful. Almost 21% said the report was too long, and only 27.4% had discussed the report with the patient's relatives. More than 80% thought the circumstances of the patient's death were clearly summarized, and for 48.1% the report was the first indication of how the patient had died. The cause of death was a complete surprise to almost 20% of practitioners, and the patient's death was a complete surprise to 40.7%. The report was written in a helpful manner according to 91.8%, and only 5.3% complained about too much jargon. According to 88.6%, the autopsies revealed unsuspected pathologic processes, and 74.4% felt that without an autopsy their ability to monitor standards of clinical practice would be severely impaired. More than 31% felt that autopsies were unpleasant procedures, and 11.3% believed that autopsies were unacceptable mutilations of a human being.

Conclusions.—General practitioners were overwhelmingly appreciative of autopsy reports and believed that the loss of the reports would impair their ability to monitor standards of clinical practice.

► There have been several reports similar to this one[1-3] that have measured clinicians' views on the autopsy. This English study had a different method of investigation (sending out a questionnaire with each autopsy report) but came to the same conclusions. The majority of general practitioners who responded (34.2%) thought that autopsies were valuable and that the autopsy was an important means to monitor clinical standards.

There are several biases in this study that probably favored these pro-autopsy responses. First, those who did not respond may have considered that autopsies were unimportant and consequently a survey about autopsies also unimportant. Second, the questionnaires that accompanied autopsy reports generally were ordered by the coroner; this subpopulation of deaths might be expected to reveal more "relevant information," and there was no guarantee that the population of clinicians was a general sample.

It was interesting to note the range of opinions documented by the survey. For example, 12.8% of general practitioners strongly agreed that the autopsy was "a thoroughly unpleasant procedure," and a minority (4.5%) strongly agreed that the autopsy represents "unacceptable mutilation." If there truly is a general view that autopsies are useful, the next survey should be designed to discover why more autopsies are not ordered.

S.S. Raab, M.D.

References

1. McGoogan E, Cameron HM: Clinical attitudes to the autopsy. *Scott Med J* 23:19–22, 1978.
2. Cottreau C, McIntyre L, Favara BE. Professional attitudes toward the autopsy: Survey of clinicians and pathologists. *Am J Clin Pathol* 92:673–676, 1989.
3. Harris A, Ismail I, Dilly S, et al: Physicians' attitudes to the autopsy. *J R Coll Physicians Lond* 27:116–118, 1993.

Costing Pathology Services: A Practical Approach to a Difficult Problem

Bailey PE (Princess Alexandra Hosp, Wooloongabba, Australia)

Pathology 29:196–200, 1997 16–6

Objective.—Costing methods for pathology services aggregate individual test resources, requiring detailed cost information and a lot of time. A less time-consuming, more flexible model of costing pathology services was described.

Principles.—The top-down approach to costing accumulates total costs, based on basic assumptions, during a given period. Although it is quick and easy, it does not allow costing, and therefore comparison, of individual resources. The bottom-up approach, which costs each input, is dependent on detailed financial data but provides a means of comparing efficiencies. The process is time-consuming.

Procedures.—Investigations are grouped according to technology or methodology, and costs are allocated as accurately as possible. Each technology is assumed to have identical direct costs. The standard cost per WELCAN unit (1 minute of scientific, technical, pathology assistant, and clerical time) is calculated. Variable labor costs are distributed with variable A being nonmedical salaries, variable B being medical salaries, and variable C being pathology specimen collection department labor costs. All labor costs in each category are assumed to be identical. Variable consumable costs are also distributed as category A, B, or C depending on whether they are allocated to a specific technology or methodology, reagents or generic consumable, or consumables used in specimen collection. Fixed equipment, fixed direct labor, and fixed indirect labor costs are distributed. Indirect costs such as leased spaced and service costs are allocated.

Conclusions.—This model, although developed for costing pathology services, is transferable to other areas, and can be used to raise awareness of staff about the costs incurred in the work they do.

▶ Bailey provided an Australian "top down" WELCAN approach to pathology costing that could be applied in either the clinical or anatomical pathology laboratory. Costing pathology services is critical in today's environment, and even though the Australian medical system differs significantly from ours, there are advantages in recognizing how some Australian laboratories may cost analyze. One key to cost analysis is recognizing its import. Data from a laboratory cost analysis can be used to determine cost-effectiveness of laboratory services from either a patient, laboratory, or hospital perspective; where to allocate additional resources; how to compete; or how to adjust salary schedules. I recommend that you read some of the references for other views of costing non-American laboratory services.[1-3] Being able to perform cost analyses in different ways and knowing the advantages and disadvantages of different costing methods can only serve to strengthen your laboratory in the marketplace. Bailey's article is just one way of doing it, but one should know what others are doing.

S.S. Raab, M.D.

References

1. Dick H: Costing of pathology services in the United Kingdom National Health Service. *J Clin Pathol* 41:705–709, 1991.
2. Gozzard DI, Macaulay ME, Nuttall DS, et al: A pragmatist's approach to pathology costing: The data tree approach. *J Clin Pathol* 45:650–653, 1992.
3. Bernett L: A tree structure model for analyzing laboratory test costs. *Pathology* 23:172–176, 1991.

Use of Statistical Analysis of Cytologic Interpretation to Determine the Causes of Interobserver Disagreement and in Quality Improvement

Renshaw AA, Lee KR, Granter SR (Harvard Med School, Boston; Brigham & Women's Hosp, Boston)

Cancer 81:212–219, 1997 16–7

Objective.—Interobserver interpretation of cytologic specimens can differ because of differences in diagnostic threshold and diagnostic accuracy. The causes of diagnostic disagreement were distinguished and the sources of interobserver variability and differences in diagnostic accuracy were determined using the diagnosis of atypical squamous cells of undetermined significance (ASCUS) on Pap smears as a model.

Methods.—Eighty smears (74 with a diagnosis of ASCUS) with biopsy results within 90 days of smear collection were reviewed by 3 observers and classified as negative, negative and reactive, ASCUS favor reactive, ASCUS not otherwise specified, ASCUS suggestive of squamous intraepithelial lesion (SIL), low-grade SIL, or high-grade SIL. Classifications were compared with biopsy results and analyzed statistically.

Results.—There was complete agreement on only 11% of cases. Kappa values were 0.37 for observer 1 vs. 2, 0.21 for observer 1 vs. 3, and 0.15 for observer 2 vs. 3. Whereas observers 1 and 2 classified ASCUS with a sensitivity of 97%, specificities were only 23% and 15%. For observer 3, sensitivity and specificity values were 56% and 42%, respectively. When classifying SIL, sensitivities of the 3 observers were low, varying from 16% to 9%, whereas specificities ranged from 92% to 96%. These differences were the results of different selected thresholds along the receiver operating characteristic curve. Whereas observer 2 used the negative/ASCUS threshold to significantly increase sensitivity in predicting SIL on biopsy, observer 3 was significantly more specific for SIL. Observer accuracies were 0.66 for observer 1, 0.59 for observer 2, and 0.51 for observer 3. Whereas all observers were more accurate than chance at classifying cases, differences in agreement were the result of both different diagnostic thresholds and diagnostic accuracy.

Conclusions.—Differences in cytologic interpretation were the result of different diagnostic thresholds and diagnostic accuracy. This information may be used to improve quality of interpretation.

► Of course, pathologists may not all agree on the diagnosis even when they see the same fields on the same slide. This is particularly apparent in the area of cytology, which is thought to be more "subjective." In this study, Renshaw et al. have used several different statistical analyses to measure diagnostic variation in Papanicolaou smears. This article is not for the statistically faint of heart, but does provide insight in how we might track our diagnosis and our abilities using distribution, kappa, threshold, and receiver operating characteristic curve analyses. I think it is unrealistic to believe that most pathologists will want to do these analyses on their own data, without assistance. The development of computer programs that can easily perform these analyses is the next step. Then, we must decide on the meaning of these variations and what we want to do about them.

S.S. Raab, M.D.

Continuing Medical Education for Pathologists: An Evaluation of the Royal College of Pathologists' Wessex Pilot Scheme

du Boulay C (Southampton Gen Hosp, England)

J Clin Pathol 50:1022–1026, 1997 16–8

Objective.—The Royal College of Pathologists decided to replace the informal continuing medical education (CME) by providing formal and regular CME, and requiring members to collect 250 approved credits within 5 years. Wessex pathologists were invited to take part in a pilot program.

Methods.—Opinions of 103 participating pathologists were determined in a questionnaire about general issues about CME, paired peer review, and CME points. The questionnaire consisted of one-third attitudinal survey, one-third free comments, and one-third factual questions.

Results.—There were 64 responses received. Whereas 71% knew what their learning needs were, only 25% found it easy to keep up to date reading journals, and one third did not have time to go to meetings. About 50% felt it would not be easy to obtain funding for study leave. About 44% thought that College guidelines were unclear, and 35.5% strongly disagreed that CME credits would improve their practice. Approximately 85% believed that CME was academically oriented, and they wanted to see more practice-based CME. Responders wanted to see more local CME approved. Whereas 70% valued the peer review process, 66% were not able to achieve their annual learning goals. There were 68% of respondents who wanted to see an end to the paired peer review process. Responses were evenly distributed across specialties and showed good internal consistency. Free comments were consistent with answers to factual questions.

Conclusions.—Wessex pathologists view CME positively but want more individual input into content and location of CME.

► We all do things for CME credits, and this survey measures a United Kingdom viewpoint, which I don't think is different from the North American perspective. Although most find CME useful, there are considerable time and financial restraints that limit the ability of pathologists to attend national CME meetings or conferences. I believe there are several potential solutions. First, academic centers and entrepreneurs should provide CME courses for local pathologists, so that pathologists don't have to travel extensively. Second, we should use the Internet much more extensively than we do now for CME certification. If you are sick of traveling, check the Internet to find the education you may need.

S.S. Raab, M.D.

College of American Pathologists Foundation Conference VIII on Patient-centered Pathology Practice—Outcomes and Accountability: Overview, Glossary, and Bibliography

Vance RP, Elevitch FR (Wake Forest Univ, Winston-Salem, NC; Health Care Engineering, Palo Alto, Calif)

Arch Pathol Lab Med 121:1151–1162, 1997 16–9

Objective.—The conference focused on outcomes and accountability, the relationship of outcomes management in community hospital and private laboratory practice, and how traditional skills can relate to emerging roles of outcomes and accountability.

Outcomes and Accountability in Health Care.—Outcomes and accountability were linked to cost and quality. In the rush to control costs, quality has been neglected. The role of pathologists in evaluating outcomes needs to be measured in terms of the effects of diagnostic tests on health outcomes, a measure that, in the absence of randomized health outcome studies, is still primarily based on intuition. Presently the system cannot distinguish between bad data, poor statistical models, bad luck, or bad care. In the future, accreditation systems must be performance based. A new shared decision-making model should help pathologists begin to reform the health care system at the local level.

Pathologists in the Area of Outcomes Management.—Pathologists should design and conduct quality studies in the laboratory. Results should be delivered in a timely fashion and be available in an electronic format. Pathologists should lead the way toward a systematic approach because they understand how the overall care and support system works. Outcomes should be assessed while the patient is still in the hospital, and pathologists should be involved in patient management decisions. Outcomes management should assess the performance of a hospital or group of physicians relative to other hospitals or physicians, and relate staff size and mix and supply utilization to operational success. Problem solving should involve multidisciplinary groups.

Outcomes Management in Pathology Practice.—How outcomes management can be integrated into everyday pathologic practice was discussed for oncology, transfusion medicine, and microbiology and infectious disease.

Conclusions.—Outcomes management is a necessity for today's and tomorrow's health care system. Pathologists should be ready to assume their role in developing outcomes and accountability management systems. A glossary of outcomes terms was included.

▶ What is outcomes analysis and what is the role of the pathologist in this analysis? The Vance and Elevitch article and the 2 articles listed as references[1, 2] provide overviews from slightly different perspectives. The glossary of terms provided in the Vance and Elevitch article is particularly useful for those reading the outcomes literature. Outcomes analysis, these authors argue, is one of the main areas in which pathology will, or at least has the potential, to grow in the future. Although not stated, I would say that the other area is molecular diagnostics. If we do not participate in these outcomes studies ourselves, we should encourage others to do so, for they are our discipline's future. It has been said that pathology is the gatekeeper of the diagnosis, which drives so much of medicine; therefore, we should have more input on the how, where, and why these diagnoses affect patient care. Outcomes analysis allows us to do this.

S.S. Raab, M.D.

References

1. Vance RP: Outcomes management: New opportunities in a shrinking pathology market. *Arch Pathol Lab Med* 121:1183–1186, 1997.
2. Connelly DP, Aller RD: Outcomes and informatics. *Arch Pathol Lab Med* 121:1176–1182, 1997.

The Use of Digital Images in Pathology

Furness PN (Univ of Leicester, England)

J Pathol 183:253–263, 1997 16–10

Objective.—Despite the technologic advancements that have given rise to digital imaging, diagnostic histopathology still relies mainly on 2-dimensional images. Cost, quality, and limitations of digital technology were examined, and the basic elements of the technology were explained.

Technology.—Images exist as either vector diagrams (mathematically defined shapes) or bitmaps (2-dimensional images made up of dots or pixels). Images can be stored in a variety of different formats, most of which provide for file compression. Converting images from 1 format to another always results in loss of some data. Images can be acquired by video camera, framegrabber, which can convert video analog signals into a digital bitmap for storage by computer, digital camera, and scanner. Acquired images are manipulated by computer to balance color or adjust the image. Images are archived and output can be in electronic form or as hard copy.

Applications.—Digital images can be used in routine diagnostic practice, in teaching, and in telepathology in the absence of a pathologist, for obtaining expert opinions, and for external quality assessment. Advance modeling programs can stack 2-dimensional images to provide virtual 3-dimensional structures that can be rotated, viewed, and measured from any angle.

Conclusions.—The digital imaging age is here. As the technology becomes more affordable and more widely available, it can only enhance the performance of pathologists.

▶ Furness has written an excellent review article on the nitty gritty of digitalization in pathology and the basics of telepathology. Unfortunately, this article will be out of date when it appears in the YEAR BOOK. Nevertheless, if you'd like to read more about the pathology video world, read this article. As with any new technology, it is still uncertain where pathology will be moving with telepathology and how telepathology will affect us. My opinion is that education (through continuing medical education credits) will be influenced by telepathology, and ultimately, rapid consultations also will be affected.

S.S. Raab, M.D.

17 Pathology Techniques

Extension of Life-Span by Introduction of Telomerase Into Normal Human Cells

Bodnar AG, Ouellette M, Frolkis M, et al (Geron Corp, Menlo Park, Calif; Univ of Texas, Dallas)

Science 279:349–352, 1998 17–1

Introduction.—Normal human diploid cells placed in culture undergo a finite number of cell divisions before entering a nondivided state called replicative senescence, which is characterized by altered gene expression. Replicative senescence depends on cumulative cell divisions rather than chronologic or metabolic time. Decreased proliferative capacity of cells from old donors and patients with premature aging syndromes together with the accumulation in vivo of senescent cells with altered patterns of gene expression implicate cellular senescence in the aging process and age-related diseases. It is suspected that telomere shortening triggers senescence. Two telomerase-negative normal human cell types, retinal pigment epithelial cells and foreskin fibroblasts, were transfected with vectors encoding the human telomerase catalytic subunit to determine if telomerase expression increases cell life span.

Findings.—It was demonstrated earlier that telomerase-negative control clones exhibit telomere shortening and senescence. In this experiment, telomerase-expressing clones had elongated telomeres that divided vigorously and showed decreased staining for β-galactosidase, a biomarker for senescence. The telomerase-expressing clones had a normal karyotype and exceeded their normal life span by 20 or more doublings.

Conclusion.—There may be a causal relationship between telomere shortening and in vitro cellular senescence. This ability to maintain normal human cells in a phenotypically youthful state may have important applications for research and medicine.

▶ Telomeres are tandemly repeated sequences of (TTAGGG)n, and are found at the end of chromosomes. These sequences are synthesized by a specific ribonucleoprotein, telomerase, which can be assayed using a relatively straightforward PCR-based assay. At least 1 commercial kit is on the market (Oncor). The importance of telomeres and telomerase is an evolving area but it is already clear that they play a fundamental role in senescence.[1] Briefly, it has been hypothesized that telomere shortening leads to senescence via a decrease in proliferation. This article is an important advance in the field because it provides experimental proof for this proposal. Telomerase-negative cell lines were transfected with catalytically active telomerase, and these cell lines had elongated telomeres and actively divided. This finding clearly has broad and significant implications. As pointed out by the authors, the ability may exist to rejuvenate cells. With respect to cancer research, where it has generally been found that cancer cells do not show the normal pattern of telomere shortening, the implication is that telomerase regulation may play an important role in tumor progression. The cancer literature already contains a number of articles that have analyzed telomerase activity in a variety of tumors. It is likely that this will now increase exponentially.

M.B Cohen, M.D.

Reference

1. DeLange T: Telomeres and senescence: Ending the debate. *Science* 279:334–335, 1998.
▶ This reference is the accompanying commentary to this article and provides a very useful introduction to its background and significance.

Deficient Colour Vision and Interpretation of Histopathology Slides: Cross Sectional Study

Poole CJM, Hill DJ, Christie JL, et al (Central Clinic, Dudley, England; Russells Hall Hosp, Dudley, England; City Univ, London)

BMJ 315:1279–1281, 1997 17–2

Introduction.—A variety of colored stains are used by histopathologists in making diagnoses. The additional information provided by color is superfluous in some situations and diagnosis may be made by pattern recognition within a clinical context. Many stains use combinations of pigment, which could be challenging to read for persons with congenital red-green color deficiency (prevalence: 8% males, 0.5% females). If accurate color discrimination is important to the diagnostic process, it is crucial to guide physicians with color-deficient vision to avoid particular stains and techniques that could be problematic. Two hundred seventy male histopathologists and medical laboratory scientific officers from 45 hospitals in the United Kingdom were evaluated to determine if deficient color vision affects accuracy of slide interpretation.

Methods.—Transparencies of specific features obtained from slides rather than the slides themselves were used to standardize observation and ensure that each participant saw the same features. The slides were in pairs consisting of a true and false answer. Each slide correctly identified was worth ½ a point, and subjects were marked on a maximum of 10 points.

The number of slide-pairs correctly identified were noted. The Ishihara, City University, and Farnsworth-Munsell 100 hue tests were used to test color vision.

Results.—Of 132 physicians, 15 (13%) had color deficient vision; 13 (10%) of 138 scientific officers were color deficient. Mean length of time in histopathology was 16.9 years for participants with color-deficient vision and 17.0 years for those with normal vision. Using 10 slide-pairs, the mean score for participants with normal vision was 9.6; for those with color-deficient vision, the mean score was 8.6. The difference was highly significant. Mean scores for physicians with normal and deficient color vision were 9.9 versus 9.4, respectively, a significant difference; for scientific officers, scores were also significantly different—9.4 versus 7.5, respectively. Participants with color-deficient vision were categorized as having mild, moderate, or severe deficiency. There was a significant trend for those with severe color deficiency to make more mistakes.

Conclusion.—Histopathologists and medical laboratory scientific officers must be evaluated for deficiencies in color vision. Those with severe protan or deutan deficiency need to adopt a safe system of working.

▶ In this somewhat unusual study, the authors attempted to objectively determine whether surgical pathologists who are "color blind" make more errors than those who are not. Participants were asked to examine 20 projected 35-mm slides, not glass slides under the microscope; they were by and large special stains. Their results indicate that there was a direct correlation with the degree of color vision deficiency and the numbers of errors. In addition, they recommended testing of medical students and others to aid them in making career decisions. It is hard to really know the validity of these findings. I, and others, certainly know excellent diagnostic, but visually color challenged, diagnostic pathologists. This study reminds me of another published by Berbaum and Platz.[1] In their study a form of the Facial Recognition test was administered to pathology residents. The results correlated well with overall faculty ratings of the resident but poorly with the ASCP in service examination. In summary, ancillary tools, such as identified in these 2 studies, may be useful in helping medical students and residents identify appropriate specialties.

M.B. Cohen, M.D.

Reference

1. Berbaum KS, Platz C: Perception testing in surgical pathology. *Hum Pathol* 19:1127–1131, 1988.

The Effect of Decalcification on In Situ Hybridization

Arber JM, Weiss LM, Chang KL, et al (City of Hope Natl Med Ctr, Duarte, Calif)

Mod Pathol 10:1009–1014, 1997 17–3

Introduction.—The detection of DNA and RNA nucleic acid sequences by in situ hybridization (ISH) has been diagnostically useful in detecting viral genomes and mRNAs, such as immunoglobulin light chains. Air-dried cellular smears or paraffin-embedded tissues may be used to perform ISH. Reduced mRNA detection by ISH has been demonstrated when tissues are decalcified in prepared solutions containing nitric and formic acids. The effect of 3 commercially available decalcifying agents on the ability of ISH to detect mRNA was assessed in 25 non-neoplastic and neoplastic paraffin-embedded tissues.

Methods.—A poly d(T) oligonucleotide probe was used to assess the efficacy of ISH on decalcified tissue samples. The decalcifying agents included 1 EDTA-based solution (Versenate) and 2 hydrochloric acid-based solutions (S/P Decal, RBD). The tissues were fixed in formalin for 6, 24, and 72 hours, respectively, before decalcification. The outcome of ISH performed on decalcified tissues was compared with that of nondecalcified control tissues. A numeric system was used to score tissues: 0, negative; 4, strong positivity equal to control; 5, stronger than control.

Results.—Reactivity was usually excellent, when using Versenate (mean 4.15); good, with S/P Decal (mean, 3.17); and fair-to-poor, with RBD (mean, 1.69). The result was not affected by length of time in formalin.

Conclusion.—Decalcification was not contraindicated when performing ISH. The S/P Decal and RBD hydrochloric acid-based solutions may yield accurate results but they could also produce false-negative results. Versenate produces good-to-excellent results and is recommended as the decalcification agent of choice in tissues undergoing ISH.

► Molecular biological techniques are being used with increasing frequency by anatomic pathologists both for research but now also for clinical activities. Among these is ISH, which is typically used to assess the level and localization of mRNA expression in tissue sections. Most of its use has been related to the identification of viral transcripts, particularly HPV (human papilloma virus). The procedure is long and fraught with technical pitfalls. In this article, the pathology group from the City of Hope, has investigated the effect of various decalcification procedures ("gentle": EDTA and "harsh": HCl-based). A single oligonucleotide probe was tested on 25 different tissues after formalin fixation (3 times) and decalcification. The results indicate that (1) the length of formalin fixation did not affect detection, and (2) that certain commercially available decalcifying products did affect reactivity, for example, RBD, whereas others, that is, the EDTA-based Versenate and S/P Decal, did not.

M.B. Cohen, M.D.

Tissue Preparation for Immunocytochemistry

Williams JH, Mepham BL, Wright DH (Southampton Gen Hosp, England)

J Clin Pathol 50:422–428, 1997 17–4

Introduction.—The most frequent causes of poor immunostaining in paraffin wax-embedded tissue are not a result of the technique itself, but instead are the result of alteration of the antigenic sites by the initial process of tissue preparation, including fixation, processing, and the preparation of the tissue sections. Establishing a tissue preparation schedule for optimal immunostaining has been challenging ever since the start of immunocytochemical staining of paraffin-embedded tissue. The effect of all aspects of tissue preparation on subsequent immunostaining was assessed to determine a standard tissue preparation schedule that could allow optimal staining of all antigens.

Methods.—Blocks of fresh tonsil tissues were subjected in a number of variations to standard fixation, processing, and section preparation. Each block underwent variation of only 1 of 3 components of tissue preparation, and the other 2 components remained standard. Five antibodies were used for staining using the streptavidin-biotin immunostaining technique: L26 (CD20), UCHL1 (CD45RO), CD3, vimentin, and anti-kappa light chain. When weak staining resulted with antibodies not usually requiring heat retrieval, staining was repeated using microwave pretreatment. Stained sections were examined and rated independently by 2 investigators.

Results.—Fixation factors affecting immunoreactivity included pH of the fixative, period of fixation, and type of fixative used. Immunoreactivity was improved by increased temperature and duration of dehydration and wax infiltration in tissue processing. Of all factors assessed, temperature and duration of section drying had the greatest effect on reactivity. Long-term storage of cut sections before immunostaining did not affect reactivity of tested antibodies. Alterations in tissue preparation affected antibodies by varying degrees. The most susceptible to changes in fixation were UCHL1 and vimentin; L26 was most affected by changes in processing. Microwave pretreatment usually eliminated the problem of weak staining.

Conclusion.—No standard tissue preparation schedule was determined for the optimal demonstration of all antigens. Factors from all aspects of tissue preparation may affect immunoreactivity. Precise details of the preparation table should be given when reporting immunocytochemical findings.

▶ This article describes the impact of fixation, processing, and sectioning on immunohistochemical staining. The conclusion is on the one hand somewhat disconcerting and on the other hand quite realistic: "There is no standard tissue preparation schedule for the optimal demonstration of all antigens." However, according to the authors, the key elements that impacted immunoreactivity were at the time of section drying. This is typically a step that does *not* receive a lot of attention from pathologists. Rather, the focus is usually on fixation and the use of 1 (or more) antigen retrieval methods. In addition, it is worth noting that the panel of antibodies studied (L26, UCHL1, CD45, CD3, vimentin and kappa light chain) is relatively narrow and were all obtained from Dako (Carpenteria, CA). Careful attention to details, by written protocols, will go a long way. In particular, adequate details should be provided in published manuscripts to allow other investigators to assess their methodology in relation to what has been reported.

M.B. Cohen, M.D.

Microdissection of Stained Archival Tissue

Gupta SK, Douglas-Jones AG, Morgan JM (Univ of Wales College of Medicine, Cardiff)

J Clin Pathol 50:218–220, 1997 17–5

Objective.—It is possible to extract DNA sequences of up to 200 base pairs from wax-embedded formalin-fixed tissue for the study of preinvasive neoplastic tissue uncontaminated by inflammatory or stromal cells using the polymerase chain reaction (PCR) assay.

> *Technique.*—A 5–µm section is dewaxed and stained with hematoxylin and eosin. After drying, the tissue is covered with tape and examined under a dissecting microscope. The area under investigation is excised, lifted off the glass slide, and transferred to an eppendorf tube; DNA is extracted and assayed by the PCR method.

Conclusion.—Microdissection is a valuable technique for studying genetic events involved in carcinogenesis.

► An understanding of the biology of neoplasia is of particular interest to pathologists. More specifically, the identification of putative precursor lesions has been a major focus of study. In this regard, the analysis of molecular genetic alterations of such lesions is of prime interest. In this article the authors describe another approach for obtaining microdissected tissue for such analysis. There are obviously other published and unpublished methods, but success with one technique or another may vary among laboratories. The approach described here is relatively straightforward and may prove useful for some investigators. One aspect, among others, that is not fully discussed, however, is the impact of fixation.

M.B. Cohen, M.D.

PART II

LABORATORY MEDICINE

18 Transfusion Medicine and Hemostasis

Activation of Platelets by Sera Containing IgG1 Heparin-dependent Antibodies: An Explanation for the Predominance of the FcγRIIa "Low Responder" (his_{131})-Gene in Patients With Heparin-induced Thrombocytopenia

Denomme GA, Warkentin TE, Horsewood P, et al (Hamilton Health Sciences Corp, Ont; McMaster Univ, Hamilton, Ont; Canadian Red Cross Society, Hamilton, Ont)

J Lab Clin Med 130:278–284, 1997 18–1

Background.—Heparin-induced thrombocytopenia results from heparin-dependent IgG that recognizes a heparin and platelet factor 4 (PF4) complex, which causes platelet activation by means of the platelet FcγIIa receptors (FcγRIIa). However, heparin-induced thrombocytopenia does not develop in all patients who produce heparin-dependent–IgG in response to heparin. This may be because of differences in the ability of platelets from healthy individuals to be activated by heparin-induced thrombocytopenia sera. It has been shown that a polymorphism in the platelet FcγRIIa has a key role in determining platelet reactivity to murine platelet-activating monoclonal antibodies of the IgG1 subclass: homozygous arg_{131} platelets (high responder platelets) respond well and homozygous his_{131} platelets (low responder platelets) respond poorly to murine monoclonal antibodies.

This study investigated whether preferential activation by heparin-induced thrombocytopenia–IgG of platelets with a certain FcγRIIa phenotype could explain the different risks of developing heparin-induced thrombocytopenia seen in different patients given heparin, and whether it could explain the variable platelet reactivity to heparin-induced thrombocytopenia sera.

Patients.—Samples were obtained from 84 patients with heparin-induced thrombocytopenia. Samples were also obtained from 67 control subjects with thrombocytopenia who had been given heparin but with no clinical evidence of heparin-induced thrombocytopenia; from 102 control subjects who had received heparin but did not have thrombocytopenia; and from 95 control subjects who were not given heparin.

Findings.—In 84 patients with heparin-induced thrombocytopenia, the low responder FcγRIIa gene frequency was significantly overrepresented compared with 264 control subjects. The subclass distribution of heparin-dependent–IgG was analyzed against its major antigen, heparin/PF4 complexes. This analysis showed that 55 of 61 heparin-induced thrombocytopenia sera samples expressed IgG1 antibodies alone (47 samples), combined with IgG2 (5 samples), or combined with IgG3 (3 samples).

The platelet-activating profile of heparin-induced thrombocytopenia sera was compared with that of murine platelet-activating monoclonal antibodies. This comparison predictably showed that the murine IgG1 monoclonal antibodies preferentially activated platelets from homozygous high-responder individuals. However, the low-responder homozygous platelets showed the greatest reactivity to heparin-induced thrombocytopenia sera with primarily anti-heparin/PF4 antibodies of the IgG1 subclass.

Discussion.—These findings indicate that the significant overrepresentation of the low-responder gene in patients with heparin-induced thrombocytopenia may result from the preferential activation of low-responder FcγRIIa platelets by heparin-induced thrombocytopenia antibodies of the IgG1 subclass. This IgG1 subclass is the primary immunoglobulin subclass generated in heparin-induced thrombocytopenia. However, this genetic risk factor only partially explains a patient's risk for heparin-induced thrombocytopenia.

► One of the adverse reactions of heparin therapy is thrombocytopenia caused by antibodies that bind to heparin complexed to platelet factor 4 (HIT-IgG). Previous studies have demonstrated that many patients who form HIT-IgG do not become thrombocytopenic.[1] This study provides a potential explanation for this phenomenon. The authors report that the presence of a histidine residue at position 131 of the platelet receptor for antibody (FcγRIIa) is associated with the ability of serum containing HIT-IgG to activate platelets in the presence of heparin.

The frequency of this gene is significantly higher in patients with a history of heparin-induced thrombocytopenia than in controls who do not have the antibody or other heparinized patients whose antibody status is unknown. Unfortunately, the study did not compare gene frequencies in these patients with a group who had HIT-IgG but in whom thrombocytopenia did not develop.

Based on the reported gene frequencies in the various groups, it is unlikely that the presence of the histidine residue provides the entire explanation for the development of thrombocytopenia in these patients; however, it is a first step in understanding which patients might be at risk for the development of thrombocytopenia after the administration of heparin. It also suggests that the sensitivity of testing for HIT-IgG by assays dependent on platelet function might be enhanced if platelets containing his_{131} were used in these tests.

A.J. Schlueter, M.D., Ph.D.

Reference

1. Amiral J, Peynaud-Debayle E, Wolf M, et al: Generation of antibodies to heparin-PF4 complexes without thrombocytopenia in patients treated with unfractionated or low–molecular-weight heparin. *Am J Hematol* 52:90–95, 1996.

Long-term French Experience in INR Standardization by a Procedure Using Plasma Calibrants

Houbouyan LL, Goguel AF (Hosp Ambroise Paré, Boulogne, France; Medical School, Faculty of Paris-Ouest, Garches, France)
Am J Clin Pathol 108:83–89, 1997 18–2

Objective.—There are continued problems with the use of the International Normalized Ratio (INR) for expressing prothrombin time (PT). These include problems with calibration precision in the International Sensitivity Index (ISI), the choice of normal plasma value for the PT ratio, and the instrument-dependency of the ISI. For many years, the French national external quality assurance surveys have been using plasma calibrants (PPC) for PT standardization. The PPC was compared with the use of the manufacturer's ISI. In addition, the PPC's efficiency was evaluated in 2 calibration systems: anti–vitamin K-calibrated plasmas from patients receiving oral anticoagulants or artificially depleted calibrated plasmas.

Methods.—In 2 surveys, an equivalent INR value was assigned to each plasma calibrant. The PTs were then assessed in individual French expert laboratories; by the use of different reagents and instruments in the study institution's laboratory; and at a central laboratory in a thrombosis research center. For each set of calibrants, mean INR values were calculated.

Results.—Compared to the conventional procedure, the PPC considerably reduced laboratory dispersion. In all surveys, the PPC decreased reagent and instrument effects. The artificially depleted calibrated plasmas did not improve INR dispersion. With anti–vitamin K-calibrated plasmas, dispersion was lowered to an even greater extent. The PPC avoided the need for commercial thromboplastin ISI values, recalculation of a specific ISI for local thromboplastin instruments, or a normal control plasma value for the PT ratio.

Conclusions.—Long-term experience shows the validity of PPC for PT standardization. The use of the PPC offers some key advantages over the conventional procedure and other recent proposals, though the use of lyophilized plasmas for calibration purposes has been questioned. Other problems include the assignment of an INR value to the calibrated plasmas; which thromboplastin, reagents, and values to use; and the number of calibrators needed, the reproducibility of calibration, and the minimum number of days of calibration required for optimal reliability of the PPC.

▶ Interlaboratory variation in PT improved dramatically with the institution of INR reporting. The ISI provided by the manufacturer of each thromboplastin reagent ideally would remove all interlaboratory variability from INR values. However, variability introduced by instrumentation continues to cause imprecision in the INRs reported by different laboratories on the same plasma sample. These authors and others[1] demonstrate that much of the remaining variability can be removed by local standardization of the INR or ISI using PPCs. They demonstrate decreased dispersion in INR results when laboratories perform this standardization. The authors do not address the costs that laboratories would incur should they choose to standardize their INR values in this way. They compare PPCs artificially depleted of vitamin K-dependent clotting factors and those collected from patients receiving warfarin anticoagulation and conclude that the latter are more effective in limiting test result dispersion. However, they do not speculate as to how large volumes of high quality PPC could be generated if such standardization should become accepted practice. Whether the more precise test results generated as a result of local calibration lead to improved clinical outcome remains to be determined.

A.J. Schlueter, M.D., Ph.D.

Reference

1. Poller L, Triplett DA, Hirsh J, et al: The value of plasma calibrants in correcting coagulometer effects on International Normalized Ratios: An international multicenter study. *Am J Clin Pathol* 103:358–365, 1995.

IgG Anticardiolipin Antibody Titer >40 GPL and the Risk of Subsequent Thrombo-occlusive Events and Death: A Prospective Cohort Study

Levine SR, Salowich-Palm L, Sawaya KL, et al (Henry Ford Hosp, Detroit)
Stroke 28:1660–1665, 1997 18–3

Background.—Previous studies have linked anticardiolipin antibodies (aCL) to an elevated risk of stroke. However, there are few data on the effects of aCL on recurrent thrombo-occlusive events. In the Antiphospholipid Antibodies and Stroke Study, patients with an IgG aCL positivity cutoff of more than 10 IgG phospholipid units (GPL) did not have a significant increase in recurrent thrombo-occlusive events or death. An IgG aCL cutoff of less than or greater than 40 GPL—previously used to stratify risk of miscarriage in obstetric patients and risk of thrombotic events in patients with systemic lupus erythematosus—was used in assessing the risk of thrombo-occlusive events and death.

Methods.—The prospective cohort study included 132 consecutive patients with focal cerebral ischemia: 112 with stroke and 20 with transient ischemic attack (TIA). The IgG aCL titer, measured within 1 week of the index event, was 40 or less in 111 patients and greater than 40 in 21. The effects of this cutoff point on time to and risk of thrombo-occlusive events, including stroke, TIA, deep venous thrombosis, pulmonary embolism, and myocardial infarction, were assessed. Overall mean follow-up was nearly 2 years.

TABLE 2.—Frequency of Subsequent Thrombo-occlusive Events and Death Based on Baseline IgG Anticardiolipin Antibody Titer

Event	GPL ≤40, %	GPL>40, %	*P*
None	54	29	.045
Stroke only	9	14	.434
TIA only	5	29	.003
MI only	3	0	—
DVT only	1	0	—
Death only	15	19	.608
Multiple	13	10*	NS

*All 10% of patients with GPL greater than 40 in this group had at least 1 stroke, half with transient ischemic attacks and half subsequently died.

(Reproduced with permission, from Levine SR, Salowich-Palm L, Sawaya KL, et al: IgG anticardiolipin antibody titer >40 GPL and the risk of subsequent thrombo-occlusive events and death: A prospective cohort study. *Stroke* 28:1660–1665, 1997.)

Results.—The rate of recurrent thrombo-occlusive events was 71% in the GPL greater than 40 group vs. 46% in the GPL 40 or less group. However, the absolute risk of stroke in the GPL greater than 40 group was only 4%; most events in this group were TIAs (Table 2). Median time to events was 1.9 vs. 7.4 months. Receiver operating characteristic curve analysis found no specific IgG aCL value that accurately differentiated between patients with and without subsequent events. This analysis did not consider time to events. Patients in the GPL greater than 40 group were more likely to have been taking aspirin, with or without other agents, at the time of their index event. None of the GPL greater than 40 group vs. 5% of the GPL 40 or less group were taking anticoagulants at baseline. Patients in the GPL greater than 40 group were more likely to take anticoagulants in combination with other therapeutic agents. Titers of IgM aCL were of no prognostic significance.

Conclusions.—After an index focal cerebral ischemic event, patients with an IgG aCL titer of greater than 40 GPL are at higher risk of subsequent thrombo-occlusive events and death than those with a titer of 10–40 GPL. The study is limited by its relatively small size and short follow-up, and the fact that aCLs were the only antiphospholipid antibodies systematically measured. Recurrent events are common even in patients receiving antiplatelet or anticoagulant agents or both. Randomized, controlled trials with standardized treatments are needed to clarify the effects of treatment on the natural history of focal cerebral ischemic events.

▶ aCL, one category of antiphospholipid antibodies, have been shown to be associated with thrombosis and are a risk factor for stroke. This study evaluated the risk of recurrent thrombosis in 132 patients with at least one previous thrombotic event and aCL. The patients were prospectively divided into those with high levels of IgG aCL (greater than 40 GPL) and those with IgG aCL between 10 and 40 GPL. Subsequent thromboembolic events occurred sooner and more frequently in the patients with high levels of aCL, despite the fact that this group was more likely to receive antithrombotic therapy after the initial thrombotic event. More than two thirds of the patients with high levels of aCL had recurrent events during the study period, despite a relatively short mean follow-up time of 1.9 years. β_2-Glycoprotein 1 was not measured in this study; thus, the role of this cofactor in predicting thrombotic risk was not assessed. Immunoglobulin M aCL was not a significant prognostic variable in this group of patients. This study reinforces the importance of evaluating patients with thrombotic events for IgG aCL, and suggests that continuing efforts are needed to improve management of these patients.

A.J. Schlueter, M.D., Ph.D.

Polymerase Chain Reaction Determination of RhC, Rhc, and RhE Blood Types: An Evaluation of Accuracy and Clinical Utility

Yankowitz J, Li S, Weiner CP (Univ of Iowa, Iowa City)
Am J Obstet Gynecol 176:1107–1111, 1997 18–4

Objective.—Because the Rh complex on chromosome 1 has been sequenced, it is possible to use polymerase chain reaction (PCR) to determine RhC/c/E blood type after a single amniocentesis. The accuracy of PCR determination of RhC/c/E blood type was evaluated using leukocyte-derived DNA samples from individuals of known RhC/c/E type in comparison with the gold-standard blood-banking serologic technique.

Methods.—Analysis by PCR was performed on 655 samples of leukocyte-derived DNA. Indications for fetal blood sampling included maternal or paternal antibodies against a red blood cell antigen, an indirect Coombs' titer of 1.8, or a previously sensitized pregnancy.

Results.—There were 479 RhC-positive, 176 RhC-negative, 524 Rhc-positive, 131 Rhc-negative, 131 RhE-positive, and 524 RhE-negative individuals. Eight of the RhC-positive patients, 10 Rhc-positive patients, and 4 RhE-positive patients were antigen negative by PCR. The respective sensitivities and specificities produced by using PCR to detect RhC typing were 98.3% and 91.5%, to detect Rhc typing they were 98.1% and 94.7%, and to detect RhE they were 96.9% and 99.2%. Whereas the accuracy of detecting RhE by PCR was consistent with serologic values found in the published literature, accuracies of detecting RhC or Rhc were significantly lower than the better than 98.8% accuracy obtained by the serologic technique. Database errors may have contributed to these lower accuracy values. Results of PCR using 1 set of primers and testing only the fetus should be viewed cautiously. If a serologically positive father does not show the expected PCR bands, the PCR test cannot be used for that family. Performing the PCR test on the father when the fetus is antigen negative can rule out polymorphism as a cause of a false negative result. The PCR test has been used for Kell, MN and Ss, and Fy (Duffy) antigens and can be used to help in the management of erythrocyte sensitization in 96% or more of patients. Using PCR to test fetal blood antigen type could lower the death rate from complications and could reduce the number of serial amniocenteses used. When used, they now average 3.1 per pregnancy.

Amniocentesis could replace cordocenteses for initial evaluation of the at-risk pregnancy, which has a procedure-related fetal loss of 1% or greater.

Conclusion.—Polymerase chain reaction can be used to establish RhC/c/E type. However, it gives higher false negative results than the serologic technique for RhC and Rhc.

▶ Hemolytic disease of the newborn caused by maternal sensitization to non-RhD erythrocyte antigens continues to be a cause of fetal and neonatal morbidity. Serologic evaluation of at-risk fetuses requires cordocentesis to obtain fetal erythrocytes for antigen typing, or intensive monitoring of the pregnancy on the assumption that the fetus is positive for the antigen in question.

This study evaluates the sensitivity and specificity of PCR technology for determining the presence or absence of RhC, Rhc, and RhE genes in DNA derived from individuals whose Rh phenotype was determined serologically (gold standard). In this case, leukocyte DNA was used but similar technology has been shown to be accurate with the use of DNA derived from amniocytes.[1] The sensitivity and specificity of PCR testing was equivalent to serologic testing for RhE determination, but the PCR test produced a higher number of false negatives for RhC and Rhc determination.

False negatives in this clinical setting have potentially devastating consequences for the fetus. The study abstracted here was done using a single set of primers, and the authors recommend using additional primers, additonal molecular techniques, and/or testing of the father by the same methods to rule of familial polymorphisms when the fetal sample is antigen negative.

The cost of PCR testing relative to serologic testing is not discussed; however, the authors point out that definitive diagnostic testing could be performed on a single amniocentesis rather than multiple amniocenteses (required to monitor a pregnancy assumed but not proven to be at risk) or cordocentesis. Primers are available for the erythrocyte antigens responsible for more than 95% of the sensitized pregnancies. Fetal erythrocyte antigen determination by PCR may have a place in selected at-risk pregnancies.

A.J. Schlueter, M.D., Ph.D.

Reference

1. Van Den Veyver IB, Subramanian SB, Hudson KM, et al: Prenatal diagnosis of the RhD fetal blood type of amniotic fluid by polymerase chain reaction. *Obstet Gynecol* 87:419–422, 1996.

Leukocyte Reduction and Ultraviolet B Irradiation of Platelets to Prevent Alloimmunization and Refractoriness to Platelet Transfusions

Slichter SJ, for the Trial to Reduce Alloimmunization to Platelets Study Group (Puget Sound Blood Ctr, Seattle)

N Engl J Med 337:1861–1869, 1997 18–5

Background.—Antibodies against alloantigens on donor platelets are a major reason that patients with thrombocytopenia become refractory to platelet transfusions. There are usually limited supplies of HLA-compatible platelets for patients who are refractory to platelet transfusions from random donors. Up to 60% of transfusions of platelets thought to be HLA-compatible do not increase the platelet count in patients with thrombocytopenia refractory to transfusions. The results of studies that sought to determine ways of preventing alloimmunization in patients with thrombocytopenia have been inconclusive.

Methods.—In a multi-institutional, randomized, blinded trial, it was determined whether platelets with the leukocytes removed by a filter or treated with ultraviolet B irradiation could prevent the formation of antiplatelet alloantibodies and refractoriness to platelet transfusions. All patients had untreated acute myeloid leukemia. Patients receiving induction chemotherapy were randomly assigned to platelet transfusion with (1) unmodified, pooled platelet concentrates from random donors (control group); (2) filtered, pooled platelet concentrates from random donors (F-C); (3) ultraviolet B–irradiated, pooled platelet concentrates from random donors (UVB-PC); or (4) filtered platelets obtained by apheresis from single random donors (F-AP). Filtered, leukocyte-reduced red blood cells were used in all patients. Refractoriness was defined as a corrected count increment of less than 5,000 after each of 2 consecutive transfusions of ABO-compatible platelets.

Results.—Of 530 patients at baseline with no alloantibodies, 51 were classified as refractory. Estimates for the development of refractoriness during the 8-week study period were 16% in the control group, 10% in the UVB-PC group, 7% in the F-PC group, and 8% in the F-AP group. Lymphocytotoxic antibodies developed in 45% of patients in the control group, 21% of patients in the UVB-PC group, 18% of patients in the F-PC group, and 17% of patients in the F-AP group. There were no significant differences among groups in the rates or causes of mortality or withdrawal. Remission rates were similar in all groups; 60% of patients had complete remission.

Discussion.—Transfusion with treated platelets benefited patients with no detectable lymphocytotoxic antibodies at baseline, but not patients who had such antibodies. Transfusion with leukocyte-reduced or ultraviolet B–irradiated platelets is recommended only for patients who are antibody negative. It was hypothesized that the filtered platelets obtained by apheresis from single random donors might lower the incidence of alloimmunization even further than ultraviolet B–irradiated pooled platelet concentrates or filtered pooled platelet concentrates from random donors because of exposure to fewer donors, but there was no evidence of this. The low rate of refractoriness to platelet transfusion was unexpected. The development of antiplatelet alloantibodies did not necessarily result in refractoriness to platelet transfusion in all patients. Lymphocytotoxic antibodies were often first detected 3–4 weeks after baseline, after some patients had stopped receiving platelet transfusion. Interestingly, lymphocytotoxic antibodies were seen in 19% of the 36 patients with no previous alloantigen exposure and who were given treated transfusion according to all study guidelines.

▶ This paper presents the results of a large, multicenter study evaluating 3 methods of platelet unit modification to prevent alloimmunization to platelets in the recipient, and ultimately to prevent the development of refractoriness to platelet transfusion. The study group found that ultraviolet B irradiation of pooled platelet concentrates, or leukoreduction of pooled or apheresis platelet concentrates were equally effective in preventing alloimmunization as measured by the development of leukocytotoxic antibodies and refractoriness to platelet transfusions. These data support the hypothesis that modification of platelet concentrates in one of these ways is warranted to reduce alloimmunization and its consequences, despite the fact that there was no significant difference in overall clinical outcome in this patient group. No difference was noted between leukoreduced apheresis and pooled platelet concentrates in terms of alloimmunization; thus the study group concludes that there is no reason to preferentially use apheresis units to avoid alloimmunization as long as they are leukoreduced. The majority of units were leukoreduced at the time of transfusion rather than at collection, and this fact should be considered when extrapolating the data to the latter situation. Finally, there was a subset of patients who subsequently had lymphocytotoxic antibodies despite receiving platelets modified to reduce this risk, and the stimulus for this immune response remains to be determined.

A.J. Schlueter, M.D., Ph.D.

Prevalence of Hepatitis G Virus and Its Strain Variant, the GB Agent, in Blood Donations and Their Transmission to Recipients

Roth WK, Waschk D, Marx S, et al (Inst for Chemotherapy, Georg-Speyer-Haus, Frankfurt am Main, Germany; Johann Wolfgang Goethe-Univ, Frankfurt am Main, Germany; Red Cross Blood Donor Service, Hesse, Frankfurt am Main, Germany)

Transfusion 37:651–656, 1997 18–6

Background.—Several new viruses were identified that may be associated with hepatitis non-A through non-E. Hepatitis G virus (HGV) and its strain variant, the GB agent (GBV-C), are independent isolates of these recently identified viruses. The incidence in blood donors in the United States is 1.5% to 1.9%, but there is no information on the incidence in

European blood donors. Epidemiologic studies indicate a parenteral transmission route. The prevalence of HGV/GBV-C in European blood donors and the efficiency of transmission to individuals who receive blood transfusion were examined.

Methods.—Plasma samples from German blood donors were tested for HGV/GBV-C by reverse transcription–polymerase chain reaction. Positive donors were retested and interviewed about parenteral transmission risks. Amplification products were sequenced and analyzed by phylogenetic methods. Individuals who received positive donations were tested for HGV/GBV-C infection.

Results.—Of 1,048 blood donors with an alanine aminotransferase of less than 45 IU/L, 14 were positive, resulting in a prevalence of 1.34%. Ten of the 14 recipients of these positive donations were located; 4 were positive for HGV/GBV-C 6 months after transfusion. Homology was 98% to 100%. Of 635 samples from donors in a rural area, 5 samples, or 0.78%, were positive. Of 413 samples from donors in a metropolitan area, 9 samples, or 2.18%, were positive. All positive donors except one reported parenteral transmission risks. Transmission of HGV/GBV-C occurred in 4 of 9 individuals who received transfusion. There was a 3% prevalence of HGV/GBV-C in donors with an alanine aminotransferase level greater than 45 IU/L. There were 2 mother/child pairs with highly homologous isolates.

Discussion.—Hepatitis G virus/GBV-C has a very high prevalence compared with hepatitis C virus and other agents that are chiefly transmitted through parenteral routes. Hepatitis G virus/GBV-C may be more efficiently transmitted through parenteral routes than hepatitis C virus, or there may be unknown routes of transmission. The isolates of the donation recipients and the respective donors were highly homologous, strongly suggesting transmission. Only 1 recipient was negative at the first testing, 35 days after transfusion, but positive at the second testing, 140 days after transfusion, which confirms reports of prolonged time to conversion. The high prevalence in blood donors and the low rate of posttransfusion hepatitis after the introduction of anti–hepatitis C virus screening is inconsistent with HGV/GBV-C as a transfusion-relevant hepatitis virus.

▶ The recent isolation of HGV and the high incidence of this virus in individuals from risk groups with a high likelihood of parenteral virus transmission (e.g., hemophiliacs, IV drug abusers) has raised concerns about transmission of this virus via blood component transfusions. This study, along with several others,[1–3] assesses the prevalence of HGV in the blood donor population. The rate of infection in first-time donors is quite high, at least twice the rate observed for hepatitis C. Furthermore, these authors conducted a look-back evaluation of recipients of blood products from donors demonstrated to be infected with hepatitis G. They found that 4 of 10 recipients (40%) were positive for hepatitis G, and the sequence homologies of the viruses in the donor-recipient pairs approached 100%, suggesting that the recipients acquired the virus by transfusion. These data would be of significant concern to the blood banking community, and would call for immediate exclusion of hepatitis G–positive individuals from the donor pool if this agent could be demonstrated to cause clinical disease. However, attempts to date to link the presence of this virus with clinical hepatitis have resulted in minimal support for this hypothesis. The risk of clinical sequelae from hepatitis G infection is therefore likely to be small, and large population studies may be necessary to determine whether the risk is sufficient to warrant screening of the blood supply for this virus.

A.J. Schlueter, M.D., Ph.D.

References

1. Alter HJ, Nakatsuji Y, Melpolder J, et al: The incidence of transfusion-associated hepatitis G virus infection and its relation to liver disease. *N Engl J Med* 336:747–754, 1997.
2. Yoshikawa A, Fukuda S, Itoh K, et al: Infection with hepatitis G virus and its strain variation, the GB agent (GBV-C), among blood donors in Japan. *Transfusion* 37:657–663, 1997.
3. Loiseau P, Mariotti M, Corbi C, et al: Prevalence of hepatitis G virus RNA in French blood donors and recipients. *Transfusion* 37:645–650, 1997.

Comparison of Mean Normal Prothrombin Time (PT) With PT of Fresh Normal Pooled Plasma or of a Lyophilized Control Plasma (R82A) as Denominator to Express PT Results: Collaborative Study of the International Federation of Clinical Chemistry

D'Angelo A, for the IFCC Working Group Standardization of Coagulation Tests (Scientific Inst HS Raffaele, Milano, Italy; et al)

Clin Chem 43:2169–2174, 1997 18–7

Background.—The mean normal prothrombin time (MNPT) is currently recommended as the denominator in PT ratios and International Normalized Ratio values. Unfortunately, the collection and assessment of sufficient healthy samples for calculation of the MNPT may be difficult, especially for small laboratories. The Verband der Deutschen Geräte-Hersteller has a preparation of lyophilized normal pooled plasma from 101 healthy donors, R82A, which could be used as a substitute for MNPT. The equivalence of this lyophilized pooled plasma with fresh normal plasma is not known. An International Federation of Clinical Chemistry (IFCC) collaborative project was initiated to examine the calibration of plasma R82A with MPNT and corresponding fresh normal pooled plasma (FNPP).

Methods.—Fifteen laboratories, utilizing at least 2 different thromboplastins and end point detectors each, for an overall total of 58 PT systems, were involved in this international collaborative study. Plasma samples from 30 healthy volunteers were used to calculate MNPT, FNPP was obtained from these same donors, and both were compared to lyophilized plasma R82A.

Results.—Total and between-day variations were significantly greater with FNPP than with plasma R82A. When MNPT was used as the denominator, mean PT ratios of healthy volunteers were not different from 1.00. Mean PT ratios were significantly greater than 1.00 when FNPP was used and significantly less than 1.00 when R82A was used (Fig 1). There was no effect of reagents, end point detectors, or plasma citrate concentration on PT results of healthy volunteers when MPNT was used as the denominator. End point detectors significantly affected PT ratios when FNPP was used. Reagents, end point detectors and plasma citrate concentration all had independent significant effects on PT results when R82A was used.

Conclusions.—In this international collaborative study, MNPT was compared with the PT of fresh normal pooled plasma and lyophilized control plasma, R82A, as the denominator in the expression of PT ratios and INR values. Prothrombin time ratios were underestimated when R82A was used and overestimated when FNPP was used, as compared with MNPT. Reagents affected the PT ratios when plasma R82A was used. There was also a significant difference between MNPT and FNPP-PT obtained from the same donors. These results underscore the differences in the PT derived from lyophilized plasma R82A, FNPP and MNPT. Mean

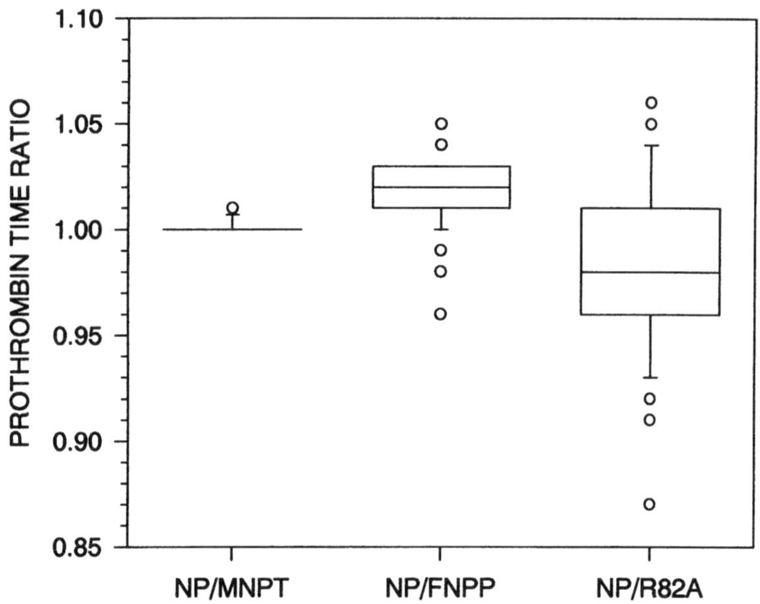

FIGURE 1.—Box plots of mean prothrombin time (PT) ratios obtained with the 58 prothrombin time systems in the 30 apparently healthy subjects examined in each laboratory and expressed with the use of the mean normal prothrombin time, fresh normal pooled plasma PT, or plasma R82A-PT as the denominator term. The 10th, 25th, 50th, 75th, and 90th percentiles of the distribution are shown. *Circles* indicate mean PT ratios outside the 10th and 90th percentiles of the distribution. *Abbreviations*: *NP/MNPT*, normal plasma/mean normal prothrombin time; *FNPP*, fresh normal pooled plasma. (Courtesy of D'Angelo A, for the IFCC Working Group Standardization of Coagulation Tests: Comparison of mean normal prothrombin time [PT] with PT of fresh normal pooled plasma or of a lyophilized control plasma [R82A] as denominator to express PT results: Collaborative study of the International Federation of Clinical Chemistry. *Clin Chem* 43:2169–2174. Copyright 1997, The American Association for Clinical Chemistry [1–800–892–1400].)

normal prothrombin time should be used as the index of normal PT in the calculation of International Normalized Ratio values whenever possible.

▶ Presently, the recommended way to determine the denominator of the International Normalized Ratio (INR) is the geometric mean of the PTs of a healthy reference population. Determination of this number may prove difficult for small laboratories, and the use of the PT determined from a lyophilized calibrant plasma as a substitute has been suggested. These plasmas are currently available, and are used to provide quality control for laboratory test systems.

This study analyzed the variation introduced to the INR calculation by the current method of MNPT, pooled fresh plasma PT, and lyophilized plasma PT. The study was conducted in 15 laboratories with a variety of instruments and thromboplastin reagents. The lyophilized plasma tended to underestimate the PT ratio and the pooled fresh plasma overestimated the PT ratio when compared to the mean of the reference range. The reasons for this are not investigated in the study. Arguments for utilizing such reagents with the addition of a correction factor provided by the manufacturer of the reagent have been made; however, the degree of variation of the PT ratio changed significantly with different instrument and reagent combinations. The degree of variation was greatest with the lyophilized plasma reagent (see Fig 1). Therefore, this solution was not thought to be practical. The use of MNPT to calculate the PT ratio for the INR continues to be the most reliable method of minimizing interlaboratory variability in oral anticoagulation management.

A.J. Schlueter, M.D., Ph.D.

Comparison of Anti–factor Xa Heparin Activity and Activated Partial Thromboplastin Time in 2,773 Plasma Samples From Unfractionated Heparin–Treated Patients

Rosborough TK (Abbott Northwestern Hosp, Minneapolis, Minn)
Am J Clin Pathol 108:662–668, 1997 18–8

Background.—The patient response to unfractionated heparin (UH) therapy is not consistent. Although monitoring is necessary, there is no agreement on the best methodology. The most common monitoring assay is the activated partial thromboplastin time (APTT). The measurement of heparin activity (HA) in antithrombin units or anti-factor Xa units, is more accurate than APTT, but more expensive and technically difficult. Technology that allows rapid, reliable and cost-effective measurement of anti-factor Xa heparin activity has become available. To examine the optimal method of determining the therapeutic range of APTT, APTT values and anti-factor Xa values were compared in a large group of plasma samples.

Methods.—A total of 2,773 blood samples were collected from patients during UH therapy. Within 2 hours of collection, plasma samples were assessed for APTT and HA with the STA Hemostasis System. There were no differences in technician time between these 2 assays. The approximate cost was $0.35 per APTT assay and $1.50 per HA assay. Of the 2,773 patients, 55 were being treated by IV nonstandardized UH infusions by their own physicians. These samples were used to develop a lean weight-based UH treatment protocol. This protocol was then used in the treatment of the remaining 694 patients during a 4-month period in 1996. Linear regression analysis of paired HA and APTT values was performed.

Results.—The best-fit linear regression equation was obtained with logarithmically transformed APTT values. With the use of this equation, the HA predicted by APTT was within 0.39 U/mL of actual HA with a 95% confidence interval. The total clinical error rate of the APTT therapeutic range selected using a best-fit regression equation was 10%. Selecting the therapeutic range based on minimization of APTT errors improved the clinical error rate to 8%.

Conclusions.—The predictive ability of the APTT for HA is limited. Even when a criterion of limiting clinical errors is used in selecting the therapeutic range with this assay, the error rate is too high for optimal clinical results. A clinical trial is required to determine the best way may be to monitor UH therapy.

► UH therapy has historically been monitored in numerous ways. Presently, the most popular assay is the APTT, which shows poor correlation wih the amount of HA in the sample as measured by factor Xa inhibition or protamine titration. Despite the lack of clinical trials comparing rates of thrombosis and bleeding complications using the APTT or HA assay to monitor heparin therapy, the current consensus is that heparin dosing should ultimately be based on HA assays and APTT assays should be standardized to equivalent HA units in each laboratory.

In this study, this standardization process was undertaken in 1 laboratory with patient populations of 2 different sizes. In both cases, a therapeutic range for APTT was determined by comparison to factor Xa inhibition. The process was first performed using 55 specimens from patients receiving heparin therapy, and was then repeated with a second set of 2,718 specimens (from 694 patients). Not surprisingly, the data yielded 2 different therapeutic ranges for APTT. The data were analyzed using a minimization of error techinique that was based on the number of samples that would have been within the therapeutic range by 1 of the 2 methods (Xa inhibition or APTT monitoring) and out of range (high or low) by the other method. Using this method to establish a therapeutic range for the APTT, the frequency with which errors of over- or under-anticoagulation would occur (which might lead to thrombosis or bleeding) was reduced to 8% (from 10% by the routine standardization method).

These data confirm once again that the APTT is limited in its ability to predict heparin concentration. It is not reasonable for each laboratory to study thousands of specimens to determine therapeutic heparin ranges for the APTT, and even with the minimization of error technique, the error rate is still quite high. The ultimate answer to this problem lies in a well-constructed clinical trial to determine the true rate of clinical complications using Xa inhibition or APTT tests as monitors of heparin therapy.

A.J. Schlueter, M.D., Ph.D.

HSV-TK Gene Transfer Into Donor Lymphocytes for Control of Allogeneic Graft-Versus-Leukemia

Bonini C, Ferrari G, Verzeletti S, et al (Istituto Scientifico HS Raffaele, Milan, Italy)

Science 276:1719–1724, 1997 18–9

Background.—Allogeneic bone marrow transplantation (allo-BMT) is the treatment of choice for many hematologic cancers but is limited by the occurrence of the potentially life-threatening complication of graft-vs.-host disease (GVHD). There is no specific treatment for GVHD. The genetic manipulation of donor lymphocytes was attempted to incorporate a "suicide gene" that could be activated in the event of GVHD, to make allo-BMT safer and more effective for a wider range of patients.

Methods.—Donor lymphocytes were transduced with a viral vector carrying a selectable marker and the herpes simplex virus thymidine kinase (HSV-TK) suicide gene, which confers sensitivity to ganciclovir. After transduction, the cells were subjected to 1 round of selection to ensure that virtually 100% were carrying the suicide gene. Twelve patients participated in this study, and this report describes follow-up on 8 of them who were treated with the donor lymphocytes.

Results.—The transduced cells survived for at least 12 months and could be detected in the patients' circulation, marrow aspirates, and tissue biopsy specimens. In 5 of the 8 patients, graft-vs.-leukemia activity could be detected, with 3 patients having complete responses. In three patients GVHD developed and was treated with ganciclovir, which resulted in elimination of all symptoms and signs of the disease without any toxicity. Two of these patients, who had achieved complete remission before the development of GVHD, remained in complete remission after ganciclovir treatment.

Conclusions.—The transfer of suicide genes to donor lymphocytes before allo-BMT provides a new therapeutic tool that combines the benefits of allo-BMT with the possibility of eliminating GVHD without toxicity. Genetic manipulation of donor lymphocytes has the potential to increase the number of patients who can benefit from allo-BMT, as well as to increase its safety and efficacy.

▶ Patients who experience relapse or have posttransplant lymphoproliferative disease (PTLD) after allogeneic bone marrow transplantation have been successfully treated in recent years with infusions of lymphocytes from their bone marrow donor. These cells are able to eliminate recipient tumor cells or Epstein-Barr virus–transformed recipient lymphocytes and result in elimination of disease. One of the side effects of such therapy is the development

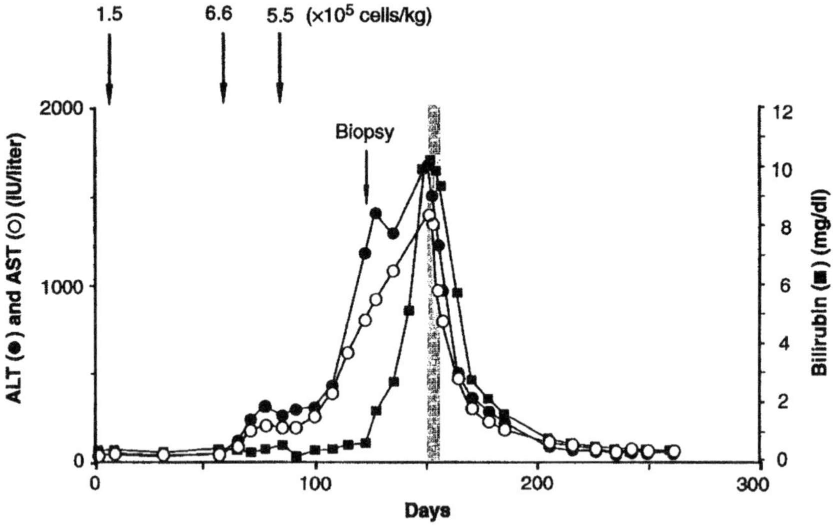

FIGURE 4.—Values of bilirubin and liver function enzymes in patient 2, who developed acute GVHD after the infusion of transduced donor lymphocytes. *Long arrows*, infusions of transduced donor cells; *short arrow*, timing of the liver biopsy performed to detect acute GVHD (biopsy). *Gray area* indicates the period of the four infusions of ganciclovir (10 mg/kg/day). (Reprinted with permission from Bonini C, Ferrari G, Verzeletti S, et al: HSV-TK gene transfer into donor lymphocytes for control of allogeneic graft-versus-leukemia. *Science* 276:1719–1724. Copyright 1997, American Association for the Advancement of Science.)

of GVHD, which may be severe and protracted because of continued proliferation of large numbers of donor T cells in the host. Ideally, one might treat relapse or PTLD with T cells of a limited life span, present long enough to result in a cure but eliminated before the development of GVHD. The treatment presented here does not quite achieve this goal but comes much closer than any treatments to date. The authors introduced two genes into the donor lymphocytes: a thymidine kinase gene and a gene for a nerve growth factor receptor (expressed on the cell surface). The second gene product was used to select transfected cells for transfer into the patient, and the first gene was used to confer ganciclovir sensitivity to the lymphocytes. When the patients experienced GVHD after infusion of donor lymphocytes, they were treated with ganciclovir to kill these cells. Resolution of GVHD symptoms after ganciclovir infusion was rapid and complete in 2 of the 3 patients who required this therapy; thus, the morbidity associated with protracted GVHD was avoided (Fig 4). The third patient had partial resolution of symptoms, correlated with partial elimination of the donor lymphocytes. Until bone marrow transplantation is completely successful in curing the underlying indication for transplant in the absence of PTLD, this sort of therapy holds great promise for successful treatment of relapse or PTLD while providing excellent quality of life by the absence of GVHD.

A.J. Schlueter, M.D., Ph.D.

Variability and Determinants of Total Homocysteine Concentrations in Plasma in an Elderly Population

Clarke R, Woodhouse P, Ulvik A, et al (Radcliffe Infirmary, Oxford, England; Addenbrooke's Hosp, Cambridge, England; Univ of Bergen, Norway; et al)

Clin Chem 44:102–107, 1998 18–10

Background.—A moderate increase in total homocysteine (tHcy) is a strong, independent risk factor for occlusive vascular disease. A previous meta-analysis of observational studies of tHcy and vascular disease demonstrated that a prolonged 1 µmol/L lower tHcy concentration was associated with a 10% decrease in the risk of coronary heart disease through a range of 10–15 µmol/L. In the current study, the variability and determinants of tHcy levels in plasma were determined in an elderly population.

Methods and Findings.—Ninety-six healthy volunteers, aged 65–74, were assessed for 1 year. Blood tHcy levels ranged from 7.1 µmol/L in the bottom quintile to 14.5 µmol/L in the top quintile. Mean tHcy was 10.4 µmol/L. Little seasonal variation was noted. The reliability coefficient was 0.88. Mean tHcy concentrations were associated inversely with mean plasma folate and B_{12} levels. Median tHcy concentrations were about 1 µmol/L greater in men than in women and in persons 70–74 years than in those 65–69 years. Concentrations were also higher in persons with TT and CT genotypes for the methylenetetrahydrofolate reductase polymorphism than in those with the CC genotype.

Conclusions.—Substantial variations in tHcy concentrations were noted among individuals in this elderly population but the intraindividual variability was minimal. The reliability coefficient, 0.88, compared favorably with that for total cholesterol and was somewhat greater than that for systolic blood pressure.

▶ Elevated plasma homocysteine levels have been demonstrated to be a risk factor for several types of vascular occlusive disease, including myocardial infarction and stroke. Most patients with this risk factor have a mutation in an enzyme used to regenerate the form of folate necessary to convert homocysteine to methionine. This leads to elevated homocysteine levels under conditions of relative folate deficiency. The risk factor is reduced by dietary supplementation with folate. Because of the relationship between homocysteine and folate, a significant influence of diet on homocysteine levels might be anticipated. These investigators studied the intraperson variability in homocysteine levels over a 13 month period to determine if a single plasma homocysteine measurement was reliable in detecting this risk factor and examined whether any seasonal variability (potentially based on diet) could be identified. In a group of 96 healthy volunteers, minimal intraperson and seasonal variability were identified. Approximately half of the study population possessed the risk factor of elevated homocysteine levels. Because dietary folate supplementation is simple, inexpensive, and has no known detrimental effects, some individuals have argued for folate treatment in patients with other thrombotic risk factors without measurement of plasma homocysteine. For those who wish to assess this risk factor directly, this study indicates that a single measurement is sufficient.

A.J. Schlueter, M.D., Ph.D.

Inhibition of Erythroid Progenitor Cells by Anti-Kell Antibodies in Fetal Alloimmune Anemia

Vaughan JI, Manning M, Warwick RM, et al (Queen Charlotte's Hosp, London; Royal Postgraduate Med School, London)

N Engl J Med 338:798–803, 1998 18–11

Background.—In infants with alloimmune anemia, less hemolysis is caused by antibodies to antigens of the Kell blood-group system than by antibodies to the D antigen of the Rh blood-group system. For the degree of anemia present, the former infants have inappropriately low numbers of reticulocytes and normoblasts. Thus sensitization to Kell antigens could lead not only to hemolysis but also to suppression of fetal erythropoiesis. This study sought to determine whether inhibition of erythroid progenitor cell growth is partly responsible for fetal anemia caused by anti-Kell antibodies.

Methods and Findings.—The in-vitro study compared the growth of Kell-positive with Kell-negative hematopoietic progenitor cells from cord blood, cultured in the presence of monoclonal anti-Kell antibodies anti-D antibodies, and sera from women with anti-Kell antibodies. Monoclonal IgG and IgM anti-Kell antibodies inhibited the growth of Kell-positive erythroid progenitor cells from cord blood in dose-dependent fashion. No inhibitory effect was noted with monoclonal anti-D antibodies. None of the 3 antibodies altered the growth of erythroid progenitor cells from Kell-negative cord blood. Growth of granulocyte or megakaryocyte progenitor cells from cord blood was unaffected by monoclonal anti-Kell antibodies or monoclonal anti-D antibodies.

Growth of Kell-positive erythroid burst-forming units and colony-forming units was inhibited by sera from 22 women with anti-Kell antibodies; growth of Kell-negative erythroid burst-forming units and colony-forming units was unaffected. The mothers' anti-Kell antibodies had no inhibitory effect on cord blood granulocyte-macrophage or megakaryocyte progenitor cells.

Conclusions.—Growth of Kell-positive erythroid burst-forming units and colony-forming units is specifically inhibited by both monoclonal and naturally occurring anti-Kell antibodies. The results add to the evidence that anti-Kell antibodies contribute to fetal anemia by suppressing erythropoiesis at the level of the progenitor cell. The results have important implications for the clinical management of pregnancies identified as having Kell alloimmunization.

▶ Maternal alloimmunization to erythrocyte antigens continues to be a source of fetal and neonatal morbidity and mortality despite the introduction of Rh immune globulin. Alloimmunization to the Kell antigen is the second most common cause of this disease and can result in severe anemia. The parameters used to predict severity of hemolytic disease of the newborn, such as bilirubinemia in amniotic fluid, were initially developed for patients with Rh alloimmunization. These parameters are much less accurate in predicting severity of Kell alloimmunization, and these authors present evidence that help to explain this phenomenon. They demonstrate that anti-Kell antibodies are capable of inhibiting proliferation of early erythroid precursors, whereas anti-D antibodies do not possess this characteristic. There was no correlation between maternal titers of anti-Kell antibodies and ability to inhibit erythroid progenitor proliferation, which parallels the observation that maternal titers frequently do not correlate with severity of fetal disease. The authors did not directly investigate the relationship between clinical outcome of affected fetuses and ability of maternal serum to inhibit erythropoiesis. The findings also provide a possible explanation for the observation that affected infants often remain anemic for up to 6 weeks after birth.

A.J. Schlueter, M.D., Ph.D.

Prestorage Inline Filtration of Whole Blood for Obtaining White Cell-reduced Blood Components

Riggert J, Schwartz DWM, Wieding JU, et al (Univ Clinic, Göttingen, Germany; Univ Clinic and Blood Donation Ctr for Vienna)

Transfusion 37:1039–1044, 1997 18–12

Background.—Adverse effects associated with white blood cells (WBCs) in blood products include alloimmunization with subsequent refractoriness to platelet transfusion, febrile reactions to transfusion, immunosuppression, and transmission of cell-associated viruses such as cytomegalovirus and human T-lymphotropic virus type I and II. Inline filtration of whole blood may be a good way to obtain WBC-reduced red blood cells (RBCs) and fresh-frozen plasma (FFP) using only 1 filter.

Methods.—A specially designed inline WBC-reduction filter was used in the preparation of 24 units of WBC-reduced RBCs (RBC-F) and FFP (FFP-F). Each of two transfusion centers in Germany and Austria used the filter. Each unit was assessed for WBC contamination with the Nageotte chamber. Several coagulation measures were assessed by standardized test systems.

Findings.—Median WBC contamination in RBC-F was 27,000 and 50,000 per unit at the 2 centers, respectively. Median WBC contamination in FFP-F was 13,000 and 31,000 per unit, respectively. Coagulation factors I, V, VIII, and XI in FFP-F did not differ from those in conventionally prepared FFP. Markers for coagulation and fibrinolysis activation (factor XIIa, prothrombin fragments, thrombin-antithrombin complexes, and fibrinogen degradation products) were not higher in FFP-F.

Conclusions.—Preparation with inline-filtered whole blood results in blood components that meet the standards for WBC-reduced RBCs and

FFP. Such preparation does not change the protein profile of FFP-F. Markers for the activation of coagulation and fibrinolysis are not increased.

► The demand for leukoreduced components continues to increase, as adverse effects resulting from leukocyte contamination of blood components continue to be identified. These effects range from the well-characterized risks of infectious disease transmission and alloimmunization to more recently identified potential risks such as increased susceptibility to infection following transfusion. Filtration during collection of whole blood units (inline filtration) is attractive as a way to accomplish leukoreduction without adding to the time required to process blood components for transfusion. However, it is important to establish that no harm is done to the products during this filtration process. This paper is one of several[1, 2] that assess the quality of components made from whole blood products following inline filtration. These authors demonstrate that packed red blood cell units prepared from inline filtered whole blood actually have lower free hemoglobin and lactate dehydrogenase levels after 35 days of storage than do units prepared without filtration. Coagulation factors in fresh frozen plasma were not significantly different in the filtered compared to the unfiltered units. One disadvantage of this method of preparing leukoreduced products is that platelets are trapped in the filter and therefore this component of the product is lost. Inline filtration has been licensed for use in the United States and is already being used in several blood collection centers.

A.J. Schlueter, M.D., Ph.D.

References

1. Riggert J, Simson G, Dittmann J, et al: Prestorage leukocyte depletion with in-line filtration of whole blood in comparison with blood component leukocyte depletion. *Vox Sang* 69:201–205, 1995.
2. Rider JR, Moore G, Payrat JM, et al: Evaluation of a new, integral, whole blood filter (RS2000) system for prestorage leucodepletion of SAG-M red cells. *Br J Haematol* 94:184–190, 1996.

Comparison of Functional Testing for Resistance to Activated Protein C and Molecular Biological Testing for Factor V R506Q in 370 Patients

Montes MA, Fox EA, Longtine JA, et al (Harvard Med School, Boston)

Arch Pathol Lab Med 122:325–329, 1998 18–13

Background.—Resistance to activated protein C (APC) is the most common cause of familial thrombosis, occurring in 20% to 50% of patients with inherited thrombophilia. Individuals heterozygous for factor V R506Q have a seven-fold increase in the risk for thromboembolic events, and those who are homozygous have an 80-fold increase in risk. Functional and molecular biologic tests for resistance to APC/factor V R506Q were compared.

Methods.—Functional and molecular biologic tests for resistance to APC/factor V R506Q were developed. In the functional method, exogenous APC was added to an activated partial thomboplastin time-based assay. A sensitivity ratio was calculated from the activated partial thromboplastin time (aPTT) with exogenous APC divided by the aPTT without the exogenous APC. The molecular biologic method involved polymerase chain reaction followed by endonuclease digestion. The results of the tests in 370 patients were compared.

Findings.—Using the molecular biologic test as the definitive technique for detecting factor R506Q mutation, the functional assay had a sensitivity and specificity of 100% and 74%, respectively when a cutoff sensitivity ratio of 0.84 was used. Its positive predictive value was 34%. The population studied had a factor V mutation prevalence of 12%. Though a normalized sensitivity ratio of less than 0.84 is taken as evidence of APC resistance in functional testing, all patients with factor V R506Q were found to have an nAPC-SR of 0.71 or less. With the use of this cut-off value, the functional test had a specificity of 87% and a positive predictive value of 52%. Patients with factor V R506Q had a higher incidence of hypercoagulability than those without factor V R506Q. The former patients also had fewer additional risk factors for hypercoagulability.

Conclusions.—The functional assay for resistance to APC is an excellent screening tool for factor V R506Q. However, findings must be confirmed by molecular biologic testing when the results are positive, because the false positive rate with functional testing is high. The false-positive rate can be decreased by lowering the cutoff for the funcational test based on comparison with molecular results.

▶ Resistance to APC, a common cause of inherited thrombophilia, most often results from a point mutation in the factor V molecule (R506Q). Either functional or molecular testing has been used to identify this risk factor for thrombosis. Functional testing is generally faster and less expensive, but is subject to false negative and false positive results when compared to the gold standard of molecular testing. Functional test results are reported as the ratio of activated partial thromboplastin times before and after the addition of APC. These authors performed both molecular and functional tests on 370 patients, and determined false negative and false positive rates for 2 different APC normalized sensitivity ratio thresholds. Both thresholds identified all of the patients with disease, providing 100% sensitivity. The lower threshold improved the specificity and positive predictive value. The authors do not state how the higher threshold was determined. The lower value was determined retrospectively as the highest ratio obtained from a patient determined (by molecular methods) to carry the mutant gene. These results demonstrate that it is reasonable to establish a testing algorithm in which only specimens with abnormal functional assay results would be subjected to molecular confirmation, and emphasizes that the threshold for the functional assay is best determined within each laboratory by comparing molecular and functional test results for a number of specimens during validation of the assay.

A.J. Schlueter, M.D., Ph.D.

Recombinant Factor VIIa Corrects Prothrombin Time in Cirrhotic Patients: A Preliminary Study

Bernstein DE, Jeffers L, Erhardtsen E, et al (Univ of Miami, Fla; NovoNordisk, Copenhagen)

Gastroenterology 113:1930–1937, 1997 18–14

Background.—Cirrhotic patients with low platelet counts and/or prolonged prothrombin times (PTs) usually do not bleed spontaneously but are at increased risk for severe bleeding episodes from routine procedures. The efficacy of recombinant factor VIIa (rFVIIa) in nonbleeding patients with the coagulopathy of cirrhosis was investigated in a preliminary study.

Methods and Findings.—Thirteen consecutive cirrhotic patients were enrolled in the dosage-escalation trial. All had a PT exceeding 2 seconds above the upper limit of the reference value. On intramuscular injection of vitamin K, 10 patients had a PT that did not correct to within 2 seconds above the control of the upper limit of the reference value. These patients were given 3 successive dosages of rFVIIa (5, 20, 80 µg/kg) over 3 weeks. In all 3 dosage groups, mean PT transiently corrected to normal. There were no adverse effects nor evidence of induction of disseminated intravascular coagulation.

Conclusions.—These preliminary findings show that rFVIIa is effective for transiently reversing the prolonged PT in a selected group of nonbleeding cirrhotic patients. A large-scale efficacy study is warranted.

► Cirrhotic patients have numerous abnormalities which predispose them to episodes of uncontrollable bleeding. One of these abnormalities is decreased synthesis of vitamin K–dependent clotting factors. Factor VII deficiency is generally the most severe, because of its short half life. This study found rFVIIa to be effective in correcting the PT in a group of nonbleeding Child's class B and C cirrhotic patients. At high doses of rFVIIa, the PT remained normal for up to 12 hours after bolus infusion. Use of similar preparations in hemophiliacs with inhibitors to factor VIII or IX has been associated with increased risk of inappropriate thrombosis or disseminated intravascular coagulation. No clinical evidence of these complications occurred in this group of patients, although increased concentrations of D-dimer and fibrinopeptide A were observed at the highest dose of rFVIIa. These preliminary results are promising, but cannot be extrapolated to the bleeding cirrhotic patient without further study. Advantages to using such preparations in place of fresh frozen plasma include markedly smaller volumes of fluid administered as well as decreased risk of infectious disease transmission. These advantages must be weighed against the significantly higher cost of such preparations. Recombinant FVIIa may ultimately find a place in the treatment of a subset of bleeding cirrhotic patients.

A.J. Schlueter, M.D., Ph.D.

Evaluation of Changes in Hemoglobin Levels Associated With ABO-incompatible Plasma in Apheresis Platelets

Mair B, Benson K (Univ of South Florida, Tampa)

Transfusion 38:51–55, 1998 18–15

Background.—Though most medical centers try to provide ABO-identical platelets for transfusions, it is not always possible to do so. Minor ABO incompatibility may lead to acute hemolysis. The current study was done to identify possible hemolysis associated with the transfusion of plasma-incompatible apheresis platelets.

Methods.—Sixteen patients were included in the retrospective study. All were of non-group O type, receiving apheresis platelets. The patients were given both ABO-identical and plasma-incompatible platelet transfusions within 24 hours. No red cells were transfused between the collection of the pretransfusion and posttransfusion hemoglobin samples.

Findings.—Twenty-four paired platelet transfusions able to be evaluated were available for analysis. Mean change in hemoglobin after transfusion of the ABO-identical platelets was −0.50 g/dL, and after transfusion of plasma-incompatible platelets, it was −0.11 g/dL.

Conclusions.—These patients had no significant changes in hemoglobin concentration associated with the transfusion of plasma-incompatible apheresis platelets. At the authors' hospital, the risk of clinically significant acute hemolysis following ABO-incompatible platelet transfusion is about 1 in 9,000.

▶ The transfusion of ABO-nonidentical platelets carries the risk of hemolytic transfusion reaction resulting from anti-A (or anti-B) antibodies in the plasma of the platelet unit. Although there is no requirement by regulatory agencies for transfusion of ABO-identical platelets, it is common practice to provide ABO-identical units, if available, to avoid this risk. Because of the short shelf life of platelet units and the high cost associated with discarding unused units, most institutions will transfuse ABO-nonidentical platelets when ABO-identical units are not available. This study was initiated following an index case of well-documented hemolytic transfusion reaction, which occurred after group O platelets were transfused to a group A patient. It retrospectively addressed the frequency of hemolytic transfusion reactions following the transfusion of ABO-incompatible plasma in platelet units. All 16 patients in the study were autologous bone marrow transplant recipients, and had recieved both ABO-identical and -nonidentical platelet transfusions. This allowed the patients to serve as their own controls. The change in hemoglobin following platelet transfusion was used as the indicator of hemolysis. No episodes of hemolysis were identified. These data support a previous study[1] which also identified a very low risk of hemolytic transfusion reactions following ABO-nonidentical platelet transfusions. Several methods exist to further decrease this risk, such as determining the anti-A (or anti-B) titers of all platelet donors, or reducing the volume of platelet units prior to transfusion. The expense of these maneuvers, and the potential decrease in quality of the product, do not justify their use at present.

A.J. Schlueter, M.D., Ph.D.

Reference

1. Shanwell A, Ringden O, Weichel B, et al: A study of the effect of ABO incompatible plasma in platelet concentrates transfused to bone marrow transplant recipients. *Vox Sang* 60:23–27, 1991.

19 Microbiology

Surreptitious Hepatitis C Virus (HCV) Infection Detected in the Majority of Patients With Cryptogenic Chronic Hepatitis and Negative HCV Antibody Tests

Schmidt WN, Wu P, Cederna J, et al (Univ of Iowa, Iowa City)
J Infect Dis 176:27–33, 1997 19–1

Background.—Although chronic hepatitis has many causes, in a small group of patients no etiologic agent can be identified. These patients are considered to have cryptogenic liver disease or non-A, non-B, non-C (NANBNC) chronic hepatitis. These authors have previously reported a methodology for the detection of hepatitis C virus (HCV) RNA in whole blood (WB). This method was used to screen 15 patients previously diagnosed with NANBNC chronic hepatitis for HCV RNA.

Methods.—Fifteen patients from the University of Iowa Liver Clinic with a diagnosis of NANBNC chronic hepatitis were identified from a review of medical records. All patients had been seronegative for HCV antibody by EIA.2 on at least 2 samples obtained at least 6 months apart. Whole blood and plasma were collected for reverse transcription-polymerase chain reaction (RT-PCR) assays for HCV RNA.

Results.—HCV RNA was detected in the WB samples from 10 of these 15 NANBNC chronic hepatitis patients. Hepatitis C virus RNA was only detected in the plasma samples from 5 patients, indicating that the plasma assay has lower sensitivity. Nucleic acid hybridization and HCV genotypic analysis confirmed the specificity of the HCV assay. Liver biopsies revealed histopathologic differences between the HCV RNA-positive and HCV RNA-negative patients in the study group.

Conclusions.—The results of screening patients with unexplained chronic hepatitis with a method to detect HCV RNA in whole blood revealed that HCV infection is not uncommon in these patients. Assays to detect HCV RNA in WB appear to be more sensitive than plasma assays.

▶ The extent of the HCV problem in this country was unrealized until the early 1990s when a specific assay for antibody was introduced. Since that time, the test has been improved by the addition of several more antigens from the virus. It is estimated that there are between 2 and 4 million people in this country infected with the virus; and because a large proportion of those infected go on to chronic disease, there is fear of an epidemic of chronic liver disease and its consequences in the future.

This paper describes 15 patients with chronic, unexplained hepatitis who were negative for the HCV antibody test on at least 2 occasions. Using both whole blood and plasma RT-PCR, the authors were able to identify HCV RNA in a majority of these patients. The whole blood assay detected more patients than the plasma assay. Because the HCV antibody assay performed on serum is usually the initial test and determines whether additional tests are run, the implications of this paper are to be noted. The prevalence of hepatitis C may be even greater than previously thought, and the effectiveness of blood donor screening using the antibody test is reduced.

R. Feld, Ph.D.

Cross-Reactivity in *Histoplasma capsulatum* Variety *capsulatum* Antigen Assays of Urine Samples From Patients With Endemic Mycoses

Wheat J, Wheat H, Connolly P, et al (Indiana Univ, Indianapolis; Univ of Arkansas, Little Rock; Johns Hopkins Univ, Baltimore, Md; et al)

Clin Infect Dis 24:1169–1171, 1997 19–2

Background.—Detection of a specific polysaccharide antigen in patient urine has been used as a rapid technique in the diagnosis of histoplasmosis. Although the antigen assay was initially believed to be highly specific, cross reactions have subsequently been reported in patients with blastomycosis and paracoccidiomycosis. The cross-reactivity of the *Histoplasma capsulatum* var. *capsulatum* assay to antigens of other fungal pathogens in patient urine was more fully evaluated.

Methods.—Urine samples of patients with *Penicillium marneffei* (*n* = 18), *Coccidioides immitis* (n = 6), *Blastomyces dermatitidis* (n = 19), *Paracoccidioides brasiliensis* (n = 9), *H. capsulatum* var. *duboisii* (n = 1), and 2 control urine samples were tested using a previously described solid-phase enzyme immunoassay for *H. capsulatum* var. *capsulatum*.

Results.—Positive assay results occurred for urine samples of 17 patients (94.4%) infected with *P. marneffei*, 12 (63.2%) with blastomycosis, 8 (88.9%) with paracoccidioidomycosis, and in the single patient infected with *H. capsulatum* var. *duboisii*. Cross reaction was not noted for any urine samples collected from patients with coccidioidomycosis.

Conclusion.—Cross reactions may be expected with disseminated infections by *H. capsulatum* var. *capsulatum*, *P. marneffei*, *B. dermatitidis*, *P. brasiliensis*, and *H. capsulatum* var. *duboisii*. Although the immunoassay may be useful in the rapid diagnosis of disseminated disease caused by one of these organisms, further evaluation is required before a specific diagnosis can be made.

▶ Detection of polysaccharide antigen in urine has proven useful in the diagnosis of histoplasmosis. Earlier studies demonstrated the high specificity of the *H. capsulatum* antigen assay when applied to specimens from individuals infected with *Candida*, *Aspergillus*, or *Cryptococcus* species. Limited data suggest that cross-reaction may be observed in cases of blastomycosis, paracoccidioidomycosis and coccidioidomycosis.

This study was designed to more fully explore the possible cross-reactivity of the *H. capsulatum* antigen test in patients infected with a variety of endemic fungal pathogens. Cross-reactivity was noted in samples from patients with blastomycosis, paracoccidioidomycosis, disseminated *P. marneffii* infection, and African histoplasmosis (*H. duboisii*). Cross-reaction was not observed in samples from patients with coccidioidomycosis. Although such extensive cross-reactivity is disturbing, it does not negate the value of the *Histoplasma* antigen test for rapid diagnosis. In fact, such cross-reactivity may expand the usefulness of the assay to include diagnosis of the other endemic mycoses, depending on the geographic location and travel history of the patient.

The epidemiologic and clinical differences between these mycoses are important considerations when using this test. Because treatment with either amphotericin B or itraconazole is indicated for disseminated or extensive pulmonary infections with any of the endemic mycoses, detection of urinary antigen remains a useful aid in rapid diagnosis. It should be noted that the sensitivity of the test has been optimized for diagnosis of histoplasmosis and requires further evaluation for the other endemic mycoses.

M.A. Pfaller, M.D.

Macrophages as a Source of HIV During Opportunistic Infections

Orenstein JM, Fox C, Wahl SM (George Washington Univ, Washington, DC; Molecular Histology Inc, Gaithersburg, Md; NIH, Bethesda, Md)

Science 276:1857–1861, 1997 19–3

Background.—Infection with HIV-1 results in progressive loss of CD4 T lymphocytes and concurrent increase in host susceptibility to opportunistic infections (OIs). Unexpectedly, the incidence of OIs is positively correlated with HIV-1 expression, even in the presence of severe lymphoid involution. The source of free HIV-1 during this advanced stage of the disease has been puzzling. Monocytes or macrophages have not been thought responsible because infected monocytes/macrophages are rarely seen in blood or lymphoid tissue; however, productive infection of CD4+ macrophages does occur in the central nervous tissue, and infected monocytes/macrophages can produce large amounts of the virus without succumbing to the infection. The potential role of macrophages in enhanced HIV-1 replication in the presence of decreasing CD4+ T cell numbers was evaluated.

Methods.—Lymph nodes infected with *Pneumocystis carinii* and *Mycobacterium avium* complex collected from patients infected with HIV-1 were probed for HIV-1–specific RNA by in situ hybridization, and the distribution of message within the tissues and the strength of the signals were determined. Production of HIV-1 was then compared between lymph nodes from 11 HIV-1–positive patients with OIs and lymph nodes from 11 HIV-1–positive patients without OIs.

Results.—HIV-1–positive cells in the *P. carinii*–infected lymph nodes were far more numerous than the expected number of infected lymphocytes in an OI-free lymph node. Human immunodeficiency virus–1 RNA was associated with mononuclear and multinuclear cells and in apparently cell-free areas. Transmission electron microscopy revealed virions budding from plasma membranes of mononuclear cells and multinucleated macrophages, but not lymphocytes, with virus production apparently not associated with death in these cells. Production of HIV-1 in the *M. avium*–infected nodes was intense and was associated with mononuclear cells and multinucleated giant cells which were coinfected with the bacterium. Between fivefold and 100-fold more HIV-1–producing cells were identified in lymphoid tissue from 11 patients with OIs, compared with those without OIs, with cells of monocyte/macrophage lineage accounting for a major proportion of infected cells. The number of HIV-1 transcripts per cell was also notably greater in lymphoid tissue from OI-infected patients than in those without OIs.

Conclusions.—Macrophages may produce HIV-1 when CD4 lymphocyte numbers have become low. This apparently occurs in the presence or absence of OIs. Opportunistic infections, however, profoundly alter HIV-1 expression within macrophages, apparently by recruiting macrophages to sites of infection and stimulating expression of the virus. The mechanism of this upregulation has yet to be established. Control of OIs may benefit patients as much by reducing HIV-1 expression as by controlling direct damage caused by the opportunistic pathogen.

► The latter stages of HIV infection are characterized by steadily declining CD4 T lymphocytes, quantitative and qualitative impairment of lymphoid tissue, an increasing level of viremia, and frequent infection with opportunistic pathogens such as *M. avium* complex, *P. carinii*, and *Cryptococcus neoformans*. Given the tremendous loss of lymphoid tissue, the source of increased circulating HIV-1 has been puzzling.

In this study, the authors demonstrate that tissue macrophages are highly productive sources of HIV. Furthermore, they show that co-infection with opportunistic pathogens results in a dramatic increase in the production of virus. The authors used in situ hybridization, immunohistochemical, and electron microscopic techniques to show differences in virus production in lymph nodes from patients with and without OIs. It is postulated that in patients with OIs, foci of HIV-1 production are established by recruitment of HIV-1–infected and infectible macrophages and stimulation of their viral expression.

The mechanism of upregulation of HIV-1 RNA expression by OIs remains to be determined. These findings suggest that in addition to eliminating the direct pathogenicity of OIs, treatment and prevention of these infections in HIV-infected individuals may also be important in controlling HIV production.

M.A. Pfaller, M.D.

Molecular Epidemiology of *Enterobacter aerogenes* Acquisition: One-Year Prospective Study in Two Intensive Care Units

Davin-Regli A, Monnet D, Saux P, et al (Hôpital Salvator, Marseille, France; Hôpital Ste Marguerite, Marseille, France; Centre de Coordination de la Lutte contre les Infections Nosocomiales Sud-Est, France)

J Clin Microbiol 34:1474–1480, 1996 19–4

Background.—*Enterobacter aerogenes* infection has newly risen to the third most common cause of gram-negative nosocomial infection, replacing *Klebsiella pneumoniae* in this position. The epidemiology of the bacterium, however, including mode of transmission, has not been well described. The genetic diversity of the bacterium, means of patient exposure, and the role of clinical and environmental factors on disease transmission were evaluated in this prospective epidemiologic study.

Methods.—All clinical *E. aerogenes* isolates collected from patients in a surgical ICU and a medical ICU in 2 separate hospitals in Marseille, France between 1994 and 1995 were evaluated for antimicrobial susceptibility and epidemiologic type. Environmental isolates from the 2 ICUs were similarly evaluated. Epidemiologic typing was performed by random amplification of polymorphic DNA (RAPD) and by genomic fingerprinting based on a polymerase chain reaction technique using enterobacterial repetitive intergenic consensus sequences (ERIC-PCR).

Results.—One hundred sixty four of the 175 isolates collected from patients in the ICUs and all of the 10 environmental isolates produced an extended-spectrum β-lactamase and were resistant to the majority of antimicrobials tested, with the exception of cefepime, colistin and imipenem, and, with the exception of 4 isolates, to moxalactam and gentamicin. Analysis by RAPD and ERIC-PCR allowed identification of 25 types from the 130 surgical ICU clinical isolates and 15 from the 45 medical ICU clinical isolates. Up to 4 types were identified from each infected patient. A single clone comprised 41% to 58% of clinical isolates and 9 of 10 environmental isolates. Three related types, specific to each ICU, comprised 17% to 24% of clinical isolates. Small clusters of other types represented 6% to 8% of clinical isolates, and unique types comprised 17% to 29%.

Conclusion.—*E. aerogenes* may be acquired by transmission of a prevalent or related strain of the organism between patients, emergence of a strain from the natural flora of a patient, or by acquisition and subsequent transmission between patients of a nonendemic strain. More than two thirds of pathogen acquisition in this study was apparently caused by patient-to-patient transmission. Earlier studies have implied that transmission of the bacterium between patients is rare, suggesting a possible change in the ecology of strains of the organism endemic to hospitals over the past decade.

► Antimicrobial resistance among gram-negative and gram-positive bacteria is an increasing problem affecting both hospitalized and nonhospitalized patients. Among hospitalized patients, *E. aerogenes* is an important cause of serious nosocomial infection, particularly in the ICU setting. *Enterobacter aerogenes* strains are frequently resistant to a broad array of penicillins and cephalosporins as the result of an inducible chromosomal cephalosporinase.

In this study, the authors investigated the acquisition of *E. aerogenes* by patients hospitalized in 2 ICU settings. Their results confirmed the fact that 94% of the isolates were resistant to a majority of the antibiotics and combinations of antibiotics tested. They found that *E. aerogenes* was acquired in the ICU in 3 different ways: (1) patient-to-patient spread of a prevalent strain; (2) acquisition de novo of a strain from the patients' own endogenous flora; and (3) acquisition of a nonendemic strain followed by limited patient-to-patient transmission.

These findings point to selection of resistant strains within the hospital environment after broad-spectrum antibiotic therapy and also to cross-transmission from critically ill, heavily colonized patients who require prolonged and intense nursing and medical care. Isolation of the prevalent *E. aerogenes* strains from the environment and from the hands of care providers suggests that cross-contaminations are not caused by direct contact between patients, but by contact with nursing personnel either by direct patient-personnel contact or after the care giver has touched a contaminated surface. Control of antibiotic-resistant organisms, such as *E. aerogenes*, in the hospital requires limiting the overuse of broad-spectrum antimicrobials and also rigorous infection control policies. Simple hand washing between patients is a critical step in this process.

The laboratory may assist in this process by providing accurate and timely identification and antimicrobial susceptibility-testing results. In selected instances, detailed molecular typing results, performed on-site or in a reference laboratory, may also be useful.

M.A. Pfaller, M.D.

HIV Antibody Assay That Gave False Negative Results: Multicentre Collaborative Study

Evans BG, for the Multicentre Collaborative Study Group (Public Health Lab Service, London)

BMJ 315:772–774, 1997 19–5

Background.—In 1995, Abbott Laboratories changed its assay kit for HIV antibody to increase its sensitivity, but in 1996, it announced that there had been reports of false negative results associated with this assay. The laboratory advised customers to stop using the assay or to evaluate each specimen both undiluted and at a 1:4 dilution. An investigation was made to identify false negative results arising from the use of this kit to detect HIV1 and HIV2 antibody.

Methods.—All laboratories in the United Kingdom that had used the Abbott Laboratory assay between July 1995 and March 1996 were asked to retest all specimens that had been tested with the assay and had produced a negative result. The serum samples that had a false negative result underwent further analysis.

Results.—The assay had been used in 24,181 individuals who had been given negative results for HIV antibody and in 497 individuals who had been given positive results. Re-testing was done in serum samples from 20,973 individuals. It was found that 4 individuals had false negative results associated with the kit and 3 other individuals had false negative results associated with other laboratory testing. These 7 individuals were of a diverse risk group and HIV1 subtype. In 4 individuals, there was evidence of recent HIV infection.

Discussion.—These results showed that the commercial kit for detecting HIV antibody had a sensitivity of 99.2%, or less than 99.2% if the 3 additional individuals with false negative results were considered. This incident appeared to decrease public confidence in HIV testing, which is assumed to be 100% sensitive. Steps must be taken to avoid false negative results in HIV testing. Laboratories must retain samples, 2 screening assays should be used for individuals with a higher risk of infection, and even single HIV assay failures should be reported.

▶ Two reportedly recurring nightmares are being late for a final examination or falling off a cliff. Luckily when the person awakens, reality takes over. This paper, however, reports on a nightmare that is real. Abbott Laboratories modified their HIV 1/HIV 2 antibody assay in 1995 to make it more sensitive to subtypes that had been reported to not react in the then-current assay. On the face of it, this would seem good because it would prevent false negative results.

After the assay had been evaluated with numerous serum samples of known reactivity, it was released in Europe in July 1995. In March 1996, Abbott wrote to all laboratories using the test stating that there had been reports of false negative results, that the test should be discontinued, and that previously analyzed specimens should be rescreened. The defect was later identified as complement activity in fresh sera and was corrected by the addition of ethylenediaminetetraacetic acid.

In rescreening over 20,000 samples, 7 false negative results were identified. No common feature in these patients was identified. The authors make several recommendations including long-term storage of samples in case retesting is necessary. They also recommend testing by 2 different assays if the patient is at increased risk. Although these are good recommendations in light of their experience, they would present an additional burden for laboratories now performing this testing. Although improvements in assays are considered positive outcomes, assays such as the HIV antibody assay, whose results are so critical, should not be tampered with lightly. In this case, an assay modification introduced to decrease false negatives in fact gave just the opposite result.

R. Feld, Ph.D.

Performance of Three Generations of Anti-Hepatitis C Virus Enzyme-linked Immunosorbent Assays in Donors and Patients

Vrielink H, Reesink HW, van den Burg PJM, et al (Red Cross Blood Bank Amsterdam)

Transfusion 37:845–849, 1997 19–6

Objective.—The third generation hepatitis C virus (HCV) antibody test, now being used routinely in Europe for blood-donor screening, is not required in the United States because it is recognized as an improvement over the second generation product rather than a third-generation test. The sensitivity and specificity of first-, second-, and third-generation anti-HCV enzyme-linked immunosorbent assays (ELISAs) were compared using serial samples from patients with well-documented acute posttransfusion HCV infection.

Methods.—Between May 1990 and January 1996, 99,394 blood donations were screened with ELISA-1, 167,999 donations were screened with ELISA-2, and 262,090 donations were screened with ELISA-3. Sequential samples from 9 patients with HCV were tested with the 3 assays before and at 2, 4, 6, 8, 10, 12, 16, 20, 26, and 32 weeks after transfusion. Recombinant immunoblot assay (RIBA) and complementary DNA–polymerase chain reaction (cDNA-PCR) were used as confirmatory tests. Sensitivities and specificities of the 3 assays were compared statistically.

Results.—Eight repeat donors (37%), who were positive in ELISA-2 and positive in the RIBA-2 and/or cDNA-PCR tests, were negative in ELISA-1. The ELISA-2 had a specificity of 99.7%. The 20 patients who were positive in ELISA-1, RIBA-2, and cDNA-PCR were also positive in ELISA-2. Of first-time donors, 0.4% were positive in ELISA-3, and 21% of these were RIBA-3- and cDNA-PCR–positive. The ELISA-3 had a specificity of 99.7%. The ELISA-1, -2, and -3 detected HCV antibodies in serial samples from infected patients. In 2 patients, ELISA-3 detected HVC antibodies significantly earlier than the first- and second-generation assays.

Conclusion.—The ELISA-2 and ELISA-3 had similar specificities, although ELISA-3 detected HCV antibodies significantly earlier in some patients. The ELISA-2 and ELISA-3 were significantly more sensitive than RIBA-2 and RIBA-3.

▶ The 1990 introduction of a test for antibodies to HCV has significantly reduced the incidence of posttransfusion hepatitis and allowed us to identify a growing epidemic of HCV in the American population. As with software, there is an expectation of improvement in succeeding generations. The anti-HCV test is currently in its third generation. This has been accomplished by increasing the number and kind of antigens that are used in the test. Although the third-generation test is widely used in Europe, it is not required by the Food and Drug Administration in United States testing facilities.

This report from the Netherlands looks at donor screening using each of the 3 generations of tests. The authors also compared the tests in patients in whom posttransfusion HCV developed. This testing was done on sequential samples up to 32 weeks after transfusion.

Although the previously noted problems with the first-generation test, such as a high false positive rate, were confirmed, the authors found little difference between the second- and third-generation tests with regard to donor screening. The third-generation test did detect antibody sooner in 2 patients with transfusion-related HCV than did the second-generation test. It seems that the third-generation test may not represent an improvement in donor screening but may identify infected patients earlier in the course of the disease.

R. Feld, Ph.D.

Immunohistologic Identification of *Aspergillus* spp. and Other Hyaline Fungi by Using Polyclonal Fluorescent Antibodies

Kaufmann L, Standard PG, Jalbert M, et al (Natl Ctr for Infectious Diseases, Atlanta, Ga)

J Clin Microbiol 35:2206–2209, 1997 19–7

Background.—The best way to diagnose infection with *Aspergillus* or *Fusarium* is to demonstrate the pathogens from clinical materials. However, isolation and identification may be difficult to achieve. The hyphae of the 2 molds appear very similar in vivo, while their manifestations in situ are not specific. Polyclonal fluorescent-antibody reagents to *Aspergillus fumigatus* and *Fusarium solani* were developed and tested.

Methods and Results.—The new reagents were based on the finding that *A. fumigatus* and *F. solani* shared epitopes with each other, with other *Aspergillus* and *Fusarium* species, and with *Paecilomyces lilacinus* and *Pseudallescheria boydii.* The reagents were formed by adsorption of the *A. fumigatus* conjugate with cells of *Fusarium proliferatum* and *F. solani* and *F. solani* antiserum with cells of *Aspergillus flavus.* While capable of differentiating between *Aspergillus* and *Fusarium,* the reagents still cross-stained *P. lilacinus* and *P. boydii.* The polyclonal fluorescent antibodies were applied to formalin-fixed tissue specimens from patients with culture-confirmed mycotic infections. With adjunctive use of a specific *P. boydii*-conjugate, the reagents were able to identify *Aspergillus* and *Fusarium* organisms, as well as *P. lilacinus* and *P. boydii.*

Conclusions.—Polyclonal fluorescent antibody reagents to *A. fumigatus* and *F. solani* were described for use in identifying infections caused by these and other mycotic pathogens. Immunohistologic studies may be useful when no diagnosis can be made on histologic grounds. The use of the study reagents would be complicated by the time-consuming immunization schedules and adsorptions needed to produce the 3 reagents.

▶ Despite its importance clinically, the diagnosis of filamentous fungal infection remains inadequate. Infections caused by hyaline fungi such as *Aspergillus, Fusarium,* and *Paecilomyces* spp. are increasingly common in immunocompromised patients and carry an excessive morbidity and mortality. Accurate diagnosis of these infections is essential for delivery of appropriate therapy. Histopathologic examination of infected tissue is a mainstay in the diagnosis of such infections, but frequently is of limited use because of the inability of the pathologist to differentiate among the various fungi that produce hyaline hyphae in tissue.

In this study, the authors provide preliminary data suggesting that polyclonal fluorescent-antibody reagents can be developed that will enable the identification of *Aspergillus* spp., *Fusarium* spp., *P. lilacinus*, and *P. boydii* in formalin-fixed tissue sections. Although this report is promising, the procedure described is cumbersome and the reagents are not available commercially. Commercial development of immunologic and molecular reagents for diagnosis of fungal infections is overdue and will be necessary if we are to realize any progress in this area of clinical diagnosis.

M.A. Pfaller, M.D.

Morphologic Criteria for the Preliminary Identification of *Fusarium, Paecilomyces,* and *Acremonium* Species by Histopathology

Liu K, Howell DN, Perfect JR, et al (Duke Univ, Durham, NC; Veterans Affairs Med Ctr, Durham, NC)

Am J Clin Pathol 109:45–54, 1998 19–8

Background.—*Fusarium, Paecilomyces,* and *Acremonium* are unusual fungal pathogens that cause infection predominantly in immunocompromised patients. These infections are characterized by the formation of colorless, septate fungal hyphae in the host cells. Although laboratory culture is necessary for definitive identification, initial diagnosis can be made through the examination of stained biopsy sections for fungal reproductive structures, such as phialides and phialoconidia, attributable to adventitious sporulation in host cultures. Rapid diagnosis is important, because these organisms are often resistant to common antifungal agents. The records of 19 patients with culture-documented infections with one of these unusual pathogens were reviewed to determine histologic characteristics that would be helpful in diagnosis.

Study Design.—A review of the records of 19 patients seen from 1985 to 1996 who had cultures positive for *Fusarium, Paecilomyces*, or *Acremonium* was performed. All histologic sections were stained with hematoxylin and eosin, Gomori methanamine silver, or periodic acid-Schiff method.

Findings.—All specimens from these 19 patients contained septate, hyaline hyphae. The hyphae were usually irregular. Hyphal branching was detected in 17 of 19 specimens. Phialoconidia were detected in 16 of 19 specimens, including all cases involving closed spaces. Phialides were detected in 15 of 19 cases. Phialides appeared as tapering structures on hyphae with a terminal orifice and a periclinal wall thickening. The periclinal wall thickenings stained more intensely than other regions. Necrosis and acute inflammation were detected in 14 cases. Most of these infected patients were immunosuppressed. All 6 deaths were in patients with disseminated infection. Those infections that occurred in patients who were not immunosuppressed were all cases of keratitis.

Conclusions.—This retrospective study of 19 patients infected with *Fusarium*, *Paecilomyces*, or *Acremonium* revealed that the histopathologic characteristics that can be used to identify these infectious agents are their reproductive structures, phialides and phialoconidia, and their hyaline septate hyphae. Early recognition of these unusual pathogens is important in prompt initiation of appropriate therapy.

▶ The anatomical pathologist often plays an essential role in the diagnosis of invasive fungal disease. Histopathologic examination of clinical material often can establish a presumptive or definitive diagnosis rapidly, detect and identify unculturable pathogens, evaluate the clinical significance of a cultured organism, and establish a diagnosis when cultures are either negative or unavailable. In some instances, subtle morphological clues may allow one to distinguish among several different mycotic pathogens. Although *Candida* and *Aspergillus* species are by far the most common fungal pathogens, we are faced with an ever-increasing array of emerging opportunistic fungal pathogens, many of which produce in tissue, nonpigmented (hyaline), branched, septate hyphal structures that may be difficult to distinguish from those of aspergilli. Among the more important emerging mycotic pathogens are *Fusarium, Paecilomyces*, and *Acremonium* species. The ability to distinguish these emerging pathogens from *Aspergillus* (or even *Candida*) has important therapeutic implications because many of the emerging fungi are resistant to standard antifungal therapy and may require surgical intervention and/or prolonged therapy with one or more antifungal agents.

The article by Liu and colleagues describes several subtle morphological features exhibited by *Fusarium, Paecilomyces*, and *Acremonium* species that may allow the pathologist to distinguish them from *Aspergillus* and other hyaline fungi. The authors note that invasive tissue infection with these organisms often demonstrates irregular hyphae with both 45- and 90-degree angle–branching. Furthermore, they describe specialized structures resulting from adventitious sporulation in tissue that may allow one to distinguish *Fusarium, Paecilomyces*, and *Acremonium* from *Aspergillus* species. Detection of phialides and phialoconidia through careful histological examination of GMS- or PAS-stained material may allow presumptive identification of these organisms. This approach has merit; however, there are numerous confounding issues such as integrity of the specimen, the plane of section, and development of unusual or misleading structures by other fungi that can be confusing and result in an incorrect diagnosis. It is always necessary to correlate histopathologic findings with those of culture. In the future, techniques such as immunohistochemistry and in situ hybridization may serve to augment our diagnostic capabilities for invasive mycoses.

M.A. Pfaller, M.D.

Effects of Storage Temperature and Time on Qualitative and Quantitative Detection of Cytomegalovirus in Blood Specimens by Shell Vial Culture and PCR

Roberts TC, Buller RS, Gaudreault-Keener M, et al (Washington Univ, St Louis)

J Clin Microbiol 35:2224–2228, 1997 19–9

Introduction.—Blood samples obtained to detect and quantitate cytomegalovirus (CMV) are often stored or transported to a virology laboratory, resulting in a delay of 1–2 days or more before processing and testing. A study was conducted to examine the effects of storage temperature and sample processing time on the detection of CMV in blood samples by shell vial culture (SVC) and polymerase chain reaction (PCR).

Methods.—Blood samples were collected from 10 renal transplant recipients who were CMV positive and suspected of having CMV viremia. Tubes containing 20 mL of whole blood were transported immediately to a virology laboratory, then divided into 2-mL aliquots. One aliquot was processed immediately and 2 were stored at either 4°C or room temperature (RT), then processed after 6, 24, 48, or 72 hours of storage.

Results.—All specimens tested positive by SVC and PCR at baseline. After cold storage, 75% of aliquots were still SVC positive at 6 hours, 50% were positive at 24 hours, and 10% were positive at both 48 and 72 hours. After RT storage, 75% were still SVC positive at 6 hours, 60% at 24 hours, 10% at 48 hours, and 0% at 72 hours. Although the sensitivity of SVC declined progressively over time, all samples remained PCR positive at all time points. Quantitative DNA levels remained stable over time.

Conclusion.—Culture should not be used to detect or quantitate CMV if a 24-hour delay occurs between specimen collection and processing. Samples can be transported or stored at RT, however, without adversely affecting the results of PCR.

► CMV is an important cause of morbidity and mortality among immunocompromised hosts. Among the rapid diagnostic tests for detection of CMV, SVC, antigenemia detection, and PCR are most common. PCR is attractive because it is rapid and sensitive and may be performed quantitatively. In this study, the authors demonstrate that detection of CMV DNA by PCR is also stable and is relatively unaffected by delays in processing and suboptimal storage conditions. In contrast, SVC sensitivity is negatively affected by processing delays and storage conditions.

A similar lack of stability has been noted for detection of CMV antigenemia in buffy coat specimens. The PCR may be performed qualitatively or quantitatively. The quantitative DNA levels did not decline over time and were not affected by storage temperature. For diagnosis of CMV infection, DNA is a stable analyte.

M.A. Pfaller, M.D.

Determination of Hepatitis C Virus Genotypes in the United States by Cleavase Fragment Length Polymorphism Analysis

Marshall DJ, Heisler LM, Lyamichev V, et al (Third Wave Technologies Inc, Madison, Wis; Univ of Pittsburgh, Pa)

J Clin Microbiol 35:3156–3162, 1997 19–10

Background.—Most assays for the detection and quantification of hepatitis C virus (HCV) are aimed at the 5'-noncoding region (5'NCR). Genotyping techniques focus on a limited number of diagnostic sequence polymorphisms located throughout this region, but these approaches are limited in the number of types and subtypes they can identify. A new DNA-based technique for HCV genotyping, termed Cleavase Fragment Length Polymorphism (CFLP), can identify unique collections of cleavage products, or structural fingerprints, that permit identification of different DNA sequences.

Methods.—The CFLP method was applied to 251–bp cDNA products generated by reverse transcription-polymerase chain reaction (RT-CPR) of the 5'NCR of HCV. Confirmatory DNA sequencing data were available in 87 samples.

Results.—The isolates identified reflected 98% of the types commonly encountered in the United States, namely types 1a, 1b, 2a/c, 2b, 3a, and 4. On blinded analysis, the CFLP findings agreed 100% with the DNA sequencing results, and could identify viral genotypes different by no more than a single nucleotide. Genotypes that were closely related showed patterns of strong familial resemblance; more divergent genotypes showed patterns with marked dissimilarities. The aggregate patterns reflected genotypic groupings, whereas the finer changes were consistent with subgenotypic differences. Analysis of different isolates within a single subtype and repeated analysis of a single sample suggested that CFLP analysis was highly reproducible.

Conclusions.—The CFLP technique appears highly appropriate for use in HCV genotyping. The assay can be completed on RT-PCR products within 2 hours or less. It may provide a less expensive, high-throughput alternative to DNA sequencing or other less advantageous genotyping techniques, thus improving the effectiveness and timeliness of patient care.

► Determination of the genotype of HCV has proven to be a useful prognostic marker in the management of patients with HCV infection. Although DNA sequencing is the "gold standard" for genotyping, more simple techniques have been employed to identify HCV genotypes. These techniques include restriction fragment length polymorphism (RFLP) analysis of the 5'NCR and the use of allele-specific oligonucleotide analysis. These approaches are considered simpler than direct sequence analysis, but are limited in the number of types and subtypes that they can discriminate. CFLP analysis is a new DNA-based technique that allows determination of genotype through the use of CFLP technology. CFLP technology uses the Cleavase I enzyme to identify unique secondary structures in DNA and generates a specific set of cleavage products for a given DNA fragment. The structural fingerprint that results from CFLP analysis allows one to identify the extent to which sequences of different DNA strands are related to one another. Thus, it may be useful in establishing genotypes. CFLP technology may be applied to identify genotypes among HCV. CFLP proved to be sensitive, specific, and reproducible, and compared favorably to DNA sequencing for identification of different HCV genotypes. CFLP structural fingerprinting was capable of distinguishing sequence changes as subtle as a single nucleotide. Thus, it may be useful in identifying emerging genotypes. The CFLP assay can be applied to the analysis of RT-PCR products and carried out in 2 hours or less. The total material cost is reportedly less than other genotyping methods, including DNA sequencing. This is an exciting new technology that may have broad applicability in the area of DNA analysis.

M.A. Pfaller, M.D.

An Epidemic of *Malassezia pachydermatis* in an Intensive Care Nursery Associated With Colonization of Health Care Workers' Pet Dogs

Chang HJ, Miller HL, Watkins N, et al (Ctrs for Disease Control and Prevention, Atlanta, Ga; Univ of Chicago; Dartmouth–Hitchcock Med Ctr, Lebanon, NH; et al)

N Engl J Med 338:706–711, 1998 19–11

Background.—Lipophilic yeasts of the genus *Malassezia* have become important nosocomial pathogens. Numerous outbreaks have been reported in low–birth weight newborns receiving lipid emulsions. The authors' intensive care nursery recently had an outbreak of *Malassezia pachydermatis*, an organism linked to otitis externa in dogs. The results of an investigation of that outbreak were reported.

Methods and Findings.—Fifteen infants had positive skin cultures for *M. pachydermatis* during a 15-month period. There were 8 cases of bloodstream infection, 2 of urinary tract infection, and 1 of meningitis; the other 4 patients had asymptomatic colonization. In a cohort study, 23% of patients weighing 1,300 g or less were infected or colonized, compared with none of 419 heavier infants. On multivariate analysis, independent risk factors were severity of underlying illness, odds ratio (OR) 19.7; arterial catheterization for 9 days or longer, OR 29.5; and exposure to 1 nurse on the unit. A point-prevalence survey found positive cultures for *M. pachydermatis* in 9 additional infants, 1 health care worker, and 12 dogs owned by the health care workers. Restriction-fragment–length polymorphisms showed that all the affected infants, the health care worker, and 3 of the dogs had the same *M. pachydermatis* isolate. A survey revealed inadequate hand-washing practices on the unit. With correction of hand-washing practices, all staff cultures became negative and there were no further cases.

Conclusions.—This outbreak of *M. pachydermatis* infection in an intensive care nursery appears to have resulted from colonization of health care workers from pet dogs at home. Once established in the nursery, the organism persisted through patient-to-patient transmission. Careful hand washing by health care workers on entering the unit and before and after all patient contacts is necessary to prevent the introduction and nosocomial transmission of pet-related pathogens.

▶ Approximately 11% of nosocomial fungal infections are caused by fungi other than *Candida* and *Aspergillus* spp. Among these miscellaneous opportunistic fungal pathogens are the *Malassezia* species. The *Malassezia* genus is a group of lipophilic yeasts containing 7 known species, including *M. furfur* and *M. pachydermatis. Malassezia* pachydermatis is an emerging pathogen that has been reported to cause infections in both animals and humans. It is a well-known cause of otitis and skin infections in dogs and has been reported to cause catheter-related fungemia in the neonatal intensive care unit (NICU) setting.

Chang et al. describe an epidemic of *M. pachydermatis* infection in an NICU. Investigation identified 8 patients with bloodstream infection, 2 with positive urine cultures, and 1 with meningitis. An additional 4 patients were colonized. Cultures of personnel revealed 1 nurse with positive hand cultures. In addition, *M. pachydermatis* was cultured from the ears of 12 of 39 dogs belonging to health care workers. Molecular typing studies found a single strain shared by all patients, the colonized nurse, and 3 of the dogs. This evidence coupled with documented poor hand-washing practices strongly suggested transmission of *M. pachydermatis* from patient to patient via the hands of health care workers. The colonized patients in the NICU likely served as a reservoir for the epidemic strain, as did the pets of the health care workers. Improved hand-washing practices in the NICU resulted in termination of the epidemic.

This remarkable report serves to emphasize the vast array of opportunistic pathogens that must be detected and identified by the laboratory. In this instance, accurate identification of this unusual yeast was key to defining the outbreak and to identifying the mode of transmission and the potential reservoir. A laboratory report of "yeast detected, not *Candida*" would simply not suffice. The importance of simple hand washing as the cornerstone of infection control efforts is also emphasized.

M.A. Pfaller, M.D.

Antimicrobial Susceptibility Testing of a Clinical Isolate of Vancomycin-dependent Enterococcus Using D-Alanine-D-Alanine as a Growth Supplement

Sng L-H, Cornish N, Knapp CC, et al (Cleveland Clinic Found, Ohio)
Am J Clin Pathol 109:399–403, 1998 19–12

Background.—Many centers have seen the emergence of vancomycin-resistant enterococci (VRE), often occurring with high-level aminoglycoside and ampicillin resistance. Some of these vancomycin-resistant strains have even proved to require vancomycin for growth. In susceptibility studies of vancomycin-dependent enterococci (VDE), the use of vancomycin as a growth supplement could affect the in vitro activity of other antimicrobial agents. D-alanine-D-alanine (DADA)—a substance required for cell-wall synthesis—was used instead of vancomycin as a growth supplement in susceptibility studies of a VDE isolate.

Methods and Results.—A VDE was isolated as the cause of bacteremia in a renal transplant patient receiving long-term vancomycin. The patient had underlying pancreatitis and a wound infection and bacteremia caused by VRE. The VDE grew in culture only when vancomycin and DADA were present. After 48 hours of incubation, colonies beyond the periphery of VDE growth around a vancomycin disk showed vancomycin-independent revertant mutants. On pulsed-field gel electrophoresis, the VDE, revertant mutant, initial VRE isolate, and an autopsy isolate were all identical.

A standard macrobath dilution susceptibility test of the VDE isolate was performed using DADA as a growth supplement. The VRE isolate and VDE revertant showed similar minimum inhibitory concentrations (MICs). Both isolates were resistant to ampicillin, high-level gentamicin, ciprofloxacin, imipenem, vancomycin, and daptomycin; both were susceptible to fusidic acid, high-level streptomycin, rifampin, and quinupristin-dalfopristin. The clinical VRE isolate had a 2 µg/mL or less MIC of teicoplanin, compared with 16 µg/mL for the VDE revertant isolate. The autopsy isolate was not susceptible to any of the antimicrobials tested. Its MIC for quinupristin-dalfopristin was 4 times greater than that of the original blood isolate. Except for vancomycin, the VDE showed susceptibility to all drugs tested.

Conclusions.—The patient in this study had a VDE isolated during vancomycin treatment for vancomycin-resistant enterococcal bacteremia. On genotyping studies, all isolates identified—the original VRE, the VDE, a revertant mutant strain, and an autopsy isolate—were related. Using DADA as a growth supplement for VDE avoids the problems associated with vancomycin for susceptibility testing.

▶ VRE are now widely recognized as important nosocomial- and community-acquired pathogens. As a group the enterococci are highly ubiquitous and have demonstrated a remarkable capacity to survive in the environment and to become resistant to numerous antimicrobial agents. It is well recognized that the development of glycopeptide resistance among enterococci has been linked to the tremendous utilization of glycopeptides in both medical and agricultural settings. Now in addition to becoming resistant to vancomycin, we have reports of enterococcal strains that require vancomycin for growth. Sng and colleagues report the sixth such case and also provide useful methods for isolation of the organism and for performing in vitro susceptibility testing of these strains. They demonstrate that the original VRE, the VDE, the revertant mutant, and an autopsy isolate were all the same strain. They also show that the revertant mutant and the autopsy isolate were both significantly more resistant to several antimicrobial agents than the original isolate or the VDE. These data emphasize the extreme adaptability of the *Enterococcus* and its ability to develop increased resistance in vivo. Thus, laboratories must remain vigilant and flexible and be willing to use growth supplements for both detection and susceptibility testing of enterococci in selected situations. This amazingly successful pathogen will continue to provide a challenge to laboratories and clinicians alike.

M.A. Pfaller, M.D.

Optimal Screening and Diagnosis of *Microsporida* in Tissue Sections: A Comparison of Polarization, Special Stains, and Molecular Techniques

Lamps LW, Bronner MP, Vnencak-Jones CL, et al (Vanderbilt Univ, Nashville, Tenn; Univ of Washington, Seattle)

Am J Clin Pathol 109:404–410, 1998 19–13

Introduction.—Infection with *Microsporida* is an increasingly important clinical problem, particularly in patients with AIDS. Several different diagnostic methods have been proposed, but there is no "gold standard." Confirmation of the presence of *Microsporida* has become increasingly important with advances in treatment protocols. The best screening technique was determined for the detection of *Microsporida* in biopsy specimens.

Methods.—The analysis included 42 small intestine biopsy specimens from 31 immunocompromised patients. Sixty-eight percent of the patients had AIDS. Each specimen was evaluated by polarization and a battery of stains, including hematoxylin-eosin (H & E), modified trichrome, Warthin-Starry, and Brown-Brenn. This was followed by polymerase chain reaction and Southern blot assays in all positive cases.

Results.—The modified trichrome stain detected *Microsporida* in 21% of specimens, all from patients with AIDS. Seven of these 9 specimens were positive on Brown-Brenn staining, and 5 were positive on Warthin-Starry staining. Two cases were associated with focal weak polarization on H & E staining and 3 with special stains. The molecular studies confirmed the presence of *Microsporida* in 4 of 9 cases (Table 2). Several findings on routine H & E staining were nonspecifically associated with microsporidian infection, including focal villous blunting, loss of goblet cell mucin at the epithelial surface, and a patchy lymphoplasmacytic infiltrate in the lamina propria.

Conclusions.—Polarization is not a sensitive screening method for *Microsporida* in tissue sections. The most sensitive stain for screening purposes is the modified trichrome stain. The combination of the Brown-Brenn or Warthin-Starry stain with the trichrome stain helps to exclude false-positive results related to granular artifacts.

▶ Intestinal microsporidian infection is a frequent cause of chronic diarrhea, abdominal pain, and weight loss in individuals with AIDS. Although the success of treatment regimens is quite variable, modest advances in this

TABLE 2.—Microsporidian Detection by Light Microscopy and Molecular Methods

Case No.	*Trichrome*	*Gram*	*Silver (WS)*	*Polarization H & E*	*Polarization Special Stains*	*Coinfection Detected*	*CD 4 T cells/mm³*	*Microsporidian PCR/SB*	*Clinical Manifestation*
1	+	+	+	−	−	Cyclo/crypto	Unknown	−	Unknown
2	+	+	−	−	+	CMV	12	+	Diarrhea
3	+	+	−	−	+	−	12	−	Diarrhea
4	+	−	+	−	−	CMV	16	+	Abdominal pain
5	+	+	+	−	+	MAI	16	+	Diarrhea
6	+	−	−	+	−	−	3	−	Diarrhea
7	+	+	+	−	−	−	Unknown	+	Abdominal pain
8	+	+	−	+	−	Crypto	4	−	Diarrhea
9	+	+	+	−	−	*Candida* species	9	NA	Diarrhea
Percentage Detection	100	78	56	22	30	67	—	44	—

Abbreviations: WS, Warthrin Starry; *H & E*, hematoxylin-eosin; *PCR/SB*, polymerase chain reaction/Southern blot analysis; +, positive; −, negative; *Cyclo, Cyclospora* species; *Crypto, Cryptosporidium* species; *CMV*, cytomegalovirus; *MAI, Mycobacterium avium intracellulare* complex; *NA*, not applicable; unable to extract DNA from sample.

(Courtesy of Lamps LW, Bronner MP, Vnencak-Jones CL, et al: Optimal screening and diagnosis of *Microsporida* in tissue sections: A comparison of polarization, special stains, and molecular techniques. *Am J Clin Pathol* 109:404–410. Copyright 1998 by the American Society of Clinical Pathologists. Reprinted with permission.)

area have placed an emphasis on improved diagnosis. Diagnostic approaches include light microscopic examination of stool specimens using the modified trichrome stain, Gram stain with and without polarization, and the calcofluor white stain. Detection of *Microsporida* in gastrointestinal biopsy specimens has used the above stains plus silver stains (Warthin-Starry, Steiner), electron microscopy, (EM), and molecular (polymerase chain reaction [PCR]-based) methods.

In this study, the authors examined the use of several of these approaches (trichrome, polarization, Gram, silver, PCR, EM) in an attempt to determine the optimal light microscopic method for screening and diagnosis of microsporidian infections. They examined 42 small bowel biopsy specimens (68% from AIDS patients), only 1 of which was known previously to contain *Microsporida*. *Microsporida* were detected in 9 of 42 cases (21.4%), with modified trichrome proving to be the most sensitive (100%), followed by Gram (78%) and silver stains (56%). Polarization detected only 22% of infections, and PCR followed by Southern hybridization confirmed the diagnosis in 50%. Coinfection with other intestinal pathogens (cyclospora, cryptosporidia, cytomegalovirus, mycobacteria) was observed in 67%. All the microsporidial infections were in patients with AIDS. These findings emphasize the difficulty in diagnosing microsporidiosis and confirm the utility of the modified trichrome stain as a useful screening measure for examination of both stool smears and small bowel biopsy specimens. The Brown-Brenn or Warthin-Starry stains can serve as useful confirmatory stains. Pathologists and microbiologists should be aware of the frequent occurrence of co-infections in patients with AIDS and realize that the detection of one gastrointestinal pathogen in such patients should not preclude the search for others such as *Microsporida*.

M.A. Pfaller, M.D.

An Outbreak Involving Extensive Transmission of a Virulent Strain of *Mycobacterium tuberculosis*

Valway SE, Sanchez MPC, Shinnick TF, et al (Ctrs for Disease Control and Prevention, Atlanta, Ga; Colorado State Univ, Fort Collins; Tennessee Dept of Health, Upper Cumberland Region, Cookeville; et al)
N Engl J Med 338:633–639, 1998 19–14

Background.—Variability in transmission of tuberculosis outbreaks has been attributed to environment or source patient characteristics but not usually to variations in virulence between strains. This report describes a large 1994 outbreak of tuberculosis in a small rural community with a population at low risk of tuberculosis. The extent of transmission and the virulence of the outbreak strain were studied.

Methods.—The index patient was a 21-year-old, HIV-negative, American white man, who lived in a small rural community. The patient's list of contacts were cross-matched with state tuberculosis registries and county health department pharmacy logs. Patients with tuberculosis were interviewed, and their medical records were reviewed. Family, co-workers, and social contacts of the index patient underwent tuberculin-test screening. Strains from this outbreak were sent to the Center for Disease Control for DNA-fingerprint analysis. Strain virulence was assessed in C57BL/6 mice and compared with the virulent laboratory strain *Mycobacterium tuberculosis* Erdman.

Results.—The index patient, the source patient, and another patient infected 18 other individuals. In 5 patients, active disease developed after casual exposure. Of 429 contacts, 72% had positive skin test reactions. There were 86 documented skin-test conversions. Mice infected with the virulent laboratory standard Erdman strain had approximately 1,000 bacilli per lung after 10 days and 10,000 after 20 days. Mice infected with the outbreak strain had approximately 10,000 bacilli per lung after 10 days and 10 million per lung after 20 days.

Conclusions.—This report documents extensive tuberculosis transmission in a rural population with low risk factors. The strain involved in the outbreak appears to have a much higher growth rate than that encountered in typical virulent strains, which may have contributed to its increased transmission rate. The outbreak strain was selected for the tuberculosis genome-sequencing project, which may permit identification of important virulence genes.

▶ The rise in tuberculosis in the United States and worldwide over the past 10-15 years has prompted a great deal of concern and has resulted in considerable attention to clinical, epidemiologic, and microbiologic aspects of *M. tuberculosis*. In many instances the increase in cases of tuberculosis in the United States was associated with active transmission of antibiotic-resistant *M. tuberculosis* among the homeless and those with AIDS. Aside from drug resistance, there was little evidence of an increase in virulence or transmissibility among strains of *M. tuberculosis*. The outbreak of tuberculosis investigated in this study is remarkable because of the extensive transmission of a single strain of *M. tuberculosis* among individuals with little or no risk factors for acquiring tuberculosis. The fact that even a brief exposure to an infected patient resulted in transmission of the outbreak strain suggested that the increased rate of transmission may have been due to particular features of the organism rather than to environmental or patient characteristics. Notably, the epidemic strain was not drug resistant. Increased virulence, marked by the ability to replicate extensively in a murine model of tuberculosis, was demonstrated for the epidemic strain. Rapid investigation and aggressive tuberculosis-control efforts limited the number of active cases but may not have identified the entire reservoir of infected individuals. This report serves as a sobering reminder of the continuing threat of *M. tuberculosis* in both highly developed and underdeveloped nations. Continued attention to rapid and accurate diagnosis and ongoing programs of surveillance and control are essential.

M.A. Pfaller, M.D.

Comparison of ATB Staph, Rapid ATB Staph, Vitek, and E-Test Methods for Detection of Oxacillin Heteroresistance in Staphylococci Possessing *mecA*

Frebourg NB, Nouet D, Lemée L, et al (Hôpital Charles Nicolle, Cedex, France)

J Clin Microbiol 36:52–57, 1998 19–15

Background.—Oxacillin-resistant staphylococci, major nosocomial pathogens, often have multiple resistance, resulting in the overuse of glycopeptide treatment. This strong antibiotic pressure can be reduced by optimizing the detection of oxacillin resistance in clinical laboratories. The performance of the E-test system and 3 automated systems currently used in France—the ATB Staph, Rapid ATB Staph, and Vitek systems—were compared.

Methods and Findings.—Testing was performed on 64 *Staphylococcus aureus* strains and 76 coagulase-negative staphylococcal strains. All strains were *mecA*-positive and characterized by the oxacillin agar screen plate test. Fifty-four percent were heterogeneous by a large-inoculum oxacillin disk diffusion assay. Oxacillin minimal inhibitory concentrations (MICs) for 63.6% were 32 µg/mL or less. On the E-test, 4.7% of *S. aureus* strains and 32.9% of the coagulase-negative strains were classified as susceptible, as defined by the National Committee for Clinical Laboratory Standards (NCCLS) oxacillin breakpoint. In 11% of *S. aureus* isolates and 42.1% of coagulase-negative isolates, the ATB Staph method did not detect oxacillin resistance. All but 6 of the discrepant isolates had MICs of 16 µg/mL or less. The Rapid ATB Staph method, tested against *S. aureus* strains only, yielded 23.4% false susceptible results for strains with MICs of 32 µg/mL or less. The Vitek system had the best performance. This system failed to detect oxacillin resistance in only 4.7% of *S. aureus* strains and 19.7% of coagulase-negative strains, all with MICs of 2 µg/mL or less.

Conclusions.—When the prevalence of borderline-heteroresistant staphylococci is high, the performance of the 2 ATB Staph systems can be limited. The unreliability of the E-test and the Vitek technique may be decreased by the potential revision of the oxacillin breakpoint currently recommended by the NCCLS.

► The availability of molecular methods for detection of antibiotic resistance genes in bacteria has refined our ability to validate commercial methods for determining antibiotic resistance phenotypes. This is especially true for the detection of the *mecA* gene, which encodes for methicillin and oxacillin resistance among staphylococci. Whereas phenotypic detection of oxacillin resistance has been difficult, especially among the coagulase-negative staphylococci (CoNS), polymerase chain reaction-based methods for detecting *mecA* have been shown to be sensitive, accurate, and clinically valid. Thus, detection of *mecA* may serve as a "gold standard" for the evaluation of commercial products designed to detect oxacillin resistance among staphylococci. In this study, the authors evaluated 4 different commercial test systems—ATB Staph, Rapid ATB Staph, Vitek, and E-test—for their ability to classify isolates of *S. aureus* and CoNS as resistant to oxacillin. All of the isolates were positive for *mecA* by polymerase chain reaction. Both E-test and Vitek performed reasonably well in testing *S. aureus*, but none of the test systems performed satisfactorily with the CoNS. A large number of false susceptible results were observed with both of the ATB Staph systems. It is notable that several of the *mecA*-positive CoNS isolates that were misclassified by E-test and Vitek as susceptible were inhibited by 0.125–2 µg/mL of oxacillin. This suggests that the National Committee for Clinical Laboratory Standards interpretive breakpoint for oxacillin and CoNS (susceptible as 2 µg/mL or less) may be incorrect. Modification of this phenotypic breakpoint to reflect the molecular data (susceptible as 0.25 µg/mL or less) would improve the accuracy of both E-test and Vitek to greater than 95%. Thus, this combined molecular and phenotypic analysis has revealed major deficiencies among the ATB and Rapid ATB Staph systems, and has pointed out a flaw in the interpretive breakpoints currently recommended by the NCCLS.

M.A. Pfaller, M.D.

Apparent Increased Prevalence of High-level Aminoglycoside-resistant *Enterococcus durans* Resulting From False Identification by a Semiautomated Software System

Tsakris A, Woodford N, Pournaras S, et al (Aristotelian Univ of Thessaloniki, Greece; AHEPA Univ Hosp, Thessaloniki, Greece; Central Public Health Lab, London)

J Clin Microbiol 36:1419–1421, 1998 19–16

Background.—An apparent increase in the prevalence of high-level aminoglycoside-resistant *Enterococcus durans* was recently noted at the authors' institution. The possibility that this increase was the result of false identification by a semiautomated software system was investigated.

Methods and Findings.—A high proportion of *E. durans*, especially among isolates highly resistant to gentamicin and streptomycin, was noted in a university hospital in Thessaloniki, Greece. The semiautomated system PASCO had been used to identify the enterococci. Fourteen isolates identified as *E. durans* between November 1996 and April 1997 were further studied by a conventional biochemical scheme and polymerase chain reaction to determine the accuracy of the identification. All of these isolates were reclassified as *Enterococcus faecalis*. Antibiotic resistance and pulsed-field gel electrophoresis revealed that unrelated strains had also been incorrectly identified.

Conclusions.—Laboratories using the PASCO system should inspect by eye the typical reactions of the enterococcal species. The system database should be based on such typical reactions. Misidentification of isolates with properties typical of another species suggests that the system database needs to be modified. Additional panel tests would probably allow the system to discriminate more clinically relevant *Enterococcus* species.

▶ Enterococci are extremely important nosocomial pathogens, both because of their frequency of occurrence and because of their propensity to exhibit significant antimicrobial resistance. The most common species causing infections in hospitalized patients are *E. faecalis* and *E. faecium*. Other species have been described; however, problems with the accuracy of available commercial identification systems cast doubt on the significance of some of these reports. Misidentification of vancomycin-resistant *E. faecium* as *E. durans* by the Vitek System has been reported. Likewise, the Vitek System has been shown to misidentify *E. raffinosis* as *E. avium*. Such misidentifications may be quite misleading and result in unwarranted clinical and epidemiologic investigations. In this study, the authors report another instance of false identification of *E. durans* by a different commercial identification system, the PASCO MIC/ID gram-positive panel. The isolates were ultimately identified as *E. faecalis* by polymerase chain reaction and conventional biochemicals. This and other examples in the literature underscore the need for manufacturers of commercial systems to improve the database of their system. Furthermore, users of these systems should be aware of the systems' shortcomings and continue in-use monitoring as part of their validation process. In particular, laboratories should question the accuracy of identification of enterococcal species other than *E. faecium* or *E. faecalis* when rendered by a commercial identification system. Specifically, an identification of *E. durans* by the Vitek or PASCO systems is likely to be incorrect and should be confirmed by alternative methods.

M.A. Pfaller, M.D.

Interpretation of Trailing Endpoints in Antifungal Susceptibility Testing by the National Committee for Clinical Laboratory Standards Method

Revankar SG, Kirkpatrick WR, McAtee RK, et al (Univ of Texas, San Antonio; South Texas Veterans Health Care System, San Antonio)

J Clin Microbiol 36:153–156, 1998 19–17

Objective.—The National Committee for Clinical Laboratory Standards (NCCLS) method of antifungal susceptibility testing of yeasts has become the standard for use in testing of HIV-infected patients with oropharyngeal candidiasis. However, in the testing of certain yeast isolates, there are ongoing problems with trailing endpoints in the NCCLS method. For these isolates, minimal inhibitory concentrations (MICs) of 1 µg/mL or less at 24 hours and of greater than 64 µg/mL at 48 hours are commonly seen. Three HIV-positive patients with recurrent oropharyngeal candidiasis with multiple serial isolates and trailing endpoints observed with fluconazole were described.

Methods.—The patients all had multiple serial isolates for which trailing endpoints were encountered when the NCCLS method was used for antifungal susceptibility testing with fluconazole. Agar dilution susceptibility testing and restriction fragment length polymorphism analyses were performed for each strain. The fluconazole dose was increased as necessary to achieve a clinical response.

Results.—The 24-hour MICs, by both macrodilution and microdilution approaches, were usually 1 µg/mL or less. By 48 hours, the MICs had increased to greater than 64 µg/mL; however, agar dilution testing continued to show susceptibility to fluconazole. Most episodes of recurrent oropharyngeal candidiasis associated with trailing-endpoint isolates responded clinically to fluconazole dosages as low as 100 mg/day. In 2 of the 3 patients, NCCLS broth macrodilution and microdilution testing showed both susceptible and trailing-endpoint isolates. Pulsed-field gel electrophoresis using restriction fragment length polymorphisms showed that both of these isolates were of the same strain. The third patient had 2 different strains: 1 showed trailing endpoints, while the other was susceptible at 48 hours.

Conclusions.—In HIV-infected patients with recurrent oropharyngeal candidiasis, yeast isolates showing trailing endpoints at 48 hours are still shown to be susceptible by agar dilution techniques. Most such isolates respond to fluconazole doses similar to those effective on susceptible isolates. Isolates showing trailing endpoints with fluconazole thus appear to be susceptible, and the NCCLS result obtained at 24 hours may be more appropriate. Isolates with MICs of greater than 64 µg/mL at both 24 and 48 hours by the standard NCCLS method should be confirmed by agar dilution or other alternate methods. This is particularly important for cultures showing other yeast isolates with trailing endpoints and/or MICs indicating susceptibility.

► Standardization of antifungal susceptibility testing for yeasts has resulted in the development of interpretive breakpoints for fluconazole and itraconazole and a broader application of this method. One of the problems encountered with the performance of broth dilution testing of fluconazole has been that of incomplete growth inhibition resulting in trailing endpoints. Despite published criteria for reading these endpoints (80% inhibition of growth relative to control), this remains a difficult area. Extensive trailing is observed with some, but not all, strains of *Candida albicans* and may result in the organism being classified as resistant (MIC ≥ 64 µg/mL) to fluconazole. This is especially true when the test is read after 48 hours of incubation. Agar-based testing using fixed concentrations of 8 and 16 µg/mL of fluconazole may minimize the difficulty in interpreting MIC endpoints and allow characterization of isolates as "susceptible" (≤8 µg/mL) or "resistant" (MIC > 16 µg/mL) to fluconazole.

In this study, the authors use NCCLS broth dilution, agar dilution, and molecular typing methods to attempt to clarify the significance of trailing endpoints for fluconazole when testing *C. albicans* isolates from AIDS patients with oropharyngeal candidiasis. The results indicate that the trailing phenomenon may be variable among genotypically identical isolates, but in some individuals it may be genotype specific. Broth dilution MICs read after

24 hours of incubation agreed with agar-based test results and were consistent with clinical results. Those isolates with low fluconazole MICs at 24 hours but high MICs at 48 hours appeared to be responsive clinically to fluconazole. Reading the fluconazole MIC endpoint at 24 hours may be more appropriate clinically. Alternatively, an agar-based method may be quite useful in screening isolates for decreased susceptibility to fluconazole.

M.A. Pfaller, M.D.

20 Clinical Chemistry and Toxicology

Ascertaining Hypoglycorrhacia in an Acute Patient
Skipper BJ, Davis LE (Univ of New Mexico, Albuquerque)
Am J Emerg Med 15:378–380, 1997 20–1

Background.—Hypoglycorrhacia or lower than normal glucose content in the CSF can be a sign of meningitis. In a fasting state, CSF glucose has been determined to be 60% to 70% of blood glucose. The problem is that fasting levels cannot usually be obtained in the emergency room when infectious meningitis is suspected. Under these conditions, hypoglycorrhacia is diagnosed if the CSF to blood glucose ratio is below 0.5. An analysis was done to determine whether the use of a CSF/blood glucose ratio was appropriate for the diagnosis of hypoglycorrhacia in the emergent setting.

Methods.—The study group consisted of 79 men, aged 15–85 years, undergoing diagnostic lumbar puncture, who voluntarily permitted blood to be drawn. These patients did not fast. Blood and CSF glucose levels were determined by the glucose oxidase method within 1 hour of samples being obtained. All CSF samples were sterile with normal laboratory tests.

Results.—The intercept for the regression line of the relationship between CSF and blood glucose values did not pass through the origin, indicating that the relationship between these 2 values was not a ratio. These data were similar to those obtained from 4 previously published studies.

Conclusions.—The relationship of CSF to blood glucose is not a ratio, as has been assumed for clinical purposes. The relationship between these 2 values is only in the expected 0.6–0.7 range when blood glucose is between 89 and 115 mg/dL. The relationship is less than 0.6 when blood glucose is greater than 125 mg/dL. The relationship is less than 0.5 when blood glucose is greater than 192 mg/dL. If CSF glucose is below the lower 95% normal limit, hypoglycorrhacia can usually be diagnosed.

► Decreased glucose in CSF along with other measurements such as elevated protein have been used for years by physicians to help diagnose meningeal infections. The problem with using this measurement is that CSF glucose concentrations are dependent on the blood concentration. Therefore, a CSF glucose value cannot be correctly interpreted without a concomitant blood level. The usual relationship quoted for these 2 values is that the CSF glucose should be 60% to 70% of the blood glucose value and that any value below a ratio of 0.5 indicates hypoglycorrhachia.

By comparing CSF and blood glucose values, these authors found that the regression line did not bisect zero, which would indicate a constant ratio of CSF to blood glucose. Instead the 0.6 to 0.7 ratio only held when blood glucose was between 89 and 115 mg/dL. The ratio was less than 0.5 when the blood glucose was greater than 192 mg/dL. Because CSF puncture for the diagnosis of meningeal infection is usually an emergency procedure, the patient is rarely fasting. These data indicate that interpreting a CSF glucose in the face of an elevated blood glucose may be a difficult task.

R. Feld, Ph.D.

Instrumental Variability of Respiratory Blood Gases Among Different Blood Gas Analysers in Different Laboratories

Kampelmacher MJ, van Kesteren RG, Winckers EKA (Univ Hosp Utrecht, The Netherlands)

Eur Respir J 10:1341–1344, 1997 20–2

Background.—Analysis of arterial oxygen tension (PO_2) and carbon dioxide tension (PCO_2) are useful in both clinical care and research. If differences in blood gas analyzer (BGA) performance exist, research and clinical conclusions may be confounded by the performance characteristics of the BGAs used in the study. Interinstrument variability of BGAs was tested.

Methods.—Fresh venous blood was obtained from a single volunteer. Samples of tonometered blood (PO_2 8.1 kPa and PCO_2 5.3 kPa) were placed in airtight glass syringes and transported in ice water to 10 hospitals. Blood gas analysis was performed within 3.5 hours by 17 analyzers, including 10 different models, on the same day.

Results.—The mean differences between the measured and target values of PO_2 was -0.01 ± 0.19 and for PCO_2 was 0.21 ± 0.13 kPa. The mean of the difference between 2 samples on 1 analyzer was 0.06 ± 0.06 and 0.04 ± 0.03, respectively. The interinstrument standard deviations were 0.18 and 0.13 kPA, respectively. The intrainstrument standard deviations were 0.06 and 0.03 kPA, respectively.

Conclusions.—Both for oxygen tension and carbon dioxide tension, there is more inter- than intrainstrument variability in blood gas measurement. However, this variability in the measurement of blood gas values is insignificant. Variability in blood gas values predominantly depends on errors in the preanalytical phase of sample manipulation.

► When I first entered the laboratory (too many years ago), blood gas measurements were one of the most temperamental analyses. Patient care areas had to schedule gases at least 15 minutes in advance so that the technologist could calibrate and set up the instrument. This was necessary because the calibration stability was notoriously fickle. The only quality control we had for PO_2 was a syringe full of air.

Few analytic methods have advanced as far in the intervening time. Although the principle of the ion-selective electrode measurement has not changed, the size of the electrodes and sample has decreased considerably, and instrument design and electronics have advanced. We now have excellent quality control specimens that span the analytic range. The effects of these advancements can be seen by scanning a copy of the College of American Pathologists blood gas survey.

This paper uses tonometered blood to test between and within instrument variance for PO_2 and PCO_2. They conclude that there is excellent agreement between instruments regardless of manufacturer and that the preanalytical phase of blood gas analysis still accounts for the majority of variability in blood gas values.

R. Feld, Ph.D.

Lowering Cutoffs for Initial and Confirmation Testing for Cocaine and Marijuana: Large-scale Study of Effects on the Rates of Drug-positive Results

Wingert WE (Lab Corp of America, Raritan, NJ)

Clin Chem 43:100–103, 1997 20–3

Background.—The Substance Abuse and Mental Health Services Administration (SAMHSA), a federally regulated, civilian drug-testing program, tests urine samples for cocaine (COC) and marijuana (THC). A large-scale study was performed to determine whether it was possible to lower the initial testing and confirmation cutoffs accurately and whether this would significantly affect the number of positive samples detected.

Methods.—Initial urine screening was performed with Abu-screen OnLine reagents. Cocaine specimens that had readings of at least 100 µg/L were retested by GC-MS. Marijuana specimens with readings of at least 20 µg/L were retested with the Cannabinoid 20 Assay. Positive specimens were retested with GC-MS.

Results.—Of the 4911 urine samples screened, 59 were COC-positive according to the SAMHSA-mandated cutoffs. Use of a 100 µg/L screening cutoff and a confirmation cutoff of 50 µg/L, detected 105 positive specimens. If the cutoff was lowered to 30 µg/L, 119 positive specimens were detected. At the 1 µg/L limit of detection, 139 samples were positive. The chromatography was acceptable with no interfering peaks and adequate peak areas for quantification. Of the 6,427 urine samples screened for THC at the SAMHSA-mandated cutoff, 179 samples were positive. Lowering the screening cutoff to 20 µg/L, identified 262 positive samples. If the confirmation test was also lowered to 5 µg/L, the number of positive samples was 281. The chromatography was acceptable, without interfering peaks and with peak areas adequate for quantification.

Conclusions.—Using current SAMHSA-mandated screening guidelines, many urine specimens containing low levels of COC or THC metabolites are being reported as negative specimens. Use of current technology permits these standards to be lowered without sacrificing accuracy. Use of lowered standards would increase the detection window and permit the identification of a larger number of truly positive specimens.

▶ In the continuous war between drug takers and drug testers, the battle line of the positive cutoff can mean victory or defeat. This paper examines the effect of lowering the cutoffs for the screening and confirmation test to levels lower than those advocated by SAMHSA or the Department of Defense. A total of nearly 5,000 urines were screened using both current and lower cutoffs. The lower cutoffs produced nearly a doubling of drug-positive urines. This was accomplished with only minor modifications to the analytic techniques employed. The question of whether an innocent person could achieve values greater than the cutoffs by passive inhalation was addressed. The author, citing literature, felt that this was highly unlikely. Of course the question must be asked what society should do for the people currently escaping detection who would be identified by the lower limits.

R. Feld, Ph.D.

Candidate Reference Methods for Hemoglobin A_{Ic} Based on Peptide Mapping

Kobold U, Jeppsson J-O, Dülffer T, et al (Research Ctr Tutzing, Germany; University of Lund, Malmö, Sweden; Groot Wezenland, Zwolle, The Netherlands)

Clin Chem 43:1944–1951, 1997 20–4

Purpose.—Hemoglobin A_{1c} is a proven measurement for monitoring of glycemic state in patients with diabetes. The measurements must be reliable and reproducible, because the difference between patients at high and low risk of complications is a small one. As part of efforts to achieve international standardization of Hb A_{1c}/glycohemoglobin, a reference method specific for Hb A_{1c} is needed. A new method for quantification of Hb A_{1c}, based on capillary electrophoresis, has been developed.

Technique.—The new method relies on the specific N-terminal residue of the hemoglobin β-chains. The technique optimized enzymatic cleavage of the intact hemoglobin molecule using the endoproteinase Glu-C, to produce the β-N-terminal hexapeptides of Hb A_{1c} and Hb A_0. The peptides were then separated by reversed-phase high-performance liquid chromatography and quantitated by electrospray ionization-mass spectrometry or capillary electrophoresis. These techniques avoided the problems with insufficient resolution associated with current protein separation systems. The mass spectrometry technique was more specific and thus a better candidate for the Hb A_{1c} reference method; however, the capillary electrophoresis method also had potential to be classified as a reference method.

Discussion.—Potential new reference methods for Hb A_{1c}, based on the principle of peptide mapping, were developed. With either of the 2 potential reference methods, the Hb A_{1c} values found will be lower than with current routine methods.

▶ Truth is elusive, especially in some analytical methods. Hemoglobin A_{1c} has been found to be extremely useful for monitoring the extent of glucose control over long periods. The usefulness of this assay was emphasized by the publication of the Diabetes Control and Complications Trial,[1] which demonstrated dramatic reductions in the complications associated with diabetes in patients whose average glucose as measured by A_{1c} was kept as normal as possible by intensive treatment.

To date there has not been a reference method available for A_{1c}. This is especially important because of the myriad of assays that are available and the lack of agreement between differing methodologies. High pressure liquid chromatography has been used as the de facto reference method, but it has shortcomings in that several molecular forms of hemoglobin which are not A_{1c} co-elute with the desired analyte.

These authors begin by first using enzymatic cleavage to obtain β-N-terminal peptides of hemoglobin. It is only those hemoglobin molecules that are irreversibly glycated at one or both of N-terminal valines of the β-chain that qualify for A_{1c} status.

The peptides are then separated by either high pressure liquid chromatography with quantitation by either electrospray ionization-mass spectrometry or capillary electrophoresis. The availability of a reference method for A_{1c} will allow companies and laboratories to achieve better standardization and accuracy for this important analyte.

R. Feld, Ph.D.

Reference

1. Anonymous: The effect of intensive treatment of diabetes on the development and progression of long-term complications in insulin-dependent diabetes mellitus: The Diabetes Control and Complications Trial Research Group. *N Engl J Med* 329:977–986, 1993.

Heterophilic Antibodies Remain a Problem for the Immunoassay Laboratory

Ward G, McKinnon L, Badrick T, et al (Princess Alexandra Hosp, Woolloongabba, Australia; Nicolaides & Partners, Brisbane, Australia)

Am J Clin Pathol 108:417–421, 1997 20–5

Objective.—To avoid interference of nonspecific antibodies in immunoassays, manufacturers are now adding small amounts of serum or immunoglobulin from animals of the same species as the immunoglobulins used in the assay to adsorb interfering antibodies. Some patients still have inappropriate results because of the presence of very high concentrations of heterophilic antibodies. Hence, the prevalence of heterophilic antibody interference in the patient population served was assessed in a commercially available thyrotropin immunoassay.

Methods.—The number of cases of interference was determined by measuring thyrotropin in serum samples from 295 consecutive patients using an assay with zero blocker (protocol A), routine blocker concentration (protocol B), and extra blocker (protocol C).

Results.—By protocol A, 6 patients had thyrotropin levels more than 600% greater (more than 13 standard deviations [SD]) than protocol B, and 4 patients had levels more than 150% greater (more than 9 SD). Protocols B and C yielded similar results. In another series of 21,000 patients, 7 had a concentration of heterophilic antibodies so high that inappropriate results were obtained, even with extra blocker.

Conclusion.—In 3.4% of the study population inappropriate results were obtained by thyrotropin assays without added blocker. When heterophilic antibody concentrations are extremely high, they can overwhelm added blocker and yield inappropriate results. Assayists must be alert to this possibility.

▶ Monoclonal antibodies quickly found their way from the research laboratory to the clinical laboratory. The ability to produce large quantities of a single antibody that has very high specificity for a particular ligand makes them very attractive as reagents in clinical testing.

Soon after the introduction of these reagents, reports appeared of patients whose results were inconsistent with the clinical situation. Further investigation revealed antibodies in the patients' serum that could bind the monoclonal antibodies. As most monoclonal antibodies are produced in mice, the name *HAMA* (human antimouse antibody) was given to these interferents. However, interference was described in assays which use antibodies produced in other species, and the broader term "heterophilic" antibodies is also used. Manufacturers countered by adding serum or immunoglobulins from the animal species as blocking agents. In most cases, this is sufficient to negate this problem. However, there are occasional patients who have such high concentrations of these heterophilic antibodies that they exceed the capacity of the blocking agents and produce false results. This is especially true in 2-site immunometric assays, in which any molecule that can link the capture and repartee antibody will give a positive signal.

The use of monoclonal antibodies in diagnostic and treatment regimens can also lead to large levels of heterophilic antibodies in patients. Without sufficient clinical history, the laboratory is dependent on the clinician to report these discrepancies to the laboratory. The laboratory can then use additional animal sera or use other methods to reduce the interference.

Our laboratory had a problem with a patient who consistently had elevated troponin I values. We interpreted normal creatine kinase values with elevated Troponin I values as a late infarction. When notified by the clinician that this was unlikely, we were able to demonstrate very high levels of heterophilic antibodies. It is also important to remember that in these patients, there will be erroneous results in almost any 2-site immunometric assay.

R. Feld, Ph.D.

Glucose Measurements in Patients With Diabetes Mellitus With Dermal Interstitial Fluid

Bantle JP, Thomas W (Univ of Minnesota, Minneapolis)

J Lab Clin Med 130:436–441, 1997 20–6

Background.—Measurement of capillary blood glucose from a blood sample obtained by a finger prick is the standard method of self-monitoring for individuals with diabetes mellitus. A less invasive method would be desirable. Tamada et al. recently reported that a glucose flux obtained transdermally with a low-level electric current was quantitatively related to serum glucose. Measuring dermal interstitial fluid glucose concentrations may be an alternative means of monitoring blood glucose.

Methods.—Plasma glucose, capillary blood glucose, and dermal interstitial fluid glucose were measured in 17 individuals with type I diabetes mellitus. Samples were collected during a 5-hour preprandial and postprandial period of rapid change in plasma glucose. The ability of dermal interstitial fluid glucose to predict plasma glucose in a range of glucose concentrations was determined.

Results.—There was high correlation between dermal interstitial fluid glucose and plasma glucose (Fig 1). The mean absolute difference between dermal interstitial fluid glucose and plasma glucose was 1.2 mmol/L. The mean percent difference between dermal interstitial fluid glucose and plasma glucose was 10.6%. There was no significant difference between the kinetics of dermal interstitial fluid glucose and plasma glucose. Mean glucose excursion, peak glucose concentration, and time to peak glucose concentration were similar in dermal interstitial fluid glucose and plasma glucose. The relation between dermal interstitial fluid glucose and plasma glucose was as strong as the relation between capillary blood glucose and plasma glucose.

Discussion.—These preliminary results show that measurement of dermal interstitial fluid glucose can predict plasma glucose. It may be possible

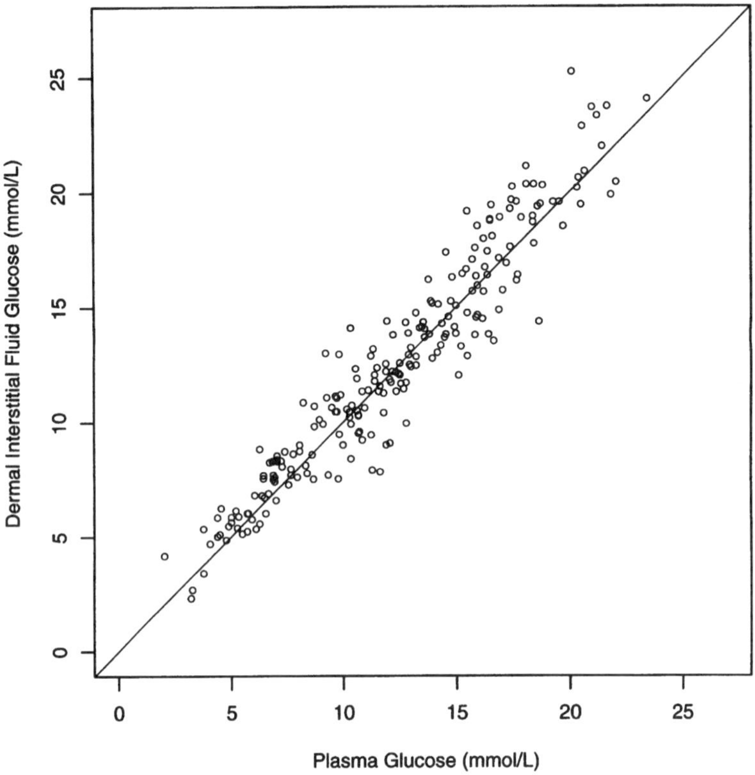

FIGURE 1.—Plasma glucose versus dermal interstitial fluid glucose concentrations for all observations of all subjects (n = 223); the *line* shown is the line of identity (x = y). (Courtesy of Bantle JP, Thomas W: Glucose measurement in patients with diabetes mellitus with dermal interstitial fluid. *J Lab Clin Med* 130:436–441, 1997.)

to use this technique in patients with diabetes mellitus to monitor blood glucose if the performance issues in this study can be resolved and if the collection techniques can be performed by patients.

► There have been many changes in the diagnosis, monitoring , and treatment of diabetes in the last decade. Recently the criteria for the diagnosis of diabetes has been changed to 2 fasting glucose values of 126 mg/dL or greater. This change is estimated to reclassify 2 million additional patients as diabetics and to increase the number categorized as having impaired glucose tolerance. The introduction of HbA_{1c} and home glucose monitoring has helped greatly in achieving good control. The Diabetes Complications and Control Trial has shown that good glucose control can greatly reduce the complications that are common in the disease. Home glucose monitors allow the diabetic to adjust insulin dosage to achieve blood glucose values that are as close to normal as possible. However, frequent monitoring comes at the price of frequent fingersticks. This mildly painful procedure is annoying to adults and terrorizing to children.

This paper evaluates a device that painlessly collects a small sample (0.5 µL) of dermal interstitial fluid. By measuring the glucose of the fluid, the authors were able to show that there was a strong correlation between dermal interstitial fluid glucose levels and plasma and capillary blood glucose levels. Another group tested the same device with similar conclusions.[1] The next step is to combine the sampling device with a measurement of interstitial fluid glucose in a hand-held device. As an interim method between the capillary blood glucose and the totally noninvasive methods in development, this sampling device may eliminate the bother and pain of the lancet.

R. Feld, Ph.D.

Reference

1. Service FJ, O'Brien PC, Wise SD, et al: Dermal interstitial glucose as an indicator of ambient glycemia. *Diabetes Care* 20:1426–1429, 1997.

Improved Detection of Minor Ischemic Myocardial Injury With Measurement of Serum Cardiac Troponin I

Apple FS, Falahati A, Paulsen PR, et al (Univ of Minnesota, Minneapolis)

Clin Chem 43:2047–2051, 1997 20–7

Background.—Acute myocardial infarction is biochemically confirmed by a serial rise and fall in serum creatine kinase (CK) and its MB isoenzyme (CK-MB). Although these enzyme markers are commonly used, they can be problematic. Recently, cardiac troponin I and cardiac troponin T have become available for detecting myocardial injury. They have higher sensitivity for detection of acute myocardial injury than CK-MB in cases of suspected acute myocardial injury. The diagnostic accuracy of serum cardiac troponin I was compared with CK-MB mass measurements in patients with minor myocardial injury and a measured total CK activity that was not more than twice the upper reference limit (300 U/L for men and 200 U/L for women).

Methods.—A total of 48 consecutive patients with acute minor ischemic myocardial injury were studied. There were 27 men and 21 women, and the mean patient age was 65 years. During a period of 36 hours after admission, ECG, echocardiogram, and serial serum CK-MB mass, serum cardiac troponin I, and total CK were measured.

Results.—In 58% of patients, peak total CK activity was within normal limits. The mean peak CK-MB mass was 16.4 µg/L, and the mean peak cardiac troponin I concentration was 132 µg/L. From 7 to 36 hours, the peak biochemical marker index was significantly higher for cardiac troponin I than for CK-MB (Fig 1). Sensitivity for detection of myocardial injury was 100% for cardiac troponin I and 81.8% for CK-MB.

Discussion.—In these patients, cardiac troponin I was more sensitive than CK-MB for detecting myocardial injury in cases of small increases of total CK. These results support cardiac troponin I as the preferred marker for detecting minor ischemic cardiac injury. The use of a twofold increase

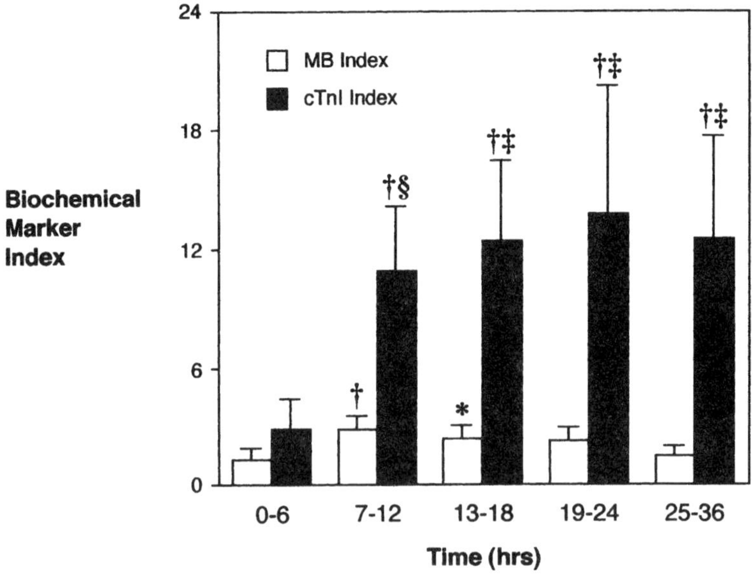

FIGURE 1.—Mean (95% confidence *error bars*) biochemical marker index values for CK-MB mass and cardiac troponin I (*cTnI*) after onset of chest pain in 48 patients with minor ischemic cardiac injury. Within group comparisons: *$P < 0.05$ vs. 0–6 hours; † $P < 0.01$ vs. 0–6 hours. Between group comparisons: ‡ $P < 0.001$ vs. CK-MB; §$P < 0.05$ vs. CK-MB. (Courtesy of Apple FS, Falahati A, Paulsen PR, et al: Improved detection of minor ischemic myocardial injury with measurement of serum cardiac troponin I. *Clin Chem* 43:2047–2051. Copyright 1997, The American Association for Clinical Chemistry [1–800–892–1400].)

in total CK activity as an indicator of acute myocardial infarction should be reevaluated.

▶ One of the advantages of the troponins, both T and I, is their ability to detect minor myocardial damage. This damage is often referred to as microinfarction, although no one has placed a number on how many cardiac myocytes must die to qualify for this term. This is supposedly why the troponins can stratify patients with unstable angina into those who are at great risk for a myocardial event and those who are at low risk. This allows aggressive treatment by surgery or drugs to modify the outcome of the group with elevated troponin.

In this paper, Apple et al. studied patients with minor myocardial injury as defined by CK activity of less than twice normal, or ECG evidence of minor injury. The phenomenon of normal CK and elevated CK-MB has been well described and is not uncommon in the elderly. These patients are often classified as non–Q-wave infarction, although there is debate whether this condition is different from unstable angina. Serum CK-MB had a sensitivity of 82% in these patients, whereas troponin I had a sensitivity of 100% and was more sensitive than CK-MB at every period from 0 to 36 hours. Because CK-MB is the de facto gold standard, confusion can arise when comparing a better test to it. The troponins continue to demonstrate their superiority to

CK-MB, and it is just a matter of time before they supplant this test, which has served us well but now deserves a well-earned retirement.

R. Feld, Ph.D.

Troponin I Is Released in Bloodstream of Patients With Acute Myocardial Infarction Not in Free Form But as Complex

Katrukha AG, Bereznikova AV, Esakova TV, et al (HyTest Ltd, Turku, Finland; Moscow State Univ, Russia; Inst of Med Ecology, Moscow, Russia; et al)

Clin Chem 43:1379–1385, 1997 20–8

Background.—Troponin, a protein that is involved in cardiac muscle contraction, is composed of troponin C (TnC), troponin I (TnI), and troponin T (TnT). Serum cardiac TnI (cTnI) is a highly sensitive and specific marker of myocardial tissue damage. Immunoassays for cTnI vary widely in their results. The serum of patients with acute myocardial infarction (AMI) was examined with a series of monoclonal antibodies (mAbs) generated against purified cTnI to analyze whether cTnI is released into the blood stream as an isolated protein or as a complex with other proteins.

Methods.—Blood samples were collected from patients with AMI. Fourteen monoclonal antibodies were generated to purified cTnI and their

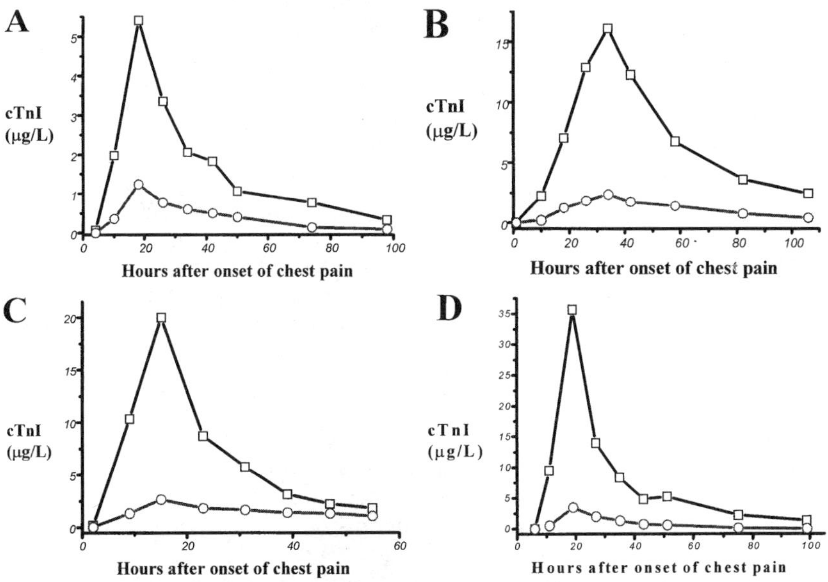

FIGURE 4.—Time course of liberation of total cardiac troponin I (cTnI) measured by 10F4–7F4 assay in the presence of ethylenediaminetetraaceticacid (*squares*) and free cTnI measured by 7F4–414 assay (*circles*) in the serum of 4 representative patients with AMI. (Courtesy of Katrukha AG, Bereznikova AV, Esakova TV, et al: Troponin I is released in bloodstream of patients with acute myocardial infarction not in free form but as complex. *Clin Chem* 43:1379–1385. Copyright 1997, The American Association for Clinical Chemistry [1–800–892–4100].)

specificity was confirmed by Western blot. Antibody 414, specific for cTnI, was supplied by HyTest. A 2-step immunofluorescence assay was performed to detect cTnI in the samples from patients with AMI.

Results.—The formation of a TnI-TnC complex was associated with a significant decrease in the interaction of the majority of cTnI-specific mAbs with cTnI. Using an mAb that only recognized free cTnI and another that recognized both free and complexed cTnI, it was determined that the majority of cTnI in serum samples from patients with AMI existed in complexed form (Fig 4).

Conclusions.—Studies of cardiac troponin I in the bloodstream of patients with AMI has demonstrated that the majority of this protein exists in complexed form. The formation of this complex significantly affects the interaction of cTnI with specific monoclonal antibodies and may explain the difference between immunoassays used to detect this protein. Reliable immunologic detection of cTnI in serum samples from patients with AMI requires antibodies that recognize both free and complexed cTnI.

▶ Yogi Berra is supposed to have said, "It's like deja vu all over again," and that is the feeling one gets after reading this article. Just as the prostate-specific antigen story has progressed to free and bound, we learn that TnI is released mostly complexed with TnC. This is not surprising because they have a high affinity interaction with each other in the myofibril and this interaction is dependent on the saturation of calcium-binding sites of TnC. By using 196 combinations of mAbs in the presence of calcium or ethylenediaminetetraacetic acid, the authors were able to measure both total complexed TnI and free TnI. Using these assays, the authors demonstrate that in patients who have had a myocardial infarct, the majority of the TnI in the circulation is in the complexed form. Furthermore, the ratio of bound to free varies in the time course of the observations and varies among patients. This has implications for assays in regard to the reactivity of the antibodies chosen with regard to free and bound troponin. It also explains the great variation among troponin assays when measuring the same sample as is observed in the trial College of American Pathologists proficiency samples. Laboratories that perform TnI assays should inquire of the manufacturer as to the specificity of the antibodies toward bound vs. free.

R. Feld, Ph.D.

Alternative Sequences of Thyrotropin and Free Thyroxine Assays for Routine Thyroid Function Testing: Quality and Cost

Nordyke RA, Reppun TS, Madanay LD, et al (Straub Clinic and Hosp Inc, Honolulu; Univ of Hawaii, Honolulu; Queen's Med Ctr, Honolulu; et al)

Arch Intern Med 158:266–272, 1998 20–9

Introduction.—Guidelines for thyroid function testing issued by professional societies have varied, largely because of tradeoffs between quality and cost. Patient billing changes and Medicare reimbursement are usually higher for thyrotropin (TSH) than for free thyroxine (FT_4) tests, despite similar direct costs. The recent reduction in laboratory costs prompted a reconsideration of the effectiveness and cost of alternative test sequences.

Methods.—Four laboratories took part in the study: a multispecialty fee-for-service group practice, an HMO, a military hospital, and a large private laboratory. Each performed TSH and FT_4 tests on 500 consecutive patients during a 3-month period in 1993. For each of the laboratories, direct costs of reagents and personnel per reportable test were calculated. Three alternative test sequences were evaluated: the TSH first, followed by the FT_4 test if results proved abnormal; the FT_4 test first, followed by the TSH test; and both tests done together.

Results.—The 2 tests had similar sensitivities for detecting clinical hyperthyroidism and hypothyroidism. The TSH test was better at detecting subclinical function and at monitoring thyroxine treatment. The FT_4 test proved to be better at detecting central hypothyroidism and monitoring rapidly changing function. Although direct costs were equal, charges for the TSH test were higher. Average direct costs per patient of the alternative test sequences were $4.61 when starting with the FT_4 test, $5.90 when starting with the TSH test, and $6.50 when using both tests together. There were substantial discrepancies between Medicare reimbursements and direct costs of laboratory tests. Reimbursement was $13.06 for the FT_4 test vs. $24.12 for the TSH test.

Discussion.—The recommended protocol starts with the TSH test, followed by an FT_4 assay if the TSH test result is abnormal. Although this approach has a slightly higher cost, the cost difference is offset by greater clinical effectiveness. Doing both tests together results in a slightly higher direct cost but increases efficiency and diagnostic accuracy.

▶ Thyroid function testing has come a long way since the basal metabolic rate and protein-bound iodine. Unfortunately, the new Health Care Finance Administration (HCFA)–approved thyroid panels were suggested by those who obviously do not understand the newest thyroid function tests. This paper looks at 2 popular tests for screening thyroid function and seeks to answer the question of the most efficient sequence: TSH followed by FT_4 if the first test is abnormal, the opposite sequence, or both tests at the same time.

The authors correctly point out that Medicare reimbursement for TSH is significantly greater than FT_4, probably because of the historically higher direct cost for this assay. However, advances in technology have made possible cheaper TSH assays so that the current direct costs for the 2 assays are nearly equal. This allows the ordering pattern to be determined on clinical, rather than financial, grounds.

The arguments for beginning the sequence with FT_4 include diagnosis of central hypothyroidism and the avoidance of subclinical hyperthyroidism and hypothyroidism whose treatments are of uncertain benefit. The arguments for beginning with TSH are that subclinical hyperthyroidism and hypothyroidism are important conditions and there is benefit in treating them and that TSH in the reference range best defines the euthyroid state. Performing both tests together circumvents the limitations of either test; also the combination test is best in patients with changing thyroid function. The higher direct costs for both tests are not much greater than for the sequence. Someone should send this paper to the HCFA and tell them to redo the thyroid panel.

R. Feld, Ph.D.

Ethylene Glycol Poisoning: Toxicokinetic and Analytical Factors Affecting Laboratory Diagnosis

Eder AF, McGrath CM, Dowdy YG, et al (Univ of Pennsylvania, Philadelphia; Univ of British Columbia, Vancouver)

Clin Chem 44:168–177, 1998 20–10

Background.—Early diagnosis and aggressive treatment are essential for patients with severe ethylene glycol poisoning. The challenges of diagnosing ethylene glycol intoxication were illustrated in the case reports of 4 patients.

Patients and Findings.—The patients were 4 men, aged 18–58. The first 2 patients reported a clear history of ethylene glycol ingestion. These 2 patients had several of the classic signs and symptoms of poisoning. Appropriate treatment was begun promptly, preventing neurologic, cardiac, and renal damage. The third patient was initially seen with a confusing picture of unexplained metabolic acidosis and renal failure. He repeatedly denied ingesting ethylene glycol. Results of serum ethylene glycol measures were repeatedly negative. Renal biopsy was needed to diagnose ethylene glycol poisoning in this patient. The fourth patient also denied ingesting ethylene glycol. However, his initial signs and symptoms were consistent with ethylene glycol poisoning, including a laboratoy test positive for serum ethylene glycol. However, this result was found to be the result of serum component interference in the ethylene glycol enzymatic assay (Table 2).

TABLE 2.—Toxicokinetic Parameters for Ethylene Glycol*

Lethal dose†	1.4–1.6 mL/kg
V_d	0.5–0.8 L/kg
$t_{1/2}$	3–8.6 h
$t_{1/2}$ during ethanol infusion	17–18 h
$t_{1/2}$ during hemodialysis	2.5–3.5 h
Mean renal clearance‡	0.75–27.5 mL/min
Mean dialyzer clearance	156–210 mL/min

*Data compiled from references 18, 23, 26, 27, and 33.

†Although the lethal dose is considered 100 mL for a 70 kg adult, survival has been reported after ingestions of 0.27 to 2 L. Also, death has been reported after ingestion of 30 mL.

‡Lower value obtained in patient with renal failure; upper value obtained in patient with normal renal function.

Conclusions.—Ethylene glycol, ingested in the form of antifreeze or other automotive products, results in CNS depression, cardiopulmonary compromise, and renal insufficiency. The metabolism of this substance to organic acids leads to metabolic derangement and organ damage. Laboratory findings indicating ethylene glycol poisoning are increased anion gap metabolic acidosis, increased osmolal gap, calcium oxalate crystalluria, and detectable levels of ethylene glycol in serum.

▶ Ethylene glycol along with methanol are two toxins that produce an osmolal gap not explained by ethanol and when metabolized to oxalate and formate will produce an anion gap acidosis. This paper presents four patients that are representative of the various presentations of ethylene glycol poisoning. The paper covers the metabolism of ethylene glycol, the sensitivity and specificity of osmolal and anion gaps, as well as the toxicokinetics under various conditions and the laboratory analysis of the toxin. We have found this paper very useful in two recent cases at our institution with regard to scheduling the frequency of ethylene glycol determinations during dialysis. The gas chromatography technique that we employ is labor intense and uses significant technologist time, and therefore minimizing the number of analyses is helpful.

Prompt treatment with either ethanol or the newly approved alcohol dehydrogenase inhibitor, 4-methylpyrazole, can present the metabolism of ethylene glycol to its total metabolite and prevent the consequences such as renal failure. Any laboratory that aids in the diagnosis and treatment of overdose patients should have a copy of this article at the ready.

R. Feld, Ph.D.

Point of Care Testing: Randomised Controlled Trial of Clinical Outcome

Kendall J, Reeves B, Clancy M (Bristol Royal Infirmary, England; Univ of Bristol, England)

BMJ 316:1052–1057, 1998 20–11

Background.—Point-of-care testing is defined as any laboratory test done outside a hospital central laboratory. Faster test results may expedite diagnosis and start of treatment, and may shorten the time that patients spend waiting in emergency departments. An evaluation of point-of-care testing is needed to determine its value to patients and its cost-effectiveness.

Methods.—The percentage of patients treated in an emergency department whose treatment was changed after blood analysis at the point of care was determined, as well as the effect of point-of-care testing on clinical outcome. Blood samples of patients treated in an accident and emergency department were randomly sent to the hospital laboratory for testing, or allocated to point-of-care testing. Mortality, length of hospital stay, admission rate, time patients spent waiting for results of blood tests,

TABLE 6.—Comparison of the Mean Total Time Patients Spent in the Emergency Department, Length of Stay in Hospital, Number of Admissions, and Mortality for Patients Whose Samples Were Allocated to Point of Care Testing or to Laboratory Testing

	Point of care testing		Laboratory testing		Point of care *v* laboratory testing	
	No of patients*	Mean (95% CI) or No (%)	No of patients	Mean (95% CI) or No (%)	Difference (95% CI)	P value
Mean (95% CI) time spent in emergency department (min)	859	188 (181 to 194)	868	193 (186 to 200)	5 (−5 to 15)	0.30
Mean (95% CI) length of stay in hospital (days)†	730	7.8 (6.9 to 8.6)	720	8.3 (7.5 to 9.1)	0.5 (−1 to 2)	0.37
No (%) admissions	860	733 (85.2)	868	725 (83.5)	1.7 (−1.7 to 5.1)	0.33
No (%) deaths‡	859	55 (6.4)	867	48 (5.5)	0.9 (−1.4 to 3.1)	0.45

*One patient discharged himself before test results became available.

†Information on length of stay in hospital was not available for 3 point of care patients and 3 patients allocated to laboratory testing who were transferred to other hospitals. Information was missing from the hospital information system for 2 additional patients allocated to laboratory testing.

‡Information was not available for 1 point of care patient and 1 patient allocated to laboratory testing, because they were transferred to other hospitals.

(Courtesy of Kendall J, Reeves B, Clancy M: Point of care testing: Randomised trial of clinical outcome. *BMJ* 316:1052–1057, 1998. This table was first published in the *BMJ* and is reproduced by permission of the *BMJ*.)

time taken to decide on patient management, and time patients spent in the emergency department were compared between the 2 groups.

Results.—Blood samples were obtained from 1,728 patients. In the point-of-care testing group, changes in patient management in which timing was considered critical were made in 59 of 859 patients. When point of care testing was used, management decisions were made 74 minutes earlier for blood tests, 86 minutes earlier for biochemical tests, and 21 minutes earlier for arterial blood gases analysis. No differences in mortality, length of hospital stay, admission rates, or time spent in the emergency department were seen between groups (Table 6).

Conclusion.—These results indicate that point-of-care testing shortens the time it takes to make decisions about patient management that depend on the results of blood tests. In almost 7% of patients, point-of-care testing resulted in faster changes in treatment in which timing was critical. Clinical outcome and the time that patients spent in the emergency department were not affected by these changes.

▶ By now, most people know the arguments both for and against point-of-care testing. Although it is true that point-of-care tests provide results sooner than do central laboratories, few studies have tried to address the question of whether this benefits the patient. Patients seen in the emergency department were randomized to receive laboratory data either from the central laboratory or from a point-of-care instrument. Two sets of tests, blood gases and electrolytes with urea, glucose, and calculated hemoglobin were evaluated. Over 1,700 patients were evaluated. Outcome measurements investigated included length of time waiting for results, and the proportion of patients in whom point-of-care testing resulted in a critical change in diagnosis or treatment. As would be expected, the time needed to obtain results from the point-of-care instrument was significantly shorter than that needed to obtain results from the central laboratory. The mean differences varied from 21 to 86 minutes. Physicians interviewed after the patient was admitted or discharged felt the more rapid results resulted in a critical diagnostic or treatment change in about 7% of patients. Surprisingly, though, the 2 groups did not differ in length of inpatient stay, mortality, admission rates, or time spent in the emergency facility. These results imply that laboratory results were not the rate-limiting step in the disposition of these patients. These results were obtained in 1 area and 1 facility and are not applicable to other situations, such as intensive care units. Still, it is interesting that in spite of faster availability of results, and physicians' perception of benefit, no benefit to the patient could be demonstrated.

R. Feld, Ph.D.

21 Hematopathology and Immunopathology

Reticulocyte Hemoglobin: An Integrated Parameter for Evaluation of Erythropoietic Activity

Brugnara C, Zelmanovic D, Sorette M, et al (Harvard Med School, Boston; Bayer Corp, Tarrytown, NY; Jefferson Med College, Philadelphia)

Am J Clin Pathol 108:133–142, 1997 21–1

Background.—Conventional reticulocyte counts can only partially estimate erythropoietic bone marrow activity and do not explain qualitative variations in reticulocyte cellular indices or hemoglobin (Hb) content. Reticulocyte Hb (retHb) is a new, integrated parameter for evaluating erythropoietic activity. Reticulocyte Hb measures the Hb in the circulating reticulocyte compartment in grams per liter.

Methods.—Complete blood cell and reticulocyte counts were studied in patients with various hematologic disorders and normal control subjects (Table 2). The retHb was obtained by multiplying the absolute reticulocyte count and reticulocyte cell Hb content.

Results.—In control subjects, the retHb values were lower in patients who were double heterozygotes for HbS and HbC (sickle cell disease) than in (1) patients with homozygous HbS disease and concomitant α-thalassemia, and (2) patients with sickle cell disease but no α-thalassemia. The Hb in the red blood cell pool can also be determined by subtracting retHb values from the total Hb. The ratio between the 2 pools (red blood cell and retHb) is an estimate of red blood cell survival. This was 9.8 in patients with homozygous HbS disease, 16.2 in patients with homozygous HbS disease and 3 normal α-genes, 14.7 in patients with homozygous HbS disease and 2 normal α-genes, and 36.6 in patients with sickle cell disease and no α-thalassemia. retHb was also examined in patients undergoing hydroxyurea therapy for homozygous HbS disease, receiving IV or oral iron for iron deficiency, or undergoing recombinant human erythropoietin therapy. These conditions involve changes in reticulocyte counts and substantial variation in reticulocyte cellular Hb content that can be integrated into the retHb values.

Discussion.—It may be possible to estimate the reduction in red blood cell survival and severity of hemolysis in anemia by determining retHb and

TABLE 2.—Reticulocyte Indices, Reticulocyte Hemoglobin, and the Mature Red Blood Cell Hemoglobin/Reticulocyte Hemoglobin Ratio in Healthy Pediatric Subjects and Children with Hematologic Disorders

	Hemoglobin (g/L)	rbcHb (g/L)	Reticulocytes ($\times 10^9$/mL)	CHr (pg)	retHb (g/L)	rbcHb/retHb Ratio
Healthy control subjects (n = 212)	113 ± 9.0	111.3 ± 9.3	61 ± 22.5	26.5 ± 2.1	1.6 ± 0.6	78.5 ± 30.4
Sickle cell disease (n = 17)	73.9 ± 15.3	65.8 ± 14.4	306.2 ± 118.1	26.0 ± 2.4	8.1 ± 3.4	10.6 ± 7.3
Hereditary spherocytosis (n = 12)	100.8 ± 29.8	91.4 ± 30.8	336.1 ± 94.4	28.2 ± 2.7	9.4 ± 2.4	10.8 ± 5.5
Iron deficiency (n = 7)	83.0 ± 13.0	81.5 ± 13.2	91.1 ± 35.8	17.2 ± 3.1	1.5 ± 0.4	59.0 ± 21.9

Abbreviations: rbcHb, mature red blood cell hemoglobin; *CHr*, reticulocyte cell hemoglobin content.

(Courtesy of Brugnara C, Zelmanovic D, Sorette M, et al: Reticulocyte hemoglobin: An integrated parameter for evaluation of erythropoietic activity. *Am J Clin Pathol* 108:133–142. Copyright 1997 by the American Society of Clinical Pathologists. Reprinted with permission.)

the mature red blood cell Hb/retHb ratio. These measurements may also allow better monitoring of the response to hydroxyurea, iron, recombinant human erythropoietin, and other treatments.

▶ In addition to knowing the absolute reticulocyte count, knowing the amount of Hb in the reticulocyte pool can also serve as a valuable parameter in evaluating hemolysis. Newer hematology analyzers are now capable of reporting not only the reticulocyte count but also the mean corpuscular volume, the cell Hb concentration, and the Hb content in reticulocytes. Using these parameters, it is possible to determine the concentration of retHb in the blood as well as the proportion of Hb in the mature and reticulocyte pools.

These authors have demonstrated the usefulness of these new parameters in the evaluation of patients with sickle-cell disease, in terms of their diagnosis of hemolysis as well as in monitoring their therapy. They call attention to the "rough" relationship between the red cell–to–retHb ratio and the red cell survival. Correlation of these parameters with actual chromium-labeled red cell survivals has not been performed; however, the general information provided by this ratio could be of value in estimating red cell survival. Further evaluation of these parameters in other hemolytic processes will be of interest; however, the available information applied in the appropriate settings can be very useful in evaluation for hemolysis.

J.D. Olson, M.D., Ph.D.

Clinical Significance of Immature Reticulocyte Fraction Determined by Automated Reticulocyte Counting

Chang C-C, Kass L (Metro Health Med Ctr, Cleveland, Ohio; Case Western Reserve Univ, Cleveland, Ohio)

Am J Clin Pathol 108:69–73, 1997 21–2

Background.—Assessment of reticulocyte maturation is important for determining the degree of effective erythropoiesis, for studying the pathophysiologic changes in anemia, and for the differential diagnosis of anemia. The Sysmex R-3000 can determine the maturation of reticulocytes by measuring the fraction of reticulocytes in low-, middle-, and high-fluorescence intensity regions.

Methods.—Analysis was done in 132 specimens from 102 patients being evaluated for anemia. The immature reticulocyte fraction was determined by adding the fraction of high-fluorescence intensity regions and the fraction of middle-fluorescence intensity regions. The clinical significance of the immature reticulocyte fraction in the assessment of anemia was studied by (1) comparing the immature reticulocyte fraction with the absolute reticulocyte count, (2) comparing the immature reticulocyte fraction with the reticulocyte production index, and (3) reviewing medical records.

Results.—The immature reticulocyte fraction had a weak, but significantly positive, correlation with the absolute reticulocyte count and retic-

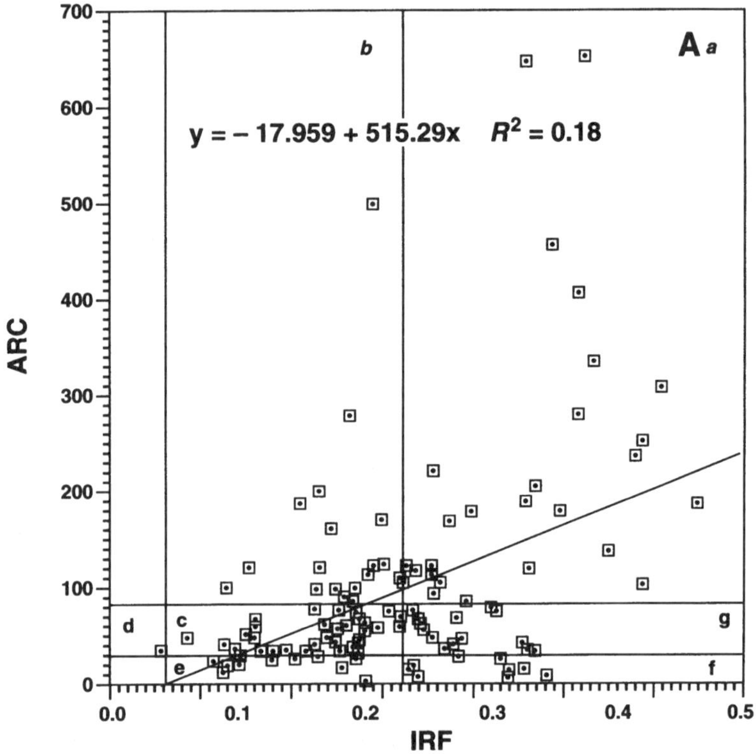

FIGURE 2, A.—Correlation between the absolute reticulocyte count (*ARC*) and the immature reticulocyte fraction (*IRF*) for samples from patients. Section *a* shows sickle disease with crisis (n = 8), physiologic anemia secondary to respiratory insufficiency (n = 1)*, pregnancy (n = 2), acute infection (n = 3), and lead poisoning (n =1). Section *b* shows sickle disease with crisis (n = 1), physiologic anemia secondary to respiratory insufficiency (n = 1)*, hypothyroidism (n = 4), sarcoidosis (n = 2), neurosyphilis (n = 1), and eating disorder with malnutrition (n = 2). Section *c* shows chronic renal failure (n = 30) and eating disorder with malnutrition (n = 3). Section *d* shows chronic renal failure (n = 1). Section *e* shows chronic renal failure (n = 8). Section *f* shows iron deficiency anemia (n = 3), HIV infection (n = 3), and acute infection (n = 2). Section *g* shows iron deficiency anemia (n = 2), HIV infection (n = 2), pregnancy (n = 1), acute infection (n = 5), sickle disease with crisis (n = 4), and myelodysplastic syndrome (n = 1). *Asterisks* indicate different specimens from the same patient. (Courtesy of Chang C-C, Kass L: Clinical significance of immature reticulocyte fraction determined by automated reticulocyte counting. *Am J Clin Pathol* 108:69–73. Copyright 1997 by the American Society of Clinical Pathologists. Reprinted with permission.)

ulocyte production index. This suggested that the immature reticulocyte fraction would be useful for evaluating erythropoietic activity in anemia. Integrating the immature reticulocyte fraction and reticulocyte enumeration (absolute reticulocyte count and reticulocyte production index) was useful in the subclassification of anemia. An elevated immature reticulocyte fraction and absolute reticulocyte count usually indicated an adequate erythroid response to anemia.

Of specimens with an immature reticulocyte fraction of less than 0.23, all but 3 had a reticulocyte production index of 2 or less. These specimens were from individuals with underlying diseases that are known to decrease erythropoietic activity. Specimens with a normal or subnormal absolute reticulocyte count, but with an immature reticulocyte fraction greater than 0.23, were from individuals with various underlying conditions such as acute infection, iron deficiency anemia, HIV infection, sickle disease with crisis, pregnancy, and myelodysplastic syndrome (Fig 2, A).

Discussion.—These findings suggest that in patients with anemia, an immature reticulocyte fraction of 0.23 or less indicates bone marrow that is nonresponsive or underresponsive to the anemia. Patients with an immature reticulocyte fraction of 0.23 or greater may require further evaluation to determine the cause of the anemia.

► The reticulocyte count has been a tried-and-true method for determining bone marrow response to anemia. It has always been fraught with the difficulty of counting very small percentages of cells, leading to significant technical error. For approximately the last decade, methods using flow cytometers have been available, allowing for greater precision in the assay. In this report, the authors have taken advantage of fluorescence intensity reported by the Sysmex R-3000 reticulocyte counter to determine the fraction of reticulocytes that are more intensly fluorescent, therefore immature. The authors did comparisons with the absolute reticulocyte count, using, for the "gold standard," the reticulocyte production index.

There are a couple of important features in this paper. In the figure, one can see the wide degree of scatter when comparing the absolute reticulocyte count with a proportion of those cells that are immature. In addition, the grids identified as g and f are of particular interest because they constitute cases in which there is hemolysis, normal or low absolute reticulocyte count with elevated immature reticulocyte fractions. In contrast, the majority of those patients in grid b—the grid in which the absolute reticulocyte count is elevated but the immature fraction is low or normal—constitute predominantly patients without true hemolytic processes but processes primarily affecting the bone marrow. In conclusion, this report calls attention to the potential importance of the most immature fraction of the reticulocyte pool in evaluating patients with possible hemolysis.

J.D. Olson, M.D., Ph.D.

Dipstick Only Urinalysis Screen for the Pediatric Emergency Room

Craver RD, Abermanis JG (Louisiana State Univ, New Orleans; Children's Hosp, New Orleans, La)

Pediatr Nephrol 11:331–333, 1997 21–3

Background.—In the authors' pediatric emergency department, most urinalyses are done to detect urinary tract infection. Although both dipstick urinalysis and complete urinalysis can detect urinary tract infection, the dipstick method is much faster and cheaper. The results of urine microscopy were examined to determine whether this method could detect infections missed by the dipstick method in pediatric patients. Eliminating urine microscopy as part of routine urinalysis would shorten testing turn-around time and save money.

Methods.—The results of dipstick and complete urinalyses were compared with results of urine cultures in 236 children treated in a hospital emergency department. The subjects were between the ages of 3 weeks and 21 years.

Results.—The ability of the dipstick method alone and complete urinalysis alone to detect urinary tract infection in these subjects was similar. Microscopic evaluation of biochemically normal (Dipstick-negative) urine added many false positive results without detecting additional infections.

Discussion.—Because of the sensitivity of the dipstick method, this hospital now uses dipstick urinalysis alone in the emergency department for children older than 2 years of age. If the dipstick results are positive, a microscopic analysis is performed automatically. When no microscopic analysis is done, the hospital charge is reduced to $12 from $32, and testing turn-around time is reduced to 12.3 minutes per test. Time and money can be saved by eliminating the microscopic portion of emergency urinalyses in children older than 2 years of age.

► Routine microscopic examination of the urine in the face of normal urine biochemistry studies, as indicated by dipstick examination, has been the subject of considerable controversy over the last 2 decades. These authors have prospectively analyzed the urine in 236 children with suspected urinary tract infection, using urine culture as the diagnostic standard. Of particular interest is their finding that microscopic examination in cases with negative dipstick findings (nitrate and blood) yielded no increase in the sensitivity of the test but significantly increased the false positives.

These findings clearly indicate that negative dipstick results in patients with suspected urinary tract infection is a sufficient screen and that performing microscopic examinations in these patients serves only to increase the false positive cases and to increase the cost of patient care. It is a very useful paper for laboratories to have in their file when discussing the issue of microscopic examinations of biochemically normal urine.

J.D. Olson, M.D., Ph.D.

Leukocytosis: A New Look at an Old Marker for Acute Myocardial Infarction

Green SM, Vowels J, Waterman B, et al (Loma Linda Univ, Calif; Orlando Regional Med Ctr, Fla)

Acad Emerg Med 3:1034–1041, 1996 21–4

Background.—Before the availability of creatine kinase testing for the diagnosis of acute myocardial infarction (AMI), the most useful diagnostic laboratory finding was leukocytosis. Now, though white blood cell (WBC) counts are routinely obtained in patients with suspected AMI, they are almost never used in the cardiac evaluation. The WBC count was reevaluated as an indicator of AMI.

Methods.—The retrospective, cross-sectional study included 832 patients admitted to a university teaching hospital to rule out AMI. Of those, 668 had nondiagnostic ECG results. Hospital laboratory data were used to define the following threshold evaluations: total creatine kinase (CK), 275 U/L; CK-MB, 7.5 μg/L; WBC count, 11.5×10^9/L; and absolute neutrophil count (ANC), 8.0×10^9. For each of these measures, sensitivity, specificity, and predictive values were calculated and receiver operating characteristic curves constructed. The WBC count was evaluated, on its own or in combination with CK and CK-MB, as a diagnostic marker of AMI.

Results.—Initial WBC count was 11.1×10^9/L for patients with AMI vs. 8.8×10^9/L for those without. Diagnostic sensitivity among patients with nondiagnostic ECG results were 39% for initial total CK, 73% for CK-MB, 35% for WBC, and 36% for ANC. Specificity values were 94%, 93%, 85%, and 86%, respectively. Leukocytosis was a significant, independent predictor of AMI on logistic regression analysis, with an adjusted odds ratio of 4.08. The finding of either an elevated CK-MB or elevated WBC count had a sensitivity of 88%, with a specificity of 79%. The combination of elevated CK-MB and elevated WBC count had a specificity of 99%, with a sensitivity of 20%.

Conclusions.—Leukocytosis is a weak but independent marker of AMI. Combining the WBC count with the CK-MB measurement may offer additional information beyond that of CK-MB alone; on their own, neither factor was sufficiently sensitive for the diagnosis of AMI. The WBC count, as a complement to other tests, may have a useful role in clinical decision making in suspected AMI.

► Leukocytosis has been a well-recognized marker of acute inflammation since early in the century. It has been well recognized for a long time that leukocytosis occurs in patients with AMI; however, it has not been a valuable diagnostic marker because of its lack of specificity. In this article, the authors have taken a new look at leukocytosis in patients with chest pain and nondiagnostic ECG results. They have evaluated sensitivity, specificity, and receiver operating characteristic curves for the CK-MB, the ANC, and the 2 parameters together. What they have found is that CK-MB alone had a specificity of 93%; however, when combined with an elevated WBC count, this specificity increased to 99%. As emergency treatment centers are evaluating patients with chest pain having information concerning the ANC in conjunction with markers of myocardial damage can be helpful. The study does not address the question of troponin, one of the newer markers for myocardial infarction. Doing so may be of interest.

J.D. Olson, M.D., Ph.D.

Automated Five-part White Blood Cell Differential Counts: Efficiency of Software-generated White Blood Cell Suspect Flags of the Hematology Analyzers Sysmex SE-9000, Sysmex NE-8000, and Coulter STKS

Thalhammer-Scherrer R, Knöbl P, Korninger L, et al (Univ of Vienna)

Arch Pathol Lab Med 121:573–577, 1997 21–5

Background.—With the introduction of newer hematology analyzers, modern hematology laboratories have become largely automated. In the automated 5-part white blood cell (WBC) differential count, cells that cannot be categorized because of abnormal features are signaled by software-generated "suspect flags." Although previous results have documented the good performance of the automated 5-part WBC differential count, studies of the quality of WBC flagging have been less consistent. Three different hematology analyzers were studied to determine the efficiency of software-generated WBC suspect flags.

Methods.—The analyzers compared were the Sysmex SE-9000, the Sysmex NE-8000, and the Coulter STKS. A random sample of 467 blood specimens were tested. The finding of any suspect WBC flag in an automated WBC differential count, reflecting the presence of blasts, myeloid precursor cells, or abnormal lymphocytes, was considered a positive result. For each sample, 400 WBCs were microscopically examined to obtain reference differential counts. Then, using the reference method for comparison, the automated differential counts were classified as true positive, true negative, false positive, or false negative. The analyzers were compared for flagging efficiency, i.e, the percentage of correctly classified subjects.

Results.—For the detection of 1% or more abnormal WBCs, flagging efficiency rates were 78% with the Sysmex SE-9000, 77% with the Sysmex NE-8000, and 72% with the Coulter STKS. Samples with normal WBC counts had the best flagging efficiency rates. All 3 analyzers were most efficient at flagging blast cells.

Conclusions.—The 3 hematology analyzers tested show comparable efficiency in their software-generated WBC suspect flags. However, even when a detection limit of 1 or more % normal WBCs is observed, more than 20% of samples are not correctly flagged. In any patient with a suspected hematologic disorder, a microscopic differential count must be performed, regardless of whether a suspect WBC flag is produced by one of these automated hematology analyzers.

► During the past 3 decades, the sophistication of automated hematology analyzers has grown remarkably. Current instruments are capable of providing more than 3 dozen different measured and calculated parameters of the cellular elements in the blood. In this article, the authors have examined the ability of 3 automated analyzers to detect the presence of abnormal WBCs. The "gold standards" used in this study were a manual differential count done of 400 cells. They defined the level of significance as being greater than 1%.

There are 3 important points about this particular article:

1. It's unfortunate that the authors did not include in the study one of the Bayer instruments, which differentiates cells by a different methodology, using enzymatic staining of the cells; the 3 instruments compared used similar methodologies for the differential counting:
2. Although the 400-cell differential is a useful parameter for finding the 1% threshold of abnormal cells, this number of cells is rarely counted in production in most clinical laboratories. It's unfortunate that information concerning the sensitivity of the 100-cell manual differential was not also included:
3. Despite the two previous mentioned shortcomings, there is important information provided, namely, that in 20% of cases in which abnormal cells were present by the manual differential standard, the instruments failed to flag the abnormality. This information is particularly worrisome. Hospital and commercial laboratories doing high volumes of WBCs with differentials rely upon the instruments to flag cases that are abnormal so that they can be examined by alternate methodology, examination of the blood film in most cases. It is unfortunate that the study did not also include any abnormal flag that could lead to a review of the blood film. This would more closely approximate actual practice. However, the fact that 20% of these cases were never detected is particularly alarming.

This article points out the importance of all laboratories knowing the sensitivity of the particular instrumentation they use as they create criteria for the examination of peripheral blood films.

J.D. Olson, M.D., Ph.D.

Polycythemia Vera: A Retrospective and Reprise

Berlin NI, Wasserman LR (Univ of Miami, Fla; Mount Sinai School of Medicine, New York)

J Lab Clin Med 130:365–373, 1997 21–6

Introduction.—The disease now known as polycythemia vera was first described by Vaquez in 1892. Osler recognized it as a new clinical entity in 1903 and classified polycythemias into 3 groups. A new era in treatment was opened in 1939, when John H. Lawrence used ^{32}P to treat a patient with polycythemia vera. The subsequent history of polycythemia vera can be traced through the development of an algorithm (Fig 1) for evaluating an elevated hematocrit and the development of the first protocol of the Polycythemia Vera Study Group (PVSG). This retrospective analysis described the changing diagnostic methods and treatments of polycythemia vera.

Methods of Diagnosis.—The first procedure in the decision tree is to measure total red cell volume (TRCV) with isotopically labeled red cells. A substantial number of patients with hematocrit values from 50% to

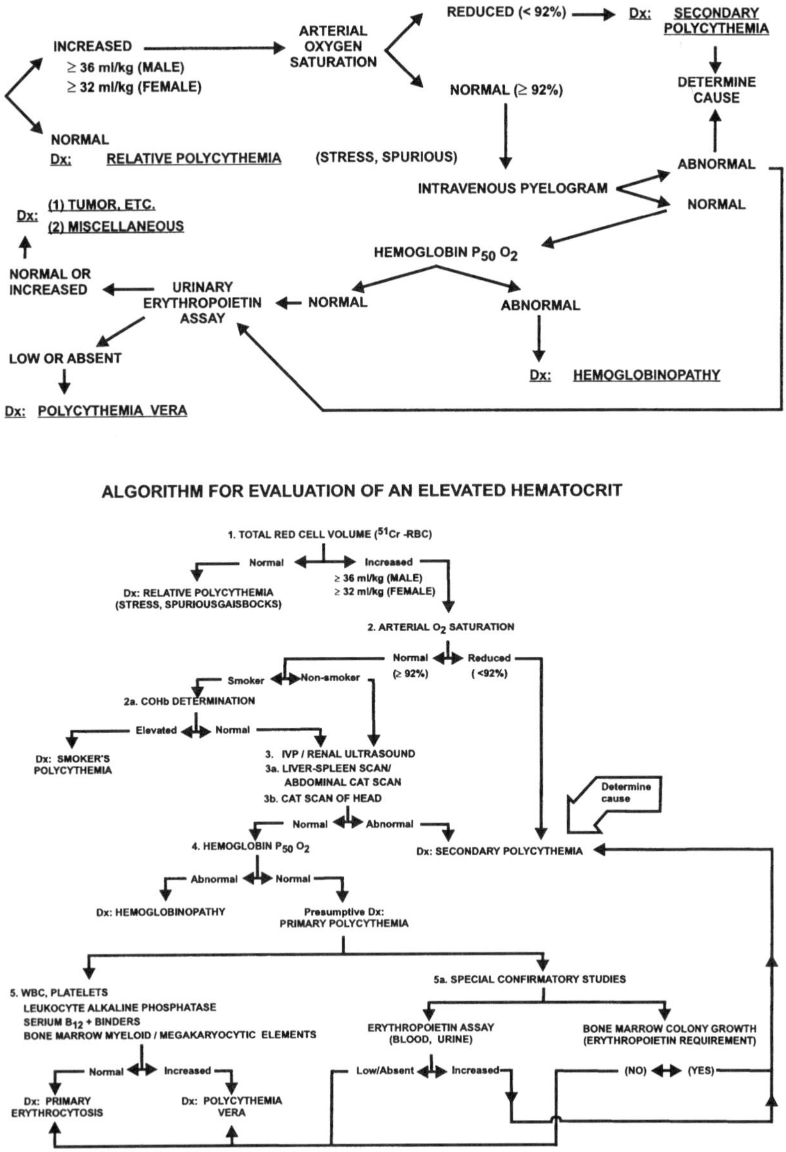

FIGURE 1.—The original and the latest iteration of the Polycythemia Vera Study Group decision tree (algorithm) for the evaluation of an elevated hematocrit. *Abbreviations*: *Dx*, diagnosis; $P_{50}O_2$, partial pressure of oxygen measurement at which hemoglobin is 50% saturated; *RBC*, red blood cell count; *COHb*, carboxyhemoglobin; *WBC*, white blood cell count. (Courtesy of Berlin NI, Wasserman LR: Polycythemia vera: A retrospective and reprise. *J Lab Clin Med* 130:365–373, 1997.)

60% have a normal TRCV. The upper limit of a normal TRCV was selected by the PVSG on the basis of TRCV determinations in large series of normal men and women. Patients with an elevated hematocrit and a normal TRCV are considered to have relative polycythemia; when both measures are elevated, the patient has absolute polycythemia. Reduced blood oxygen saturation indicates that the patient may have secondary polycythemia. "Smokers" polycythemia may be present in patients with increased carboxyhemoglobin.

Treatment.—Three types of treatment are used: repeated phlebotomy, destruction of circulating red cells with a hemolytic agent, and suppression of erythropoiesis with either ionizing radiation or chemotherapeutic drugs that are toxic to the bone marrow. The use of hydroxyurea is coming into question, as is the ability to maintain patients with phlebotomy alone.

Discussion.—Although the PVSG lost support from the National Cancer Institute and no longer exists as an operational group, French and Italian polycythemia study groups remain active and some members of the PVSG continue to explore new treatment approaches. The disease must be considered a chronic disorder; median survival is approximately 10–12 years.

► This paper is an enjoyable review of the history and the evolution of understanding of the disorder known as polycythemia rubra vera. The authors are students of the late John H. Lawrence who, in 1939, first treated a patient with polycythemia vera using radioactive phosphorous. They have, in a brief but concise article, laid out the highlights in the development of our understanding of polycythemia vera through key individuals involved in the early study of the disorder and the formation of the PVSG in 1966.

The PVSG developed diagnostic criteria for polycythemia vera and carried out randomized trials of the available therapies. The group still exists today, receiving data concerning the disorder; however, it does not develop new, prospective clinical protocols. Individual investigators are reporting the use of interferon and anagrelide for treating polycythemia vera. It seems to this reviewer unfortunate that the efforts of the PVSG to organize randomized, controled trials with these newer therapies will not be available.

J.D. Olson, M.D., Ph.D.

Endotoxin as a Factor in Adverse Reactions to Latex Gloves

Williams PB, Halsey JF (IBT Reference Lab)

Ann Allergy Asthma Immunol 79:303–310, 1997 21–7

Introduction.—Endotoxins can cause reactions that include skin rashes, fever, respiratory congestion, asthma, and anaphylactoid shock. Because similar clinical sequelae occur with latex glove use, researchers hypothesized that some of the gloves are contaminated with endotoxin.

Methods.—Extracts prepared from natural latex gloves and synthetic control gloves from different manufacturers were examined for endotoxin content, the distribution and origin of endotoxin, and its association with latex proteins. An Anderson multistage air sampler was used to determine particle size and density associated with the release of endotoxin. Endotoxin was measured by a quantitative kinetic Limulus assay, protein by a modified Lowry assay, and allergen by radioallergosorbent test inhibition.

Results.—The latex gloves varied considerably in their protein content, from below the assay detection limit (less than 25 μg/g) to 1,150 μg/g of glove. In contrast to latex surgical gloves, which had an average protein content of 74.7 μg/g of glove, latex examination gloves had an average protein content of 460 μg/g. Powdered latex gloves and nonpowdered latex gloves also differed considerably in average protein content (444 vs. 47 μg/g of glove). Endotoxin levels ranged from 0.09 ng/g to 2.8 μg/g of glove, and more than 70% of the endotoxin was associated with particles in the less than 7 μm aerodynamic diameter range. Nonsterile examination gloves had the highest levels of endotoxin. There was a tendency for both endotoxin and protein to be found at higher levels in powdered gloves. The rate of endotoxin and allergen release into an aqueous buffer from the latex gloves was quite rapid.

Discussion.—The finding of variable and, at times, very high amounts of endotoxin in natural latex gloves supports the hypothesis that endotoxin is the cause of reactions associated with the gloves. The amounts were greater in powdered gloves than in nonpowdered gloves and in nonsterile examination gloves than in sterile surgical gloves. Release of the endotoxin and protein from the interior of some gloves suggests that contamination occurred during manufacture while the gloves were inside-out on their molds. The contaminants can be removed by washing.

▶ Although precautions have been taken by health care workers for decades to prevent transmission of infection either to themselves or to patients, the practice of universal precautions has recently become the standard of care. This has, of course, created demand for appropriate low-cost disposable gloves that can be used in both the clinical and laboratory setting. Originally, a large proportion of the gloves used were made of latex. Many institutions discovered that both health care workers and patients had hypersensitivity reactions when contacted by the gloves. These reactions are occasionally anaphylactic and fatal.

In an effort to help understand these reactions, these authors have examined natural latex gloves for a variety of potential mediators: endotoxin; protein; allergen. They also examined particle size and density. Their data demonstrate that nonsterile examination gloves are often actually contaminated with significant amounts of endotoxin and protein. The finding lends support to the hypothesis that endotoxin may be a factor in the tissue irritation that occurs in response to these gloves in patients and health care workers and may help to explain the disproportionate severity of the reactions seen. The fact that both protein and endotoxin can be significantly reduced by washing should be a signal to manufacturers to include or increase washing in the production of these gloves.

J.D. Olson, M.D., Ph.D.

Capillary Isoelectric Focusing and High-Performance Cation-Exchange Chromatography Compared for Qualitative and Quantitative Analysis of Hemoglobin Variants

Mario N, Baudin B, Aussel C, et al (Hôpital Saint-Antoine, Paris; UFR Pharmacie Université René Descartes-Paris V)

Clin Chem 43:2137–2142, 1997 21–8

Objective.—Electrophoretic approaches are still widely used for the investigation of hemoglobinopathies, although their use is declining due to various shortcomings. High-performance liquid chromatography (HPLC) is regarded as a sensitive, specific, and reproducible alternative to electrophoresis. Capillary electrophoresis, based on various separation principles including capillary isoelectric focusing (CIEF), has given encouraging results in hemoglobin (Hb) separation. This study compared 2 techniques—a CIEF assay and an HPLC assay—for complete routine Hb analysis.

Methods.—The assays, both developed by the authors, were an HPLC assay on the weak cation-exchanger Poly Cat A and a 2-step CIEF assay on the neutral-coated capillary from Beckman. The 2 techniques were used to analyze adult and neonatal samples sent from the maternity ward for routine Hb analysis.

Results.—The assays required comparable separation times of 20 minutes or less. Both assays provided satisfactory resolution, separating the normal and common abnormal Hbs Hb A, Hb F, HB A_2, Hb S, Hb C, and Hb E. They differed somewhat in the resolution for Hb C-Harlem, Hb D-Punjab, and other uncommon variants. Both assays showed satisfactory reproducibility of retention times, with CVs or 3.3% for HPLC and 4.9% for CIEF. The assays quantified Hb A_2, Hb F, and Hb S with imprecision of less than 5%, although imprecision was greater when the CIEF technique was used to quantify low concentrations of Hb A_2. The 2 assays were highly correlated in the quantitative data obtained for these 3 Hb forms.

Conclusions.—Both HPLC on Poly Cat A columns and CIEF on a neutral capillary are appropriate for routine evaluation of hemoglobinopathies. Either assay can identify and quantify major and minor forms of Hb in small volumes. They can also be used to detect hemoglobinopathies in newborns, such as in screening settings. The 2 assays have many qualities in common although they are based on different separation principles, and could become complementary or competitive in Hb analysis.

▶ Laboratories that deal with the issue of abnormal Hbs on a regular or irregular basis most frequently use electrophoresis on cellulose acetate and citrate auger for identification. Many Hbs, because of their charge characteristics, co-migrate in these media. The consequence is frequent cases in which exact diagnosis is precluded. Isoelectric focusing and ion-exchange chromatography have been used for some time for Hb identification. These authors describe the comparison of a new, capillary isoelectric focusing method to HPLC for the identification of Hb variants. The description of the validation of these methods is vigorous and their conclusion that the two methods are comparable is justified. The capillary isoelectric focusing method offers high resolution and specificity of identification based on the isoelectric point. It shares with HPLC the benefits of direct, online detection, and automation of results. In laboratories where Hb identification is performed with regularity, this new methodology would appear to be an accurate method for Hb identification and quantification. Unfortunately, the authors have not addressed the issue of the costs involved, an extremely important issue in these times of capitated care.

J.D. Olson, M.D., Ph.D.

Application of the 'APT Test' in Prenatal Diagnosis to Evaluate the Fetal Origin of Blood Obtained by Cordocentesis: Results of 30 Pregnancies

Ogur G, Gül D, Özen S, et al (GATA Med Faculty, Ankara, Turkey; GEN-MED Centre for Genetic Diseases and Prenatal Diagnosis, Ankara, Turkey)

Prenat Diagn 17:879–882, 1997 21–9

Introduction.—Several disorders can be diagnosed during the prenatal period by cordocentesis under US guidance. Current methods used to discriminate between maternal and fetal blood require special equipment and experience and are time consuming. A modified version of the hemoglobin alkaline denaturation test (Apt test), reported by Moir and Holbrook in 1993, was evaluated in 30 cases of cytogenetic prenatal diagnosis.

Methods.—After the blood samples were obtained and just before the set-up of cultures for cytogenetic analysis, 0.05 mL of blood was added to 5.0 mL of distilled water plus 1.0 mL of 0.25 sodium hydroxide in a test tube. The mixture was gently agitated for a few seconds. As a control, known adult blood was tested simultaneously for each sample. The persistence of a bright pink color after 60 seconds indicated fetal blood; a change from pink to dark green-brown was accepted as an adult hemoglobin reaction. All 30 pregnancies were followed to delivery.

Results.—Cordocentesis was performed for US abnormalities in 23 cases, for advanced maternal age in 6, and for Rh incompatibility in 1. Two separate samples were withdrawn in 1 case, providing 31 samples for analysis. Twenty-eight samples yielded a fetal hemoglobin reaction, and cytogenetic results correlated well with the gender of the fetus. There was 1 discrepancy in gender of the fetus, the cytogenetic result, and the result of the Apt test. In the case with 2 samples, a male with Down syndrome, the first sample yielded adult hemoglobin reaction and a karyotype of 46,XX; the second ended as fetal blood with a karyotype of 47,XY, +21. A test with mixtures of both fetal and adult blood suggested that mixed samples could also yield a fetal blood reaction.

Discussion.—The modified Apt test is a rapid and inexpensive method of determining the origin of blood samples obtained by cordocentesis. Samples containing a mixture of both fetal and adult blood could yield a fetal hemoglobin reaction. A sample showing strong discoloration in less than 6 minutes may have maternal contamination; in such cases, at least 30 metaphases from different slides should be counted.

► In 1955, a pediatrician named Apt developed a simple and rapid test for the differentiation of adult from fetal hemoglobin. The original test was applied primarily to the study of bloody diarrhea and emesis in newborn infants. The debate, of course, regarded whether the infant had swallowed maternal blood during the delivery or whether gastrointestinal hemorrhage had developed from other pathology. The test is still commonly used by obstetricians and neonatologists for its original purpose.

In the reviewer's experience, it is, when performed at the bedside, frequently used to test inappropriate specimens and can be inappropriately interpreted. As with other laboratory tests, performance by trained personnel using well-controlled reagents and test protocols is of value, even in the most simple test. These authors have described the use of the Apt test in the determination of the fetal or maternal origin of blood obtained at cordocentesis.

It is, of course, important for cytogenetic laboratories to verify the fetal source of specimens submitted for karyotype. The authors have found, in 30 cases, that the Apt test is an excellent method for validating the origin of the specimen.

J.D. Olson, M.D., Ph.D.

Chromosome Aberrations in Atypical Chronic Lymphocytic Leukemia: A Cytogenetic and Interphase Cytogenetic Study

Bigoni R, Cuneo A, Roberti MG, et al (Università di Ferrara, Italy; Thomas Jefferson Univ, Philadelphia)

Leukemia 11:1933–1940, 1997 21–10

Purpose.—Appreciation of the cytologic heterogeneity associated with B cell chronic lymphocytic leukemia (CLL) is growing. This has led to the development of criteria for the related forms of typical CLL and atypical CLL (aCLL). It has been suggested that aCLL may have a relatively more aggressive course; however, its cytogenetic profile is ill defined. This study, using a combination of conventional chromosome analysis and fluorescence in situ hybridization, sought to clarify the chromosomal profile of aCLL.

Methods.—Cytogenetic and interphase cytogenetic studies were performed in 43 patients with aCLL, diagnosed by standard criteria. The investigation used mitogen-stimulated cultures and DNA probes to detect +12 and 13q14 deletions, which are the most common anomalies in CLL.

Results.—All 43 patients had monoclonal CD5/CD19–positive lymphocytosis. Findings included greater than 10% large lymphocytes or prolymphocytes in peripheral blood smears and reactivity with FMC7. Some cases showed bright expression of surface immunoglobulins. Sixty-three percent of patients showed karyotype abnormalities, including +12 in 9 cases, 13q14 aberrations in 5, 11q anomalies in 3, 6q21–q23 abnormalities in 2, and 4q anomalies with different breakpoints in 2. Further chromosome abnormalities were apparent in 4 cases with +12, 3 cases with 13q14 anomalies, 2 cases with 11q anomalies, and 1 case with 6q and 4q anomalies. Three patients had trisomy 12 associated with 13q14 anomalies; 1 of these patients also had an 11q abnormality. One patient had a 13q14 deletion with a 6q anomaly, 1 had an 11q anomaly with 13q− and 7q−, and 1 had a 6q anomaly with 7q− and +12.

The results of interphase cytogenetic studies were comparable to those of chromosome banding analysis. Of 6 patients with an apparently normal or with no mitosis, 4 actually showed concomitant +12 and 13q14 deletion, 1 had isolated +12 deletion, and 1 had isolated 13q14 deletion. Thus, 76% of patients overall had cytogenetic abnormalities. Nineteen patients had +12, 13q14 deletions, 11q, and 6q21–q23 anomalies. This group had a median 2-month interval between diagnosis and treatment, compared with 24 months for 14 patients with a normal karyotype or nonrecurrent chromosomal changes.

Conclusions.—Patients with aCLL appear to have a high incidence of chromosomal abnormalities. Recurrent chromosome changes may be present, involving chromosomes 12, 13q14, 6q21q23, 11q, and possibly, 4q. Sequential chromosomal changes can occur, as evidenced by the finding of complex karyotypes with concomitant 13q, +12, 6q, and 11q. These sequential changes could be the basis of leukemogenesis in patients with aCLL, helping to explain its relatively aggressive clinical course.

► Chromosomal analysis has been a frequently used tool in the identification of clones in primary bone marrow disorders, such as the acute leukemia, myeloproliferative, and dysmyelopoietic syndromes. More recently, the results of chromosomal analysis have been reported in the lymphocytic leukemias. In this study, the authors performed cytogenetic analysis on 43 patients in which more than 10% of cells are enlarged or prolymphocytic in character. Cases of de novo prolymphocytic leukemia were excluded. A substantial percentage, 62.8%, demonstrated karyotypic changes. The authors carefully described a variety of recurrent changes, such as the 12+, 13q14 and 11q anomalies that occurred in more than one patient. In addition, six patients with normal karyotype or no mitosis in fact had concomitant +12 and 13q14 deletion or isolated +12 or 13q14 deletion detected by FISH, resulting in a total of 76% with cytogenetic abnormalities. These abnormalities were associated with aggressive clinical behavior. These findings are important because they document the high frequency of cytogenetic abnormalities in these atypical CLLs and demonstrate the possibility of sequential chromosomal changes, rather than single specific anomalies, that may underlie leukemogenesis in these patients.

J.D. Olson, M.D., Ph.D.

Eosinophilia Detected by Automated Blood Cell Counting in Ambulatory North American Outpatients: Incidence and Clinical Significance

Brigden M, Graydon C (Penticton Regional Hosp, BC)

Arch Pathol Lab Med 121:963–967, 1997 21–11

Introduction.—With current hematologic instruments, including automated 5-part white blood cell differentials, many new cases of eosinophilia—defined as an absolute eosinophil count of greater than 0.7×10^9/L—are being detected. The physician who orders the test is frequently not expecting the finding of eosinophilia, and there is debate as to whether further investigation is warranted. A group of patients with eosinophilia detected on automated blood cell counting, but with an otherwise normal hematologic profile was reviewed.

Methods.—The study included all patients with eosinophilia detected as part of an instrument-generated 5-part white blood cell differential count over a 1-year period. The results of the hematologic profile, including the absolute eosinophil count, were reviewed, along with the probable cause of the eosinophilia. The impact of the eosinophilia on patient management or clinical outcome was evaluated by physician surveys.

Results.—Eosinophilia was detected in 225 of 195,300 patients undergoing a hematology profile, for an overall incidence of 0.1%. In 85% of the cases, eosinophilia was not detected; in 36%, there was no apparent cause for the abnormal finding. For most patients in whom the cause of eosinophilia was known, various allergic diseases were present. Eosinophilia marked parasitemia or a serious systemic condition in fewer than 9% of patients (Table 2). In 69% of the cases, the detection of eosinophilia was followed by additional clinical follow-up. This included further laboratory testing in 59% of the patients, and most commonly a repeat

TABLE 2.—Etiologic Factors Responsible for Eosinophilia

Etiologic Factor	No. of Patients (n = 225)	Percent of Total
Unknown	80	36
Seasonal allergy/allergic rhinitis	66	29
Asthma	31	14
Eczema/dermatitis	21	9
Cancer	7	4
Drug allergy	7	3
Collagen disease	8	3
Parasitic disease	5	2

(Courtesy of Brigden M, Graydon C: Eosinophilia detected by automated blood cell counting in ambulatory North American outpatients: Incidence and clinical significance. *Arch Pathol Lab Med* 121:963–967, 1997.)

TABLE 3.—Physician Follow-up in Patients With Eosinophilia

Follow-up/Action	No. of Patients (n = 225)	Percent of Total
Clinical follow-up		
Repeat office visit	156	69
None	69	31
Laboratory follow-up		
Further laboratory testing	132	59
None	93	41
Individual tests ordered		
Repeat hematologic profile	118	52
Stool examinations for ova and parasites	46	20
Allergic skin testing	14	6
Chest radiograph	11	5
Throat culture	7	3
Urinalysis	5	3

(Courtesy of Brigden M, Graydon C: Eosinophilia detected by automated blood cell counting in ambulatory North American outpatients: Incidence and clinical significance. *Arch Pathol Lab Med* 121:963–967, 1997.)

hematology profile or stool tests for ova or parasites (Table 3). The detection of eosinophilia led to a significant alteration in patient management or outcome in just 2 cases, both involving gold therapy.

Conclusions.—For most outpatients with eosinophilia detected on automated blood cell counting, the abnormality reflects an allergic condition. The finding of eosinophilia per se does not justify extensive further testing, unless indicated by the history and physical examination findings. In most cases, the incidental discovery of eosinophilia does not significantly affect patient management or outcome.

► In this interesting paper, investigators in British Columbia, Canada, have audited, for the finding of eosinophilia, more than 195,000 patients for whom automated blood cell counts were performed. They were able to find 225 cases of absolute eosinophilia (greater than 0.7 × 109/L), a rate of less than 0.1%. The finding was not anticipated in the majority of patients. Of importance, the investigators found that for approximately 70% of these patients there were additional office visits, including laboratory tests performed to pursue the cause of the eosinophilia. The results of these additional studies were largely nonrevealing. In the largest proportion of patients there was no known cause for the eosinophilia, and in fewer than 9% of the patients a cause other than allergy or allergic complications of medication was identified. In only 2% of the patients were parasites identified. The authors' conclusions merit some comment. They state: "An extensive investigation of eosinophilia in ambulatory North American outpatients does not appear to be warranted unless specifically indicated by the results of history and physical examinations." The first comment would be that these findings are valuable, and in the Canadian population and in most of the population of the northern tier of the United States these findings may be generally applicable.

They properly demonstrated that all additional testing should be driven by the history and physical examination findings in these patients. The second comment, however, concerns extension of these findings beyond the populations in the northern reaches in North America. These findings would need to be confirmed in other regions where the prevalence of parasitic infection, and other etiologic factors may be significantly higher such as the southern reaches of the United States as well as, of course, Central America and the tropical regions in the world. Even in North American and European urban centers, where emigration is now common, the prevalence of parasitic infestation could be substantially higher. Similar studies in other regions would certainly be of value.

J.D. Olson, M.D., Ph.D.

Use of Urine Specific Gravity to Improve Screening for Albuminuria

Moore RR, Hirata-Dulas CA, Kasiske BL (Mayo Health System, Eau Claire, Wis; Univ of Minnesota, Minneapolis)

Kidney Int 52:240–243, 1997 21–12

Background.—Screening for albuminuria is a valuable tool for clinicians. Timed urine collections can be difficult to use in outpatient clinics because of the inconvenience, cost, and problems with incomplete collection. Other screening techniques only estimate albumin concentration and can be inaccurate because of differences in urine volume. Urine specific gravity, or relative density, can be easily measured and may be a good alternative to the albumin-to-creatinine ratio.

Methods.—Urine specific gravity, as an alternative to urine creatinine to correct albumin concentration for differences in urine volume was tested in 50 men and women from a nephrology and hypertension clinic.

Results.—Urine specific gravity accurately calculated urine creatinine concentrations. In a random spot urine sample, the albumin estimated-creatinine ratio, as well as the albumin-to-creatinine ratio, were correlated with urine albumin excretion in a 24-hour urine collection. The sensitivity and specificity of the albumin estimated-creatinine ratio for determining microalbuminurina were comparable to those of the albumin-to-creatinine ratio. The sensitivity of the Micral-Test was poor, and improved only slightly after correcting for urine specific gravity.

Conclusion.—These findings suggest that combining urine specific gravity with more precise, rapid techniques of estimating urine albumin concentration might result in more convenient and less expensive methods than the albumin-to-creatinine ratio for screening for albuminuria and microalbuminuria.

▶ The albumin-to-creatinine ratio has been used clinically to evaluate excretion rates for albumin in the urine. Currently available methods must be performed in central laboratories and have the usual difficulties (although minimal) of performing 2 separate evaluations and merging the data. Methods for measuring urinary albumin at the bedside are now evolving, and specific gravity measurement at the point of care is available. These authors have demonstrated a method of using a measurement of urine specific gravity in place of creatinine to extrapolate a urinary albumin creatinine ratio and therefore determine the albumin excretion rate. The data from 50 patients, 31 men and 19 women, (a somewhat limited sample) indicate a good correlation between the laboratory measured urinary creatinine and the urine creatinine histomated from the specific gravity. The authors then use estimated creatinine to create an albumin estimated-creatinine ratio, and correlated that with actual measurements of albumin excretion, compared with the conventional albumin creatinine ratio measurements. The data are convincing. They indicate that the estimation of albumin excretion can be made with enough accuracy for clinical work, using methods that are available at the bedside. The data are likely to be helpful for clinicians managing patients with a real insufficiency.

J.D. Olson, M.D., Ph.D.

Comparative Evaluation of Unfixed and Fixed Human Neutrophils for Determination of Antineutrophil Cytoplasmic Antibodies by Indirect Immunofluorescence

Yang P (Örebro Med Centre Hosp, Sweden)
J Clin Pathol 50:677–680, 1997 21–13

Background.—Patients with vasculitides and ulcerative colitis have antineutrophil cytoplasmic antibodies (ANCAs) in the sera. On indirect immunofluorescence on ethanol fixed neutrophils, these antibodies yield either a cytoplasmic staining pattern (C-ANCA) or a perinuclear staining pattern (P-ANCA).The latter may be an artefact of alcohol fixation. The current study looked for changes in the ANCA staining pattern, using indirect immunofluorescence on unfixed neutrophils or neutrophils fixed by ethanol, acetone, or paraformaldehyde.

Methods.—Serum samples were obtained from 21 patients with ulcerative colitis and 19 healthy participants. Sera were also obtained from 17 patients with vasculitides, including 8 with proteinase 3 positive C-ANCA and 9 with myeloperoxidase positive P-ANCA. Indirect immunofluorescence on unfixed neutrophils or cells fixed by ethanol, acetone, or paraformaldehyde was used to analyze ANCAs.

Findings.—All ulcerative colitis-associated ANCA-positive sera showed a perinuclear staining pattern on unfixed and fixed cells. Acetone and paraformaldehyde fixation reduced the ulcerative colitis P-ANCA titers, and paraformaldehyde fixation reduced myeloperoxidase positive P-ANCA titers. No changes were seen in the staining patterns of the proteinase 3 positive C-ANCA sera, or in 8 of the 9 myeloperoxidase positive P-ANCA sera, whether the cells were fixed or unfixed.

Conclusions.—The fixation method does not affect the ANCA staining patterns. Thus the P-ANCA pattern is apparently not an artefact of alcohol fixation. The antigen of ulcerative colitis-associated P-ANCA is exposed better on ethanol fixed neutrophils than on acetone or paraformaldehyde fixed cells.

► ANCAs are commonly identified in patients with vasculitis and chronic ulcerative colitis. Patterns of staining in direct immunofluorescent tests allow for the ANCA to be classified as C-ANCA or P-ANCA staining. There has been discussion in the literature concerning the optimal target cells for ANCA testing. This author has compared the reactivity of the ANCA in a total of 57 patients, 21 of whom have ultra ulcerative colitis, 17 of whom have vasculitis, and 19 of whom are healthy controls. Antineutrophil cytoplasmic antibody staining was performed, using unfixed cells and cells fixed in ethanol, acetone, or paraformaldahyde. The P- and C-ANCA reactivity were compared. The findings in this study, despite the relatively small number of patients involved, do demonstrate that unfixed cells and ethanol fixed cells perform comparably in the test, and that acetone fixation and paraformaldahyde fixation tend to decrease the sensitivity of the cells to patient antineutrophil cytoplasmic antibodies. This study failed to demonstrate [previously reported false positively that has been attributed to ethanol fixation]. The findings merit further comment. The challenge in performing ANCA tests is to be able to distinguish the various types of reactions and, therefore, the conditions that caused them. No single method can accomplish this; it requires examining cells fixed by more than 1 method, and merging the results. Reactions vary because of both disorder and the fixation method used for the target cells. Therefore, many immunopathologists advocate performance with both ethanol fixed and paraformaldehyde fixed cells to classify the reactions more accurately.

J.D. Olson, M.D., Ph.D.

Case-Control Study of Childhood Acute Lymphoblastic Leukemia and Residential Radon Exposure

Lubin JH, Linet MS, Boice JD Jr, et al (Natl Cancer Inst, Bethesda, Md; Univ of Southern Calif, Los Angeles; US Environmental Protection Agency, Washington, DC; et al)
J Natl Cancer Inst 90:294–300, 1998 21–14

Background.—Mean indoor radon concentrations have been positively associated with risk of leukemia at all ages. The relationship between acute lymphoblastic leukemia (ALL) among children younger than 15 years and indoor radon exposure was further investigated.

Methods.—This case-control study included 505 case patients and 443 control participants. Radon detectors were placed in the current and previous homes in which the children had lived for 6 months or longer. Radon levels could be estimated for 97% of the exposure period (5 years before diagnosis).

Findings.—Mean radon levels were lower for the patients than for members of the control group. Relative risks based on matched case-control pairs were 1.00 for less than 37 Bqm^{-3} of radon exposure, 1.22 for 37–73 Bqm^{-3}, 0.82 for 74–147 Bqm^{-3}, and 1.02 for 148 or more Bqm^{-3}. No association was found between radon exposure and ALL in subgroups defined by age, income, birth order, birth weight, sex, type of residence, magnetic field exposure, parental age at participant's birth, parental occupation, or parental smoking status.

Conclusions.—In contrast to previous ecologic studies, this study found no evidence of a relationship between indoor radon exposure and childhood ALL. This was true in various subgroups as well as in the overall group.

▶ Epidemiologic linkage of radon to malignancy began with studies of mine workers, who had a substantially increased incidence of lung cancer following inhalation of a high cumulative dose of radon. Subsequent epidemiologic studies directed at the risk of the inhalation of residential, low-level radon, have also linked radon to lung cancer, as well as to a number of other adult and childhood malignancies. In contrast to the studies of mine workers, who had been exposed to very high levels, studies of these low-level exposures have not led to convincing evidence of linkage. In addition, the discussion in the press and the scientific literature has led to considerable general concern, and an industry devoted to the measurement of radon in residences. Earlier studies have implied a generalized increased risk of childhood malignancy, including leukemia, with increased residential-level radon exposure.

These investigators have, very usefully, undertaken an age-matched case-control study of childhood ALL in the United States to determine the risk of radon exposure. This study is large, including more than 900 participants (505 cases and 443 age-matched controls). The results failed to demonstrate any relationship between increased radon inhalation and risk of ALL.

The population had a variety of radon concentrations analyzed within subgroups by categories of age, income, birth order, birth weight, sex, type of residence, magnetic field exposure, parental age at participant's birth, parental occupation, and parental smoking habits. None of these subgroups demonstrated increased risk of ALL associated with radon exposure. Similar studies will be useful in other disease categories to help to define more accurately whether there is a radon-related risk for various diseases, and, if so, what the precise magnitude of that risk might be.

J.D. Olson, M.D., Ph.D.

Analysis of Prognostic Factors in Newly Diagnosed Acute Promyelocytic Leukemia Treated With All-*trans* Retinoic Acid and Chemotherapy

Asou N, for the Japan Adult Leukemia Study Group (Kumamoto Univ Hosp, Japan; et al)

J Clin Oncol 16:78–85, 1998 21–15

Background.—All-*trans* retinoic acid (ATRA) has been shown to result in high rates of complete remission (CR) in patients with acute promyelocytic leukemia (APL), a distinctive subtype of acute myeloid leukemia. The efficacy of differentiation therapy with ATRA, followed by intensive chemotherapy, in patients with newly diagnosed APL was tested in the current multicenter trial, and the prognostic factors for CR, event-free survival (EFS), and disease-free survival (DFS) were determined.

Methods.—One hundred ninety-eight patients were enrolled in the trial. All were given ATRA until CR. Those with an initial leukocyte count exceeding 3×10^9/L received doxorubicin and behenoyl cytarabine as well. During treatment, patients with blast and promyelocyte counts exceeding 1×10^9/L were given additional doxorubicin and behenoyl cytarabine. After entering CR, patients were given 3 courses of consolidation and 6 courses of maintenance/intensification chemotherapy.

Findings.—One hundred ninety-six patients were evaluated at the end of the study. Eighty-eight percent had entered CR. In a multivariate analysis, favorable factors for achieving CR were no or minor purpura at diagnosis, and age younger than 30. The predicted 4-year overall survival rate was 74%, and the EFS rate, 54%. The 4-year predicted DFS rate for 173 patients in CR was 62%. Prognostic factors for longer EFS were age younger than 30, and initial leukocyte count of less than 10×10^9/L. Initial leukocyte count of less than 10×10^9/L was the only significant predictor of longer DFS.

Conclusions.—These patients with newly diagnosed APL had a high CR rate and superior survival with ATRA, given alone or combined with chemotherapy, followed by intensive consolidation and maintenance/intensification chemotherapy, when results were compared with those in patients receiving chemotherapy alone. Age, hemorrhagic diathesis, and initial leukocyte count are prognostic indicators in patients given ATRA and intensive chemotherapy.

▶ The diagnosis of acute promyelocytic leukemia requires typical morphologic characteristics of promyelocytes (or microgranular promyelocytes) and the t (15; 17) translocation identified cytogenetically. This is a translocation that fuses the promyelocytic leukemia gene to the retinoic acid receptor a gene. Since the advent of the use of ATRA, there has been considerable improvement in both the induction of remission and long-term survival in patients with promyelocytic leukemia. This article from the Japan Adult Leukemia Study Group evaluates 198 patients with acute promyelocytic leukemia, 196 of whom could be assessed. The authors have performed both a univariate and a multivariate analysis of a variety of potential prognostic factors to determine which factors can predict outcome, induction of remission, overall survival, event-free survival, and disease-free survival. The overall survival of 74% and event-free survival of 54%, with a 4-year predicted disease-free survival of 62%, demonstrates the significant improvement of therapy including ATRA or ATRA followed by chemotherapy. In their studies the authors have found that age younger than 30, the absence of hemorrhagic diathesis as evidenced by the absence of purpura at the time of diagnosis, and initial leukocyte count less than 10 × 109 L are all favorable prognostic factors. These findings are particularly useful not only in determining prognosis for individual patients but also in the continued design of studies, partitioning patients with less favorable prognostic factors for alternative, therapeutic approaches.

J.D. Olson, M.D., Ph.D.

22 Molecular Pathology

Parity Among the Randomly Amplified Polymorphic DNA Method, Multilocus Enzyme Electrophoresis, and Southern Blot Hybridization With the Moderately Repetitive DNA Probe Ca3 for Fingerprinting *Candida albicans*

Pujol C, Joly S, Lockhart SR, et al (Univ of Iowa, Iowa City; Laboratoire de Génétique Moléculaire des Parasites et des Vecteurs, Montpellier, France)

J Clin Microbiol 35:2348–2358, 1997 22–1

Background.—*Candida albicans* is the most common fungal pathogen. Of the different methods that have been used to measure the genetic distances between strains, Southern blot hybridization with the probe Ca3, randomly amplified polymorphic DNA (RAPD) analysis, and multilocus enzyme electrophoresis (MLEE) appear to be especially effective. These 3 methods were compared for their ability to identify related isolates, to cluster weakly related isolates, to distinguish unrelated isolates, and to evaluate microevolution within a strain.

Methods.—Twenty-nine American *C. albicans* isolates were assessed by RAPD analysis, MLEE, and DNA fingerprinting with midrepetitive species-specific probes, Ca3 and CARE2. Similarity coefficients were calculated.

Results.—There was strong concordance of the results from RAPD analysis, MLEE, and Southern blot hybridization with probe Ca3 and weaker concordance of the results with those from Southern blot hybridization with probe CARE2. All methods could resolve microevolution within a strain. The Ca3 probe method had the greatest resolving power. Clustering capability was also demonstrated by all methods. Both RAPD analysis and MLEE provide evidence for linkage disequilibrium and a clonal population structure.

Conclusions.—These results demonstrate that RAPD analysis, MLEE, and Southern blot hybridization with midrepetitive probes are all effective methods for the analysis of genetic relatedness of *C. albicans*. The RAPD method was quickest, but least reproducible; MLEE was reproducible, but time-consuming. Southern hybridization was reproducible and fast, and the Ca3 probe was the best for analyzing microevolution within a strain. Southern blot hybridization with the midrepetitive probe Ca3 appears to be the best all around analytic tool for epidemiologic studies of *C. albicans*.

► Fungal infections, especially those attributable to *C. albicans*, are assuming a prominent role in modern medicine. For this reason, there is an acute need for better understanding of the epidemiology and pathogenesis of candidiasis. These studies are facilitated by the use of DNA fingerprinting methods that can be used to identify and monitor specific strains and assess the genetic relatedness of strains. Several methods have been used to fingerprint *C. albicans*, including electrophoretic karyotyping, restriction fragment length polymorphism (RFLP) analysis, Southern blot hybridization with a variety of moderately repetitive DNA probes, and multilocus enzyme electrophoresis. An effective fingerprinting method must (1) discriminate between unrelated strains; (2) identify the same strain or highly related strains in independent isolates; (3) generate a pattern that is complex enough to provide a quantitative measure of genetic relatedness between 2 isolates; (4) generate a pattern amenable to automatic computer-assisted analysis; (5) be highly reproducible within a laboratory and between laboratories; (6) be verified by an independent method of measuring genetic distance (i.e., an unrelated fingerprinting method); and (7) reveal microevolutionary changes between isolates in an infecting population. Unfortunately, the vast majority of studies of *Candida* epidemiology do not utilize fingerprinting methods that have been characterized for their level of discrimination and the methods have not been verified by other unrelated methods for their capacity to measure genetic distance between independent isolates.

Pujol and colleagues present an elegant analysis of 4 DNA fingerprinting methods for *C. albicans*. They show strong concordance of the results for RAPD analysis, MLEE, and Southern blot hybridization with Ca3 and weaker concordance with these 3 methods and Southern blot hybridization with CARE2. They also demonstrate the ability of all 4 methods to resolve microevolution within a strain. With this validation, DNA fingerprinting with Ca3 encompasses all of the characteristics of an effective fingerprinting method as outlined above. This method is highly reproducible, relatively fast, and is an excellent indicator of microevolution. It is highly amenable to computer-assisted analysis. Application of DNA fingerprinting with Ca3 will prove to be a powerful tool to improve our understanding of *C. albicans* epidemiology and pathogenesis.

M.A. Pfaller, M.D.

Molecular Evidence and Clinical Significance of Herpesvirus Coinfection in the Central Nervous System

Tang Y-W, Espy MJ, Persing DH, et al (Mayo Clinic, Rochester, Minn)
J Clin Microbiol 35:2869–2872, 1997 22–2

Introduction.—Although herpesviruses are an important cause of CNS infections, conventional laboratory diagnosis of CNS infections caused by these viruses is not always successful. Previous reports suggest that polymerase chain reaction (PCR) may be the new standard for the diagnosis of herpes simplex virus (HSV) in patients with CNS disease. Using PCR, 60 CSF specimens from patients with symptoms of viral CNS disease were examined for 5 herpesviruses and 2 bacterial pathogens. The specimens were previously determined to be positive or negative for HSV DNA.

Methods.—Sixty CSF specimens were HSV DNA positive; patients had a mean age of 44.1 years and a male-female ratio of 3:7. The 30 control samples were HSV DNA negative and were matched for age and gender to HSV DNA–positive specimens. All specimens were tested by PCR for DNA specific for cytomegalovirus (CMV), Epstein-Barr virus (EBV), varicella-zoster virus (VZV), human herpesvirus 6 (HHV-6), *Borrelia burgdorferi,* and *Tropheryma whippelii.*

Results.—Among the 30 HSV-positive CSF samples, 2 were also positive for HHV-6 DNA and 1 was positive for EBV by PCR. One of the 30 HSV DNA-negative samples was positive for EBV. None of the CSF specimens tested positive by PCR for CMV, VZV, *B. burgdorferi,* or *T. whippelii.* In the 3 specimens positive for more than 1 herpesvirus, amplicons generated with virus-specific primer sets hybridized specifically to the corresponding virus-specific probe. Eight of the 30 patients who had HSV DNA detected in the CSF had a clinical diagnosis of meningitis; all recovered fully. Twenty-two patients were treated with acyclovir after receiving a clinical diagnosis of viral encephalitis. Of the 19 patients with only HSV DNA in CSF, 1 died, 12 recovered partially, and 6 recovered fully. Two patients with HSV and HHV-6 died. The HSV-negative control patient with EBV had an underlying T-cell lymphoma. Other diagnoses in the HSV-negative group were noninfectious CNS disease, autoimmune diseases, aseptic meningitis, and meningoencephalitis. No control patient died.

Discussion.—The laboratory diagnosis of CNS infections can be achieved by PCR detection of viral nucleic acid targets. Whereas target genes of organisms responsible for CNS infections are usually present in the acute phase of the disease, CSF samples from patients without an infectious cause do not contain the signature nucleic acid sequences.

► Herpesvirus is an important cause of CNS infection. These viruses include HSV type 1, HSV type 2, EBV, VZV, CMV, and HHV-6, -7, and -8. Conventional methods such as culture and serology have proven to be inadequate for the diagnosis of CNS infections caused by these viruses.

Detection of viral DNA in CSF by PCR has brought a new dimension to the laboratory diagnosis of viral CNS infections. It is now clear that the diagnosis of CNS infection caused by HSV is markedly improved by PCR, allowing the administration of specific antiviral therapy early in the course of the disease. The availability of specific primers and probes for other herpesviruses makes it possible to test for coinfection in patients suspected of HSV encephalitis.

In the study abstracted here, the authors used PCR to examine CSF from 60 patients with symptoms suggestive of viral encephalitis for the presence of HSV, HHV-6, EBV, CMV, VZV, *B. burgdorferi,* and *T. whippelii* DNA. They found coinfection with HSV and HHV-6 in 2 patients and HSV and EBV in 1 patient. Two of these 3 patients died, suggesting that coinfection may influence the disease course adversely.

The diagnosis of viral coinfection is considered rare but, until now, has been limited by highly insensitive conventional methods. Molecular methods for viral diagnosis provide rapid, sensitive, and specific testing capabilities and allow for prompt confirmation of viral CNS disease. This is certainly an advantage with HSV infection. Detection of other herpesviruses may be important for prognosis and in directing the medical management of such patients. Further study is required.

M.A. Pfaller, M.D.

A Comparative Analysis of FISH, RT-PCR, and Cytogenetics for the Diagnosis of *bcr-abl*–Positive Leukemias

Cox MC, Maffei L, Buffolino S, et al (Univ of "Tor Vergata," Rome; Univ of "La Sapienza," Rome)

Am J Clin Pathol 109:24–31, 1998 22–3

Background.—The prognosis associated with Philadelphia (Ph) chromosome-positive leukemias with the *bcr-abl* gene translocation is dismal. Identifying Ph-positive patients is essential, because only aggressive treatments, such as allogeneic bone marrow transplantation, permit long-term, disease-free survival. The current study compared the efficacy of fluorescence in situ hybridization (FISH), reverse transcriptase-polymerase chain reaction (RT-PCR) analysis, and cytogenetics in the diagnosis of *bcr-abl* translocation–positive leukemias.

Methods and Findings.—Seventy-five patients with leukemia or other myeloproliferative syndromes were tested. The FISH technique was done with BCR and ABL double-color probes. The sensitivities of RT-PCR and FISH in identifying Ph-positive patients were 100% and 97%, respectively. A Ph-positive case that was fusion-negative by RT-PCR was identified as positive by FISH. Five percent of RT-PCR results were false positive (Table 2).

Conclusions.—The FISH technique is a simple, reliable method for diagnosing *bcr-abl*-positive leukemias, detecting *bcr-abl* fusion in the pres-

TABLE 2.—Comparison of Cytogenetic, RT-PCR, and FISH Results

	FISH		RT-PCR		Ph	
Results	Positive	Negative	Positive	Negative	Positive	Negative
Ph positive (n = 34)	34	0	33	1	—	—
FISH positive (n = 38)	—	—	37	1	34	3*
RT-PCR positive (n = 37)	37	0	—	—	34	2*

*Not determined in 1 case.

Abbreviations: RT-PCR, reverse transcriptase-polymerase chain reaction; *FISH,* fluorescence in situ hybridization; *Ph,* Philadelphia.

(Courtesy of Cox MC, Maffei L, Buffolino S, et al: A comparative analysis of FISH, RT-PCR, and cytogenetics for the diagnosis of *bcr-abl*–positive leukemias. *Am J Clin Pathol* 109:24–31.

ence of all types of molecular junctions. It can be used alone or to validate RT-PCR results.

► The treatment of chronic myelogenous leukemia, particularly in younger patients, commonly includes bone marrow transplantation. During recovery and remission following bone marrow transplantation, it is common practice to analyze specimens for the presence of the chromosome and the *bcr-abl* gene translocation. Methods have included classical cytogenetics looking for the Ph chromosome, southern blot analysis, RT-PCR, and FISH. These authors prospectively performed cytogenetic, RT-PCR, and FISH analyses on 75 patients with leukemia and other myeloproliferative syndromes to evaluate the relative sensitivity and specificity of the methods. The authors found that FISH's sensitivity and specificity are equal to and may exceed those of RT-PCR. Both RT-PCR and FISH are more sensitive than cytogenetics alone, a phenomenon which has been previously described. The authors have concluded, and their data support, the contention that the use of PCR methods alone continues to have the problem of cross-contamination, and that the use of FISH for the identification of the *bcr-abl* gene translocation is equally and possibly more effective in the clinical setting.

J.D. Olson, M.D., Ph.D.

Panfungal PCR Assay for Detection of Fungal Infection in Human Blood Specimens

Van Burik J-A, Myerson D, Schreckhise RW, et al (Fred Hutchinson Cancer Research Ctr, Seattle; Univ of Washington, Seattle)

J Clin Microbiol 36:1169–1175, 1998 22–4

Background.—A polymerase chain reaction (PCR) assay for detecting fungal nucleic acids may be the best approach for diagnosing fungal infections. Such an approach has the potential for being more sensitive than current culture-based methods, for encompassing multiple fungal genera, and for being applicable to a variety of specimen types. In the current study, a novel panfungal PCR assay that detects the small-subunit rRNA gene sequence of the 2 major fungal organism groups was used to assess whole-blood specimens from a series of blood or bone marrow transplant recipients.

Methods and Findings.—The 580–bp PCR product was detected after panfungal primer amplification and hybridization to a 245–bp digoxigenin-labeled probe. The assay's lower limit of detection was about 4 organisms per milliliter of blood. Findings of the PCR were negative in multiple whole-blood specimens obtained from 5 patients without fungal infection or colonization. The findings were positive in specimens from 11 infected patients and from 3 patients with pulmonary aspergillosis. In 1 patient, blood drawn the week before infection was diagnosed by bronchoalveolar lavage fluid culture was positive by PCR. Blood specimens obtained from 2 patients 1–2 days after lung biopsy and which were sterile by culture, were positive by PCR. Positive PCR signals were also found in the blood of 4 patients with candidemia, 3 with mixed fungal infections, and 1 with fusariosis.

Conclusions.—The panfungal PCR assay is able to detect multiple fungal genera. It may serve as an adjunct to conventional techniques for detecting fungal infection or for describing the natural history of fungal infection. Additional research is needed to define the sensitivity and specificity of this assay for diagnosing fungal infection before the existence of other clinical or laboratory indications.

▶ The early diagnosis of invasive fungal infection is considered essential to optimal therapy in severely immunocompromised patients. Unfortunately, culture is often negative or too slow to be of use in directing therapy. Histopathology is clearly more rapid and definitive but is often negative or not obtainable because of the condition of the patient. Molecular detection of circulating nucleic acids, using amplification-based methods such as PCR, has proved useful in many infectious processes, including fungal infections. In this study, the authors describe the use of a novel panfungal PCR assay which detects the small-subunit rRNA gene sequences of *Candida* and *Aspergillus* species. The authors applied this technology to whole-blood specimens obtained from bone marrow transplant patients with and without invasive fungal infections. The panfungal PCR assay appeared capable of detecting multiple fungal genera, and, although not superior to more conventional forms of diagnosis, appeared to be useful as an adjunctive method for diagnosis of invasive fungal infection. This conclusion is similar to that of previous studies indicating that a combination of antigen detection, PCR, culture, and histopathology provided better diagnostic yield than any individual approach. This makes sense, given the highly complex nature of invasive fungal infection in severely immunocompromised patients. This article shows that yet another amplification-based method can provide additional and useful diagnostic information. Further studies of sensitivity, specificity, and early diagnostic capabilities are warranted.

M.A. Pfaller, M.D.

Computerized Analysis of Restriction Fragment Length Polymorphism Patterns: Comparative Evaluation of Two Commercial Software Packages

Gerner-Smidt P, Graves LM, Hunter S, et al (Statens Seruminstitut, Copenhagen; Ctrs for Disease Control and Prevention, Atlanta, Ga)

J Clin Microbiol 36:1318–1323, 1998 22–5

Background.—Electrophoresis-based fingerprinting techniques are commonly used for the epidemiologic typing of bacteria and fungi. The development of computer-based pattern analysis has enabled a comparison of a large number of patterns generated in the same or different laboratories. Two computerized restriction fragment length polymorphism pattern analysis systems, the GelCompar and the BioImage systems, were compared in the current study to determine whether their results are similar.

Methods.—These systems differ in their approaches to comparing patterns from various gels. GelCompar uses a standard reference pattern in 1 gel to normalize subsequent gels containing lanes with the same reference pattern, whereas, in the BioImage system the fragments' molecular sizes are determined from size standards in each gel.

Findings.—The molecular size estimates for 12 restriction fragments of phage λ ranged from 97% to 101% of their actual sizes, with a standard deviation of less than 1% of the mean estimated size for most fragments. At the window sizes used for analysis, the GelCompar system was somewhat better than BioImage at identifying visually identical patterns produced by electrophoretic separation of *Hha*I-restricted DNA of *Listeria monocytogenes.* With both systems, the user must also make critical decisions in the analysis. The user must visually confirm that the systems are finding all bands in each lane and that there are no artifacts. Manual editing can be done in both systems. The user must verify results obtained in pattern matching or clustering parts of the analysis.

Conclusions.—Two commercial software packages for analysis of restriction fragment length polymorphism patterns were evaluated. In both programs, the molecular size estimates for most test fragments were within 98% of their actual size. Additional features, such as statistical, combining, printing, exporting, and program linkage capabilities, may also be important to consider when purchasing such a program.

▶ Analysis of restriction fragment length polymorphism (RFLP) patterns is a necessary aspect of many approaches to molecular diagnostics and molecular epidemiology. Comparison of similarities and differences among patterns may be done manually if only a few samples are to be analyzed. Comparison of patterns obtained from a large number of samples run on different gels may become quite difficult, and usually requires some degree of computer-assisted analysis. Several software packages designed to aid in analysis of RFLP patterns are now available. These packages generally allow one to build databases of RFLP patterns and to perform identity searches and comparisons of new patterns with those already stored in the database. In this study, 2 such software packages, GelCompar and BioImage, are compared for their ability to analyze RFLP patterns obtained from isolates of *L. monocytogenes.* Both systems proved to be quite useful as aids in comparing these complex profiles. The GelCompar System performed slightly better than the BioImage System in finding identical profiles within the collection; however, the BioImage System was easier to use. It is important for the prospective user of any of these systems to realize that they all have limitations and require considerable input by the user to ensure accurate analysis of RFLP patterns. Both of these systems require the user to make critical decisions regarding band finding and comparison. Manual editing is almost always required, and the user should visually verify that the systems are finding all of the bands. User verification of the results obtained in pattern matching or clustering portions of the analysis is also required. Although these systems are far from being foolproof, they are a significant advance, and are essential for analysis of large numbers of patterns.

M.A. Pfaller, M.D.

23 Laboratory Management

Errors, Mistakes, Blunders, Outliers, or Unacceptable Results: How Many?

Witte DL, VanNess SA, Angstadt DS, et al (Lab Control Ltd, Ottumwa, Iowa; Univ of Iowa, Iowa City)

Clin Chem 43:1352–1356, 1997 23–1

Background.—Managing quality is a primary goal of any clinical chemistry laboratory, but little has been published on the frequency of unacceptable results. A review of discrepant analytic results from multiple prospective method evaluation studies is presented.

Study Design.—The methods comparison studies included in this survey involved mature systems with well-characterized reagents that were completed between March 1977 and September 1995 in 5 locations. These studies included at least 14 operators and 16 analyzers. Each result had at least 2 associated results with which it could be compared, including replicate sample analysis results, comparison method results or quality-control specimen results. Results suggesting internal instrument problems or sample mix-ups were not included in this analysis.

Findings.—Of 219,353 separate analyses, 98 were greater than 7 standard deviations from the expected value. Of these 98 outliers, 43 were controls and 55 were samples. Although no patient harm occurred, 9 results had the potential to cause errors in patient management.

Conclusions.—These data demonstrate that significant analytic errors that contribute to patient management errors are rare, but that improvement is possible.

► Many studies have shown that the majority of laboratory errors occur in the preanalytic or postanalytic portions of the process. In spite of this, most of the effort and financial resources for quality assurance of laboratories are directed toward the analytic portion of the process. This is probably because it is the only part of the process that is completely under laboratory control and is subject to government and other regulation.

By reviewing more than 200,000 clinical chemistry results that were used for methods comparison studies, the authors were able to identify the number of results that differed by more than 7 standard deviations. This translated to an error rate of 447 parts per million. The authors also reviewed the clinical relevance of these errors and concluded that few would have had a detrimental effect on the patient. They also discuss what an acceptable error rate may be. Although vigilance of the analytic process is necessary and there is always room for improvement, it is obvious that emphasis on improving the preanalytic and postanalytic processes may reap greater rewards.

R. Feld, Ph.D.

How Fast Is Fast Enough for Clinical Laboratory Turnaround Time? Measurement of the Interval Between Result Entry and Inquiries for Reports

Winkelman JW, Tanasijevic MJ, Wybenga DR, et al (Brigham and Women's Hosp, Boston)

Am J Clin Pathol 108:400–405, 1997 23–2

Background.—The value of clinical laboratory test results is strongly dependent on the timeliness of delivery. At the Brigham and Women's Hospital, the Hospital Information System (HIS) permits measurement of the time between test completion and result inquiry by the requesting clinician. Report inquiry behavior for the complete blood cell count (CBC), as a surrogate for frequently requested tests, was evaluated.

Study Design.—All CBC were performed with an automated analyzer linked to the HIS, so that results were downloaded as soon as available. This study included all 10,569 CBC results requested by clinical services from October 1 to October 13, 1995. The report inquiry was defined as the first time the end-user accessed result look-up options on the HIS. The data were stratified into routine or stat reports and further divided into inpatient and outpatient reports.

Findings.—The median time to report inquiry was 90 minutes for routine inpatient tests, 35 minutes for stat inpatient tests, and 30 minutes for stat outpatient tests. Most reports were requested within 4 hours of entry of the results into the HIS. Of the routine outpatient test reports, 31% were requested within 8 hours.

Conclusions.—The majority of inpatient routine and stat test results, outpatient stat test results, and many outpatient routine test results, are required rapidly after sample submission to the laboratory. These tests cannot be moved off site without compromising current standards of medical practice.

▶ Few subjects provoke as much discussion between laboratorians and clinicians as the turnaround time of laboratory results. The event that triggers the stopwatch to start is viewed differently by these 2 groups. Clinicians tend to use the time when the sample is drawn or when they give the order to get the test, whereas laboratorians tend to start the clock when the sample arrives at the laboratory. When physicians are polled about desired turnaround times, they inevitably respond with times that are frequently unattainable by centralized laboratories. This is 1 reason given for the growing popularity of bedside or point-of-care testing, which of course bypasses the transportation and reporting part of the analytic cycle.

These authors used the CBC as a model test to see if physicians accessed the data in a timely manner. The turnaround time from the laboratory for the CBC was excellent, ranging from 23–28 minutes for a stat order to 30–44 minutes for a routine order. The authors then monitored the interval between the time the result was available on the computer system to the time of physician look-up on the system. For inpatients, median time to report inquiry was 90 minutes for routine tests and 35 minutes for stat tests. For outpatients, the stat orders had median times similar to inpatients, but routine orders had a much longer time to inquiry. The authors use these data to justify keeping laboratory services on-site to provide the reporting time needed by physicians. The larger question left unanswered was would patient care suffer if reporting times were lengthened, either by reducing staff in the laboratory or sending analyses off-site.

R. Feld, Ph.D.

An Erbium: YAG Laser to Obtain Capillary Blood Samples Without a Needle for Point-of-Care Laboratory Testing

Fonseca V, Hinson J, Pappas A, et al (Univ of Arkansas for Med Sciences, Little Rock)

Arch Pathol Lab Med 121:685–688, 1997 23–3

Background.—Transmission of infectious disease via needlestick injuries represents a considerable occupational hazard to health care workers. Although education and safer needle and lancet devices have decreased the incidence of needlestick injuries, the possibility has not been eliminated, and increasing point-of-care testing will likely increase the use of lancet devices and the resulting risk of disease transmission. A technique of capillary blood collection using a portable pulsed erbium:yttrium-aluminum-garnet (Er:YAG) laser was described, and the effect of the Er:YAG laser on the properties of the collected blood was evaluated.

Methods.—Capillary blood was collected from the fingertips of 100 patients with diabetes mellitus, at a single hospital, by either a Er:YAG laser alone or a conventional lancet with a second sample taken by laser. Blood was analyzed for blood glucose, carbon dioxide, sodium, potassium, urea nitrogen and glycosylated hemoglobin concentrations.

Results.—Blood was successfully collected in 98% of participants using either technique. Greater blood flow was obtained using the laser than the lancet. For the first 60 patients, significantly greater immediate pain was reported for the laser than the lancet. After modification of the laser tip to lower the energy output for the final 40 patients, however, pain scores for the 2 techniques did not differ. Phlebotomists preferred the Er:YAG laser to the conventional lancet, probably because of the greater blood flow attained. The plasma potassium concentration was significantly higher in blood collected with the laser than with the lancet, at 5.3 and 4.5 mEq/L, respectively, probably as a result of hemolysis. No other blood parameters differed between the 2 techniques.

Conclusion.—The Er:YAG laser is a safe alternate to the lancet for collecting capillary blood. It is hoped that lasers causing less hemolysis and pain will be developed through further research. The occupational hazard posed by needlestick injuries may ultimately be eliminated through laser use in blood collection. A reduction in biologically hazardous waste is a secondary advantage of this technique.

▶ The increase in point-of-care testing has also led to an increase in the number of capillary blood samples that must be obtained from patients. The usual method for obtaining capillary blood involves the use of a lancet. As with any sharp object used to obtain blood, the risk of disease transmission is always present. The spring-action lancet has been responsible for the transmission of hepatitis because the stage that rests on the finger was not changed between patients.

The laser technique uses a pulsed infrared laser to puncture the skin and produce a sample. In this study, blood flow was greater with the laser compared with the lancet and was, therefore, preferred by phlebotomists. After modification of the energy output of the laser, patients had no preference between the laser and the lancet with respect to pain. There was an increase in hemolysis with the laser, as judged by an increase in potassium values, vs. the lancet. Serum hemoglobin values were, unfortunately, not measured. The increased tendency of the laser to produce hemolysis could limit its usefulness.

Cost is always an issue in today's environment. I was told at the booth at the American Association for Clinical Chemistry meeting that the laser costs about 40¢ per use. This is more expensive than the lancet, but that fact must be weighed against the advantages of increased safety and less biological waste.

R. Feld, Ph.D.

Implementation of a Successful On-Call System in Clinical Chemistry

Hobbs GA, Jortani SA, Valdes R Jr (Univ of Louisville, Ky)

Am J Clin Pathol 108:556–563, 1997 23–4

Introduction.—The successful clinical pathologist must make a broad range of laboratory, clinical, and managerial decisions. The best way to learn these decision-making skills is by a service-oriented, on-call approach. An on-call beeper system is used in a postdoctoral training program in clinical chemistry with the goals of educating trainees, providing clinicians with consultations to help solve laboratory-related problems, and enhancing laboratory quality assurance. The implementation and growth of this beeper on-call system were reviewed.

Beeper On-call Program.—The system follows a laboratory-initiated approach to linking laboratory results to patient care. A digital pager and cellular phone are issued to the clinical chemistry fellow or pathology resident on call. Beeper calls are activated by specified extreme values measured, unusual situations that cannot be managed by the technologist or supervisor, and consultation requests by medical staff. All beeper calls are recorded, and selected calls are discussed in weekly on-call report sessions. A written report is made using a specified form, which is reviewed by the faculty. The system is operative 24 hr/day 7 days/week, thus covering all laboratory shifts.

Findings.—Over a 5-year period, the number of weekly beeper calls increased to between 8 and 20 per week. Sixty-three percent of responses were clinical in nature, 42% were analytical, 13% were consultations, and 12% each were administrative or quality assurance-related. As illustrated by case reports, individual calls fell into multiple categories. Contact with clinicians was required in nearly one fourth of the calls. The on-call report sessions were useful in teaching the investigative skills needed by an effective laboratory director. For medical staff, the systems helped to establish the laboratory as an integral part of patient care.

Conclusions.—An on-call service in the clinical chemistry laboratory can enhance education, improve clinical services, and increase laboratory efficiency. It exposes residents and fellows to opportunities to sharpen their skills in solving real-world problems. Although calls initiated by laboratory personnel are the mainstay of the system, there are a growing number of direct or consultation-type calls. This experience may be useful to other institutions wishing to implement on-call systems.

▶ Many clinicians view the laboratory as a source of numbers, only occasionally turning to the pathologists, clinical chemists, or microbiologists for knowledge and helpful information. The laboratory enables this perception by transmitting most of the results electronically, as numbers with reference ranges. A large number of clinicians never use a more sophisticated laboratory interpretive model than "normal" or "abnormal."

Valdes started a Clinical Chemistry consult service at Kentucky when he arrived in 1990. What is unique about this service is its proactive nature. It is the postdoctoral fellow or resident that initiates the interaction with the clinician. Trigger points for a call are critical values, an unusual situation, or consults by medical staff. This system has received acceptance by the clinical staff as judged by the increase in calls. Interesting cases are shared in weekly report sessions so that learning is disseminated. The authors describe several cases where the laboratory-initiated consult led to benefit for the patient and education for both the clinician and laboratory. The laboratory must be proactive in initiating consults with clinicians if it is to be recognized by the medical staff as more than a number generator.

R. Feld, Ph.D.

Mistakes in a Stat Laboratory: Types and Frequency

Plebani M, Carraro P (Azienda Ospedaliera di Padova, Italy)

Clin Chem 43:1348–1351, 1997 23–5

Introduction.—The goal of total quality management in laboratory medicine is to reduce or eliminate mistakes in the total process, including preanalytical and postanalytical phases. A mistake can occur anywhere along the way, from test ordering to test reporting. The frequency and types of mistakes made in the Stat Service of a teaching hospital laboratory service were analyzed.

Methods.—Stat laboratory tests performed for 4 departments—internal medicine, nephrology, surgery, and ICU—were closely monitored for 3 months. A mistake was defined as any defect throughout the testing process that had any effect on the quality of the laboratory service.

Results.—The total number of analyses was 40,490. Of those, 359 were cited as questionable and 189 confirmed as mistakes. The relative frequency of mistakes was 0.47%, higher in the department of internal medicine. Sixty-eight percent of the mistakes took place in the preanalytical phase, 13% in the analytical phase, and 19% in the postanalytical phase. The most common type of mistake in the preanalytical phase was inaccurate procedures for sample collection. Although three fourths of the mistakes did not affect patient outcome, 19% led to additional, inappropriate laboratory tests. In 6% of cases, the mistake led to inappropriate care or inappropriate modification of care.

Conclusions.—Although the frequency of mistakes in a stat laboratory service is low, this is subject to underestimation and may vary from center to center and from time to time. Laboratory quality control efforts must include the preanalytical and postanalytical phases, as well as the analytical phase itself.

▶ Tremendous time and money is spent in laboratory medicine controlling the analytical process. The Clinical Laboratory Improvement Act (CLIA) specifically targets this portion of the laboratory process with mandated proficiency testing. However, numerous studies have demonstrated that most laboratory "errors" occur in the preanalytical phase of laboratory testing.

This study was conducted by 4 clinical areas using data generated by a stat laboratory. Questionable laboratory results were noted by the clinical staff and were then reviewed by the laboratory. Once again the preanalytical and postanalytical phases of the laboratory process accounted for the majority of the errors detected. Most of the preanalytical problems were accounted for by errors in patient identification and sample procurement.

The preanalytical phase is frequently not under total laboratory control as compared to the analytical phase. This makes error detection and, more important, process improvement more difficult. Phlebotomy service that is offered 24 hours a day is expensive and is likely to be closely scrutinized by hospital administrators when money must be conserved. True quality assurance involves all phases of the laboratory process and a cooperative effort between the patient care staff and the laboratory could eliminate many of the laboratory errors attributable to the preanalytical phase.

R. Feld, Ph.D.

Quality Assessment of Blood Glucose Testing in General Practitioners' Offices Improves Quality

Stahl M, Brandslund I, Iversen S, et al (Vejle County Central Hosp, Denmark; Fredericia Hosp, Denmark)

Clin Chem 43:1926–1931, 1997 23–6

Background.—Blood glucose is frequently measured in the offices of Danish general practitioners. The average number of blood glucose measurements performed each year by each general practice office is 350. In Denmark, there are no recommendations for quality control of blood glucose analysis or for relevant use of such analysis. A new quality assurance system was designed to assess the quality of glucose measurements in general practice, as well as the results of the new quality control program.

Methods.—Fresh, unstabilized samples of whole blood were analyzed by office methods and a hospital laboratory comparison technique. This quality assurance system was used in 98 offices of 171 general practitioners for 5 years.

Results.—Initial results in 1992 showed that the quality assurance system did not meet the criterion that the difference between a single result from the physician's office and the laboratory should not exceed ± 20% of the laboratory result. A consultation and assistance program was initiated, and in 1994 and 1996, the proficiency testing rounds improved considerably. The percentage of values outside the acceptance limits was 12% in 1992, 4% in 1994, and 3% in 1996. This probably resulted from better choice of technology, procedures, and handling of specimens.

Discussion.—The use of bedside instruments should be reserved for the diagnosis of severe hypoglycemia or hyperglycemia and for the monitoring of glucose greater than 5 mmol/L in individuals who already have a diagnosis of diabetes. This quality assurance system is different from previous systems and may be useful for in-house proficiency testing in large hospitals.

► Ever since the Clinical Laboratory Improvement Act of 1988 (CLIA) brought physician office laboratories into the regulatory fold, there has been a terrible outcry from physicians about the adverse effects that this legislation has had on the practice of medicine, as well as the inconvenience and detriment it has caused their patients. However, many surveys have disputed this and have showed an improvement in the quality of these laboratories attributable to the required inspections and proficiency testing.

This paper describes a program for the quality assessment of whole blood glucose measurements using bedside instruments in physician office laboratories. The study involved 98 of 120 practices in the county of Vejle,

Denmark. Whole blood samples supplemented with glucose were prepared, stabilized, and assayed at the local hospital and were then delivered to the practices. In addition, capillary blood samples collected from several patients at the practice were stabilized and brought to the hospital for analysis. The first survey in 1992 demonstrated unsatisfactory performance, with 12% of the laboratories outside the ±20% limit vs. the hospital laboratory. A program of consultation by a technologist and advice on instrument selection was instituted, resulting in significant improvement in the subsequent surveys in 1994 and 1996. The program was well accepted by the office physicians. While impractical on a large scale, this paper demonstrates that effective proficiency testing and education can have a positive effect on laboratory performance.

R. Feld, Ph.D.

Variation in Proficiency Testing Performance by Testing Site

Stull TM, Hearn TL, Hancock JS, et al (Ctrs for Disease Control and Prevention, Atlanta, Ga)

JAMA 279:463–467, 1998 23–7

Background.—In the United States, the Clinical Laboratory Improvement Act (CLIA) of 1988 were enacted to promote uniform standards and quality among all laboratory testing sites in the United States. The 2 quality indicators specified in these amendments are proficiency testing performance and periodic inspection of testing sites. The variability in proficiency testing among traditional and alternative testing sites during the first year of mandatory proficiency testing was investigated.

Methods.—An analysis was conducted of all 1994 proficiency testing score data reported to the Health Care Financing Administration. These data were classified into 2 groups: group 1 included hospitals and independent laboratories, and group 2 included all other testing sites. The main outcome measures were satisfactory and unsatisfactory performance ratings for the 2 testing site groups for each analyte or test, according to the criteria in the 1988 regulations.

Results.—The data included more than 1 million proficiency testing event scores from more than 17,000 testing sites. Analysis showed that the overall rates of satisfactory event performance for all regulated analytes, tests, and specialties were 97% for hospitals and independent laboratories and 91% for all other testing sites. The overall odds ratio for unsatisfactory proficiency testing event performance for alternative testing sites compared with hospitals and independent laboratories was 2.89; for individual analytes, the range was 2.19 to 7.51.

Discussion.—These findings show a consistent difference in proficiency testing event performance between types of testing facilities during the first year of mandatory proficiency testing under the CLIA regulations. Higher rates of satisfactory performance were seen in traditional testing sites, such as hospitals and independent laboratories, than in alternative testing sites.

The history, attributes, limitations, and functions of proficiency testing were also discussed.

▶ CLIA was greeted by physicians about as warmly as finding a nest of rattlesnakes in your bedroom closet. For the first time, this act—passed in response to articles in the Wall Street Journal describing isolated horrors in cytopathology—brought all laboratories under regulation, regardless of the place of testing. Those laboratories performing tests of moderate or high complexity were required to participate in proficiency testing which consisted of 15 challenges per analyte divided into 3 shipments of 5 each year.

This paper and an accompanying paper[1] and editorial[2] explore the results of proficiency testing in the entire country, and in California in particular. In both instances, physician office laboratories (POLs) did worse on proficiency testing than hospital and independent laboratories. The performance of POLs has improved on subsequent challenges and the number of deficiencies cited by inspectors has been reduced.

Although this improvement has come at a cost of reduced access of patients to laboratory tests in some instances, the growing list of waived tests and new technology should alleviate this problem. As the editorial states, it is time for organized medicine to accept CLIA and time for members of Congress (Archer-Hutchison) to stop introducing legislation to repeal it. It is ultimately the patients who will benefit as quality improves.

R. Feld, Ph.D.

References

1. Hurst J, Nickel K, Hilborne LH: Are physicians' office laboratory results of comparable quality to those produced in other laboratory settings? *JAMA* 279:468–471, 1998.
2. Bachner P: Is it time to turn the page on CLIA 1988? (editorial). *JAMA* 279:473–475, 1998.

How Promptly Are Inpatients Treated for Critical Laboratory Results?

Kuperman GJ, Boyle D, Jha A, et al (Brigham and Women's Hosp, Boston)

JAMIA 5:112–119, 1998 23–8

Objective.—The goal of laboratory testing is not met until the clinician receives the results and takes the indicated action. There is evidence to suggest that responses to laboratory results showing serious abnormalities may be inappropriate or delayed. The frequency of critical laboratory results (CLRs), as well as the frequency with which they are acted on, was determined.

Methods.—The retrospective study, carried out in the laboratory of a large, academic hospital, examined the proportion of chemistry and hematology test results meeting criteria for CLRs over a 13-day period. In

TABLE 5.—Findings for Time Until Treatment Ordered and Time Until Condition Resolved

	Time until treatment ordered (hours)			Time until condition resolved (hours)		
	Median	Range	Interquartile range	Median	Range	Interquartile range
All CLRs (n = 99)	2.5	0–32.7	0.6–5.3	14.3	0.3–145.9	7.4–22.6
CLRs meeting BWH criteria (n = 56)	1.8*	0–15.6	0.5–4.0	12.0†	0.3–66.7	6.5–17.1
CLRs meeting Tate's criteria only (n = 43)	2.8*	0.2–32.7	0.8–6.1	20.9†	2.7–145.9	9.7–27.7

*$P = 0.07$ Wilcoxon.
†$P = 0.006$ Wilcoxon.
(Courtesy of Kuperman GJ, Boyle D, Jha A, et al: How promptly are inpatients treated for critical laboratory results? *JAMIA* 5:112–119, 1998.)

addition, a random sample of patients with CLRs for sodium, potassium, and glucose measurements were reviewed to determine how long it took before appropriate treatment was ordered, and how long until the patient's critical condition resolved. Sodium, potassium, and glucose were selected for study because of the particular importance of critical results. The study of treatment timeliness addressed such factors as a rapid change in sequential laboratory results, or a result that was serious in light of the patient's medications.

Results.—The study found 1,938 CLRs in a series of 201,037 laboratory results. The rate of CLRs was 0.96%, or 0.44 per patient-day. Ninety-nine patients with CLRs met inclusion criteria for the chart review study. Median time to appropriate treatment in the 99 patients was 2.5 hours overall, 1.8 hours for CLRs meeting laboratory criteria and leading to a phone call, and 2.8 hours for CLRs meeting more complex criteria that did not require a phone call. The delay to treatment was 5 hours or longer in 27% of CLRs. Median time to resolution of the critical condition was 14.3 hours overall, 12.0 hours for CLRs meeting hospital criteria, and 20.9 hours for CLRs meeting more complex criteria (Table 5).

Conclusions.—Critical laboratory results are a common occurrence. Appropriate treatment for the critical condition is often delayed. Treatment delays are more likely for results that do not meet hospital criteria for a CLR but still reflect a serious clinical situation. At least some of the treatment delays probably result from problems in communicating the critical results directly to the treating clinician. Computers and other technologies should be investigated for their ability to reduce treatment delays related to CLRs.

▶ Few subjects strike fear into the hearts of laboratorians more than panic or critical values. Physicians always feel that the critical value should be 1 unit less than the value chosen by the laboratory to initiate a telephone call. The messages are frequently not delivered to the appropriate caregiver. Most critical values are called in to the physician; the time of the call and person given the value are noted in case there is any question of notification at a later date. When the system breaks down and blame must be assessed, nobody involved benefits, least of all the patient.

This paper examines the physician response to critical values for sodium, potassium, or glucose. Two outcomes were examined: (1) the time from filing the critical value until treatment was ordered, and (2) the time between filing and the resolution of the critical condition. This was determined by the time of arrival in the laboratory of a follow-up specimen for analysis that demonstrated resolution of the critical value. The median time until treatment was ordered for 99 critical values was 2.5 hours. This time was considered by the authors to be unacceptable. Even though the critical result is called in, the treating physician may not be available to receive the information. Frequently the value is given to another person (nurse, secretary, etc.), and it is not immediately communicated to the treating physician. The authors also discuss the limitations of the study. They express the view that this is a problem that begs a technological solution. I concur!

R. Feld, Ph.D.

Subject Index

A

B

C

D

E

F

G

H

I

J

K

L

N

O

P

S

T

U

V

W

X

Y

Author Index

A

B

C

D

E

W

X

Y

Z